T5-BYH-926

CHILD HEALTH
BEHAVIOR

CHILD HEALTH BEHAVIOR

A BEHAVIORAL PEDIATRICS PERSPECTIVE

Editors

NORMAN A. KRASNEGOR
National Institute of Child Health
and Human Development

JOSEPHINE D. ARASTEH
National Institute of Child Health
and Human Development

MICHAEL F. CATALDO
The John F. Kennedy Institute

A Wiley-Interscience Publication

John Wiley & Sons

New York   Chichester   Brisbane   Toronto   Singapore

Library of Congress Cataloging in Publication Data:

Main entry under title:

Child health behavior.

   Wiley series on health psychology/behavioral
medicine.
   "A Wiley-Interscience publication."
   1. Pediatrics—Psychological aspects—Addresses,
essays, lectures.   2. Sick children—Psychology—Addresses, essays, lectures.   I. Krasnegor, Norman A.
II. Arasteh, Josephine D., 1925-   .   III. Cataldo,
Michael F.   IV. Series.   [DNLM: 1. Behavior Therapy—in
infancy & childhood.   2. Behavioral Medicine—in
infancy & childhood.   3. Child Behavior. WS 105 C533809]

RJ47.5.C442   1986   618.92'00019   85-20347
ISBN 0-471-82261-2

Printed in the United States of America

10 9 8 7 6 5 4 3 2 1

To Daniel Gideon and Joshua David
NAK

To Dariush and Roya
JDA

To Marilyn and the future
MFC

Contributors

ROBERT ADER, Ph.D.   Director, Department of Psychiatry, University of Rochester, School of Medicine & Dentistry, Rochester, New York

FRANK ANDRASIK, Ph.D.   Associate Professor & Associate Director, Center for Stress & Anxiety Disorders, SUNY at Albany, Albany, New York

LINA BABANI, M.A.   Doctoral Student Behavioral Pediatrics Program, Orthopaedic Hospital, Los Angeles, California

DONALD M. BAER, Ph.D.   Ray A. Roberts Distinguished Professor, Department of Human Development, University of Kansas Medical Center, Lawrence, Kansas

DUDLEY D. BLAKE   Doctoral Student, Department of Psychology, SUNY at Albany, Albany, New York

JOSEPH V. BRADY, Ph.D.   Professor, Department of Behavioral Biology, The Johns Hopkins Hospital, Baltimore, Maryland

KELLY D. BROWNELL, Ph.D.   Associate Professor, Department of Psychiatry, University of Pennsylvania, School of Medicine, Philadelphia, Pennsylvania

ANN F. BRUNSWICK, Ph.D.   Director, Young Adult Health Unit, School of Public Health, Columbia University, New York, New York

EDWARD R. CHRISTOPHERSEN, Ph.D.   Professor, Department of Pediatrics, University of Kansas, College of Health Sciences, Kansas City, Kansas

THOMAS J. COATES, Ph.D.   Associate Professor, Division of General Internal Medicine, University of California, School of Medicine, San Francisco, California

LINDA DARNELL   Research Dietician, Diet Modification Clinic, Baylor College of Medicine, Houston, Texas

ROBERT A. DERSHEWITZ, M.D.   Pediatrician, Harvard Community Health Plan, Braintree, Massachusetts and Attending Physician, Massachusetts General Hospital and Brigham Women's Hospital, Boston, Massachusetts

CRAIG K. EWART, Ph.D.   Assistant Professor, Department of Health Education, The Johns Hopkins University, School of Hygiene and Public Health, Baltimore, Maryland

STEPHEN B. FAWCETT, Ph.D.   Director, Center for Community Development and Social Policy and Associate Professor, Department of Human Development & Family Life, University of Kansas, Lawrence, Kansas

JACK W. FINNEY, Ph.D.   Associate Director, Project HEALTH, Columbia, Maryland and Instructor, Department of Psychiatry and Behavioral Sciences, The Johns Hopkins University, School of Medicine, Baltimore, Maryland

JOHN FOREYT, Ph.D.   Director, Diet Modification Clinic, Baylor College of Medicine, Houston, Texas

PATRICK C. FRIMAN, Ph.D.   Intern in Behavioral Pediatrics, University of Kansas, College of Health Sciences, Kansas City, Kansas

KEN GOODRICK   Research Associate, Diet Modification Clinic, Baylor College of Medicine, Houston, Texas

LAWRENCE GREEN, Dr. P.H.   Director, Center for Health Promotion and Development, University of Texas Health Science Center, Houston, Texas

MORRIS GREEN, M.D.   Lesh Professor & Chairman, Department of Pediatrics, Indiana University, School of Medicine, Indianapolis, Indiana

ROBERT J. HAGGERTY, M.D.   President, William T. Grant Foundation, New York, New York

JANET R. HANKIN, Ph.D.   Research Scientist, Johns Hopkins Center for Metropolitan Planning & Research, The Johns Hopkins University, Baltimore, Maryland

DELLA M. HANN   Doctoral Student, Department of Psychology, University of Tennessee, Knoxville, Tennessee

FRANCES DEGEN HOROWITZ, Ph.D.   Professor, Department of Human Development and Family Life, University of Kansas, Lawrence, Kansas

BARBARA J. HOWARD, M.D.   Co-Director, Developmental & Behavioral Pediatrics, Sinai Hospital at Baltimore, Baltimore, Maryland

ISMET KARACAN, M.D., (Med) D.Sc.   Director, Sleep Disorders & Research Center, Baylor College of Medicine, Houston, Texas

LLOYD J. KOLBE, Ph.D.   Associate Director, The University of Texas, Health Science Center at Houston, Houston, Texas

A.S. KORTON, Ph.D.   Assistant Director, Sleep Disorders & Research Center, Baylor College of Medicine, Houston, Texas

EDWARD LICHTENSTEIN, Ph.D.   Professor & Research Scientist, University of Oregon, Oregon Research Institute, Eugene, Oregon

MEREDITH STEELE McCARRAN   Doctoral Student, Department of Psychology, SUNY at Albany, Albany, New York

CHERYL R. MERZEL, M.P.H.   Research Assistant, School of Public Health, Columbia University, New York, New York

MARION O'BRIEN, Ph.D.   Research Associate, Lawrence Day Care Program, University of Kansas, Lawrence, Kansas

JOHN M. PARRISH, Ph.D.   Director of Training & Outpatient Services, The John F. Kennedy Institute and Assistant Professor of Psychiatry, The Johns Hopkins University, School of Medicine, Baltimore, Maryland

DENNIS C. RUSSO, Ph.D.   Director, Behavioral Medicine Program, Department of Psychiatry, Children's Hospital Medical Center, Boston, Massachusetts

THOMAS SEEKINS, Ph.D.   Research Associate, Center for Public Affairs, University of Kansas, Lawrence, Kansas

HERBERT H. SEVERSON, Ph.D.   Director & Research Scientist, Oregon Research Institute, Eugene, Oregon

JEAN SMITH, M.D.   Staff Physician, Primary Care Center and Coordinator, Behavioral Pediatrics Teaching Program, Sinai Hospital at Baltimore, Baltimore, Maryland

GENE STAINBROOK   Research Associate, Center for Health Promotion, Research and Development, University of Texas Health Science Center, Houston, Texas

Barbara H. Starfield, M.D.   Professor of Health Policy Management, Johns Hopkins Center for Metropolitan Planning and Research, The Johns Hopkins University, Baltimore, Maryland

Karen L. Thompson, M.A.   Doctoral Student, Behavioral Pediatrics Program, Orthopaedic Hospital, Los Angeles, California

James W. Varni, Ph.D.   Co-Director, Behavioral Pediatrics Program, Orthopaedic Hospital, Clinical Associate Professor of Psychology, Pediatrics & Psychiatry, University of Southern California, Los Angeles, California

Robert G. Wahler, Ph.D.   Professor, Department of Psychology, University of Tennessee, Knoxville, Tennessee

Diane Ward   Research Associate, Department of Physical Education, University of South Carolina, Columbia, South Carolina

William E. Whitehead, Ph.D.   Associate Professor of Medical Psychology, The Johns Hopkins University, School of Medicine, Baltimore, Maryland

Roger Widmeyer   Editorial Assistant, Sleep Disorders and Research Center, Baylor College of Medicine, Houston, Texas

Harriet Williams, Ph.D.   Director, Motor Development and Motor Control Laboratory, Department of Physical Education, University of South Carolina, Columbia, South Carolina

Modena Wilson, M.D., M.P.H.   Assistant Professor, Department of Pediatrics, The Johns Hopkins University, School of Medicine and School of Hygiene and Public Health, Baltimore, Maryland

Series Preface

This series is addressed to clinicians and scientists who are interested in human behavior relevant to the promotion and maintenance of health and the prevention and treatment of illness. *Health psychology* and *behavioral medicine* are terms that refer to both the scientific investigation and interdisciplinary integration of behavioral and biomedical knowledge and technology to prevention, diagnosis, treatment, and rehabilitation.

The major and purposely somewhat general areas of both health psychology and behavioral medicine which will receive greatest emphasis in this series are: theoretical issues of bio-psycho-social function, diagnosis, treatment, and maintenance; issues of organizational impact on human performance and an individual's impact on organizational functioning; development and implementation of technology for understanding, enhancing, or remediating human behavior and its impact on health and function; and clinical considerations with children and adults, alone, in groups, or in families that contribute to the scientific and practical/clinical knowledge of those charged with the care of patients.

The series encompasses considerations as intellectually broad as psychology and as numerous as the multitude of areas of evaluation treatment and prevention and maintenance that make up the field of medicine. It is the aim of the series to provide a vehicle which will focus attention on both the breadth and the interrelated nature of the sciences and practices making up health psychology and behavioral medicine.

THOMAS J. BOLL

The University of Alabama in Birmingham
Birmingham, Alabama

Preface

This book rose out of a conference sponsored by the Human Learning and Behavior Branch of the National Institute of Child Health and Human Development, held at the Xerox Center, Leesburg, Virginia in September 1983. Although the volume is based upon the proceedings of the conference, its contents do not mirror them. Rather, the individual contributions are presented in the form of chapters that provide overviews of the topics on which they focus. As such they give the reader a scholarly and, in most instances, an in-depth coverage of the subject discussed.

What is unique about the book is its emphasis upon both clinical issues and research domains that are germane to the field of children's health behavior.

In addition the book exposes the reader to the ideas, perspectives, and data generated by pediatricians and psychologists who are currently working on aspects of behavioral pediatrics. Previously published works on this topic have dwelt on either biomedical or psychological aspects of children's health. This book can be distinguished from such other volumes by the prominence given to biobehavioral perspectives of behavioral pediatrics as a recurrent theme in each of the presentations.

The book should be of interest to a variety of readers, particularly because of the immediate practical applications that flow from its clinically oriented chapters. The practicing pediatrician, for example, will find here the latest research findings on topics highly relevant to presenting behavioral problems seen in private practice and/or clinic settings.

The work also offers an important addition to the literature for biomedical and behavioral researchers who employ biobehavioral approaches to gain an understanding of the etiology of disease and the promotion and maintenance of health. Finally, we believe that the book will also be of immediate use as a contribution to the syllabus for medical and graduate school doctoral level courses which focus upon general pediatrics, behavioral medicine, or child development.

NORMAN A. KRASNEGOR
JOSEPHINE D. ARASTEH
MICHAEL F. CATALDO

Bethesda, Maryland
Bethesda, Maryland
Baltimore, Maryland
January 1986

Acknowledgments

The editors gratefully acknowledge the assistance of Keith Slifer, who materially aided us in the scheduling of outside reviews of the chapters contained in this book. His diligence, scholarship and care for details contributed substantially to the success of our undertaking.

In addition to being subjected to the editors' scrutiny, each chapter was reviewed anonymously by other readers, whose names we make known here by way of grateful acknowledgment:

Donald Baer	Morris Green
Joseph Brady	Robert Haggerty
Norman Braveman	Barbara Howard
Kelly Brownell	Robert Kleges
Thomas Coates	Lloyd Kolbe
Edward Christophersen	Barbara Korsch
Catherine DeAngeles	Larry Ng
Jack Finney	Frank Parker
William Fordyce	Dennis Russo
Rex Forehand	Marvin Schuster
Larry Green	Jean Smith

Barbara Starfield   William Whitehead
James Varni   Barry Zuckerman
Robert Wahler

N.A.K.
J.D.A.
M.F.C.

Contents

PART VI   FUTURE DIRECTIONS

CHILD HEALTH
BEHAVIOR

PART I

CHILD HEALTH BEHAVIOR: AN INTRODUCTION

NORMAN A. KRASNEGOR

The past decade has witnessed the emergence of a developing consensus among clinicians and researchers alike concerning the necessary roles of biological and behavioral factors in the etiology of illness, the prevention of disease and the promotion of health. In the late 1970s the Academy of Behavioral Medicine Research was established. This event was followed by the founding of the Society of Behavioral Medicine in 1979. Both of these organizations are actively involved in advocating the value of an interdisciplinary perspective as the framework within which research and practice related to health should be conducted. Professional societies interested in children's health have also been formed. For example, there currently exists a research society dedicated to the study of behavioral pediatrics. Of equal importance in March 1985, a group of leading pediatricians and psychologists held a national conference on behavioral pediatrics. This meeting was organized to bring into focus a series of definitional, research, and practice issues of common interest to those clinicians and scientists who work in this new aspect of behavioral medicine.

This book is at the cutting edge of the trends noted above. Specifically, the volume incorporates the viewpoints of the leading advocates of behavioral pediatrics from the fields of pediatrics and behavioral science. The work presented provides an excellent sampling of the philosophical and scientific underpinnings of the field. It gives as well an in-depth coverage of research findings on topics that are of interest both to the practicing pediatrician and the academician/scientist. The volume is divided into five parts: (1) Perspectives; (2) Determinants; (3) Prevention; (4) Treatment; and (5) Future Directions

PERSPECTIVES

This section includes six chapters. The first by Robert Haggerty, who at the time of this writing is president of the American Academy of Pediatrics, discusses the vast changes that are taking place in the practice of pediatrics and the trends that have influenced these new directions. His chapter is followed by Morris Green's presentation, in which he outlines his viewpoint on child health in the context of his biopsychosocial model. The work is written from the perspective of a pediatrician and emphasizes the need for studying the whole child, both biologically and psychologically and in the child's social context, in order to understnd health and treat illness. Another viewpoint is provided by Joseph Brady, who advocates a behavioral biology perspective as the framework for addressing issues of child health behavior. He too emphasizes the necessity for studying the interaction between biology and behavior in the context of an organism's environment. But his focus is upon the experimental analyses of behavior under controlled laboratory conditions. His chapter elucidates the basic principles that underpin applied behavior analytic techniques employed by psychologists to intervene and treat children in pediatric settings.

Dr. Brady's chapter is followed by Donald Baer's, in which he discusses how the principles of the experimental analysis of behavior have been applied to problems associated with the health of children. More specifically he gives a perspective on how applied behavior analysts employ their scientific and clinical skills in health promotion, disease prevention and treatment of illness. His essay addresses the issues of generalization of behavior change, the social validity of methods employed by behavior analysts and behavior therapists, the medical validity of behavioral treatment approaches, and the design of placebo controls for evaluating the efficacy of behavioral interventions. The two remaining chapters provide epidemiological perspectives on the prevalence of behavioral problems in children, and health problems that occur primarily during the adolescent phase of development. The chapter by Janet Hankin and Barbara Starfield estimates the prevalence of various psychosocial problems and reviews data on who treats these problems, their duration, and the consequences for the service system. The chapter by Ann Brunswick and Cheryl Merzel provides an overview of health risk behaviors exhibited by adolescents. Their analysis highlights the importance of accidents and substance abuse in teenagers as major etiological factors involved in the morbidity and mortality rates for this age group.

DETERMINANTS

The section on determinants contains three chapters focusing respectively upon (1) Psychoneuroimmunology; (2) Developmental Factors; and (3) Behavioral Determinants in Childhood Pyschopathology.

The chapter by Robert Ader, who is one of the founders of the field of psychoneuroimmunology, discusses some of the experimental evidence that demonstrates how an organism's behavior can affect its immune system. The general implications of such findings for the developing organism are discussed; however, in keeping with his preference for staying close to the data, Ader does not venture too far down the road of speculation.

An interaction model framework forms the core of the chapter by Frances Degen Horowitz and Marion O'Brien. They discuss how behavior management and developmental determinants influence outcome and priorities for child development research. The chapter by Robert Wahler and Della Hann discusses a behavior analytic framework as a context for elucidating child behavior problems that develop in the social setting represented by the mother-father-child triad. A central feature of their exposition is the setting event. This concept is based upon the work of Kantor and appears also in the writings of Bijou. The setting event is an addition to the three factors (discriminative stimulus, response, and reinforcement) traditionally employed by behavior analysts for elucidating behavior problems in children.

PREVENTION

This section ranges over a diverse series of topics that include: health promotion, childhood injury, disease prevention by the practicing pediatrician, teenage cigarette smoking, obesity, and hypertension.

The chapter by Lloyd Kolbe and Lawrence Green and their associates provides a lucid overview of health promotion research. It includes discussions of findings on diet, exercise, sleep and stress and how these factors influence children's cognitive performance. The authors make a cogent argument for health promotion in school to help foster the learning potential of children.

The presentation by Michael Cataldo and his colleagues addresses childhood injury. This topic is of high relevance for the public health since it is the leading cause of morbidity and mortality in children. Accidental injury of children contributes more to the incidence and prevalence of health impairments than the next six leading causes combined. The review of the epidemiology of childhood injury and the research on this topic make this chapter a valuable reference for public health officials and practicing pediatricians.

The chapter by Patrick Friman and Edward Christophersen focuses upon four clinically relevant pediatric medical disorders seen by the practicing pediatrician: (1) obesity; (2) nocturnal enuresis; (3) encoporesis; and (4) testicular cancer. The authors review the incidence of each condition, its causes and correlates, treatment approaches, and strategies for prevention. They discuss the contributions that pediatricians, with their unique perspective, can make to preventive medicine.

The last three chapters in this section are devoted to specific risk factors that affect children's health. The chapter by Herbert Severson and Edward Lichtenstein provides an excellent critical overview of smoking prevention programs targeted for children. Their evaluation of the research to date provides an appraisal of what has been done and suggestions for future research directions. Kelly Brownell's chapter reviews childhood obesity research. It details the significance of obesity for the health of our nation's children and provides research findings on behavioral treatment approaches that have shown the most promise for having an impact on this risk factor. Thomas Coates and Craig Ewart focus their chapter on the prevention of hypertension in adolescents. Their contribution provides a comprehensive summary of the research literature and of approaches for modifying behaviors demonstrably involved in the etiology of elevated blood pressure.

TREATMENT

The subject of this section is the treatment of pediatric patients. Included are chapters on common behavior problems, pediatric pain and headaches, compliance, chronic illness, and biofeedback.

Dr. Edward Christophersen's chapter provides a review of the research on the identification and treatment of common behavioral problems in primary care settings. Topics of interest include anticipatory guidance, recognizing behavioral problems, educating parents, prevention of behavior problems, and referral of behavior problems to other specialists. The two chapters on pain, by James Varni and Karen Thompson, and by Frank Andrasik, Dudley Blake, and Meredith Steele McCarran, provide the practitioner with excellent perspectives on the complexities of pediatric pain and headache and the behavioral treatment approaches to these problems. The chapter by Frank Andrasik and his colleagues provides a comprehensive review of the literature and a classification scheme for categorizing different types of headaches diagnosed in children and should be of great interest to the behavioral pediatrics practitioner, who frequently deals with these presenting symptoms in the clinic.

The inclusion of the three chapters on compliance attests to the central role played by this behavioral issue in the treatment of pediatric populations. The chapter by Edward Christophersen, Jack Finney, and Patrick Friman describes a series of experiments on compliance carried out in a pediatric outpatient clinic. Studies reviewed include research on appointment keeping and on compliance for medical regimens (otitis media and vaginitis and pharyngitis). In addition, child passenger-safety compliance and home injury-control studies are discussed. The work demonstrates the feasibility of incorporating compliance protocols in a clinic setting.

The chapter by John Parrish addresses the issue of parental compliance in the medical regimens that their children are to follow. The work reviews findings concerning behavioral strategies for improving compliance and investigates how parent characteristics and other relevant factors interact with the type of disease being treated, the compliance regimen, and the parent/therapist relationship.

The third chapter on compliance, by James Varni and Lina Babani, focuses upon chronically ill children. These patients display different kinds of compliance problems than do those who have acute illness. Varni and Babani emphasize the need for more research on patient education and the treatment regimen, and a functional analysis of compliance behaviors. They assert that such research will help develop a knowledge base for effective procedures for increasing compliance among chronically ill children.

The chapter by Dennis Russo also focuses upon the chronically ill child. A central premise of his exposition on chronicity is that the child who suffers from a chronic disease should be considered a psychologically normal individual who may display aberrant behaviors as a consequence of the altered learning environment that often shapes and reinforces illness behaviors and dependency. When a chronically ill child is viewed from the perspective of being normal, it follows that the patient's behavior can be appropriately modified to enhance both adaptation and coping skills. He argues cogently that such improvements can favorably affect overall functioning of the patient.

The final chapter in this section by William Whitehead presents an elegant demonstration of the utility of biofeedback for treating fecal incontinence in children. It describes how behavioral training can ameliorate a biological process that resists usual treatments. The findings reported have general interest because of their implications for the etiology and treatment of other childhood disorders, such as asthma, epilepsy, and headache.

FUTURE DIRECTIONS

The final section of the volume contains three chapters that identify research and training needs for the future. The chapter by Michael Cataldo provides a synthesis of significant findings in the field of behavioral pediatrics and shows how such knowledge can shape the entire field of child health behavior. He identifies gap areas and proposes an agenda of research priorities to address significant aspects of child health. The chapter by Barbara Howard and Jean Smith focuses upon the training needed to provide appropriate experience and background for the professional whose goal is to provide comprehensive health care for children. They discuss the need to orient trainees toward the literature on child development, and present their viewpoints concerning the content of training and the qualities needed by the faculty who will train the next generation of researchers and clinicians in the field of behavioral pediatrics. The final contribution in this section is the chapter by Michael Cataldo and Norman Krasnegor on training. They advocate a programmatic approach that would incorporate behavior analytic training in the curriculum of pediatricians and nurses and biological training for trained behavioral scientists/clinicians. This latter aspect of training would enable nonphysicians to screen for serious medical problems and insure timely referral to physicians. Both groups of professionals would also be exposed during their education to research and practice concerning interaction of biological and behavioral processes and the relevance of such interaction for behavioral pediatrics.

This book attests to the fact that behavioral pediatrics is becoming, in the context of the new morbidity alluded to by Robert Haggerty, a multidisciplined profession. Progress in this field of endeavor is predicated upon the development of a strong alliance between pediatricians and the behavorial scientist/clinician. Each side of this emerging partnership must evaluate its own disciplinary strengths and gauge how best to collaborate to most effectively enhance the health of our nation's children. The future holds great promise for behavioral pediatrics, both as a field for practice and a focus of research. The work herein presented is a prologue for what the field can become.

PART II

PERSPECTIVES

1

The Changing Nature of Pediatrics

ROBERT J. HAGGERTY

Pediatrics, whose basic science is growth and development, or change, is itself faced with major changes in the next two decades. These changes have great implications for the increasing role of behavioral issues in pediatric practice.

MORTALITY AND MORBIDITY CHANGES

There have been striking decreases in the mortality of children of all ages, except in adolescence, during which the major causes of death are now violent: accidents, homicide and suicide (see Figure 1.1 and 1.2). This has resulted in the practicing pediatrician having considerably less involvement with problems likely to cause death in children. In addition, the increasing technology of hospital care has separated the primary care pediatrician from many of the remaining serious problems of childhood which lead to hospitalization. Children with such problems are now generally

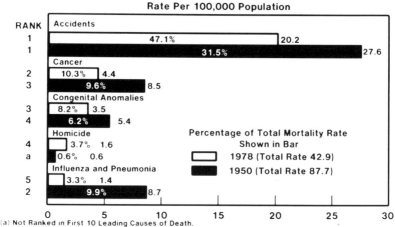

MAJOR CAUSES OF CHILDHOOD DEATHS:
1950 AND 1978
AGE GROUP 1 - 14 YEARS

Rate Per 100,000 Population

FIGURE 1.1.   Major causes of childhood deaths: 1950 and 1978. Age group 1–14 years (From NCHS. Vital Statistics-Special Report-National Summaries, 1950, Vol. 37:NCHS, "Final Mortality Statistics, 1978." Monthly Vital Statistics Report, Vol. 29, No. 6, Supplement 2, September 17, 1980.)

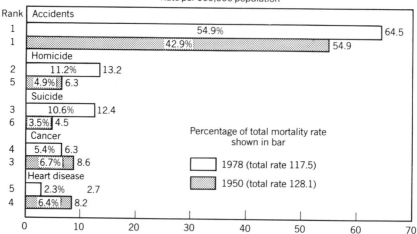

MAJOR CAUSES OF ADOLESCENT DEATHS:
1950 AND 1978
AGE GROUP 15 - 24 YEARS

Rate per 100,000 population

FIGURE 1.2.   Major causes of adolescent deaths: 1950 and 1978. Age group 15–24 years. (From NCHS. Vital Statistics-Special Report-National Summaries, 1950, Vol. 37:NCHS, "Final Mortality Statistics, 1978." Monthly Vital Statistics Report, Vol. 29, No. 6, Supplement 2, September 17, 1980.)

10

POLIOMYELITIS

POLIOMYELITIS (Paralytic) - **Reported Cases Per 100,000 Population**
by Year, United States, 1951-1981

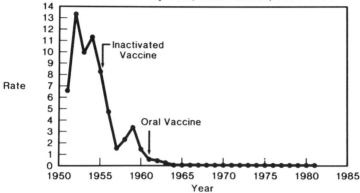

FIGURE 1.3.   Poliomyelitis (paralytic)—reported cases per 100,000 population, by year, United States, 1951–1981. (Data from Morbidity and Mortality Weekly Reports. DHHS, Public Health Service, Centers for Disease Control.)

MEASLES

MEASLES (Rubeola) - Reported Cases Per 100,000 Population,
by Year, United States, 1955-1981

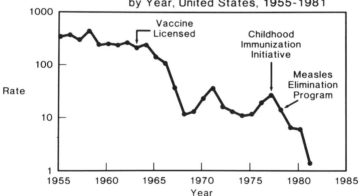

FIGURE 1.4.   Measles (rubeola)—reported cases per 100,000 population, by year, United States, 1951–1981. (Data from Morbidity and Mortality Weekly Reports. DHHS, Public health Service, Centers for Disease Control.)

cared for in a tertiary care hospital by subspecialists, leaving the office based general pediatrician a smaller role in the hospital. At the same time, *morbidity* has also changed with marked decreases in the common infectious agents, largely through immunizations (such as for polymyelitis, measles, rubella and mumps) (Figure 1.3 and 1.4) and effective antimicrobial therapy. The remaining health problems brought to the pediatrician, while no more prevalent than in the past, occupy a larger percentage of practice

TABLE 1.1.   DATA FROM COMMUNITY CHILD HEALTH
STUDIES

	% Children 0-17 Years Parent Reported Psychosocial Problems			
	Behavioral		Social	
	(1)	(2)	(1)	(2)
Genesee County	2.8	7.8	1.8	5.9
Berkshire County	6.2	18.9	2.6	13.2
Cleveland				
C. F.		28.6		6.5
C. P.		22.7		13.6
Spina Bifida		19.5		6.1
Multiple Handicap		37.0		20.0

84WTGF1.01

(1) = Random Sample
(2) = Chronic Disease Sample

today, and include the biobehavioral and psychological problems of children, and the psychosocial implications of chronic physical disease. Prevention has always been a large part of pediatrics, and now constitutes some 40 to 50 percent of the average practitioner's time. In the past, preventive services were limited largely to immunization against infectious diseases and to advice on feeding. In light of the changing morbidity and mortality, the emphasis of these preventive services will shift from a major concern with preventing infectious diseases to a concern for preventing behavioral problems and accidents. Behavior problems are far more prevalent than any single "organic" disease. Various surveys have demonstrated a frequency, in the general population of children, of between 5 to 15 percent of all children suffering from behavioral problems, and those with chronic physical disease have nearly double this rate. Table 1.1 is from a study we did in several areas: Genesee County, Michigan, Berkshire County, Massachusetts, and the city of Cleveland, Ohio. The overall fre-

TABLE 1.2.   MOST COMMON HEALTH
PROBLEMS REPORTED BY PARENTS

- School
- Behavior
- Speech
- Hearing
- Vision
- Teeth
- Allergy

From Haggerty, R. J.: The Changing Role Of The Pediatrician In
Child Health Care, Am. J. Dis. Child 127:545, 1974.   84WTGF1.05

quency of behavioral and social problems in a random sample of children was 8.8 percent in Massachusetts. In all samples, children with chronic physical disease had higher frequencies of such problems (Community Child Health Studies, 1981). Table 1.2 lists the most common problems reported by parents in a random sample of children in Monroe County (Rochester) New York. Except for allergy, no physical disease has a prevalence greater than 1 percent. Therefore because of reduced frequency of serious physical health problems, the high frequency of behavioral problems, and the emphasis on prevention, a large and increasing percent of the practicing pediatrician's time is concerned with behavioral issues.

SOCIODEMOGRAPHIC CHANGES

There has been a striking reduction in the number of births in the United States in the past two decades and, while these have now about leveled off, they are at a considerably lower rate than a decade ago. The large cohort of children born in the 1970s means that there is frequently a large proportion of the childhood population in the adolescent age range today. This age group has a high frequency of behavior problems. In addition there are a variety of other social changes, such as the large influx of immigrants, especially from southeast Asia and Latin America, who do not fit the traditional pattern of family life in America. Indeed the increasing varieties of family life in America, with more single parent families, and working mothers who have postponed child birth to their mid-thirties, resulting in highly valued and stimulated first and only children of older parents, have lead to extraordinary varieties of child rearing practices. This in turn has led to a need for alternative times for the provision of health services, such as evenings and weekends, added difficulties in communication between physicians and patients, and a challenge to pediatricians to know about a much wider range of social and behavioral issues than in the past.

PROFESSIONAL AND ECONOMIC CHANGES

The rapid increase in the number of all physicians, including pediatricians, has led to a much larger pediatrician-per-population ratio. This coupled with the stable birthrate, is leading to increased competition among providers for patients. New methods of payments, such as preferred provider organizations (PPO), HMOs, IPAs, and so on, are rapidly altering the traditional fee-for-service mechanism of paying for office practice for pediatrics. Another change in the economic scene is the current development of advertising by practitioners. Still another development in economics of practice is a marked increase in medical liability or malpractice suits. This has become a special problem for pediatrics since the period at risk in many states for the "statute of limitations" is 21 plus 3 years, rather than the 3 years traditional for the rest of medicine. This means that problems which arose in the newborn may be the subject of a malpractice suit up to 24 years later. All of this has increased the malpractice insurance rates enormously, leading to a considerable increase in defensive practice of medicine. Both young practitioners beginning practice and older practitioners who wish to slow down have difficulty doing so in the states with the highest malpractice rates, because malpractice insurance does not vary with the volume of one's practice. Thus older practitioners who wish to slow down are more inclined to quit entirely, or move out of the states with high malpractice rates. Competition for patients and the high risk of malpractice in caring for sick newborns are additional factors leading pediatricians to provide care to adolescents, and deal with issues of behavior in an office based practice, rather than for sick children in hospitals.

IMPLICATION FOR PRACTICE

Many of the implications of these changes cannot be clearly foreseen at this time. However, it is clear that pediatric practice will be more concerned in the next two decades with health promotion, care of children with behavior problems and preventions of such problems (especially biopsychosocial disorders), increased care of adolescents, and increased care of children with chronic physical disease. A special role for the pediatrician is to care for children with psychosomatic problems. An illustration of the link between physical and behavioral factors in illness is found in a study of students taking an examination (McClelland, Floor, Davidson & Saron, 1980). Tables 1.3 and 1.4 show that students who had three characteristics (high in need for power, high in need for control, and a high degree of anxiety about the test) had more respiratory illnesses following the test, had a higher amount of urinary epinephrine, and of those with an above the

TABLE 1.3.   RELATION OF POWER, STRESS CATECHOLAMINES

	HHH*	Other Subjects	
MEAN NUMBER ILLNESSES	2.08	1.26	p < .05
MEAN SEVERITY ILLNESS	10.55	5.86	p < .05
%EPINEPHRINE ABOVE MEDIAN	83.00%	40.00%	p = .07

*High inhibited power, high power, stress

TABLE 1.4.   EPINEPHRINE EXCRETION
RELATION TO S - I g A

	High	Low
Percent Subjects Above Median For Epinephrine Excretion	18%	75%

P < .01

mean urinary epinephrine, the majority had a decreased secretory IGA in their saliva. Thus we have one explanatory mechanism for why stress leads to increased susceptibility to infection. This type of interrelation between biology and behavior has led many of us to the concept of multiple causes of multiple diseases. Traditionally medicine looked for a single cause of disease, and in the biological field this was a most effective strategy. However, most of the complex diseases that remain are now recognized to be due to multiple causes. Figure 1.5 illustrates this point. When we move into the behavioral field it is clear that we are dealing not only with multiple causes of each of the problem behaviors, but that most of these problem behaviors have the *same* multiple causes (Figure 1.6). Pediatricians are beginning to approach the prevention of disease, and improvement of function, through a much more noncategorical approach than ever before. Stein and her colleagues have shown that the care of a wide variety of children's chronic illnesses includes more modalities common to all than there are special modalities for specific illnesses (Stein & Jessup, 1984). The prac-

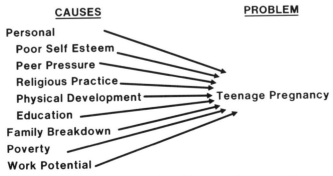

FIGURE 1.5.   Categorical approach: multiple causality of a problem model.

NON-CATEGORICAL
MULTIPLE PROBLEMS - MULTIPLE
CAUSALITY MODEL

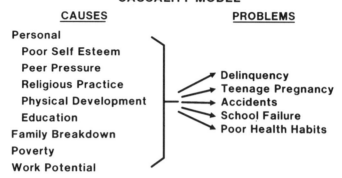

FIGURE 1.6.   Noncategorical: multiple problems—multiple causality model.

ticing pediatrician is a generalist, and must deal with general as well as specific issues of care.

There will be marked changes in the organization and practice of medicine. These will include more pediatric services being given outside of the pediatrician's office, in schools, "emergi" centers, hospitals, and greater collaboration with other health professionals, especially psychologists, social workers, and nurse practitioners. At the same time, there may be a tendency to fragment the medical profession into those who work in hospitals and those who work in offices. There will be increased competition for patients, with a possibility that services of unproven effectiveness will be offered, especially in the behavioral area. The availability of more pediatricians with time available presents the opportunity for them to begin meeting some of the unmet needs in the biobehavioral and adolescent area in the next decade. Because so little research has been done to demonstrate the effectiveness of care in this area, there is a great need for research on common problems of children seen in the office practice of pediatrics, especially the biobehavioral, and to study the effectiveness of prevention and therapy of these conditions. Behavioral pediatrics will be a major frontier of pediatrics in the remainder of this century.

REFERENCES

Community Child Health Studies—Harvard School of Public Health (1981). Printed by Harvard University, available from D.K. Walker, Harvard School of Public Health.

McClelland, D.C., Floor, E., Davidson, R.J., & Saron, C. (1980). Stressed power, motivation, sympathetic activity, immune function, and illness. *Journal of Human Stress 6*, 11–19.

Stein, R.E.K., & Jessop, D.J.J. (1984). General issues in the care of children with chronic physical conditions. *Pediatric Clinics of North America. 31*, 189–198.

2

Developmental Psychobiologic Implications for Pediatrics

MORRIS GREEN

INTRODUCTION

The pediatrician's developmental perspectives in health and disease are biologic and psychosocial, cross-sectional and longitudinal, preventive and therapeutic. They involve the child, the family and the environment or community. In addition to their long-standing interest in growth and development, pediatricians are increasingly concerned with the *adaptation* of children and families. To my mind, helping children and parents adapt and cope is a pediatric role which will be more clearly delineated over the next 10 years (Cohen & Lazarus, 1983). Psycho-neuroendocrinology, psychoneuroimmunology, developmental neuro-anatomy, psychopharmacology, developmental, behavioral and social psychology, sociology, epidemiology and cultural anthropology all constitute important parts of the knowledge base required for the expanding and changing opportunities for the pediatric practitioner and investigator (Prugh, 1983).

That biologic, psychologic and social factors are inseparably intertwined in child health and illness has long been recognized. Alan Gregg underlined the reality of this integration over thirty years ago in his statement that: "No part can be changed without changing in some way and in some measure all the others. . . . It is intellectual weakness that prompts us to ascribe a given result to only one sufficient cause. We ignore the value of suspecting that a result may be due to a convergence of several causes . . ." (Gregg, 1951).

Recent advances in psychobiology, which have helped elucidate the connections between the cerebral cortex, hypothalamus, the limbic and the reticular systems, have greatly contributed to our understanding of how psychologic stimuli associated with life experiences are translated in the brain to produce physiologic changes and how biologic alterations in the body may be transduced through endocrine and neurotransmitter channels in the brain to psychologic effects (Reister, 1980).

PEDIATRIC CLINICAL EXPERIENCES IN HEALTH AND DISEASE

Our present state of knowledge does not yet permit a psychobiologic nosology of child health or illness based on specific psychologic, physiologic or social factors, nor is such a classification likely to be forthcoming in the near future. In the meantime, several operational groupings of clinical disorders relevant to this book may be discussed, recognizing the considerable overlap in this classification.

Psychosomatic, or somatopsychic, pediatric disorders which have joint psychologic and physiologic components certainly include anorexia nervosa, bulimia, obesity, conversion reactions, depression, drug abuse, alcoholism, failure to thrive, psychogenic pain disorders (headache, chest pain, abdominal pain and limb pain), psychogenic purpura (Gardener-Diamond syndrome) and rumination. Psychosocial dwarfism, a dramatic "experiment of nature" which occurs in some emotionally deprived young children, is characterized by abnormal eating habits, understature, and deficiencies in ACTH and growth hormone secretion. These biologic and behavioral findings are impressively reversed when the affected child is removed from an emotionally disturbed home and placed in a nurturing environment (Powell, Brasel, Raiti, & Blizzard, 1967).

Chronic illness and handicapping disorders in children which are associated, at times, with psychosocial sequelae, many of a major character, include asthma, blindness, burns, cerebral palsy, craniofacial anomalies, cystic fibrosis, deafness, diabetes, iron-deficiency anemia, end-stage renal disease, epilepsy, hemophilia, inflammatory bowel disease, malignancies, migraine headaches, myelodysplasia, fecal and urinary incontinence, rheumatoid arthritis and Tourette's syndrome. Chronic illness and handicap remain high on the agenda of pediatric care and research in the 1980s.

Pediatricians are also concerned with the causes and the effects of such affects as depression, anxiety, sadness, anger, and fear—not only in children but also in their parents.

Developmental patterns and disorders, possibly with both biologic and psychosocial determinants, include attention deficit disorder, atypical behavior syndrome, autism, environmental deprivation, delayed speech, failure to thrive, learning and perception disabilities, memory dysfunction, impaired gender development, mental retardation, and sleep disorders.

Substance abuse during pregnancy has effects on the child's development and behavior. Cranial radiation and chemotherapy during pregnancy appear to be followed by learning problems at school for some offspring.

Nutritional problems of a psychobiologic character include failure to thrive, anorexia, obesity, insatiable appetite in children with the Prader-Willi syndrome and pica.

Health problems which are overrepresented in children from families of low socioeconomic status include congenital anomaly, infectious disease, intrauterine growth retardation, iron-deficiency anemia, lead poisoning, mental illness, prematurity and infant mortality—all major health problems in the 1980s.

STRESSORS AFFECTING CHILDREN

The Institute of Medicine report on *Stress and Human Health* concluded, as have many other publications, that persons experiencing emotionally disruptive situations are at increased risk of developing a physical or mental disorder (Elliott & Eisdorfer, 1982; Holmes & Rahe, 1967; Shapiro et al., 1979). Stressful events, especially those of sudden onset, which demand rapid changes in attitude or behavior are often accompanied, at least transiently, by physiological changes. Since different experiences may be perceived psychologically in about the same way by different individuals, it is understandable that the neuroendocrine and clinical responses to these dissimilar events may be similar.

Antecedent stressful events are frequently identified in many infants, children and adolescents who present the pediatrician with problems of a psychobiologic character. Most of the studies on vulnerability to stress have been performed with adult populations, but children also appear to manifest a causal relationship between important life changes and somatic complaints such as abdominal pain and headache, hyperactivity, diarrhea, encopresis, enuresis, failure to thrive, anorexia and obesity. Although these emotionally charged events do not always lead to psychologic or biologic symptoms and disease, they are frequently noted in the history of children with those presentations. Their prevalence is, of course, high in our society today. Clusters of such experiences especially seem to increase the risk. On the other hand, the reason why some children and parents appear to be strengthened in response to such events is not understood. Such stressors include:

Accidents; trauma

Entrance to new school

Family violence

Hospitalization, especially when there is insufficient time to prepare the child

Acute or chronic illness

Natural disasters; for example, floods, fires, tornados, hurricanes

Parental emotional illness; for example, depression, anxiety, alcoholism, psychosis

Parental unemployment

Physical abuse

Remarriage of parent

Separation experiences—acute or potential

   Death or anticipated death of a significant person

   Divorce or desertion

   Parental separation

   Family move

   Placement of child outside of the home

   Older sibling leaving home

Parental life-threatening illness, for example, cancer, coronary artery disease

Sexual abuse

Surgery

In addition to short-term effects, some emotionally charged experiences appear to have long-term sequelae. Children who are expected by their parents to die prematurely because of a history of a serious illness may demonstrate the vulnerable child syndrome—a fairly common clinical disorder. Such children may demonstrate continuing anxiety along with separation problems, infantilization, bodily overconcern and school underachievement (Green & Solnit, 1964). Children are also at special risk for the development of antisocial behavior following the separation or divorce of their parents (Rutter, 1974). Those who are under 11 years of age when one or both of the parents die have an increased susceptibility to depression (Brown & Harris, 1978).

The nature of the clinical disorder associated with stressful life events also differs depending upon the child's developmental stage (Green, 1975). Rumination and failure to thrive, for example, occur in infants; sleep disorders and anorexia appear in the toddler; hyperactivity and psychosocial dwarfism are seen in the preschool child; and somatic complaints, conversion symptoms and depression are noted in the school age child and the adolescent. These developmental stage differences are unexplained, but they may be related to individual biologic variability, changes in the degree of the child's dependency on the mother, biologic rhythms, maturation of the brain and the endocrine system, gender, the stage of cognitive reasoning, and experience.

Children whose parents experience deleterious stressors are also at special risk if, as a result of the stress, the quality of their parenting is compromised. In addition to many other personal or environmental stressors, some adverse life events may center on the child and therefore engage the pediatrician. For example, in the perinatal period stressful events may include the birth of an infant with a congenital anomaly, a critical neonatal illness, stillbirth or death, guilt about returning to work, illness in other family members which creates a burden on the mother, an infant's difficult temperament, multiple births, prematurity, and maternal depression. In the older child serious illness, injury, or need for surgery are other causes of parental stress.

THE PSYCHOBIOLOGY OF HEALTH AND DISEASE

The daily clinical experiences of the pediatric clinician can be of great heuristic value in identifying specific research hypotheses relevant to three broad questions (modified from Weiner, 1982):

1.   Why do some children become ill while others with similar life experiences are not susceptible?

2.   Why does a specific child respond to adversity with one manifestation of disorder rather than another?

3.   Why do certain stressors or psychosocial experiences produce such a broad variety of symptoms, diseases or developmental aberrations?

It is obviously not feasible to summarize in this brief overview the very extensive psychobiologic research literature which seeks to address these difficult and complex questions. The following discussion, which is eclectic rather than exhaustive, touches upon topics of interest to the pediatrician.

Psychoneuroimmunology

Studies of the neuroendocrine mechanisms through which the immune system is regulated and modulated by the brain are of special pediatric interest (Ader, 1980, 1981; Ader & Cohen, 1975). Acute and chronic family stresses have been shown to be significant determinants of whether individual members of a family became ill with streptococcal infections. The risk of such a response increased three- to fourfold after a stressful event (Haggerty, 1980; Meyer & Haggerty, 1962). In animal studies, a number of experimental conditions, including physical restraint, unavoidable electric shock, loud noises, isolation and crowding, have been demonstrated to increase susceptibility to infectious agents (Ader, 1980). Both humoral and cell-mediated immunity may be affected by psychosocial stressors. In animal studies, disruption of the mother-infant relationship has also been reported to increase vulnerability to infection (Ader, 1980). Clinical evidence suggests that psychosocial stress may increase vulnerability in adults to immunologic disorders such as infections, autoimmune diseases and malignancies.

Mother-Infant Interactions

In addition to possible repression of immunity and an increase in vulnerability to infectious illness, the psychobiologic effects of mother-infant interaction and attachment are obviously of great pediatric relevance. In addition to the vast psychologic literature about these relationships, a growing number of biologic studies are being pursued. The enzymes tyrosine hydroxylase and phenylethanolamine N-methyltransferase have been reported to be altered in mice who are socially isolated in early life (Henry, Stephens, Axelrod, & Mueller, 1971).

Hofer has been especially interested in what he has termed the "hidden regulatory processes which usually govern the interaction between mother and infant." In a series of elegant animal studies, he found that separation of the infant from the mother led to changes in a number of variables, including rocking behavior, sleep patterns, heart rate, respiratory rate, growth hormone secretion, vocalization, motor activity and enzyme levels. Furthermore, he demonstrated that the mother's milk regulated the sleep of her infant and that sleep patterns were disrupted by maternal-infant separation (Hofer, 1976). Maternal separation also led to a fall in the cardiac and respiratory rates (Hofer & Weiner, 1972). Based on this work, Hofer concluded that a variety of components appear to be involved in the interaction between a mother and infant, each mediated by a separate input channel and a different brain circuit leading to physiologic responses and behavioral changes in the infant. The mother, in effect, externally regulates her offspring's behavior through multiple sensory input pathways, physiologic responses and brain chemistry (Hofer, 1981, 1982). These regulatory actions are interrupted by separation of the mother from the infant.

Circadian Rhythms

The biologic systems that govern patterns of sleep; levels of cortisol, growth hormone, aldosterone, estrogen, insulin and thyroid hormones;

and patterns of neurotransmitter release, eating, and body temperature have a rhythmic nature (Anders, 1982). Circadian rhythms have an effect both on the appropriate timing of diagnostic procedures in children and adults, that is, blood and urine levels, and on therapeutic interventions, that is, administration of drugs, surgery and radiation. Resistance to disease has also been thought to vary with the time of the day (Moore-Ede, Czeisler, & Richardson, 1983). Emotional stress has been shown to be capable of disrupting an individual's circadian rhythms (Stoebel, 1971). Disturbances of the circadian timing system occur at one end of the pediatric age spectrum in sleep disorders and at the other in anorexia nervosa. In the latter, the circadian patterns of luteinizing and FSH are inappropriate for the patient's age (Boyar et al., 1974).

Endocrine Effects

Hormonal influences on behavioral patterns and cognitive function in children represent another aspect of biologic investigation germane to pediatric research. The precise neural circuits and neurochemical mechanisms through which environmental stimuli lead to behavioral, endocrine, autonomic and other bodily changes, and the feedback circuits for these processes are not yet established.

A number of investigators have demonstrated the role of several peptides in the regulation of feeding behavior. Androgens are reported to affect cognitive abilities; for example, Hier and Crowley (1982) suggested that spatial skills may be influenced by an androgen effect at or before puberty; however, this hypothesis remains unproven (Kagan, 1982). Plasma androgen levels have been positively correlated with aggressive behavior and social rank in a number of species (Lloyd, 1975; Rose, Holaday, & Bernstein, 1971). Secondary amenorrhea attributable to changes in gonadotropin excretion related to stress is a well-known phenomenon.

Two of four prepubertal children with major depressive disorders of the endogenous subtype demonstrated cortisol hypersecretion during their illness. In a manner similar to that of adults, this pattern returned to normal during recovery (Puig-Antich, Chambers, Halpern, Hanlon, & Sachar, 1979). Catecholamines, corticosteroids and growth hormones are thought to account for differences in the responses of individual children to stress, including coping patterns. The level of secretion of epinephrine has also been related to the social and emotional adjustment of children (Frankenhaeuser & Johansson, 1975). One may hypothesize that temperament in infants and young children may also have a neurobiologic basis. Marked increases in plasma cortisol levels were demonstrated to occur after 20 minutes of crying in young infants, presumably owing to that activity (Anders, Sachar, Kream, Roffwarg, & Hellman, 1970). The stage of cognitive development in a specific infant, child or adolescent will also influence whether or not an environmental event is perceived as threatening. In an important clinical study, Wolff, Hofer and Mason (1964) were able to relate the level of adrenocortical excretion in the parents of leukemic children to their psychologic defenses.

Vulnerability and Invulnerability

The concept of vulnerability or invulnerability to stressful circumstances is important in understanding individual responses to stress. Many persons who would appear to be at risk of developing a disease, for example, a peptic ulcer, based on the presence of a specific biologic marker, or an elevated level of the pepsinogen isoenzymes, do not, in fact, become ill.

Since vulnerabilities represent potential precursors of disease, their identification in individual children could provide specific opportunities for prevention. The number and nature of these vulnerabilities depends on multiple factors such as genetic inheritance, psychological background, chronological and developmental maturation, environment, socioeconomic status, family constellation, past experience, life style, and the presence of disease, especially chronic illness. Environmental events appear to have their greatest negative impact when perceived as unpredictable, threatening, and outside of personal control or coping ability. Social supports or an internal rather than external locus of control may diminish susceptibility to such stressors (Rotter, 1966).

Invulnerability is analogous to what Caplan (1981) has termed *mastery,* that is, ". . . behavior by the individual that (1) results in reducing to tolerable limits physiological and psychological manifestations of emotional arousal during and shortly after a stressful event and (2) mobilizes the individual's internal and external resources and develops new capabilities in him that lead to his changing his environment or his relation to it so that he reduces the threat or finds alternate sources of satisfaction for what is lost."

Other synonyms for invulnerability include "plasticity" and "reserve". Among the resources contributing to what she has termed "resiliency," Werner has identified "adaptability on the biological, psychological, social, and cultural levels: profound ties to concrete immediate others; and formal or informal ties between the individual and his or her community" (Werner & Smith, 1981).

The preservation or reestablishment of psychobiologic homeostasis is the central purpose of pediatrics. Figure 2.1, which I have termed a Homeogram, has been clinically helpful in appraising the strengths (invulnerabilities), potentialities, vulnerabilities and problems of individual children, families and environments (Green, 1983). With such an assessment, the clinician can plan preventive or therapeutic actions for individual children and families.

Genetics

The biologic and behavioral responses to stress are also conditioned by genetic differences in endocrine responsiveness, psychoneurologic mecha-

HOMEOGRAM

		Child	Family	Environment
+	Strengths			
(+)	Potentialities			
(—)	Vulnerabilities			
—	Problems			

FIGURE 2.1.   Homeogram.

nisms and immunologic competence. Biologic markers may also permit the identification of persons at risk in a population. The further delineation of genetic influences on an individual's response to stressful experiences would facilitate preventive pediatric intervention.

IMPLICATIONS FOR PEDIATRICS

Prevention

Advances in psychobiology may permit the pediatrician to use biologic and psychologic markers to identify individuals at risk. Coupled with an awareness of high risk situations, for example, bereavement, the clinician may be able to help the individual at risk avoid or modify behavioral patterns or habits that may be health-damaging, maintain self-esteem and utilize social support systems. A major task for pediatricians in the future, perhaps in concert with the schools, will be to help children learn how to develop skills to *adapt* to, *cope* with, and at times, *master* biologic and psychosocial stressors.

Treatment

Psychoneuropharmacology has contributed to the treatment of such psychobiologic disorders as Tourette's syndrome (Golden & Hood, 1982), attention deficit syndrome with hyperactivity, depression and anxiety. The physiologic effects of biofeedback, relaxation therapy, and hypnotherapy are also open to pediatric investigation.

Opportunities for Collaboration in Research

As pediatric practice is being transformed and reinstitutionalized to meet the changing needs of the times, there are both continuing and new

opportunities for fruitful collaboration and intersectoral cooperation between pediatrics and the behavioral and biologic sciences. These include:

1.   The new prevention and health promotion in pediatrics.   In the
past, insufficient attention has been given in pediatric health supervision
visits to child development and behavior. Currently, the scope of these visits is being broadened so as to include clinically applicable information
from child development and the behavioral sciences, and to adapt their
content to the changing needs of families.

In recognition of the many changes in the American family and the need
to make fuller use of periodic pediatric assessments, the American Academy of Pediatrics Committee on the Psychosocial Aspects of Child and
Family Health is preparing content packages for Health Supervision Visits
from the prenatal period through adolescence that will include attention to
appropriate biomedical, developmental and psychosocial issues.

Operationally, the new prevention will include biomedical and psychosocial assessment of the child, the family and the environment; physical
and developmental assessment; anticipatory guidance and containment of
vulnerabilities, including accident prevention; education in and enhancement of parenting skills; promotion of positive parent-child interactions;
intervention for identified problems; and attention to health promotion, for
example, physical activity, sufficient sleep, adequate nutrition and avoidance of smoking and substance abuse.

2.   The new initiative on adaptation. The emphasis in pediatrics on
youth's *growth* and *development* is now being extended to include *adaptation*.
This change is in recognition of the multicausality of disease and the impact that a wide variety of stressors and significant life changes have on the
physical and psychological health of children.

The pediatrician must therefore be prepared to help children and parents to adapt to and cope with the stressors identified above. Much of such
help will, of course, be based on data and approaches developed in the
behavioral sciences.

3.   The increase of function, contribution to comfort and realization of
potential. The pediatrician has long been involved in increasing function
and attending to comfort in relation to children with chronic disorders,
psychologic disorders and/or pain. Behavioral scientists can help identify
therapeutic techniques, for example, in relation to weight loss in obesity, rectal incontinence in children with myelodysplasia, performance of
chronic ambulatory peritoneal dialysis and such cognitive interventions as
graded imagery, progressive muscle relaxation and self-hypnosis. There is
a need to identify clinically useful methods to promote the achievement of
children with unrealized potential, in part through the use of peer therapists.

4.   The organization of care. In my view, the organization of ambula-

tory pediatric care will evolve into a three level system based on the following determinants: (1) length of time and number of visits required for the specific service provided, (2) level of competence required to provide the service, (3) complexity of the problem, (4) professional cast, that is, the pediatrician acting alone or sharing roles with other health and nonhealth disciplines, and 5) the setting of the service, that is, pediatrician's office, school, community hospital or community agency. Other pertinent areas of potential collaboration include enhanced parent participation and compliance.

5. Pediatric psychobiologic research. The vitality of any discipline derives from its capability of renewal through continuous reassessment and extension of its knowledge base. To pursue the clinically relevant but highly complex lines of psychobiologic investigation, a new generation of pediatric investigators must be developed. Too few appropriate pediatric role models now exist in this field of potential pediatric research.

David Hamburg has termed this field "integrative biology—pulling together observations at all levels of organization from molecular to behavioral characteristics of living organisms." The pool from which such future academicians may be recruited includes pediatric endocrinology, genetics, epidemiology, pharmacology, immunology, biochemistry, molecular biology, neurology and neonatology as well as general pediatrics, especially that aspect concerned with the psychosocial aspects of child health. Investigators with combined M.D.-Ph.D. degrees would appear to be ideal candidates for such research careers. Developments in pediatric psychobiologic research could be greatly facilitated by federal or foundation support of training programs and the availability of career investigator awards.

This development will require enhanced communication and collaboration between investigators from multiple biomedical and behavioral disciplines, including child develpment; developmental, social, school and behavioral psychology; child psychiatry; sociology; cultural anthropology; nursing; and social work. The pediatrician can bring to this multidisciplinary group his or her unique perspectives and seminal hypotheses based on a wide variety of clinical experiences, including psychobiologic experiments of nature.

SUMMARY

Pediatric research will in part utilize animal models in which simultaneous attention may be directed to the whole organism at various stages of development and to events at the cellular, organ and body system levels. Animal studies also permit pure genetic strains of animals to be used, and allow control of the timing, quality and quantity of stressors.

Investigtion of the correlations between the periodicity and rhythmic function of biologic systems will further our understanding of the temporal occurrence of psychobiologic disorders. Psychoneuroimmunologic studies are needed to assess the suspected relationships between stress and immunosuppression.

Genetic and epidemiologic studies may be expected to relate biologic and psychologic markers to an individual child's and to a population's vulnerability or invulnerability to biopsychosocial disorders. Finally, epidemiologic and longitudinal clinical studies would appear to offer significant opportunities for the delineation of immediate and long-term psychobiologic causes and effects.

REFERENCES

Ader, R. (1980). Psychosomatic and psychoimmunologic research. *Psychosomatic Medicine, 42,* 307–321.

Ader, R. (Ed.) (1981). *Psychoneuroimmunology.* New York: Academic.

Ader, R., & Cohen, N. (1975). Behaviorally conditioned immunosuppression. *Psychosomatic Medicine, 37,* 333–340.

Anders, T.F. (1982). Biological rhythms in development. *Psychosomatic Medicine, 44,* 61–72.

Anders, T.F., Sachar, E.J., Kream, J., Roffwarg, H.P., & Hellman, L. (1970). Behavioral state and plasma cortisol response in the human newborn. *Pediatrics, 46,* 532–537.

Boyar, R.M., Katz, J.L., Finklestein, J.W., Kapen, S., Weiner, H., Weitzman, E.D., & Hellman, L. (1974). Anorexia nervosa: Immaturity of the 24-hour luteinizing hormone secretory pattern. *New England Journal of Medicine, 291,* 861–865.

Brown, G.W., & Harris, T. (1978). *Social origins of depression: A study of psychiatric disorders.* New York: Free Press.

Caplan, G. (1981). Mastery of stress: psychosocial aspects. *American Journal of Psychiatry, 138,* 413–420.

Cohen, F., & Lazarus, R.S. (1983). Coping and adaptation in health and illness. In D. Mechanic (Ed.), *Handbook of health, health care, and the health professions* (pp. 608–635). New York: Free Press.

Elliott, G.R., & Eisdorfer, C. (Eds.). (1982). *Stress and human health. Analysis and implications of research.* New York: Springer.

Frankenhaeuser, M., & Johansson, G. (1975). Behavior and catecholamines in children. In L. Levi (Ed.), *Society, stress and disease, Volume 2, Childhood and adolescence* (pp. 118–126). London: Oxford University Press.

Golden, G.S., & Hood, O.J. (1982). Tics and tremors. *Pediatric Clinics of North America, 29,* 95–103.

Green, M. (1975). A developmental approach to symptoms based on age groups. *Pediatric Clinics of North America, 22,* 571–581.

Green, M. (1983). Coming of age in general pediatrics. *Pediatrics, 72,* 275–282.

Green, M., & Solnit, A.J. (1964). Reactions to the threatened loss of a child: A vulnerable child syndrome. *Pediatrics, 34,* 58–66.

Gregg, A. (1951). *Multiple causation and organismic and integrative approaches to medical education.* Paper presented to the Conference on Psychiatric Education, American Psychiatric Association, Washington, D.C.

Haggerty, R.J. (1980) Life stress, illness and social supports. *Developmental Medicine and Child Neurology, 22,* 391–400.

Henry, J.P., Stephens, P.M., Axelrod, J., & Mueller, R.A. (1971). Effect of psychosocial stimulation on the enzymes involved in the biosynthesis and metabolism of noradrenaline and adrenaline. *Psychosomatic Medicine, 33,* 227–237.

Hier, D.B., & Crowley, W.F, Jr. (1982). Spatial ability in androgen-deficient men. *New England Journal of Medicine, 306,* 1202–1205.

Hofer, M., & Weiner, H. (1972). Mechanisms for nutritional regulation of autonomic cardiac control in early development. *Psychosomatic Medicine, 34,* 472.

Hofer, M.A. (1976). The organization of sleep and wakefulness after maternal separation in young rats. *Developmental Psychobiology, 9,* 189–205.

Hofer, M.A. (1981). Toward a developmental basis for disease predisposition: The effects of early maternal separation on brain, behavior, and cardiovascular system. In H. Weiner, M.A. Hofer, & A.J. Stunkard (Eds.), *Brain, behavior and bodily disease* (pp. 209–228). New York: Raven.

Hofer, M.A. (1982). Some thoughts on "The transduction of experience" from a developmental perspective. *Psychosomatic Medicine, 44,* 19–28.

Holmes, T.H., & Rahe, R.H. (1967). The social readjustment rating scale. *Journal of Psychosomatic Research, 11,* 213–218.

Kagan, J. (1982). The idea of spatial ability. *New England Journal of Medicine, 306,* 1225–1227.

Lloyd, J. (1975). Social behavior and hormones. In B. Eleft-Heriou & R. Sprott (Eds.), *Hormonal correlates of behavior.* New York: Plenum.

Meyer, R.J., & Haggerty, R.J. (1962). Streptococcal infections in families: Factors altering individual susceptibility. *Pediatrics, 29,* 539–549.

Moore-Ede, M.C., Czeisler, C.A., & Richardson, G.S. (1983). Circadian timekeeping in health and disease. *New England Journal of Medicine, 309,* 469–476.

Powell, G.F., Brasel, J.A., Raiti, S., & Blizzard, R.M. (1967). Emotional deprivation and growth retardation simulating idiopathic hypopituitarism. II. Endocrinologic evaluation of the syndrome. *New England Journal of Medicine, 276,* 1279–1283.

Prugh, D.C. (1983). *The psychosocial aspects of pediatrics.* Philadelphia: Lea & Febiger.

Puig-Antich, J., Chambers, W., Halpern, F., Hanlon, C., & Sachar, E.J. (1979). Cortisol hypersecretion in prepubertal depressive illness: a preliminary report. *Psychoneuroendocrinology, 4,* 191–197.

Reiser, M.F. (1980). Implications of a biopsychosocial model for research in psychiatry. *Psychosomatic Medicine, 42,* 141–151.

Rose, R., Holaday, J., & Bernstein, I. (1971). Plasma testosterone, dominance, rank, and aggressive behavior in rhesus monkeys. *Nature, 231,* 366–368.

Rotter, J.B. (1966). Generalized expectancies for internal versus external control of reinforcement. *Psychology Monographs: General and Applied, 80,* 1–28.

Rutter, M. (1974). *The qualities of mothering: Maternal deprivation reassessed.* New York: Jason Aronson.

Shapiro, A.P., Benson, H., Chobanian, A.V., Herd, J.A., Julius, S., Kaplan, N., Lazarus, R.S., Ostfeld, A.M., & Syme, S.L. (1979). The role of stress in hypertension. *Journal of Human Stress, 5,* 7–26.

Stoebel, C.F. (1971). The importance of biological clocks in mental health. In E.A. Rubenstein & G.V. Coelho (eds.), *Behavioral Sciences and Mental Health* (PHS Publication No. 2064). Washington, DC: U.S. Government Printing Office.

Weiner, H. (1982). The prospects for psychosomatic medicine: Selected topics. *Psychosomatic Medicine, 44,* 491–517.

Werner, E.E., & Smith, R.S. (1981). *Vulnerable but invincible: A longitudinal study of resilient children and youth.* New York: McGraw-Hill.

Wolff, C.T., Hofer, M.A., & Mason, J.W. (1964). Relationship between psychological defenses and mean urinary 17-hydroxycorticosteroid excretion rates. II. Methodologic and theoretical considerations. *Psychosomatic Medicine, 26,* 592–609.

3

A Behavioral Perspective on Child Health

JOSEPH V. BRADY

The premise of this chapter is the now commonplace observation that health-related processes interact in profound and enduring ways with environmental circumstances and behavioral activities. The analysis of these biobehavioral relationships and their application to child health has been aided by the strong empirical influence of the experimental laboratory, and it is the extensive range of these operationalized interactions which this chapter addresses.

Conceptually, the roots of this behavioral perspective on child health can be identified with the fundamentals of environmentalism, which has two main features. The first of these is that knowledge comes from experience rather than from innate ideas, divine revelation, or any other obscure source. And the second holds that action is governed primarily by consequences rather than by instinct, reason, will, cognitions, beliefs, attitudes, or any of the myriad explanatory fictions that appear to have been created out of whole cloth by the magic of human language. Taken together, these two constructs about human nature define a philosophy of social optimism, which holds that if persons want to be a certain way or to do certain things, the necessary or sufficient circumstances can be arranged. The coalescence of these two ideas took place in nineteenth-century England, and dated the emergence of modern behaviorism. Their influence upon medicine in general and child health problems in particular appears to have developed much more slowly amidst dominant biological orientations, but their impact is now finding expression in the emergence of a behavioral perspective in medicine and pediatrics that enhances these fields of scientific and professional endeavor and encompasses virtually all aspects of health and disease (Pomerleau & Brady, 1979).

The important influence of the experimental laboratory data base that now provides the empirical foundations for these assertions originated with the contributions of I. P. Pavlov, focusing on the role of behavioral activities and environmental circumstances in the physiological and biochemical adjustments and adaptations of the milieu interieur. Pavlov's work also provided the foundation for conceptualizing behavioral interactions within the context of a systematic and orderly body of scientific knowledge based on observation and experiments. The contrast between this objective approach to behavior analysis and more traditional (and lamentably, to some considerable extent, contemporary) appeals to unobserved and unobservable "mental" processes (in whatever cognitive guise they may appear) is worth emphasizing.

But what, in fact, has been learned in the laboratory about those behavioral activities at the interface between individuals and their environments, and to what extent are these findings relevant to child health problems? At the most basic level, there appear to be *two fundamental modes* that characterize this interactive process. In the *first instance,* a *reactive mode* is clearly rooted in the physiological and biochemical adaptations of the organism to a changing environment (that is, the environment acts on the organism and the organism reacts). This respondent paradigm has provided the basis for Pavlovian descriptions and experimental analysis of increasingly more complex interactions directly relevant to clinical medicine, in general, and to child health in particular. Respondent conditioning studies (Deane & Zeaman, 1958; Dykman & Gantt, 1958) have provided systematic accounts of how neutral environmental stimuli (e.g., lights and tones), which produced only minimal initial changes in somatic activity could, for example, elicit conditional physiological responses (e.g., increases in heart rate) of considerable magnitude and duration when paired repeatedly with other environmental stimulus events (e.g., electric shock or food) that could normally have elicited such changes. If such conditional light or tone stimuli (CS) are presented a number of times without the unconditional food or shock stimuli (UCS), the frequency and magnitude of the conditional response (CR; heart rate increase) elicited by the CS decrease, and respondent extinction occurs. When time intervenes between such extinction and subsequent CS presentations, however, spontaneous recovery of the CR occurs as a temporary reappearance of the response elicited by the CS.

The power to elicit a CR developed in one CS by conditioning can extend to other stimuli; the degree of this "stimulus generalization" is determined by the differences and similarities between other stimuli and the CS. Because such other stimuli differ from the CS with respect to the frequency and magnitude with which they elicit the CR, "stimulus discrimination" is also observed. Discrimination can be made increasingly more pronounced by pairing the UCS repeatedly only with a specific CS (i.e., respondent conditioning) thus insuring that other stimuli are not paired with the UCS.

These basic observations relevant to the reactive or respondent conditioning mode have been extended in numerous laboratory and clinical-experimental studies since Russian investigators first introduced this systematic approach to behavior analysis. It has been convincingly demonstrated, for example, that second- or higher-order conditioning occurs when a well-established CS is paired with a neutral stimulus. The neutral stimulus acquires eliciting properties with respect to the reactive CR. It has not been determined just how far this process can be carried; however, the development of eliciting properties by CSs two or three steps removed from the original UCS is not uncommon. And the intensive investigative effort, principally Russian in origin, to extend the conceptual framework of such classical or Pavlovian (i.e., respondent) conditioning to encompass verbal stimuli and somatic responses (Razran, 1961) suggests potentially important directions for development of theory and practice in the child-health area.

Elicited responses of the type that have provided the primary focus for such fundamental respondent or reflex conditioning analyses must nonetheless be seen to constitute only a relatively small proportion of the behavioral repertoire of higher organisms. The most prominent aspects of such advanced performances are represented by the *second basic,* and generally more *active* than reactive, *mode* characterizing behavioral interactions; this second mode focuses on the operations performed by organisms on their internal and external environments rather than on their "reflex" reactions to such environmental influences. Technically, this active mode has been explicated within the framework of a 3-term contingency analysis emphasizing the temporal relationships between *organismic performances (R), reinforcing consequences (S^R),* and the *environmental context (S^D)* in which the $R{\rightarrow}S^R$ relationship occurs. Major contributions to the experimental analysis of such "operant" (i.e., the organism "operating" on the environment) behavior interactions have been identified with the work of B. F. Skinner, his students, and his colleagues. The dominant relationship between these component terms emphasizes the governance of action (i.e., the likelihood of a response) by the contingently occurring effects of that action (i.e., its reinforcing "consequences"). Emergent relations between S^D (i.e., environmental context) and R (i.e., response) components are also specified to the extent that "response-consequence" contingency relations are dependent on contextual occasioning events (i.e., environmental stimulus). More complex interrelationships between these terms have also been elaborated (e.g., rule or schedule relations), and along with historical variables, have enhanced precise definitional accounts of such behavioral contingencies. *Within the context of these empirical referents, the likelihood, strength, and persistence of behavior can be more readily accounted for than within any other conceptual framework.*

Over the past three decades, a broad range of animal laboratory and human experimental studies has provided important insights into the principles that determine the acquisition, maintenance, and modification of operant behavior (Honig, 1966; Honig & Staddon, 1976). The basic observation is that the rate of an operant response already in an organism's repertoire can be readily increased by reinforcement (operant conditioning). Beyond this, it has been possible to make explicit the process called *"shaping,"* whereby operant conditioning can extend existing simple responses into new and more complex performances. Of critical importance for this shaping process is the observation that a reinforcer not only strengthens the particular response that precedes it, but also produces an increase in the frequency of many other similar bits of behavior, and, in effect, raises the individual's general activity level.

The shaping of behavior proceeds as reinforcers are initially presented following a response similar to or approximating the desired one. Since this tends to increase the strength of various other similar behaviors, a response still closer to the desired one can be selected from the new array and can be reinforced. Continued narrowing and refinement of the response criteria required for reinforcement leads progressively to new available behavior. In this way, by successive and progressive approximation, a new and desired performance can be shaped. The importance of this simple but fundamental and powerful shaping process for the development and modification of behavior cannot be overstated, since the weight of available evidence suggests that a careful and systematic application of such procedures with effective reinforcers is sufficient to establish or alter any operant performance of which the organism is physically capable, and a number of others of which it was thought to be incapable. This shaping process is obviously of enormous clinical importance in behavioral medicine and behavioral pediatrics, since many performances, child and adult alike, can effectively be changed only in this way. Without shaping, one might wait for inordinately long periods before performance of some critical health-related behavior could be reinforced.

The fact that some changes in behavior were not brought about by deliberate and systematic manipulation of the environment, however, has led to an analysis of *superstitious behavior*. A potentially reinforcing environmental event may, by chance, follow a response, resulting in the adventitious strengthening of that response. If this sequence of events reoccurs even infrequently (i.e., intermittent reinforcement, as described below), the individual may learn quite elaborate sequences of superstitious behavior that have absolutely nothing to do with production of the event that is influencing the frequency of the behavior. The elaborate rituals of the gambler do not produce winning dice combinations any more than native dances produce rain; they persist because they are occasionally followed by winning throws in the first instance and precipitation in the second.

The powerful effects of reinforcement in establishing and maintaining operant behavior suggest that witholding such reinforcing consequences (*extinction*) will have comparably powerful effects on the strength of previously reinforced responses. Indeed, such extinction procedures do reduce the frequency of response, although the reduction is not usually immediate. Rather, after the onset of extinction, the initial effect is often a brief increase in the frequency as well as the force and variability of the response previously followed by reinforcement. The extent to which operant responding persists in the absence of reinforcing environmental consequences (i.e., resistance to extinction) depends, of course, on the interaction of many complex influences including motivational factors (e.g., level of deprivation). But both laboratory and clinical evidence now confirm that the single most important variable affecting the course of operant extinction is the schedule of reinforcement on which the performance was previously acquired and maintained.

Whenever a reinforcing environmental stimulus follows some but not all occurrences of an operant response, a *schedule of intermittent reinforcement* is operating. Every reinforcer occurs according to some schedule or rule, although some schedules are so complicated that detailed analysis is required to formulate them precisely. Simple schedules of intermittent reinforcement can be classified into two broad categories: ratio and interval schedules. Ratio schedules prescribe that a certain number of responses be emitted before one response is reinforced, the term "ratio" referring to the relationship between the required response total (e.g., 50) and the one response followed by the reinforcing event (e.g., piecework schedule requiring 49 discrete responses before the single 50th performance is followed by payoff). Interval schedules, on the other hand, prescribe that a given interval of time elapse before a response can be followed by a reinforcing stimulus (e.g., salaried pay schedules).

Even simple ratio and interval schedules can in turn be classified into two general categories based on whether the required number of responses or lapse of time are fixed or variable, and all known schedules of reinforcement can be reduced to variations of these basic ratio and interval parameters. Virtually all operant behavior is followed by reinforcing stimuli according to multiple, compound, and concurrent schedules built from the same basic elements as the simple ratio and interval schedules. Each schedule, simple or complex, generates and maintains its own characteristic performance. When reinforcement is discontinued, the course and character of extinction are prominently influenced by the preceding schedule of reinforcement (Ferster & Skinner, 1957). Significantly, it has also become increasingly clear in the laboratory and the clinic that at least the *frequency or rate of a given operant performance can be more effectively controlled by reinforcement schedule manipulation than by any other means.*

The detailed experimental analysis of reinforcement schedules has also served to emphasize another very important set of relationships between operant performances and environmental events encompassed within the general conceptual framework of *stimulus control.* The occurrence of a reinforcer following an operant not only increases the likelihood that the response will reoccur but it also contributes to bringing that performance under the control of other environmental stimuli present when the operant is reinforced. A discriminative stimulus is thus defined by this process as one in whose presence a particular operant performance is highly probable because the behavior has previously been reinforced in its presence. It is important to recognize, however that discriminative stimuli do not *elicit* performances, as in the respondent or reflex case, but rather *set the occasion for* operant responses, in the sense that they provide the circumstances under which the performance has previously been reinforced. The control over driving behaviors by traffic signals occasioning vehicle braking and accelerating occurs because of systematic relationships between such performances and their consequences (e.g., accidents and fines), not because of any inherent or conditional eliciting properties of red, green, and yellow lights. *This controlling power of a discriminative stimulus (probably the most important proximal influence on behavior)* develops gradually, and at least several occurrences of the reinforcer following the response in the presence of the stimulus are required before the stimulus effectively controls the performance.

Discriminative stimulus control is not a completely selective process, however, since reinforcement of a performance in the presence of one stimulus increases the tendency to respond not only in that stimulus but in the presence of other stimuli with similar properties as well. This is *stimulus generalization.* Furthermore, related *response generalization* effects have also been observed to occur when following an operant with a reinforcer results not only in an increase in the frequency of that response but also in the frequency of similar responses.

This sensitivity to the differential aspects of stimulus and response complexes provides the basis for another major cornerstone of the stimulus-control process known as *discrimination.* Discrimination between two stimuli obtains when an organism behaves differently in the presence of each. Such stimulus discrimination is pronounced under conditions that provide differential reinforcement. This process is seen to operate in the formation of a discrimination when there is a high probability that a reinforcer will follow a given response in the presence of one stimulus, and a low probability that reinforcement will follow the response in the presence of another stimulus. The careful application of such differential reinforcement procedures can bring about remarkably precise control of an operant performance by highly selective aspects of a stimulus complex. This attention to specific properties of a stimulus can be facilitated and enhanced by the use of *instructional stimuli,* which tell about features of the environment that are currently relevant to the occasioning of reinforcement. A treasure map, for example, provides such instructional stimuli. In addition, *imitation* and *modeling,* considered analytically, appear to represent special case instances of such instructional control.

The continued association between discriminative environmental stimulus events and the occurrence of reinforcement endows at least some originally nonreinforcing stimuli with acquired reinforcing properties. These stimuli—fraternity pins and stock market quotations, for example—have come to be designated as *secondary or conditioned reinforcers* to distinguish them from innate, primary, or unconditioned reinforcers, which require no experience to be effective. The development or acquisition of conditioned reinforcing properties by a stimulus is usually a gradual process, as is the case with discriminative stimuli in general, and can be seen to provide the basis for *response chaining* of composed series of performances joined together by environmental stimuli that act both as conditioned reinforcers and as discriminative stimuli. The significance of this general chaining principle must of course be seen to reside in the fact that virtually all behavioral interactions occur as chains of greater or lesser length. Even performances usually treated as unitary phenomena (e.g., golf, bowling, tennis), can be usefully analyzed at various component levels for purposes of modification or proficiency enhancement.

A most important aspect of this complex analysis of environment stimulus events in relation to behavioral interactions is the clear implication that some degree of independence can be gained from the factors limiting conditioned-reinforcer potency by the formation of conditioned reinforcers based on two or more primary reinforcers. Such conditioned stimulus events (*generalized reinforcers*) gain potency from all the reinforcers on which they are based, and the most prominent operant performances in the human repertoire, as well as the most valued stimulus consequence in the social environment (money), can be seen to share these broadly based discriminative and generalized reinforcing properties.

This necessarily abbreviated overview of experimentally derived behavioral concepts and principles relevant to medicine in general and behavioral pediatrics in particular has thus far maintained the traditionally accepted differentiation between active (operant) and reactive (respondent) behavior interaction modes based principally on procedural distinctions identified in the laboratory. The independent and distinctive features of these two coextensive processes are seldom apparent, however, in the course of even detailed natural observation. In no investigative aspect of the behavioral universe is the complex interactions between these active and reactive modes more pronounced than in the experimental analysis of *aversive control* procedures represented (or misrepresented!) by the technical terms punishment, escape, avoidance, and their emotional and motivational corollaries.

Both empirical and theoretical accounts of those aspects of behavioral medicine and behavioral pediatrics concerned with disordered performances frequently assign a central role to historical and contemporary environmental interactions involving aversive events. Operationally characterized in terms of their behavioral effects, aversive stimuli decrease the subsequent frequency of operant responses that produce them and increase the subsequent frequency of operant responses that remove or postpone them. When an aversive stimulus follows an operant and decreases the likelihood that such performances will recur, *punishment* is defined. The short- and long-term effects of punishment will vary as a function of complex operant-respondent interactions, and both discriminative-stimulus control and reinforcement-schedule factors may operate to further influence the subsequent form and frequency of the performance.

Escape is defined by a response terminating an aversive stimulus after the stimulus has appeared. The interaction between operants and respondents is especially prominent in escape situations, since the aversive stimulus usually elicits reflexive responses which eventually result in or accompany an operant performance followed by withdrawal of the aversive stimulus. Strong generalization effects also appear during exposures to escape situations though extinction of an operant escape response usually occurs rapidly when presentation of the aversive stimulus is discontinued.

Avoidance is defined by the occurrence of an operant response that postpones an aversive stimulus. Avoidance performances may be established and maintained either in the presence or absence of an exteroceptive environmental event (i.e., warning stimulus) that precedes the aversive stimulus. When an exteroceptive warning stimulus precedes the aversive stimulus, respondent-conditioning effects operate to endow the warning stimulus with aversive properties, and so its termination following the operant avoidance response probably combines with the continued absence of the aversive stimulus to act as a reinforcer. In the absence of an exteroceptive warning stimulus, a temporal respondent-conditioning process provides discriminative cues, and the temporal stimulus correlated with the aversive environmental event acquires the same functions as an exteroceptive stimulus.

Such an analysis of aversive control emphasizes the simultaneous operation of active (or operant) and reactive (or respondent) conditioning processes in ongoing behavior segments. Whenever the conditioned stimulus in a respondent conditioning procedure is an appetitive or aversive reinforcer, operant conditioning occurs at the same time as respondent conditioning. Similarly, whenever the reinforcer in an operant procedure is an unconditioned stimulus, respondent conditioning proceeds at the same time as operant conditioning. To the extent then, that the eliciting and reinforcing stimulus classes are composed of the same environmental events, operant and respondent processes are coextensive.

Relevant applications of these basic behavior-analysis principles to clinical medicine in general and to child-health problems in particular have emerged in three major forms which define pertinent biobehavioral interrelationships. In the first instance, there is abiding concern with the effects of behavioral independent variables on behavioral dependent variables (e.g., the way in which behavioral shaping, maintenance, and modification procedures affect health-related performances like exercise, food intake, and compliance with medically prescribed regimens). In the compliance case, for example, several of the contributions to this volume document experimentally and clinically the potent effects of scheduling conditions, stimulus control, and chaining, which determine under what circumstances and in accordance with what behavioral requirements a valued commodity or substance, be it food, drug, money, social interactions, or whatever, can be obtained. All such events are subject to this kind of rule governance, some of which is very complex. But they all appear to be variations and/or combinations of a few basic types, and a great deal has been learned about their properties and effects, both in the experimental laboratory and in the natural ecology.

The two major classes into which such effects can be categorized appear to be those that are schedule-maintained, on the one hand, and those that are schedule-induced, on the other. The curious side effects of reward-enhancing intermittent schedules and complex historical circumstances (e.g., maintenance of shock-producing performances and great strengthening of adjunctive or ancillary behaviors) certainly provide examples of direct relevance to medicine and child health (Falk, 1971; Kelleher & Morse, 1968). But it is the power of the kind of environmental constraints imposed by such scheduling to entrain performances of remarkable persistence that seems most relevant in the present context. These properties of a behavioral interaction frequently appear as the most baffling and recalcitrant aspects of the health-related repertoire (for example, smoking, over-eating).

Figure 3.1 illustrates a typical cumulative record from an experiment in which a chimpanzee sustained performance on a ratio-schedule that required 120,000 responses on a heavy push-button manipulandum for access to food (Findley & Brady, 1965). After each 4000 responses toward the total requirement, a brief flash of light was presented—the same light that was on continuously during food access once the total ratio was completed. Of particular interest is the pause that followed each flash of light after a block of 4000 responses, illustrating the control acquired by this conditioned reinforcing stimulus event. Subsequent extension to a 250,000 response ratio and manipulations involving removal and reintroduction of

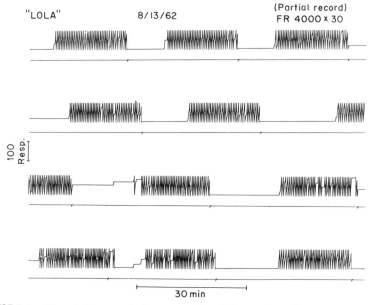

"LOLA"   8/13/62   (Partial record)
                                                      FR 4000 x 30

100 Resp.

30 min

FIGURE 3.1.   Cumulative record of responses (vertical excursion of stepping pen-reset after each 100 responses) over time (horizontal baseline-paper speed) for chimpanzee "Lola" showing pause following each flash of light (conditioned reinforcer) after a block of 4000 responses toward the total requirement of 120,000 for access to food.

the light flash after each 10,000 responses documented the critical interactions between rule-governance and stimulus control in the establishment and maintenance of such remarkably persistent performance repertoires.

While such unusual and extreme examples of schedule and stimulus-control conditions may appear to push the limits of adaptive function, they are not tricks or circus acts. They do in fact represent the orderly and lawful operation of general relationships common to all behavioral interactions, including those related to child health, and they appear to be of particular relevance to the excessive or abusive aspects of such performances.

The second major form that relevant applications of basic behavior analysis principles to clinical medicine and child health has taken emphasizes the effects of behavioral independent variables on biological dependent variables. At the laboratory level, for example, procedures have been developed for active rather than reactive behavioral control of visceral, somatomotor, and central-nervous-system processes based on the arrangement of explicit contingency relationships between specific antecedent physiological events and programmed environmental consequences. It has been convincingly demonstrated that such behavioral "biofeedback" intervention can produce reliable bidirectional control of both increases and decreases in cardiac rate (DiCara & Miller, 1969; Engel & Gottlieb, 1970) and blood pressure (Benson, Herd, Morse, & Kelleher, 1969; Pappas, DiCara, & Miller, 1970). In addition, large and enduring elevations in heart rate (Harris, Gilliam, & Brady, 1976) and blood pressure (Harris, Findley, & Brady, 1971) have also been described in more chronic behavioral conditioning studies.

The functional relations that characterize such active behavioral control of biological processes can, of course, be explicated within the same 3-term contingency framework that has provided the basis for more traditional performance analyses. The systematic application of behavioral procedures to effect biological changes differs only in that at least one of the terms (for example, the R or response term) is identified by the measurement of events that are localized within the boundary protoplasm which separates the organism from its external environment. A clinically relevant example of this second major form of behavior-analysis application to child-health problems has been convincingly provided by the work of Whitehead and his colleagues with incontinent children who have afferent or efferent neuropathology of the bowel or urinary tract. Employing manometric equipment to provide discriminative control of rectal distention and recto-sphincteric activity, it has been possible to establish continence in previously incontinent pediatric patients with myelomeningocele (Whitehead, Parker, Masek, Cataldo, & Freeman, 1981).

Of particular relevance to the application of such behavior-analysis procedures in the control of biological processes would seem to be more recent laboratory studies that document the effectiveness of operant shaping techniques in systematically altering both the amplitude and duration of blood-pressure increases in small progressive steps to extremely high levels. Figure 3.2, for example, shows the relative frequency distributions of diastolic blood pressure from an experiment in which a baboon learned to increase and maintain blood pressure elevations in order to obtain food and avoid shock (Turkkan & Harris, 1981). The shaping procedure involved delivery of food pellets for accumulation of 600 sec of time above the diastolic-pressure criterion level, and delivery of a single electric shock to the tail for accumulation of 240 sec of time below that criterion level. Experimental sessions began at noon each day, and ended at midnight. Criterion levels beginning at 65 mm Hg (i.e., pre-experimental baseline average diastolic pressure level) were progressively elevated at a rate approximating two to three mm Hg per week. The systematic shaping of diastolic pressure elevations over a 10 to 12 week conditioning period, illustrated in Figure 3.2, compares the diastolic pressure levels recorded *during* sessions (open bars) with the levels recorded during the 12-hr intervals *between* sessions (filled bars) under baseline conditions (top segment) and during successive stages of conditioning. At the highest criterion (lower right segment), diastolic pressures were elevated above 100 mm of Hg in order to maintain a food-abundant environment throughout the 12-hr experimental session, during which less than one shock per hour was delivered. It is evi-

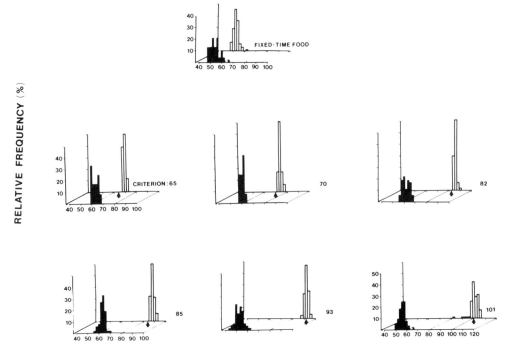

DIASTOLIC BLOOD PRESSURE (mmHg)

FIGURE 3.2.   Relative frequency distributions of 40-minute average pressures for baboon
" 82" during a baseline condition (fixed-time food), and at successively higher diastolic criteria (columns, from right to left). Open bars represent diastolic pressure levels from 4 experimental sessions, while fixed bars represent data from 4 associated postsession periods. Ar-
rows indicate the diastolic criterion level at each stage of training, with criterion values shown
numerically to the right of each graph.

dent that there was no overlap between the distributions of pressure levels
recorded at this highest criterion and those recorded during the baseline
period.

While these observations clearly reflect the participation of an active
behavioral process in the development and maintenance of biological functions traditionally considered under more reactive control, no claim to
exclusivity is implied. Multiple mechanisms, both behavioral and physiological, must be presumed operative in the mediation of such complex psychophysiological interactions. Insofar as the internal and external stimulus
events involved in these processes have common functional properties
(e.g., eliciting, reinforcing, discriminative), however, both operant and respondent conditioning, at the very least, can be considered cooperative.

The third and perhaps most familiar form in which the relevance of behavior-analysis principles to child health has been expressed involves the effects of biological independent variables (like the biochemical and physiological changes associated with drug administration) on dependent performance measures at the interface between organism and environment. Developments in the area of behavioral pharmacology over the past decade or more have revealed, for example, that pharmacologic agents can participate in behavioral interactions under the same conditions that govern the relationship between organisms and other stimulus events. As environmental stimuli, drugs can be seen to have *eliciting* properties in reactive behavioral modes, and both *reinforcing* and *discriminative* properties in more active behavioral modes. The *eliciting properties* of drugs as stimuli that *precede* biochemical, physiological, and behavioral responses in a reactive mode have traditionally provided the basis for most pharmacological and toxicological evaluations, including the development of increasingly more sensitive and reliable laboratory behavior models (Barrett, 1980; Geller, Stebbins, & Wayner, 1979; Iverson, Iverson, & Snyder, 1977). The *reinforcing properties* of drugs as stimulus events that increase the frequency of the responses they *follow* have been convincingly demonstrated with a range of pharmacologic agents that function to maintain active drug-seeking and drug-taking behaviors (Brady & Griffiths, 1977; Fischman & Schuster, 1982; Griffiths, Bigelow, & Henningfield, 1980; Yanagita, 1973). And the *discriminative properties* of drugs as stimuli that increase the probability of those responses that have previously been reinforced in their *presence* have now been extensively analyzed within the methodological framework of drug discrimination studies (Colpaert & Rosencrans, 1978; Schuster & Balster, 1977; Winter, 1978). The results of these latter experiments have shown, for example, that the occurrence of a response can be controlled (that is, occasioned) by administration of a pharmacologic agent if the response in question has previously been reinforced when (and only when) the administered drug has been "on board".

It is of course true that some biological changes, including some drugs, at some doses and at some particular times, may have no effect at all on behavior whether they precede, accompany, or follow responses. It is equally true, however, that the eliciting, reinforcing, and discriminative properties of a biological event may all participate simultaneously in complex behavioral interactions. The reinforcing and eliciting functions of alcohol, for example, have been well documented by observations and experiments involving excessive self-administration and impaired performance in both episodic and chronic abusers. But the discriminative properties of this "CNS depressant" in occasioning characteristically "drunken" behavior patterns in social situations have been vastly underrated. One can get away with a lot more "pinching and squeezing" with alcohol "on board" than when one is "cold sober!" The discriminative functions of the drug in someone else are frequently sufficient to occasion all sorts of strange behaviors in those who might be characterized as merely "participant observers" of the cocktail-party scene.

That the presence of a drug may occasion or "legitimize" behavior that might better be characterized as a concomitant of drug administration rather than as a direct result cannot be regarded as novel. The term "sick role" is in wide medical use to denote a pattern of responses occasioned or "legitimized" by prior exposure to pathogen, trauma or disorder. Indeed, these behavioral concomitants of illness are tolerated by conspecifics if, and only if, associated with illness. They are concomitants because they are not induced by pathogens. Viruses do not induce a demand to be waited on hand and foot or give license to express one's view on hospital food by throwing it at nurses. Just as prior exposure to a pathogen may license certain behaviors in the afflicted individual, those with whom the patient interacts also adjust their behavior. Illness in one individual may indirectly occasion changes in the behavior of others sometimes characterized as solicitous or care-giving. Drugs, like illness, can occasion behaviors that then serve to occasion still other changes in other individuals. This discriminative functional property is of particular importance when considering drug effects on child behavior that occurs predominantly in a social setting where the most critical relationships involve responses of other persons.

The "sick-role" notion may be used to illustrate another of the functional properties of drugs, that is, drugs as conditional reinforcers. Conditional reinforcers acquire their potency through association with already effective reinforcers and the performances that produce them. Like other reinforcers, they serve to maintain in strength responses that precede their occurrence in close temporal contiguity. In this regard, for example, it is not uncommon for pediatric patients to receive a level of attention and care seldom attained under normal conditions. Now and then, a child will appear to remain impaired far beyond the period imposed by the illness or disorder. The child behaves as though continued impairment was desirable and seeks to convince physician, nurse or family that the pathological state remains in being. Impairment appears to have acquired reinforcing properties, and behavior is directed at maintaining the condition, often at the cost of enormous losses in other parts of the child's life. In the case of human drug use, for example, there is overwhelming evidence that drugs may be ingested, not for their primary pharmacological/physiological effects but because other reinforcing events have been associated with the drug state in the past. These frequently take the form of social activity or approval. Drug self-administration itself may be no more reinforcing than laying in a hospital bed for weeks on end or ingesting goldfish at a fraternity party. Each may be seen as a behavioral strategy for inducing changes in the behavior of others.

The relevance of these basic relationships to the topic that provides the focus for these proceedings is the attention called to the *functional* interactions between behavior and biological processes in contrast to the *topo-*

graphical emphasis which has frequently characterized traditional models for the analysis of such biobehavioral effects. The distinction between topography and function is the distinction between the formal characteristics of a performance (e.g., muscle contractions and extensions involved in an arm movement) and the temporal relationships between the performance, on the one hand, and its environmental antecedents and consequences, on the other (e.g., the sighting of friend or foe, the giving of a greeting or ministering of a blow). Viewed topographically for example, the scream for help, the scream for demonstration purposes, and the child's scream for attention may, for all practical purposes, be identical, but an analysis of their functional relations to the environment (e.g., their effects on an audience) reveals differences of the greatest import. Conversely, two topographically different performances (e.g., passing one's fingers over raised letters on a cardboard and moving one's eyes over print on a page) may be functionally identical to the extent that they are both maintained by the consequences of reading.

The differences highlighted by the topographic-functional distinction would seem to be of direct relevance to critical issues involving the *generality* of this behavioral perspective on child health. Expressed concerns about the limitations on generalizing from an experimental animal's lever-pressing to the verbal performances of a human child, for example, may be quite valid when the analysis is restricted to the *topography* of responses that are so obviously different. But when events are considered *functionally* in terms of their relations to antecedents and consequences, it is quite possible to cut across performances and environmental stimuli with entirely different topographies to generalize between species and apply data from laboratory behavior models to human child-health research and practice.

In common parlance, it is the "meaning" of a behavioral assessment following a biological intervention that is so greatly enhanced by an analysis that goes beyond the topographic fetures of a performance to reveal its functional significance. The dominant relationship between a performance and its *consequences* is of course of particular importance in such an analysis, and is emphasized in behavioral models that parcel out the action of a drug, for example, as a function of the differential properties of environmental consequating events or reinforcement schedules maintaining the performance. Figure 3.3, for example, shows the differential effects of pentobarbital (20 mg/kg) on the aversive and appetitive components of a multiple-schedule performance maintained alternately by shock avoidance and food with the rhesus monkey (Brady, 1959). The animals were trained on a program that consisted of 4 alternating 15-min. cycles. During the first 15-min. portion of the record ("A," Figure 3.3), a red flashing light was presented to the animal in the presence of which a brief shock to the feet was delivered every 20 sec. unless the monkey pressed the lever within the 20-sec. interval ("Sidman" avoidance). At the end of that 15-min. period, the red flashing light and the shocks were terminated, and the animal had

Monkey M-25

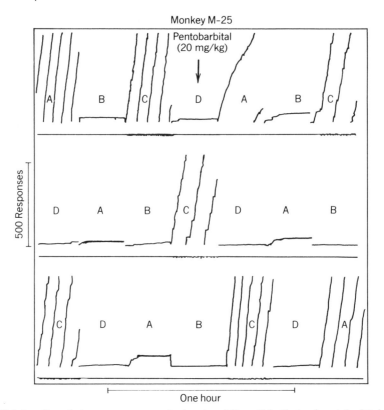

FIGURE 3.3.   Cumulative response records showing differential effects of pentobarbital upon the aversive and appetitive components of a multiple schedule performance maintained alternately by shock avoidance ("A" segments of the record) and food presentation ("C" segments of the record). There were no programmed contingencies during the "B" and "D" segments of the record which served as "time out" between the shock avoidance and food presentation components of the program. Each of the 4 components of the multiple schedule (i.e., A, B, C, D) remained in effect for 15′ and recycled repeatedly in the indicated fixed order over the course of the 6-hour experimental session.

15 min. with no stimulus light, during which lever responses were recorded but had no consequence for altering the monkey's environment ("B," Figure 3.3). After this 15-min. cycle in the absence of any signal light, a steady green light was presented to the animal in the presence of which sugar-pellet rewards could be obtained by pressing the lever on a "fixed ratio" schedule of reinforcement ("C", Figure 3.3). During this period, the animal received one sugar pellet for every 100 lever responses up to a total of 10 sugar pellet rewards (FR 100). Finally, after 10 sugar-pellet rewards or 15 min. in the presence of the green light, the cycle was terminated, and the monkey received another 15-min. period ("D," Figure 3.3) with no light stimulus and no reinforcement contingencies. Then, the entire procedure

was repeated in a cyclic program during experimental sessions of 6 to 12 hr. in length, with the 15-min. components always following each other in this same order.

The response rates of the two performances before drug administration were comparable, as shown in the first "A" and "C" sections of Figure 3.3, before drug administration, and an analysis restricted to topography (say, in different animals under separate schedules) could well have come to widely disparate conclusions about lever-pressing performances and the effect of pentobarbital. Indeed, it is clear from Figure 3.3 that pentobarbital at the indicated dose does have markedly different effects on the avoidance responding (i.e., the "A" sections of Figure 3.3 showing suppression following drug administrations) and food-maintained responding (i.e., the "C" sections of Figure 3.3 showing only slight depression following drug administration). But the interpretation of these observations in terms that appeal to differential pharmacological effects as a function of the relationship between performances and environmental consequences (i.e., aversive or appetitive properties of reinforcing stimuli) provides an account of pertinent drug-behavior interactions of far greater significance and generality than one that focuses on the topography of the lever-pressing response (Ator, 1979; Barrett, 1981).

Similar differential drug effects as a function of reinforcement schedule per se (rather than type of environmental consequating event) are shown in Figure 3.4, which illustrates performance changes following d- amphetamine (10 mg/kg) and pentobarbital (17 mg/kg) on a multiple fixed-interval (FI 10') fixed ratio (FR31) schedule of food presentation with the pigeon (McKearney, 1972). The FI and FR components of the schedule alternated throughout the experimental session. If no response was made within 60 sec. of the end of the 10-min. FI, or if 31 responses were not emitted within 60 sec. during the FR, the alternate schedule component was presented (i.e., a 60-sec. "limited-hold" was in effect). Under the FI 10 schedule there was a pause followed by an increasing rate until food presentation, whereas under the FR 31 schedule there was continuous high and steady rate until food was presented. The top section of Figure 3.4 (labeled "control"), for example, illustrates the different patterns of responding maintained by the two schedules before drug administration. The middle section of Figure 3.4 (labeled "d-amphet") shows that the FR responding was completely abolished following 10.0 mg/kg d-amphetamine, even though FI responding was little affected (or perhaps even slightly enhanced). And finally, the bottom section of Figure 3.4 (labeled "pentobarbital") shows that FR responding continued to occur normally while FI responding was markedly decreased after 17 mg/kg pentobarbital. The point to be made by both these examples is, of course, that drugs cannot be expected to have uniform effects upon behavior regardless of the circumstances under which they are administered. Their effects depend critically upon context and no context is more fundamental and inevitable than consequent/con-

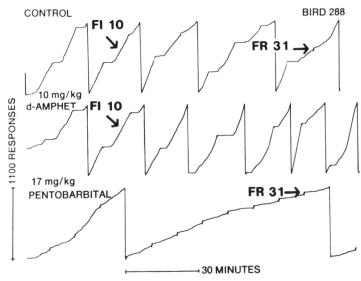

FIGURE 3.4. Cumulative records of responding under a multiple fixed-interval, fixed-ratio schedule showing the differential effects of *d*-amphetamine and pentobarbital. The FI and FR components alternated throughout the session with the 10 mg/kg dose of *d*-amphetamine completely abolishing the FR component without affecting the FI component, while the 17 mg/kg dose of pentobarbital had the exact opposite effect, markedly decreasing FI responding with no effect on the FR rate.

tingency/schedule contexts of the type illustrated in these laboratory studies.

Of equal import, say for the purpose of determining the effects of a biological intervention on sensory processes, would seem to be an analysis that focuses on the functional relations between a performance and the antecedent environmental stimuli that control its occurrence. Over the past two decades, a marriage between classical human psychophysics and basic experimental analysis of organism-environment interactions in laboratory animals has provided behavioral models of remarkable sensitivity and precision for analyzing the sensory/motor effects of drugs and other biological interventions. Figure 3.5, for example, shows the differential effects of pentobarbital (0.1–17.8 mg/kg) on auditory and visual thresholds in two baboons, based on a reaction-time procedure that required the animals to press a lever and hold it depressed for varying intervals until presentation of a light flash or tone burst lasting 1.5 sec signalled the availability of food following lever release (Brady, Bradford, & Hienz, 1979). Correct responses were defined by lever releases occurring during the 1.5 sec stimulus and were reinforced with banana-flavored food pellets. Detection thresholds were determined by systematically varying the stimulus intensity and recording the frequency of correct and incorrect responses (i.e., lever releases occurring prior to or after the 1.5 sec stimulus). In addition,

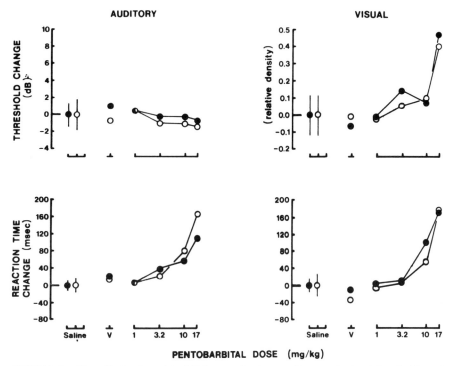

FIGURE 3.5. The effects of pentobarbital upon absolute auditory and visual thresholds and their respective median reaction times. Dose dependent elevations in visual threshold and reaction times were observed with both baboon PE (○) and baboon IK (●), though neither animal showed any change in absolute auditory threshold over the same pentobarbital dose range.

response latencies (elapsed time between signal onset and lever release) were recorded to the nearest millisecond as a measure of motor reaction time (topography?). Figure 3.5 shows that there were dose-dependent elevations in absolute-visual thresholds and reaction times in the absence of any change in absolute auditory thresholds. Only such a detailed analysis of the functional relations between the propeties of antecedent stimuli and the measured performance could have revealed this important differential behavioral effect, since the topographic features of the lever release response (for example, reaction times) were similarly affected regardless of the sensory modality involved. Moreover these results emphasize again the importance of an analysis which takes into account the inevitable contextual variations determined by differential discriminative control in assessing the behavioral effects of pharmacological interventions.

The influence of temporally more remote antecedents on the interactions between biological events and performances has also been convincingly demonstrated with behavioral models that depend critically on a functional analysis of historical variables (McKearney, 1978). When a re-

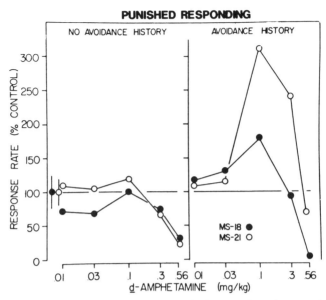

FIGURE 3.6. Effects of *d*-amphetamine upon punished responding of two squirrel monkeys before and after exposure to an avoidance (i.e., shock-postponement) training schedule. Drug produced sizeable increases in punished responding after avoidance training even though the punished performance did not change after avoidance training in the absence of *d*-amphetamine.

sponse maintained by food is punished with electric shock in squirrel monkeys (i.e., 5 sec fixed interval food-presentation schedule with every 30th response during the interval producing 5 mA electric shock to the tail), *d*-amphetamine does not typically increase (and may actually further decrease) the suppressed response rate, as shown in the left side of Figure 3.6, even though this drug usually increases low rates of responding. The effects of amphetamine on such punished behavior can be markedly altered, however, by subsequent and relatively brief training on a procedure that requires responding to avoid shock (as described above for Figure 3.3). The right side of Figure 3.6, for example, shows that *d*-amphetamine produces marked and sustained increases in punished responding even though punished performances in the absence of *d*-amphetamine were identical before and after avoidance training (Barrett, 1977). Similar historical influences have also been shown (Barrett, 1980) with regard to the rate-decreasing effects of morphine on shock avoidance responding and the effects of intervening "free shocks" (i.e., shocks occurring independently of responding). Again, this example highlights the importance (and inevitability) of historically defined contextual variables in determining the behavioral effects of drug administration.

From a broader behavior and child-health perspective, it is now becoming increasingly clear that the key to whether persons will be healthy or sick, live a long life or die prematurely, is likely to be found in the characteristics of their individual performance repertoires with regard to such common behavioral activities as eating, drinking, sleeping, exercising, smoking, and, significantly from a child-health perspective, whether speed laws and other safety measures are observed to avoid accidents and violence. Clearly, the roots of these health-related performances can be readily traced to developmental processes of obvious pediatric relevance, yet they have received surprisingly little attention from traditional medical disciplines. In a word, they have been "nobody's special business" until the expanded applications of behavior analysis to child health problems broadened the scope of potential interventions. Under such circumstances, the interaction between applied medical science and behavior analysis in the promotion of child health promises to emerge as a major movement through the remainder of this century, equal to the surgical revolution earlier in the century and the chemical revolution in the middle of the century. It will doubtless move on into the next century as a significant approach to treatment, prevention, and maintenance of child-health behaviors, just as important as any of the other systems that have come into current pediatric practice.

REFERENCES

Ator, N. A. (1979). Differential effects of chlordiazepoxide on comparable rates of responding maintained by food and shock avoidance. *Psychopharmacology, 66,* 227–231.

Barrett, J. E. (1977). Behavioral history as a determinant of the effects of d-amphetamine on punished behavior. *Science, 198,* 67–69.

Barrett, J. E. (1980, April). Behavioral pharmacology: Recent developments and new trends. *Science, April,* 215–218.

Barrett, J. E. (1981). Differential drug effects as a function of the controlling consequences. In T. Thompson & C. E. Johanson (Eds.), *Behavioral pharmacology of human drug dependence,* NIDA Research Monograph 37. Washington, D.C: U.S Government Printing Office.

Benson, H., Herd, J. A., Morse, W. H., & Kelleher, R. T. (1969). Behavioral inductions of arterial hypertension and its reversal. *American Journal of Physiology, 217,* 30–34.

Brady, J. V. (1959). Differential drug effects upon aversive and appetitive components of a behavioral repertoire. In P. B. Bradley, P. Keniker, & E. Radouco (Eds.), *Neuro-psychopharmacology.* Amsterdam: Elsevier.

Brady, J. V., Bradford, L. D., & Hienz, R. D. (1979). Behavioral assessment of risk-taking and psychophysical functions in the baboon. *Neurobehavioral Toxicology, 1*(1), 73–84.

Brady, J. V., & Griffiths, R. R. (1977). Drug maintained performance and the analysis of stimulant reinforcing effects. In E. H. Ellinwood & M. M. Kilbey (Eds.), *Cocaine and other stimulants.* New York: Plenum.

Colpaert, F. C., & Rosencrans, J. A. (Eds.). (1978). *Stimulus properties of drugs: ten years of progress.* Amsterdam: Elsevier.

Deane, G. E., & Zeaman, D. (1958). Human heart rate during anxiety. *Perceptual and Motor Skills, 8,* 103–106.

DiCara, L. V., & Miller, N. E. (1969). Transfer of instrumentally learned heart rate changes from curarized to noncurarized state: Implications for a mediational hypothesis. *Journal of Comparative and Physiological Psychology, 62* (2, Pt 1), 159–162.

Dykman, R. A., & Gantt, W. H. (1958). Cardiovascular conditioning in dogs and in humans. In W. H. Gantt (Ed.), *Physiological bases of psychiatry.* Springfield, IL: Charles C Thomas.

Engel, B. T., & Gottlieb, S. H. (1970). Differential operant conditioning of heart rate in the restrained monkey. *Journal of Comparative and Physiological Psychology, 73*(2), 217–225.

Falk, J. L. (1971). The nature and determinants of adjunctive behavior. *Physiology and Behavior, 6,* 577–588.

Ferster, C. B., & Skinner, B. F. (1957). *Schedules of reinforcement.* New York: Appleton-Century-Crofts.

Findley, J. D., & Brady, J. V. (1965). Facilitation of large ratio performance by use of conditioned reinforcement. *Journal of the Experimental Analysis of Behavior, 8,* 125–129.

Fischman, M. W. & Schuster, C. R. (1982). Cocaine self-administration in humans. *Federation Proceedings, 41,* 241–246.

Geller, I., Stebbins, W. C., & Wayner, M. J. (Eds.). (1979). *Test methods for definition of effects of toxic substances on behavior and neuromotor function.* Fayetteville, NY: ANKHO International Inc.

Griffiths, R. R., Bigelow, G. E., & Henningfield, J. E. (1980). Similarities in animal and human drug taking behavior. In N. K. Mello (Ed.), *Advances in substance abuse.* Greenwich, CT: Jai Press.

Harris, A. H., Findley, J. D., & Brady, J. V. (1971). Instrumental conditioning of blood pressure elevations in the baboon. *Conditioned Reflex, 6*(4), 215–226.

Harris, A. H., Gilliam, W. J., & Brady, J. V. (1976). Operant conditioning of large magnitude 12-hour heart rate elevations in the baboon. *Pavlovian Journal of Biological Science, 11*(2), 86–92.

Honig, W. K. (Ed.). (1966). *Operant behavior: Areas of research and application.* New York: Appleton-Century-Crofts.

Honig, W. K., & Staddon, J. E. R. (Eds.). *Handbook of operant behavior.* Englewood Cliffs, NJ: Prentice Hall.

Iverson, L. L., Iverson, S. D., & Snyder, S. H. (Eds.). (1977). *Handbook of psychopharmacology: Principles of behavioral pharmacology* (Vol. 7). New York: Plenum.

Kelleher, R. T., & Morse, W. H. (1968). Schedules using noxious stimuli. III. Responding maintained with response-produced electric shocks. *Journal of the Experimental Analysis of Behavior, 11,* 819–838.

McKearney, J. W. (1972). Effects of drugs and maintenance of responding with response-produced electric shocks. In R. M. Gilbert & J. D. Keehn (Eds.), *Schedule-effects: Drugs, drinking and aggression, schedule dependent effects.* Toronto: University of Toronto Press.

McKearney, J. W. (1978). Interrelations among prior experiment and current conditions in the determination of behavior and the effects of drugs. In T. Thompson & P. B. Dews (Eds.), *Advances in behavioral pharmacology* (Vol. 2). New York: Academic Press.

Pappas, B. A., DiCara, L. V., & Miller, N. E. (1970). Learning of blood pressure responses in the noncurarized rat: Transfer to the curarized state. *Physiology and Behavior, 5*(9), 1029–1032.

Pomerleau, O. F., & Brady, J. P. (Eds.). (1979). *Behavioral medicine: Theory and practice.* Baltimore: Williams & Wilkins.

Razran, G. (1961). The observable unconscious and the inferable conscious in current Soviet psychophysiology: Interoceptive conditioning, semantic conditioning, and the orienting reflex. *Psychological Reviews, 68,* 81–147.

Schuster, C. R., & Balster, R. L. (1977). The discriminative stimulus properties of drugs. In T. Thompson & P. B. Dews (Eds.). *Advances in behavioral pharmacology* (Vol. 1). New York: Academic Press.

Turkkan, J. S., & Harris, A. H. (1981). Differentiation of blood pressure elevations in the baboon using a shaping procedure. *Behavioral Analysis Letters, 1,* 97–106.

Whitehead, W. E., Parker, L. H., Masek, B. J., Cataldo, M. F., & Freeman, J. M. (1981). Biofeedback treatment of fecal incontinence in patients with myelomeningocele. *Journal of Developmental Medicine and Child Neurology, 23,* 313–322.

Winter, J. C. (1978). Drug-induced stimulus control. In D. E. Blackman & D. J. Sanger (Eds.), *Contemporary research in behavioral pharmacology.* New York: Plenum.

Yanagita, T. (1973). Pharmacology and the Future of Man. *Proceedings of the 5th International Congress of Pharmacology, San Francisco.* Basel: Karger.

4

Advances and Gaps in a Behavioral Methodology of Pediatric Medicine

DONALD M. BAER

A behavioral pediatrics must assume that certain behaviors of children lead to specifiable and important health outcomes. In particular, it will assume that (1) some behaviors maintain and improve health, (2) when pathologies exist, some behaviors are necessary for a cure, and (3) some behaviors cause pathologies. If these assumptions are valid, then, to that extent, a science of behavior change in children that can embrace those particular behaviors is a health science for them (Ferguson & Taylor, 1980; Russo & Varni, 1982; Varni, 1983).

A number of disciplines claim relevance to the problem of change in children. Many of them deal with the problem of changing specified cases of the child's behaviors, and very many of them also deal with the problem of changing the child as an entity. These latter disciplines, in their clinical manifestations, are often characterized by the phrase "dealing with the whole child," and they focus most often on changing the child's attitudes, motivations, feelings, relationships, personality, and world view. When they do so they assume that the child's behavior is primarily an expression of these internal organizations of the child as a whole. They propose that if these internal organizations can be changed, the child's behavior will probably change in an expression of what the child has become.

By contrast, other disciplines, and very notably behavior analysis (which often specializes in the case of children) focus primarily on changing *only* a targeted set of the child's behaviors. Behavior analysis does that because it recognizes behaviors to be not so often *expressive* of the child as a whole, as they are *instrumental* in controlling the child's environment (Skinner, 1953). In behavior analysis the probability of taking an instrumental view of behavior approaches 1.0; in the closely allied discipline of behavior therapy, instrumental logic probably informs most of its approach. In the other disciplines an expressive logic is often more probable than an instrumental one, although in recent decades instrumental concepts seem to be increasing, as do behavior-specific prescriptions of drugs and social techniques (such as seat-belt legislation), much of which has been pioneered by pediatrics.

The essence of instrumental behavior is that it accomplishes things in the child's environment that are essential, advantageous, or disadvantageous to the child as a whole. In principle, each behavior of a child can interact with the environment in different ways and can accomplish different things. Thus each behavior can lead a life of its own. Some behaviors cause good things to happen, and some behaviors prevent bad things from happening or continuing, and that is why they exist. Some behaviors cause good things to stop or diminish, and some behaviors cause bad things to happen, and that is why they rarely occur.

Obviously this view of behavior reveals that some of the mechanisms of behavior change must also be the mechanisms of environmental change. When behaviors cease to accomplish what they had in the past, and instead accomplish something different, they may well change. Then the technology of behavior change is in part the technology of:

1. Analyzing what environmental consequences of any behavior are the functional consequences that explain some of its current strength or weakness.
2. Changing those consequences into different consequences that will support a different behavior, or a different pattern of this behavior.

This strategy deserves the phrase "dealing with the child's whole environment." But since its targets are some of the child's behaviors, not the child's totality, it applies environmental contingencies rather than traditional psychotherapy. Since its targets are delimited, they are precise. Yet its analytic view is extremely broad, and because of its strong emphasis on current environmental mechanisms, always pragmatic. In fact, applied behavior analysis has produced a beginning technology of behavior change, much of it already specialized for the varieties of deviancy seen in children (Leitenberg, 1976). This technology analyzes what part of the child's environment interacts functionally with the child's behaviors that require change, and a parallel technology has learned how to change just that part of the environment (Craighead, Kazdin, & Mahoney, 1976).

The English-language journals specializing in behavior analysis or its clinical cousin, behavior therapy numbered 1 in 1957, and, conservatively counted, 15 in 1985. A graph of the growth in number of those journals, or their pages, or their data displays of control over behavior, by year, will reflect the typical exponential population-growth curve. In this context it may be useful to inquire into the conceptual and empirical origins of this discipline in order to better clarify its potential relevance to pediatrics.

Behavior analysis has its historical roots in the study of learning theory. Like many learning theories, its conceptual intent was not merely to describe the acquisition and maintenance of new behaviors and skills, but rather to analyze the control of behavior in general by the environment in general (Honig, 1966; Honig & Staddon, 1977). However, like many learning theories, its early efforts were directed primarily at the delimited problem of the acquisition of new behavior and the attachment of that behavior to new controlling stimuli. Its experiments at first concentrated on controlling behavior by stimuli in the current environment; but like most contemporary theories, it could argue that the processes it demonstrated as powerful in the organism's current environment might well have been operative in the organism's past environment, which could explain the organism's current behavior. In recent years its experiments have demonstrated repeated examples of just that.

Its early neglect of nonenvironmental factors was procedural, not conceptual: Behavior analysis, like most learning theories, acknowledged that any behavior must be attributable to some considerable extent to organismic variables, heredity prominent among them (Bijou & Baer, 1961). At the level of theory this source of causation was loosely given the same importance as environmental variables; but once having done that behavior analysis, like other learning theories, then ignored organismic variables almost entirely. The most fundamental reason for this is reliance of these theories and their practitioners on the experimental method for the data they would consider important and valid for their purposes. Because nonenvironmental variables—especially heredity—typically were not experimentable variables at that time in the case of human behavior, it was inevitable that in the early decades these variables would play no *procedural* role in the application of these theories to human behavior. Nothing could be done about those variables at that time; thus their actual roles, and the power of those roles, remained untested (not denied) and hence ignored at the level of research and practice, even while acknowledged at the level of theory (Kantor, 1947, 1959). But in recent years this has changed, and a behavior-analytic physiology as well as a physiological behavior analysis now flourish (Brady, this volume; Brady & Harris, 1977; Dunham, 1977, pp. 112–122; Satinoff & Henderson, 1977; Teitelbaum, 1977; Thompson & Boren, 1977).

Behavior analysis concentrated on what they all would call *reinforcement* mechanisms in their analysis of behavior. However, behavior analysis immediately and distinctively began the detailed, systematic codification of the contingencies between behavior and its environmental consequences within which reinforcement took place. That led promptly to the analysis of punishment and extinction contingencies as well. Any study of these contingencies shows that they have great power in the particular settings where they operate, and at the particular times they operate; yet their effects rarely extend automatically to other settings and other times. This control by setting and time over the effects of reinforcement, punishment, and extinction is so common as to deserve and require a label. It was uniformly termed *discrimination*, and its absence *generalization*, in virtually every learning theory, and it became a second-level mechanism in behavior analysis.

The effect of discrimination is to place behavior under the control of environmental cues correlated with the contingencies that fundamentally explain the behavior. Since making a behavior change through reinforcement, punishment, or extinction usually requires some repetition of these contingencies, it is most often aspects of the environment that are consistent during those repetitions that become the behavior-controlling cues. Thus the typical organization of any behavior is that it occurs, or stops occurring, in response to environmental cues whose role is to mark the time and place of the reinforcement, punishment, or extinction contingencies that are the basic analysis of the behavior.

But contingencies can vary depending on the type of behavior and organism, and their cues can be anything within the sensory capabilities of the organism. The organisms can become extraordinarily different through these mechanisms: the same event can, and indeed is likely to evoke different responses from different organisms (simply by having cued different contingencies for those responses by those organisms); and the same response of different organisms can and probably will be tied to different cues and different consequences (simply because those organisms exist in different environments).

In concentrating on reinforcement, punishment, and extinction, and on the discrimination of their effects to environmental cues, behavior analysts were quite similar to other students of environmental control of behavior. In a number of other ways, however, they were distinctively different; this distinctiveness established their discipline as a separate one, and also contributed greatly to its likelihood of producing a behavioral technology.

The most fundamental difference, and the most subtle one, was at the level of strategy. Other learning theorists began with a theory about why behavior came under the control of environmental contingencies, and pursued experiments only to confirm or disprove that theory. By contrast, behavior analysts did not start with a theory, expecting instead to finish with one. They began with a behavior—any behavior convenient for laboratory research—and asked the question: What in the current environment can control and modulate the occurrence of this behavior? Reinforcement, punishment, extinction, and discrimination mechanisms were the obvious first answers for the behavior analysts, just as they were for the other learning theorists. But whereas the other theorists typically asked *why* these mechanisms controlled behavior, behavior analysts (who operate under the control of the question, What can control this behavior?) asked *how else* these mechanisms could control behavior. In particular they asked how this control could be made more powerful, more precise, and more immediate, how many ways any of that could be done, and how it could vary from organism to organism. Implicitly they assumed that before explaining a phenomenon like behavior control, you had better see all of it, or at least a lot of it. The natural result was a descriptive, systematic exploration of the reinforcement, punishment, extinction, and discrimination mechanisms (Skinner, 1938; Honig, 1966)—an exploration that is still in progress. What has emerged is a systematic codification of these mechanisms as large families of procedures. By contrast, theory-guided research into these mechanisms is likely to find only those very selective facts that might be relevant to confirmation or disconfirmation of the theory. Yet the facts of detailed environmental control of behavior remain the same no matter which of those theories may be under pursuit at the moment.

A second crucial and distinctive characteristic of behavior analysis is its devotion to single-subject research designs. The underlying question, What can control this behavior? implies strongly that the most useful answers are those that clearly, reliably, and powerfully confer control over the behavior of a single organism at a time. This proved to be entirely possible, and its possibility became a prescription for all future research of the same analytic character: Since it could be done, it became one criterion of basic, powerful analysis (Sidman, 1960). Furthermore, the ongoing descriptive investigation of behavior-controlling mechanisms showed that a given process yielded control over many different behaviors in a variety of organisms across a broad range of settings, but only if certain parameters of the process were adjusted appropriately to the individual organism, the particular behavior, and the specific setting under study. Without adjustment of these parameters, generality of the process across organisms, behaviors, and settings could not be seen and might well be doubted; with such adjustments, generality often emerged clearly.

But the parameters of a process cannot be adjusted on the average; that must be done for the specific case under study because it may well be different—but perhaps only in detail—in the next case. Know and adjust the case, and its similarity to the previous one may emerge. But to know and adjust the case requires analysis of the case itself, not of the average of a group containing the case. Indeed, it thus became a truism for behavior analysis that averaging across different cases prior to their individual analysis and adjustment could conceal the underlying general analysis rather than reveal it. Generality is not equivalent to a large N, if each member of that large N has not been analyzed as a separate case that may or may not be an example of the same mechanism or same process as the next case. Nevertheless, in recent years group averages reflecting the actuarial outcome of a treatment technique have been recognized as essential data for wide-scale application.

A third, not so distinctive characteristic of behavior analysis is its apparent applicability to a very wide range of behavioral phenomena. Like most general behavior theories, it can be and has been applied in logic to almost every area of behavior worthy of a chapter title: learning, perception, emotion, motor skill, cognition, language, personality, intelligence, social interaction, and—the very essence of single-subject design—individual differences. These applications typically have been empirical as well. In part, this broad-scale empirical application resulted from an explicit recognition of the value and necessity of investigating the generality of any phenomenon initially studied only in single-subject designs applied to a very small sample of experimental subjects. In larger part it resulted from the character of the mechanisms revealed by behavior analysis: they are intrinsically coherent, simple, and natural. What appear to be contingencies between all these kinds of behavior and its natural environmental antecedents and consequences are abundant and inescapable in naturalistic observation. Experimentation has proven that such contingencies *can* be functional in the control of some behavior; then perhaps many, and conceivably all of these natural contingencies are similarly functional. Increasingly, research asks if they are. In other words, an experimental discipline that can see the topography of its analysis everywhere in the natural world of behavior inevitably will ask if that topography is functional in each of those cases.

Thus the character of behavior analysis has been to choose a behavior of interest—initially, as slight a target as bar-pressing in the rat; later, as grand a target as language acquisition in the child—and observe its natural contingencies with antecedent and consequent stimuli, thereby asking how much of its complexity would prove to be behavior under the control of reinforcement, punishment, extinction, and discrimination contingencies. An early tactic was to impose such contingencies on the behavior within the laboratory to see if such control was possible for that behavior and to see if it was also thorough, effective, and durable. A subsequent tactic was to take experimental control of the natural contingencies, when possible, to look for similar results. Both tactics are still in use and the underlying strategy of each is to see *how much* of the behavior can be analyzed into these mechanisms.

Often some of the behavior under study eludes explanation by these mechanisms alone. Like any research science, behavior analysis then will ask whether some other factor can account for what is still unanalyzed—not explain it, simply account for it as error variance. When such a factor is found it is usually termed a "setting event" (Kantor & Smith, 1975, pp. 46–47), and is thereby nominated not as a solution to a problem but as a problem in need of a solution: Why does the setting event account for otherwise unanalyzed variance in behavior partly analyzed by the familiar antecedent-behavior-consequence mechanisms? Obviously, the answer is to be sought both within those mechanisms and outside them, with a bias in favor of "within" explanations, but also with a systematic readiness to learn "outside" ones (as this book demonstrates).

Careful students of the approach know that its mechanisms are simple only in principle and in terminology. In their procedural detail and in the depth and breadth of their theorems they are elaborate and diverse. Thus their application to any behavioral phenomenon, from the acquisition of counting to the fullest use of language, is lengthy, detailed, and systematic in procedure. Like most general behavior theories, behavior analysis is never at first clearly inapplicable to a problem: If initial research does not find it to be applicable to the problem, for a time there will always be more procedure to be tried. The approach is distinctive, however, in that it is more procedure rather than more theory that remains to be tried, and that any try can fail, and that all tries can fail.

Behavior analysis may be said to be "fully applicable" to a behavioral phenomenon when *all* of the behavior has been experimentally accounted for as behavior under the control of some variety of reinforcement, punishment, extinction, or discrimination contingencies and their derivative procedures of scheduling, deprivation and satiation, conditional discrimination, and the organization of stimuli and responses into functionally covarying classes, plus histories of all or any of this.

ADVANCES SIGNIFICANT TO BEHAVIORAL PEDIATRICS

In the context of this book, the most significant development in behavior analysis in the past 15 years is the continuing viability of its offspring, applied behavior analysis, and its cousin, behavior therapy. They represent the application of such methods to the behaviors that constitute personal or social problems. This field began largely as a research endeavor; its practitioners were testing the generality of the mechanisms prominent in laboratory-based behavior analysis by asking if they could also analyze the behaviors identified as important human problems, without change in principle. The analysis of these behaviors, it was supposed, constituted an acid test of the generality of these principles (Baer, 1978). However, even from the start, at least a few of those practitioners were not deliberately testing the generality of behavior-analytic mechanisms; they were developing a new clinical technology in order to do socially useful things with it, whether or not that contributed to an evaluation of the scientific worth of the parent approach. This difference in intention still operates in the field, but whereas 15 years ago generality-testers outnumbered behavioral clinicians, today the reverse is true (Kazdin, 1978).

The experimentally validated accomplishments of applied behavior analysis are extremely diverse. Some sense of that diversity may be gained from the following arbitrary sample:

Motor skills
Social skills
Smiling
Compliance with instructions
Grammatical speech
Attention to task
Academic achievement of every measurable sort
Stimulus-scanning skills
Making change (as a cashier)
Self-help skills of every sort
Cleaning and maintaining the environment
Conserving energy
Sharing
Reinforcing others' good behavior
Street crossing and traffic safety
Avoiding common household dangers
Tutoring and managing others' behavior
Managing one's own behavior
Writing syntactically good sentences
Writing semantically good paragraphs
Writing letters that prompt a friendly, immediate reply
Rudimentary speech
Sophisticated speech
Rudimentary signing
Sign-board skills
Rudimentary and polished imitation skills
Nutritionally proper choice of snacks

Relaxation skills

Systematically novel behavior: inventions

Resisting behavioral control by countercontrol and many others.

See, for example, *The Journal of Applied Behavior Analysis, Behavior Therapy, Behavior Research and Therapy, Behavior Modification, Education and Treatment of Children, Child Behavior Therapy, Child and Family Behavior Therapy, Behavior Assessment, Progress in Behavior Modification, Applied Research in Mental Retardation,* and other such journals.

Furthermore, each of these constructions of a desirable behavioral repertoire implies the usually neccessary concurrent reduction or elimination of the corresponding undesirable behavior classes: inattention, disruption, aggression, self-injury, self-stimulatory behavior, hyperactivity, withdrawal, rebellion, and the like. These kinds of behavior changes have been made in normal children and in children in every currently recognized category of deviance.

Of the greatest significance for our present context, the last 10 years of effort have added to that list the behavior class of *compliance with medical regimen* (Sackett & Haynes, 1976; Stuart, 1982), some examples of which are presented in this book. The behaviors that make up compliance with medical regimen are many and diverse. They include:

Taking medicine

Sampling one's blood

Injecting one's self

Eating less

Eating more

Eating selectively

Exercise (sometimes despite pain)

Rest

Relaxation

Sanitation

Systematic defecation

Abstaining from established habits

Abstaining from substance abuse

Conflict avoidance and negotiation

Making and keeping appointments

Paced breathing

But the diversity of these behaviors is no wider than the diversity of the behaviors that have already been dealt with successfully in applied behavior analysis and behavior therapy, nor is their topography very different.

Furthermore, as we see in this volume, they are already coming under experimental control.

It seems clear that the recent advances in behavioral methodology sketched here can be and are being applied to the behavioral problems of pediatric medicine with considerable potential benefit to both disciplines. Need we do anything more systematic than continue in the same way? Emphatically, yes. We need to do considerably more than that.

GAPS IN BEHAVIORAL METHODOLOGY RELEVANT TO PEDIATRIC MEDICINE

The most significant problem remaining unsolved in applied behavior analysis and behavior therapy, which arises immediately in their application to pediatric medicine, is a frequent lack of generality. Their procedures have proven to be very powerful in accomplishing the behavior changes to which they were directed; yet that power has operated within a sharply delimited range. The directly targeted behaviors typically are changed in sufficient amount to be personally and socially useful, but this change often does not generalize to other examples of the same behavior class, or to other settings in which that behavior class needs to be changed as well; nor does it always maintain as long as desired after the experimental intervention has ended.

In other theoretical approaches to therapy, education, and human development, this lack of generality is taken as evidence that the intervention responsible for it was not profound, because generality of behavior change is presumed to be characteristic of normal human developmental processes, and is recognized as such by terms like "internalization" and "cognitive schemata." Thus a continuing lack of generality characteristic of behavior-analytic interventions may be interpreted elsewhere to mean that the mechanisms of behavior analysis are not the mechanisms operative in the important dimensions of normal human development. Any counterclaim that behavior analysis *is* a useful model of human development will require that behavior analysis henceforth contain mechanisms that accomplish thorough and longlasting generalization of its behavior changes. Alternatively, it would have to be argued that thorough and longlasting generalization, *unsupported by direct, ongoing environmental supports of the kind that behavior-analytic interventions use*, is in fact *not* characteristic of normal human development. This argument is in fact a viable one and can be supported by naturalistic observation of natural environmental events that look like ongoing behavior-analytic supports of everyday human behaviors, which means that those behaviors are thereby not *generalized* behaviors, and thus need not be thought of as "internalized" or "cognitively schematized". However, support by naturalistic observation of apparently behavior-analytic mechanisms is not the same thing as a proof. Obviously a proof will be difficult to accomplish on the necessary scale. Nevertheless, it would be theoretically significant to pursue it.

Meanwhile, the addition to behavior analysis of mechanisms that explain and accomplish more thorough and longlasting apparent generalizations of the behavior changes that it can make will enrich not only theory but application; perhaps it will enrich application more significantly, and more enduringly, than theory. However, that addition has required a shift in typical behavior-analytic logic. The early development of the behavior-analytic model recognized generalization only as a phenomenon, not as a usable mechanism. Generalization was considered epiphenomenal to the operation of the discrimination mechanism. That is, discrimination training was something that could be done; generalization was something that happened and was expected to be transitory, lasting only until discrimination training had been done more effectively. The necessary shift in logic was to recognize that generalization is also something to be taught (Baer, Wolf, & Risley, 1968), sometimes by a corresponding management of the extent and nature of discrimination training, and sometimes as if it were a skill in its own right. In either case generalization is no longer seen as something that happens, but instead as something that can be made to happen and to continue (Baer, 1981).

Several classes of procedure have already been reported to be effective in this adventure, some of them repeatedly in the experimental literature, some of them only a few times (Stokes & Baer, 1977). The generality of these solutions to the problem of generality is still at issue and is being examined. The codification of these mechanisms has begun, as has the argument about the most effective way of codifying them. Increasingly, generalization itself is targeted as the behavior change to be studied, and successes are reported steadily in the journals of the field. Thus the problem is not solved, but it appears to be on the way to a solution, with several partial solutions already in hand. To the extent that generalized behavior changes will prove essential to behavioral pediatrics, the collaboration of applied behavior analysis, behavior therapy, and pediatrics will prove salutary to all three. The behavioral disciplines already know something about the problem, and pediatrics so critically needs a solution that it may well require that any new behavioral partners either remedy the problem distinctively well or retire from the partnership. Pediatrics has a long history of dealing with behavioral phenomena, and of many alliances and collaborations with a variety of behavioral sciences.

POSSIBLE JOINT GAPS RELEVANT TO A BEHAVIORAL METHODOLOGY

Social-Validity Problems

A very recent advance in applied behavior analysis is the development of a concept of *social validity*, and the emergence of rudimentary techniques to assess it (Wolf, 1978). Social validity refers to the acceptability of an intervention to the persons most closely connected to it and its results. Experience has shown that not all effective interventions are accepted, despite their effectiveness. Some are rejected because the new behavior resulting from them is not attractive, even though the prior problem behavior has disappeared; some because the means of bringing about behavior change are not attractive, even when the behavior change is attractive; and some because the personnel bringing about the behavior change are not acceptable in the setting where the change must be made, even though the change and its means are attractive. The logic of applied behavior analysis is that an intervention must be effective to be considered applicable. If an intervention is not acceptable, even though it could be effective if it were, then it is *not* effective, and thus is not an analysis of the *entire* problem at hand and is not ready for public dissemination.

Currently social-validity methodology consists of identifying all relevant persons and groups and asking them about the acceptability of an intervention—its means, its results, and its personnel—either through interviews or questionnaires. Negative responses mean that the intervention must be changed before being used again, or that the objectors must be educated and then assessed again. For the new discipline of applied behavior analysis, with its consequent absence of social recognition as a therapeutic discipline, this new technology is essential to its extension beyond the laboratory, the university, and the research institute. Perhaps a discipline as old as medicine may, by contrast, be able to operate somewhat more on its traditional social authority and acceptance without such a cautionary technology, and may be accustomed to doing so. In forming a partnership with applied behavior analysis, though, medicine may well find that the new partner moves in with some of its old inventory, which often will include social-validity techniques and obedience to their warning messages. Considering the rate of malpractice suits now characterizing the practice of medicine in the absence of a behavioral alliance, this new acquisition may ultimately prove to be a benefit. Applied behavior analysis needs to progress beyond the rudimentary assessment techniques now characterizing its interest in social validity, and apply more of what social science knows about interview and questionnaire technique to the problem of insuring the validity of its future social-validity assessments. Poor technique could too easily allow an invalid conclusion of social validity where in fact resentment operates, resulting very likely in systematic, puzzling failures of the intervention in the future.

Medical-Validity Problems

A standing problem in applied behavior analysis is to know what behaviors to change in order to solve a problem. Some problems of course are presented essentially as behaviors to be changed—failure to discriminate *b* and *d*, or to take your medicine—and in those cases, the technology of behavior change can be applied immediately, and often successfully. But many problems are presented as nonbehavioral complaints—loneliness, for example—and before a technology of behavior change can be applied, a translation of each complaint into a list of behaviors to be changed is needed. The correct list is any one that, once changed, ends the complaint and satisfies the complainer and any others involved. In the realm of behavior this problem is recognized as disciplinary for applied behavior analysis: it is to be solved within the discipline, using the discipline's methods. In a partnership with medicine, however, it will often be the case that the problem is disciplinary for medicine. Medicine will specify what behaviors are to be changed, for example, what regimen to follow, and applied behavior analysis will obediently supply, adapt, and develop the techniques for doing so. What if medicine is sometimes wrong about those behaviors?

In the practice of medicine unsupported by such a behavioral technology, it can occasionally be quite difficult to discover that certain prescriptions do not in fact contribute to the betterment of a given condition. Suppose that a medical regimen is applied, but patients do not improve, or do so any faster than untreated patients. The regimen might be at fault, but the problem could also be that the patients did not follow the prescribed regimen. A discipline that does not know with any certainty whether patients follow their regimens or not, and cannot ensure that they do so, could be using ineffective prescriptions for a long time. However, a discipline allied to applied behavior analysis, *if* applied behavior analysis is able to operate there at its best, will more often be able to know when its regimens are being followed. Then it will be in a better position to see unambiguously if any of them is in fact the wrong regimen. On the face of it that ought to be a salutary state of affairs. On the other hand, no discipline likes to discover that one of its time-honored clinical techniques, which has seen many thousands of applications, is wrong. Perhaps applied behavior analysis, when working in medicine, should analyze the problem of surviving the occasional role of the messenger with bad news. In antiquity bad news was sometimes dealt with by killing the messenger. That was antiquity, of course.

Dissemination Problems

A momentary paradox in applied behavior analysis is that several very effective solutions to important personal and social problems that have been found or made to be socially valid (and thus are ready for widespread adoption and use as social policy and practice) remain ignored by a society that manifestly needs them. Recently the field is displaying the realization that societal adoption of a new intervention is a function of more than thorough scientific evidence of its effectiveness and attractiveness to all concerned. Indeed, proof of effectiveness is sometimes quite irrelevant to social adoption. Adoption of a new technique is itself a behavioral problem that applied behavior analysis is just acknowledging it must analyze if any of its analyses are to become applied analyses.

But medicine is itself a socially adopted delivery system for new interventions relevant to health. A partnership between applied behavior analysis and medicine may lend applied behavior analysis a piggy-back mechanism of social adoption; if so, that may be to its benefit only in the short term. If it also aborts the field's new interest in analyzing social-adoption processes, the long-term effects will be negative, for applied behavior analysis and for any change-oriented discipline needful of understanding the processes of social adoption.

The Problem of Placebo Design

Placebo designs in medical research are a longstanding recognition of the relevance of behavioral process within medical phenomena. Medicine develops agents that should cure or remediate health problems, but cannot help applying those agents with a considerable amount of behavioral wrapping. That wrapping consists of tradition, reputation, authority, titles, uniforms, special treatment settings, and instructions that the agent "will make you better." Is it in fact the supposedly curative agent that brings about the cure, or is it the wrapping? Or do they both contribute? Or do they interact? Or is each effective in the absence of the other? A common placebo design offers the curative agent with the usual wrapping, and compares the effect of that to what happens when a known noncurative agent is given with the same wrapping.

What is the placebo design when the curative agent consists of, or is wrapped in, a behavior change? Suppose that the prescription is to exercise regularly and diet to lose weight. Suppose that the considerable technology of applied behavior analysis or behavior therapy is applied to accomplish that. There may very well be a good deal of instruction and demonstration, direct and token reinforcement systems, contingency contracts, social support networks, new structurings of eating and exercise settings, participant observation, self-monitoring, and public posting of weekly outcomes. Is it the disciplinary focus on eating and exercise behaviors that produces any resultant weight losses and exercising? Or is it the fact that the patient is impressed by the procedures and is told that all this was designed to change eating and exercise patterns, *but nothing more*? If so, then the correct placebo control would be a regimen in which the patient is still told that the targets of the procedures are the same eating and exercise changes, and the procedures applied have the same topography and are equally numerous, detailed, demanding, and impressive. However, from the discipline's point of view everything was designed to alter some other behaviors entirely—say, basket-weaving and self-awareness. Comparable results would indicate that a good deal of applied behavior analysis had gone on unnecessarily and, in fact, nonanalytically—simple instructions and good theatre were sufficient. Applied behavior analysis often is good theatre.

Do we know that such designs are unnecessary when the wrapping is a solidly scientific discipline like applied behavior analysis or behavior therapy? Certainly not. Good theatre and witch-doctoring can be done in a variety of ways, including a number of ways that have excellent scientific validity in their own right. However, there is no guarantee that scientific validity is operating in any given instance. Therefore the placebo design ought to continue as a staple of all behavioral-pediatric research, even when the behavioral component is the thoroughly research-based discipline of applied behavior analysis or behavior therapy.

CONCLUSION

A partnership of pediatric medicine, applied behavior analysis, and behavior therapy has already begun. Thus this argument was not meant to recommend it so much as to characterize it. The nature of that characterization does recommend its continuing development. But it also implies a cautionary set of recommendations to recognize certain underlying interactive problems when these two disciplines are allied. Those problems must be attended to as answerable research issues, if the logical potential of the alliance is to be realized. Research can help and enrich not only the alliance, but each discipline separately as well.

Acknowledgments

The author is grateful to Drs. Norman Krasnegor, Michael Cataldo, Thomas Coates, and Ruth Baer for substantive suggestions useful in the construction of this argument (they cannot, of course, be held responsible for the argument itself). The author is also indebted to the National Institute of Mental Health for its support of research activities directly relevant to this argument during the period when it was constructed. The author acknowledges the very large qualitative and quantitative contributions to this argument resulting from its mediation by a word processor (his first) during every stage of its development. But a word processor is merely a supportive environment—a natural community of reinforcement, so to speak. Thus the author acknowledges the context within which mere supportive environments are empowered to operate: his profound love for his wife, who can, at last in his life, show him life, relationship, and profession with equal love and profundity.

REFERENCES

Baer, D. M. (1978). On the relation between basic and applied research. In A. C. Catania and T. A. Brigham (Eds.), *Handbook of applied behavior analysis: Social and instructional processes.* New York: Irvington.

Baer, D. M. (1981). *How to plan for generalization.* Lawrence, KS: H & H Enterprises.

Baer, D. M., Wolf, M. M., & Risley, T. R. (1968). Some current dimensions of applied behavior analysis. *Journal of Applied Behavior Analysis, 1,* 91–97.

Bijou, S. W., & Baer, D. M. (1961). *Child development: A systematic and empirical theory.* New York: Appleton-Century-Crofts.

Brady, J. V., & Harris, A. (1977). The experimental production of altered physiological states: Concurrent and contingent behavioral models. In W. K. Honig & J. E. R. Staddon (Eds.), *Handbook of operant behavior.* Englewood Cliffs, NJ: Prentice-Hall.

Craighead, W. E., Kazdin, A. E., & Mahoney, M. J. (1976). *Behavior modification: Principles, issues, and applications.* Boston: Houghton Mifflin.

Dunham, P. The nature of reinforcing stimuli. (1977). In W. K. Honig & J. E. R. Staddon (Eds.), *Handbook of operant behavior.* Englewood Cliffs, NJ: Prentice-Hall.

Ferguson, J. M., & Taylor, C. B. (Eds.). (1980). *Comprehensive handbook of behavioral medicine.* Holliswood, NJ: Spectrum.

Honig, W. K. (Ed.). (1966). *Operant behavior: Areas of research and application.* New York: Appleton-Century-Crofts.

Honig, W. K., & Staddon, J. E. R. (Eds.). (1977). *Handbook of operant behavior.* Englewood Cliffs, NJ: Prentice-Hall.

Kantor, J. R. (1947). *Problems in psychological psychology.* Bloomington, IN: Principia Press.

Kantor, J. R. (1959). *Interbehavioral psychology.* Granville, OH: Principia Press.

Kantor, J. R., & Smith, N. W. (1975). *The science of psychology: An interbehavioral survey.* Chicago: Principia Press.

Kazdin, A. E. (1978). *History of behavior modification: Experimental foundations of contemporary research.* Baltimore: University Park Press.

Leitenberg, H. (Ed.). (1976). *Handbook of behavior modification and behavior therapy.* Englewood Cliffs, NJ: Prentice-Hall.

Russo, D. C., & Varni, J. W. (Eds.). (1982). *Behavioral pediatrics: research and practice.* New York: Plenum.

Sackett, D. L. & Haynes, R. B. (Eds.). (1976). *Compliance with therapeutic regimens.* Baltimore: Johns Hopkins University Press.

Satinoff, E., & Henderson, R. (1977). Thermoregulatory behavior. In W. K. Honig & J. E. R. Staddon (Eds.), *Handbook of operant behavior.* Englewood Cliffs, NJ: Prentice-Hall.

Sidman, M. (1960). *Tactics of scientific research.* New York: Basic Books.

Skinner, B. F. (1938). *The behavior of organisms: An experimental analysis.* New York: Appleton-Century.

Skinner, B. F. (1953). *Science and human behavior.* New York: Macmillan.

Stokes, T. F., & Baer, D. M. (1977). An implicit technology of generalization. *Journal of Applied Behavior Analysis, 10,* 349–367.

Stuart, R. B. (Ed.). (1982). *Adherence, compliance, and generalization in behavioral medicine.* New York: Brunner/Mazel.

Teitelbaum, P. (1977). Levels of integration of the operant. In W. K. Honig & J. E. R. Staddon (Eds.), *Handbook of operant behavior.* Englewood Cliffs, NJ: Prentice-Hall.

Thompson, T., & Boren, J. J. (1977). Operant behavioral pharmacology. In W. K. Honig & J. E. R. Staddon (Eds.), *Handbook of operant behavior.* Englewood Cliffs, NJ: Prentice-Hall.

Varni, J. W. (1983). *Clinical behavioral pediatrics: An interdisciplinary biobehavioral approach.* Elmsford, NY: Pergamon.

Wolf, M. M. (1978). Social validity: The case of subjective measurement, or how applied behavior analysis is finding its heart. *Journal of Applied Behavior Analysis, 11,* 203–214.

5

Epidemiologic Perspectives on Psychosocial Problems in Children

JANET R. HANKIN AND BARBARA H. STARFIELD

This chapter presents several epidemiologic perspectives on psychosocial problems in children. We begin with the question of estimating the prevalence of psychosocial problems and describing the factors which affect those estimates. A summary of community studies and primary care studies on the prevalence of children's psychosocial problems is then provided. We next discuss three issues that arise from these epidemiologic studies: (1) who treats children with psychosocial problems, (2) the persistence of psychosocial problems in childhood, and (3) the consequences of psychosocial morbidity for the use of services. The chapter concludes with our suggestions for future research in the epidemiology of children's psychosocial problems.

Preparation of this chapter was supported in part by Grant No. MH. 33646 from The National Institute of Mental Health.

FACTORS AFFECTING THE ESTIMATES OF THE PREVALENCE OF PSYCHOSOCIAL PROBLEMS

Definitional Issues

Why is the estimated prevalence of psychosocial problems in children so imprecise, ranging from 5 to 15 percent of all children? (Gould, Wunsch-Hitzig, & Dohrenwend, 1980; Robins, 1978). One explanation is that the definition of psychosocial problems is imprecise and varies from one study to the next. Because of the frequent overlap between psychological and social problems, some investigators include within their definition of psychosocial problems phenomena that others might consider to be purely social. For example, the "new morbidity" (Haggerty, Roghmann, & Pless, 1975) includes not only affect and conduct disorders, but also learning problems, problems in development and sexual maturation, environmental hazards, poor dietary habits, drug and alcohol addiction, and venereal disease.

Other investigators restrict their concerns to a much narrower spectrum of problems. For example, the Joint Commission on Mental Health of Children (1970) defined an emotionally disturbed child as one who is impaired in (1) accurately perceiving the world around him or her, (2) controlling impulses, (3) achieving satisfying and satisfactory relations with others, (4) learning, and (5) any combination of these.

Fortunately, recent efforts to standardize psychosocial diagnoses may facilitate our understanding of the distribution and nature of these problems. In 1980 the American Psychiatric Association created specific diagnoses for children and adolescents. This effort represents the first attempt to develop a mental disorder classification system with specific criteria for this age group. The classification scheme is outlined in *The Diagnostic and Statistical Manual of Mental Disorder, 3rd Edition* (American Psychiatric Association, 1980). The DSM-III is the official manual of mental disorders. It features diagnostic criteria, multiaxial classifications, and a description of each type of disorder. Unlike previous versions of the DSM, the third edition subjected the classifications of mental disorders to extensive clinical trials before official adoption. Axes I and II of the DSM-III include all of the mental disorders. Axis III is for physical disorder, Axis IV is for severity of psychosocial stressors, and Axis V is the highest level of adaptive functioning in past year. The DSM-III has a special set of classifications for disorders that are usually first evident in infancy, childhood, or adolescence. (See Table 5.1). The American Psychiatric Association has established a task force to examine the success of this new classification scheme. In contrast to DSM-II, 1968, DSM-III omits the diagnostic class of neuroses. DSM-III has a multiaxial classification system, while DSM-II did not. Furthermore, DSM-III has a more comprehensive description of the diagnostic criteria than did DSM-II.

For the purposes of this chapter, we define psychosocial problems in a

TABLE 5.1. DEFINITION OF PSYCHOSOCIAL PROBLEMS: DIAGNOSES FROM THE DIAGNOSTIC AND STATISTICAL MANUAL OF MENTAL DISORDERS, 3RD EDITION

Diagnoses Usually First Evident in Infancy, Childhood, or Adolescence—Axis I

Mental retardation
Attention deficit disorder
Conduct disorder
Anxiety disorders of childhood
  or adolescence
Other disorders of infancy,
  childhood, or adolescence

Eating disorders
Stereotyped movement disorders
Other disorders with
  physical manifestations
Pervasive developmental
  disorders

Specific Developmental Disorders—Axis II

Developmental reading disorder
Developmental arithmetic
  disorder
Developmental language
  disorder

Developmental articulation disorder
Mixed specific developmental
  disorder
Atypical specific developmental
  disorder

Other DSM III Diagnoses

Substance use disorders
Schizophrenic disorders
Paranoid disorders
Psychotic disorders
  not elsewhere classified
Affective disorders
Anxiety disorders

Somatoform disorders
Dissociative disorders
Psychosexual disorders
Factitious disorders
Disorders of impulse control
  not elsewhere classified
Adjustment disorder
Psychological factors affecting
  physical condition

*Other Problems Which Do Not Meet DSM-III Criteria yet are
Indicative of Broad Psychosocial Problems*

Behavioral problems
Psychological problems
Parent-Child problems
Syphilis
Gonorrhea
Sexual problems

Pregnancy
Family planning
Urinary frequency
Feeding problems
Adverse effects of medicinal,
  clinical, and environmental agents
Complications of medical care

broad manner, so that we might include DSM-III mental disorders as well as milder types of problems (Table 5.1). Our definition thus incorporates all diagnoses contained in DSM-III, as well as problems which do not meet DSM-III diagnostic criteria, yet are indicative of broad psychosocial problems (Starfield et al., 1980). Clearly, studies that do not use such a broad concept could be expected to find lower prevalence rates of problems.

Measurement Issues

The second explanation for the lack of agreement on prevalence is a result of the unavailability of standardized tools for measuring deviations from the norm that have prognostic significance (Shepherd, Oppenheim & Mitchell, 1971). A variety of tools have been developed to assess psychosocial problems in children. These include inventories completed by parents or teachers, as well as direct interviews with the child (Orvaschel, Sholomaskas, & Weissman, 1979). After reviewing 44 such instruments, Orvaschel and colleagues concluded that there were relatively few adequate, well-developed, and widely used instruments to assess psychosocial problems in children. There are still no interview schedules under development for preschoolers.

One example of an inventory completed by parents is the Child Behavior Checklist (CBCL). (See Achenbach & Edelbrock, 1983.) We are using this questionnaire for a study of pediatrician's management of psychosocial problems at the Columbia Medical Plan. The CBCL consists of two parts. The Social Competence Scale includes questions on the amount and quality of the child's participation in sports, hobbies, clubs, and chores; the child's interpersonal behavior with others and his or her behavior alone; the child's academic performance and the presence of school problems. The Behavior Problems Scale includes 113 items describing a variety of behavior problems. The CBCL has been normed for males and females in three age groups: 4 to 5, 6 to 11, and 12 to 16. Achenbach and Edelbrock (1983) have also developed a similar inventory to be completed by teachers.

Comparisons of instruments that use parent ratings versus teacher ratings reveal that while each type of rater identifies the same proportion of children as suffering from psychosocial problems, they identify different children as impaired (Glidewell & Swallow, 1968; Graham & Rutter, 1977; Kellam, Branch, Agrawal & Ensminger, 1975; Rutter, Tizard, & Whitmore, 1970; Mitchell & Shepherd, 1966). Rutter (1977) explains these differences by saying, "Children tend to behave rather differently in different settings."

The National Institute of Mental Health's Center for Epidemiologic Studies has developed the Diagnostic Interview Schedule for Children (DIS-C). The DIS-C is a fully structured interview administered by lay interviewers to children 6 to 17 years old. It is designed to be compatible with the DSM-III, and takes less than one hour to administer. There is a companion instrument to the DIS-C which is administered to parents. The development and testing of the instrument has been slow. Inter-rater reliability is reportedly high, as are test-retests of the parent's version. However, test-retest reliability of the children's version is low. Radloff (1984) explains, "The major questions remaining concern (a) the meaning and validity of diagnostic information based on the current or revised computer algorithms [that are used to interpret the DIS-C] and (b) the performance of the DIS-C in non-clinical samples. Clearly, more methodologic work is needed."

Population at Risk

Another factor that influences the rates of psychosocial problems is the population at risk. Children assessed in the community have different rates than children who are seen by primary care physicians (for example, family practitioners, general practitioners, pediatricians, and internists). As Haggerty (1983) explains:

> Individual practitioner estimates then are highly variable, except for the most common illnesses. Grouping data from many practices improves these estimates, but it is also clear that not all patients with illness go to physicians, and practice estimates seriously underestimate many problems. Therefore, household surveys are needed to gain a broader view of the distribution of illness in the community. (p. 102)

In addition to the differences attributable to whether the child is assessed in a primary care practice or in the community, sociodemographic characteristics (including age, sex, and social class) influence the likelihood of pathology. For example, younger children and upper class children are likely to have lower rates of psychological problems than children who are older and poor. Generalization of the conclusions of various studies must take into account differences in the population at risk.

THE PREVALENCE OF PSYCHOSOCIAL PROBLEMS

To address these issues, our discussion of the prevalence and distribution of psychosocial problems is divided into two parts: the rates in community populations and the rates in populations seeking primary care. As noted above, the differing rates may be a result of differences in the definition of psychosocial problems as well as differences in methods of identifying these problems, and in the population under consideration.

Prevalence of Psychosocial Problems in the Community

Table 5.2 summarizes the results of community studies on the prevalence of psychosocial problems in children. Examining the most serious types of psychosocial problems, Rice and Danchik (1979) report that suicide is the fourth leading cause of death among adolescents aged 15 to 19. In 1974 two of every 1000 children aged 11 to 14 and almost 7 per 1000 of those aged 15 to 17 were arrested on suspicion of a crime of violence (murder, nonnegligent manslaughter, forcible rape, robbery, or aggravated assault). (U.S. Department of Commerce, 1980). The Joint Commission on Mental Health of Children (1970) estimated that 0.6 percent of children are psychotic, and another 2 to 3 percent are severely disturbed.

Turning to less severe problems, a national telephone survey of mothers indicated that one in seven preschoolers had a problem in growth and development, while 10 percent reported problems in behavior or discipline. Among 5-to 14-year-olds, 15 percent suffered from a behavior or discipline problem and 10 percent had problems in social relationships (American Academy of Pediatrics, 1978).

On the basis of a review of 25 U.S. community studies conducted between 1928 and 1975, Gould et al. (1980) estimated the prevalence of clinical maladjustment among persons under the age of 18 to be 11.8 percent. The majority of the studies (21 of them) relied on teachers as informants. The remainder of the studies used the parental reports. The rates vary with age, social class, ethnic group, and geographic region. While almost all psychotic children receive treatment by mental health specialists, the majority of children with other types of clinical maladjustment are not under such specialized care (Gould et al., 1980).

Specific behaviors or traits thought to be evidence of psychosocial problems are consistently prevalent in at least 10 percent of the populations studied. Tuddenham, Brooks, and Milkovich (1974) reported mothers' descriptions of approximately 3000 9-11-year-old children in a defined population of children enrolled in a prepaid group practice. Mothers were asked about the presence of 100 behavioral traits. Prevalence of the most frequent traits for boys and girls (respectively) were: outburst of temper, 19 and 10 percent; bedwetting, 15 and 16 percent; trouble getting to sleep, 12 percent for both. The authors compared their results with those of previous studies and with the findings of a national sample of children studied in the Health Examination Survey of the National Center for Health Statistics (NCHS) and found generally similar prevalence rates despite differences in study technique and passage of time. The absence of clear time trends, despite major changes over several decades in family life styles, patterns of child-rearing, and sources of tension, led the authors to conclude that stress in childhood is expressed in a finite repertoire of behavioral problems. Similar data on the prevalence of specific behavioral traits for children from 6 to 17 years of age are provided in publications of the National Center for Health Statistics (1971-1974).

A final consideration is the number of children who receive specialized mental health care. Data from the survey conducted by the Foundation for Child Development (1977) indicate that five percent of school children in the United States—more than 800,000 seven-to-eleven-year-olds—receive

TABLE 5.2.   PREVALENCE OF PSYCHOLOGICAL PROBLEMS IN THE COMMUNITY

Author	Definition of Psychosocial Problem	Population Studied	Prevalence of Psychosocial Problems
Joint Comm. on Mental Health of Children (1970)	Impaired in accurately perceiving world, controlling impulses, achieving satisfactory relationships, learning, or any combination	National estimate	0.6% psychotic 2–3% severely disturbed 8–10% other emotional problems
Task Force on Pediatric Education (1978)	Problems in growth or development, behavior or discipline, or social relationships	National telephone survey of mothers	Preschoolers: 14% problems in growth or development 10% problems in behavior or discipline 5–14 year olds: 15% problems in behavior or discipline 10% problems in social relationships

				% boys	% girls
Tuddenham et al. (1974)	Behavior traits	3000 9–11 year olds who were members of a prepaid group practice	Freq. nightmares	6	8
			Trouble getting to sleep	12	12
			Bedwetting	15	6
			Thumbsucking	6	11
			Stammering	3	1
			Worrying	12	11
			Loneliness	9	8
			Outbursts of temper	19	10
Gould et al. (1980)	Clinical maladjustment	Review of 25 community studies of under 18 year olds (y.o)	11.8%		
Foundation for Child Development (1977)	Receipt of professional help for emotional, behavioral, mental, or learning probs.	National survey of 7–11 y.o.	5%		
Roghmann et al. (1970)	Treatment by psychiatrist or psychiatric care facility	Cumulative psychiatric case register of Monroe County, N.Y. 5–17 y.o.	Lifetime: 5–9 y.o. 3.0% 10–14 y.o. 5.5% 15–17 y.o. 7.3%		

some sort of professional help during the year for emotional, behavioral, mental, or learning problems. However, it is estimated that less than one percent of all children receive care from mental health specialists in any given year (Rosen, 1979).

Using a cumulative psychiatric case register, Roghmann, Babigian, Goldberg, and Zastowny (1982) calculated the lifetime prevalence of mental disorder treated by mental health specialists. Prevalence rates were 3.0 percent for children aged 5 to 9 years, 5.5 percent for children aged 10 to 14 years, and 7.3 percent for children 15 to 17 years old.

Prevalence of Psychosocial Problems in Primary Care (See Table 5.3)

Several reports from individual practices indicate that psychosocial problems are evident in 5 to 40 percent of all visits to pediatric practices. Coleman, Patrick, and Baker (1977) studied the prevalence of emotional problems in the Community Health Care Center Plan of Greater New Haven, a comprehensive prepaid group practice. Emotional problems included adjustment reaction, behavior disorder, personality disorder, and psychosis. An overall prevalence of 8.8 percent among children under the age of 19 years old and 6.0 percent of all visits was found in this practice.

Williams, Diehr, Drucker, and Richardson (1979) compared children enrolled in a prepaid group practice and those enrolled in an independent practice plan, both in Seattle. Both groups of children lived in low-income families (defined as family incomes less than $2000 above the Federal poverty level). They counted the number of children with mental health visits, that is, any visit where the primary diagnostic code was psychoses (ICDA 290-299), neuroses (300-309), mental retardation (310-315), nervousness and debility (790) or adverse effects of psychotherapeutics (970). Low-income children in the prepaid group practice plan were more likely to have a mental health visit (5.6 percent of males 0-19 years old and 5.8 per cent of females of that age) than was the case for low-income children in an independent practice plan (2.9 percent of males and 2.0 percent of females). Both plans had liberal mental health benefits. In the prepaid plan, the physicians were salaried and employed a team approach to problems, whereas in the independent practice plan, physicians were paid a fee-for-service and emphasized individual psychotherapy.

Starfield et al. (1980) studied five different facilities (Harvard Community Health Plan–Kenmore Square, the Medical College of Virginia Family Practice Program, the Medical University of South Carolina Family Practice Program, the Columbia Medical Plan, and the Johns Hopkins Hospital Children and Youth Project) to ascertain the prevalence of psychosocial problems in children. Psychosocial problems were defined according to the broad set of criteria described earlier (DSM-III plus problems listed in Table

5.1). The frequency of diagnoses of psychosocial problems among children seen in a year's time by the pediatricians or family physicians varied from 5 to 15 percent (and as high as 30 percent in some subgroups of children). The proportion of these psychosocial problems that were psychological/behavioral varied from 10 to 25 percent, so that the variability in prevalence of behavioral problems alone was much less (1.4 to 2.3 percent) among the five facilities than was the case for the entire group of psychosocial problems. If enuresis and mental retardation or developmental failure are added, the prevalence varied from 2.3 percent to 4.8 percent. The addition of education or learning problems brings the prevalence to 3.5 to 8.1 percent.

Jacobson et al. (1980) compared the prevalence of a mental disorder diagnosis, using DSM-II and ICD-9 as the criteria, for four settings: The Columbia Medical Plan, a prepaid group practice that provides care to a predominantly middle class population in Columbia, Maryland; The Greater Marshfield Community Health Plan, a prepaid group practice serving a rural Wisconsin group of enrollees; The Marshfield Clinic Fee-For-Service, also serving rural Wisconsin; and The Bunker Hill Health Center, serving a working class, low income population in Boston. They report that between 3.3 percent and 10.1 percent of children seen in those settings received a diagnosis of mental disorder in 1975 from a health and/or mental health provider.

Goldberg, Regier, McInerny, Pless, and Roghmann (1979) asked nine pediatricians to report on all patients seen during a four-week period between January and February, 1976, in Monroe County, New York. Pediatricians were asked whether or not the child had a mental health problem, which was broadly defined as an emotional, behavioral, or school problem. Five percent of the children seen were reported to have such a problem. The prevalence rate varied by pediatrician, with a low of 1.4 percent to a high of 7.8 percent. The most frequently reported problems included adaptation reaction (22.5 percent), specific learning disorder (19.3 percent), hyperkinetic disorder (19.3 percent), psychosomatic disorder (12.8 percent) and conduct disorder (12.8 percent).

Allen, Burns, and Cook (1983) analyzed data from the 1975 and 1980 National Ambulatory Medical Care Surveys of office based physicians. The DSM-II and DSM-III definitions of mental disorder were used. From their data we calculated the proportion of visits made by 0 to 17 year-olds to primary care physicians (internists, pediatricians, family physicians or general practitioners) at which a principal diagnosis of mental disorder occurred. In 1975, 1.1 percent of visits to primary care physicians made by children were for a principal diagnosis of mental disorder; in 1980, the comparable figure was 0.3 percent—a statistically significant difference. The reason for this decline is not clear (Burns, 1983).

The studies we have reviewed suggest that while 10 to 15 percent of children in the community suffer from psychosocial problems, the range for

TABLE 5.3. PREVALENCE OF PSYCHOSOCIAL PROBLEMS IN PRIMARY CARE

Author	Definition of Psychosocial Problem	Population Studied	Prevalence of Psychosocial Problems
Coleman et al. (1977)	DSM-II (adjustment reaction, behavior disorder, personality disorder, psychosis)	Enrollees under age 19 of the Community Health Care Plan of Greater New Haven	8.8% of children 6.0% of visits
Williams et al. (1979)	Visit where primary diagnosis was psychoses, neuroses, mental retardation, nervousness and debility, adverse effects of psychotherapeutics	Low income children (0–19) in a Seattle PGP Low income children (0–19) in a Seattle independent practice plan	Percent with mental health visit: 5.6% males and 5.8% females Percent with mental health visit: 2.9% males and 2.0% females
Starfield, et al. (1980)	DSM-III and behavioral and psychological problems, parent-child problems, V.D., sexual problems, pregnancy, family planning, urinary frequency, feeding problems, adverse effects of medicinal, chemical and environmental agents, and complications of medical care	Children aged 0-17 with at *least one visit* to Harvard Community Health Plan—Kenmore Sq. (PGP) Medical College of Virginia Family Practice Program Medical University of South Carolina Family Practice Program	% children: 15.5% pediatrics, 13.6% I.M., 40.6% O.B., 2.0% triage. % visit: 6.4% peds., 7.6% I.M., 18.5% O.B., 1.9% triage 5.7% of children 3.6% of visits 14.2% of children 7.1% of visits

			% of covered child population	% of children seen
Jacobson et al. (1980)	Johns Hopkins Hospital Children and Youth Project	DSM-II and ICD-9 made by health and mental health providers	15.0% of children 6.9% of visits	
	Columbia Medical Plan (PGP)		% children: 5.4% peds., 1.1% I.M., 19.5% O.B., 0.6% urgent care. % visits: 2.0% peds., 0.6% I.M., 21.6% O.B., 0.3% urgent care	
	Columbia Medical Plan (PGP)		3.6	4.0
	Gr. Marshfield Comm Health Plan (PGP)		3.2	4.9
	Marshfield Clinics FFS		2.2	3.4
	Bunker Hill Health Center		8.2	10.1
Goldberg et al. (1979)	Children under 18 y.o. seen by 9 pediatricians in Monroe County, N.Y. during 4 week period	Emotional, behavior, or school problem	5% with range of 1.4% to 7.8% by pediatrician	
Reanalysis of data from Allen et al. (1983)	National Ambulatory Medical Care Surveys of office-based physicians. 0–17 y.o. seen in 1975 and 1980	DSM-II (1975) DSM-III (1980)	percent of visits: 1975: 1.1% 1980: 0.3%	

children treated in a primary care setting is 3 percent to 15 percent. Diagnoses of psychosocial problems occur in about 1 percent to 6 percent of all visits to primary care physicians. The range in rates reflects both the definition of psychosocial problems and measurement method used, as well as the characteristics of the population at risk. Given the level of psychosocial problems in children, the next logical question is to determine what proportion of children are treated for these problems.

WHO TREATS CHILDREN WITH PSYCHOSOCIAL PROBLEMS?

Starfield et al. (1984) examined data collected from a national survey of physician visits by children in ambulatory care settings. (Only face-to-face visits were included; telephone calls were excluded). Of all children's visits that the physicians judged to have a psychosocial focus, 20 percent were to pediatricians, 20 percent were to family physicians or general practitioners, and 60 percent were to other specialists. While the vast majority of all diagnoses of transient situational complaints were made to specialists other than pediatricians, more than 60 percent of the diagnoses of childhood behavior disorders were made by pediatricians.

Coleman et al. (1977) examined all visits for emotional problems (defined as DSM-II diagnoses) made to the Community Health Care Center Plan of Greater New Haven. They found that 64 percent of these visits were made to pediatricians, 4 percent to internists, 28 percent to mental health specialists, and the remainder (4 percent) to other types of clinicians.

Allen et al. (1983) tabulated data from the 1980 National Ambulatory Medical Care Survey on children's visits to office based physicians with a principal diagnosis of mental disorder (DSM-III). They report that 25.5 percent of these visits were made to primary care physicians, 67.5 percent to psychiatrists, and 7 percent to other types of physicians.

Data from the Columbia Medical Plan, a prepaid group practice, reveal that during 1975, 89 percent of children's visits with a diagnosis of mental disorder (DSM-II) occurred in the offices of mental health specialists, 10 percent took place in primary care departments, and 1 percent in other departments (Shapiro, Hankin & Steinwachs, 1980).

These four studies suggest that from 10 to 68 percent of children receive treatment for psychosocial problems from a primary care physician. The range reflects differences in the definitions of psychosocial problems and the nature of the health care delivery site.

Discussion

Summarizing the data obtained from primary care settings, it is possible to estimate that between 3 to 15 percent of all children seen by primary care physicians suffer from one or more psychosocial problems. In general, fewer than half of these children see mental health specialists. Since these estimates are based upon individuals seeking care and the physician then recognizing a psychosocial problem and recording the diagnosis in the chart, it is probable that the 3 to 15 percent figure is an underestimate of the true prevalence of psychosocial problems in children; this suspicion is confirmed by higher prevalence rates in community studies. Researchers have expressed concern with the amount of "hidden psychiatric morbidity" (Goldberg & Blackwell, 1970) that exists—the number of primary care patients with psychosocial problems who are not recognized by the primary care physician (Goldberg & Huxley, 1980; Starfield, 1982). In order to refer a child to a mental health specialist or treat the child within his or her own office, the primary care physician must first recognize the existence of a psychosocial problem. Studies are needed that administer standardized psychological symptom inventories to children or their parents and then ask primary care physicians to independently judge the presence or absence of psychological problems in the child. A comparison of children identified by each method would shed light on the extent of unrecognized psychiatric morbidity in medical practice. Such a study is about to be completed under the auspices of the National Institute of Mental Health.

PERSISTENCE OF PSYCHOSOCIAL PROBLEMS IN CHILDHOOD

Starfield and Hankin collected information on all children who were continuously enrolled in the Columbia Medical Plan (CMP) from January, 1974, through December, 1979, and who were under 12 years old on December 31, 1973, n = 2,591. The CMP is a prepaid group practice that serves aproximately 25,000 enrollees. Patients prepay for their medical care and then receive all necessary care. A small copayment fee is charged for each visit. During the six-year enrollment period, 25 percent of the children received at least one diagnosis for a psychosocial problem. About 55 percent of these children were seen at least once in the Department of Psychiatry. The remainder were seen only on other services, including primary care departments.

The longitudinal study of these children during 1974–1979 suggests that there are diagnostic differences between children seen by the Department of Psychiatry versus those seen by the Pediatrics Department. Children with failure to adjust to school or enuresis were more likely to be seen only in Pediatrics. Transient situational disturbances, social maladjustment, diagnosis deferred (319) and psychoses were more common in children seen by the Department of Psychiatry. Diagnoses of behavioral disorders of childhood and adolescence and learning disabilities were likely to be treated equally in Pediatrics and Psychiatry. It is not clear to what extent these differences represent divergent nomenclature used by psychothera-

TABLE 5.4.   PERSISTENCE OF PSYCHOSOCIAL MORBIDITY AMONG CHILDREN ENROLLED IN THE COLUMBIA MEDICAL PLAN FROM 1974 TO 1979, N = 2591

	Percent with a Psychosocial Diagnosis		
Any 2-year period	25.0	Two 2-year periods only	5.5
One 2-year period only	17.8	All 2-year periods	1.8

pists versus other physicians, or "true" prevalence differences between patients seen by each type of provider. Although some of the difference may reflect the referral practice of primary care physicians, this is not likely to account for most of the difference, as patients may self-refer to mental health specialists in this population.

The longitudinal nature of the data enabled us to examine the persistence of a psychosocial problem over time. Table 5.4 shows that most of the children with a psychosocial problem (71 percent) received that diagnosis during one two-year period only. A smaller proportion of children, seven per cent, received the diagnosis during each of the three consecutive two-year periods under question. In an effort to investigate the effect of aging on the likelihood of having a psychosocial diagnosis, we examined the percent of children with that diagnosis by period and age at the beginning of each period. Table 5.5 indicates that the possibility of receiving a psychosocial diagnosis peaks in preschoolers and older adolescents. These variations in rates are consistent with theories about the stresses of parental separation for preschoolers and the data on emotional turmoil experienced by some adolescents.

THE CONSEQUENCES OF PSYCHOSOCIAL MORBIDITY FOR THE USE OF SERVICES

Another important consequence of psychosocial problems is the higher use of nonpsychiatric services by children with psychosocial problems compared to those children without such problems. Jacobson et al. (1980) reported the frequency of visits for four organized health care settings. Children with a diagnosis of mental disorder (DSM-II) averaged 6.6 visits to the nonpsychiatric departments of the Columbia Medical Plan, compared to 5.1 annual visits for children without a diagnosis of mental disorder. Comparable figures were obtained for children enrolled in the Greater Marshfield Community Health Plan, a health maintenance organization (9.6 visits versus 4.0 visits), among fee-for-service patients at the Marshfield clinic (7.4 versus 3.0), and among patients in the Bunker Hill Health Center (5.6 versus 3.3).

TABLE 5.5   PERCENT OF CHILDREN WITH PSYCHOSOCIAL
MORBIDITIES BY PERIOD AND AGE AT THE BEGINNING OF THE
PERIOD. 2591 CHILDREN CONTINUOUSLY ENROLLED IN THE
COLUMBIA MEDICAL PLAN BETWEEN 1974 AND 1979

Age	Time Period			
	1974–1975	1976–1977	1978–1979	Total[a]
0	8.4			8.4
1	8.9			8.9
2	10.1	7.6		9.1
3	9.3	12.7		10.8
4	9.2	10.6	14.3	10.8
5	13.5	15.2	10.8	13.4
6	12.7	13.5	12.8	13.0
7	13.6	12.1	11.3	12.4
8	11.1	13.5	10.5	11.7
9	11.6	9.5	9.5	10.2
10	9.8	9.9	12.3	10.7
11	9.0	10.8	6.6	8.8
12		12.5	10.3	11.4
13		9.0	13.1	11.2
14			15.2	15.2
15			14.9	14.9
TOTAL	10.8	11.5	11.7	

[a]Percent of children who are that age at anytime during the six year period who received a psychosocial diagnosis. E.g., 8.8% of children who reached the age of 11 at any time during 1974 to 1979 received a diagnosis of a psychosocial problem.

The longitudinal study we conducted at the Columbia Medical Plan yielded similar results over the six-year time period. Children aged 0–6 in 1974 with a psychosocial problem anytime during the six years averaged 27 primary care visits (pediatrics, internal medical, urgent care) from 1974–1979 compared to 21 primary care visits for children without a psychosocial diagnosis. Among children aged 7 to 11 in 1974, the comparable figures were 17 and 8 visits during the six years (Hankin et al., 1984).

One reason for the greater demand on the health care system by children with psychosocial problems is the greater prevalence of diagnosed somatic problems among these children. Previous research indicates that psychiatric and physical symptoms tend to cooccur (Eastwood, 1975; Diehr, Williams, Shortell, Richardson, & Drucker, 1979; Hankin et al., 1982; Kessler, Tessler & Nycz, 1983).

Starfield et al. (1985) used the longitudinal data from the Columbia Medical Plan to investigate this possibility. We used diagnoses received during the six-year period and combined the categories of psychosocial and psychosomatic for this particular analysis.

TABLE 5.6.   COMORBIDITY AMONG CHILDREN ENROLLED IN THE COLUMBIA
MEDICAL PLAN DURING 1974–1979, N = 2591

Type of Morbidity	Percent of Children with Indicated Number of Types of Morbidity in Addition to One Listed					
Disease State	(N)	4	3	2	1	0
Psychosocial/psychosomatic	951	9.1	58.4	29.7	2.5	0.3
Chronic medical	289	30.1	49.5	17.3	2.4	0.7
Chronic specialty	1593	5.5	38.6	50.7	5.1	0.1
Acute recurrent	2337	3.7	27.9	45.5	22.2	0.8
Acute	2541	3.4	25.8	43.2	24.1	0.5

Diagnoses were grouped into five types: acute (acute self-limited, injuries, signs and symptoms); acute likely to recur (otitis media, pharyngitis, allergies, asthma, other likely to recur); chronic medical (diabetes, epilepsy, arthritis, endocrine disorders, etc); chronic specialty (dermatologic problems, hearing loss, refractions); and psychosocial/psychosomatic (any diagnosis in the DSM-III, as well as those listed in Table 5.1 and symptoms such as headache, constipation, recurrent abdominal pain.) (Starfield et al., 1984).

Table 5.6 indicates that children with psychosocial/psychosomatic illnesses are more likely to have three or more of the other types of morbidity than children with acute conditions only, acute recurrent conditions, or chronic specialty conditions, or combinations of these three types. Only children with chronic medical conditions exceed children with psychosocial/psychosomatic morbidity in proportion with comorbidities present. These data thus provide some support for the hypothesis that the higher demand for medical care by children with psychosocial problems is a function of the cooccurence of physical complaints.

WHY IS IT IMPORTANT FOR PEDIATRICIANS TO RECOGNIZE THE EXISTENCE OF PSYCHOSOCIAL PROBLEMS?

Pediatricians should recognize and deal with psychosocial problems in children because they affect the quality of a child's life, making these problems clinically important. In addition pediatricians can contribute to advances in knowledge about the distribution, cause, and management of psychosocial problems.

Children with at least some psychosocial problems are more likely to have similar problems later on in life than children without these problems. The analysis of data collected by Brunswick (Starfield, 1981) regarding the prevalence of 45 health problems reported by urban black teenagers early in adolescence (ages 12 to 17) and several years later (ages 18 to 23) showed that young adolescents with nervous or emotional problems were almost twice as likely to have them several years later than young adolescents without nervous or emotional problems in the earlier period.

In a 30-year follow-up comparison study of children with IQ's above 80, Robins (1974) showed that children referred for serious behavioral problems were more maladjusted and sicker as adults than control subjects selected from elementary school registers and matched on race, age, sex, IQ, and socioeconomic status. The great majority of the subjects (72 percent) who were evaluated as children were never treated. Only 4 percent of the control subjects had five or more adult antisocial symptoms compared with 45 percent of the patient group. Fifty-two percent of the control subjects were thought to be free of psychosomatic disease throughout their adult lives as compared with only 20 percent of the patients. At follow-up, only 8 percent of the control subjects had seriously disabling symptoms as compared with 34 percent of the patient group. Children with antisocial behavior were more likely to have problems in adulthood than were children with other behavioral problems. The more severe the antisocial behavior, whether measured by number of symptoms, number of episodes, or by arrests, the more disturbed the adult adjustment. Among the antisocial symptoms that were especially predictive of later sociopathy were pathological lying, lack of guilt, impulsiveness, truancy, runaway behavior, physical aggression, theft, incorrigibility, staying out late, "bad" associates, and recklessness or irresponsibility (Robins, 1974).

Of the 31 nonantisocial symptoms in childhood, 11 predicted later problems with alcoholism, schizophrenia, anxiety neurosis, chronic brain syndrome or hysteria. These symptoms included inattention or daydreaming, somatic symptoms, nailbiting, depression or unhappiness, worrying, fits, begging, sleep walking or talking, and "low energy." Symptoms that did not predict adult psychotic illness included reclusiveness, odd ideas, nervousness, irritability, oversensitivity, restlessness, tantrums, specific defects, fears, tics, odd food choices, insomnia, nightmares, thumbsucking, nausea, and indifference to rejection (Robins, 1974).

Gould et al. (1980) reviewed a number of longitudinal studies as part of their review of epidemiologic studies on childhood mental disorder. They reported that antisocial children have a poor longterm prognosis. Psychotic children also have a poor prognosis over time, especially if the onset of the disease is prepubertal. In contrast, neurotic children tend to become normal adults. Psychotic children, while they are more likely to receive specialized mental health care, are less likely to grow up to become normal adults (Gould et al., 1980.) Robins (1983) evaluates the data in the following way:

> Follow-up studies of children with psychiatric problems reveal no simple story concerning their future psychiatric health. With the exception of the severely retarded and the autistic who have considerable communication prob-

lems, children with diagnosable disorders frequently are psychiatrically well through much of their adult lives. On the other hand, except perhaps for those whose difficulties are limited to neurotic complaints, the risk of continuing or recurring disorder in adult life is clearly elevated in children who have had psychiatric problems. (pp. 214–215)

Psychosocial problems that do not necessarily portend problems later in life do, nevertheless, cause discomfort in childhood and disrupt family and school activities. Surveys conducted on national samples of children indicate a prevalence of 1 to 15 percent for individual problems in adjustment to everyday life; an unknown proportion of children undoubtedly have one or more of such problems. Subgroups of children, such as those who are poor, are at higher risk of having psychosocial problems, especially severe ones (Egbuonu & Starfield, 1982).

Practicing pediatricians are uniquely situated to contribute to advances in certain types of knowledge about children's illnesses. Academic researchers, especially those specialists who frequently limit their attention to certain types of childhood problems, are usually located in specialized medical centers. As a result they have inadequate knowledge about the distribution of health problems in the community, have inadequate knowledge about how problems begin, are frequently unable to observe the results of care, and are usually poorly aware of and relatively uninterested in the interrelationships among different types of health conditions, the use of health services, and the effect of these on subsequent health. In contrast practitioners, especially those who have a well defined practice population that is followed continuously over many years, are exposed to the early stages of problems. They are in a better position to take an overall view of the child, rather than focusing on particular diseases or organ systems, to observe the interrelationships among various manifestations of ill health in particular children and their ultimate outcome, and to follow the natural history of dysfunction as the child grows and develops.

DIRECTIONS FOR FUTURE RESEARCH

The potential of practitioners as researchers in general pediatrics is largely untapped. Robins (1974) provides a convincing rationale for studying the natural history of psychosocial problems in the community: Studying the natural history "means discovering the variation in its forms, the conditions out of which it arises, and its variation over time." A natural history approach not only points out precursors specific to the development of antisocial behavior, but it also shows which events in the history are not predictive of subsequent problems. In addition it enables the development of theories about social factors that contribute to disease that cannot be obtained from cross-sectional studies and are tenuous in retrospective ones.

Studies of the frequency, distribution, severity, and impact of different strategies of management on the natural history of these problems also can provide information necessary for the planning of more adequate services for children. An understanding of their impact on utilization and care cost will help to structure benefit packages and financing mechanisms to facilitate the organization and reimbursement of public and private approaches to dealing with these problems.

Another area of high priority for research concerns the identification of children who are at greatest risk for problems of various types. There is evidence that utilization of services does not distribute randomly in the population; a relatively small proportion of children contributes a relatively large proportion of total visits to health professionals. In contrast little is known about the extent to which individuals at risk for one type of morbidity cluster in the population of children, or the extent of overlap between psychosocial and somatic health problems.

The challenge to become involved in research in these common but important problems in primary care requires that practitioners organize their methods of collecting data on children under their care. Computerized systems are now available for use in office-based practice, but those developed only for administrative purposes may not be suitable for research purposes. Professional associations interested in research in ambulatory and primary care, such as the Ambulatory Pediatric Association, can provide advice, guidance, and even a mechanism for the development of collaborative research among interested practitioners. As a start pediatricians should become aware of methods to classify and categorize problems seen in their practices.

Development of a classification of psychosocial problems in children presents an even greater challenge than it does for adults (Burns et al., 1982). A different type of classification is required because so many of the problems are associated with stages of normal development and the dependent status of children. Moreover the adverse consequence of labeling in childhood may have a greater impact than is the case for adults. Also the children must be viewed in the context of relationships with key adults providing their care and in the context of an environment that exerts an even greater control over them than is the case for adults.

The International Classification of Diseases (ICD), a coding scheme developed and used to classify causes of death, is not useful for categorizing problems in ambulatory care, many of which are undifferentiated and nonspecific. Although the ICD is under continuous revision to make it more suitable for a wide variety of uses, other classification schemes are now being used to great advantage.

These classification schemes include the International Classification of Health Problems in Primary Care (ICHPPC) of the World Organization of National Colleges, Academies, and Academic Associations of General Practitioners/Family Physicians (WONCA), which includes codes specific for educational and social problems (WONCA, 1979). WHO and NIMH have developed a multiaxial classification system for primary care which is currently being field tested. As part of this effort, classification schemes for children have been developed for three types of problems: physical and mental disorders, psychological symptoms, and social problems (Burns et al., 1982). The physical and mental disorders section is compatible with DSM-III and ICD-9. It has been modified for children by Burns and her colleagues. This part of the classification system is based on descriptive categories, avoids the use of terms such as "neurosis" and "personality disorders," considers the child's developmental status, and codes categories (Burns et al., 1982).

The classification of psychological problems, adapted from Regier et al. (1982), includes developmental delays and disturbances which are inappropriate for the child's age or development period (Burns et al., 1982). This axis allows the primary care physician to record the presence of a learning problem, despite the fact that the child may not meet the diagnostic criteria of DSM-III for a learning disorder, or that the clinician may not have access to school records. The scheme to classify social problems, also a revision of Regier et al. (1982), includes major areas of the child's functioning, such as school, peers, parents, or heterosexual relationships (Burns et al., 1982).

Another issue concerns where children should be screened for psychosocial problems: in the community, the pediatrician's office, or in the school? Each setting may identify children with different psychosocial problems. It is important to design research which would examine the advantages and disadvantages of screening children in each of the three settings. For example, it may be easier to screen for specific developmental disorders in the schools rather than in the pediatrician's office, as the parents may not always be aware of school related problems. On the other hand, the pediatrician may be in an ideal situation to assess eating disorders. Research would be designed to determine whether specific problems are best identified in one setting rather than in another.

A final priority for research is evaluating the effectiveness of treatment for psychosocial problems. When does the child need to be seen by a mental health specialist, and how much can the primary care physician be expected to manage? Should the child be treated in the school system? Researchers need to design intervention studies, including some in which children with psychosocial problems are randomly assigned to groups distinguished by the ease of referral to mental health specialists. In addition the relative effectiveness of different modes of treatment for different groups of children has to be established. The site for treatment (school versus medical practice versus the community) may also be an important experimental variable. Various types of outcomes need to be examined. The results of such research will shed light on what types of psychosocial problems are best treated by a referral to a specialist, what types can be easily managed by primary care physicians or school psychologists, and the extent to which the persistence of certain types of psychosocial problems and their attendant somatic problems can be alleviated by various types of medical care intervention.

REFERENCES

Achenbach, T. M., & Edelbrock, C. (1983). *Manual for the child behavior checklist and revised child behavior profile.* University of Vermont, Burlington, VT.

Allen, G., Burns, B. J., & Cook, W. A. (1983). The provision of mental health services in the health care sector—United States. In C. A. Taube, & S. A. Barrett (Eds.), *Mental health in the United States, 1983.* DHHS Pub. No. (ADM)83-1275. Rockville, MD.

American Academy of Pediatrics Task Force on Pediatric Education. (1978). *The future of pediatric education.* Evanston, Illinois.

American Psychiatric Association. (1980). *Diagnostic and statistical manual of mental disorders* (3rd ed.). Washington, D.C.

Burns, B. J. (1983, June). Personal Communication. Division of Biometry and Epidemiology, National Institute of Mental Health. Rockville, MD.

Burns, B. J., Burke, J. D., Jr., Regier, D. A. (1982). A child oriented psychosocial classification for primary care. In M. Lipkin, & K. Kupka (Eds.), *Psychosocial factors affecting health* (pp. 185–208). New York: Praeger.

Coleman, J. V., Patrick, D. L., Baker, S. M. (1977, July). The mental health of children in an HMO program. *Journal of Pediatrics, 91,* 150–153.

Diehr, P., Williams, S. J., Shortell, S. M., Richardson, W. C., & Drucker, W. L. (1979). The relationship between utilization of mental health and somatic health services among low income enrollees in two provider plans. *Medical Care, 17,* 937–952.

Eastwood, M. R. (1975). *The relation between physical and mental illness.* Toronto: University of Toronto Press.

Egbuonu, L., & Starfield, B. (1982). Child health and social status. *Pediatrics, 69,* 550–557.

Foundation for Child Development. (1977, March). National Survey of Children: Preliminary Report. Press Release.

Glidewell, J. C., & Swallow, C. S. (1976). The Prevalence of Maladjustment in Elementary Schools: A Report Prepared for the Joint Commission on the Mental Health of Children. Unpublished Manuscript.

Goldberg, D., & Blackwell, B. (1970). Psychiatric illness in general practice. A detailed case study using a new method of case identification. *British Medical Journal, 2,* 239–243.

Goldberg, D., & Regier, P. (1980). *Mental illness in the community.* London: Tavistock.

Goldberg, I. D., Huxley, D. A., McInerny, T. K., Pless, I. B., & Roghmann, K. J. (1979). The role of the pediatrician in the delivery of mental health services in children. *Pediatrics, 63,* 898–909.

Gould, M. S., Wunsch-Hitzig, R., & Dohrenwend, B. P. (1980). Formulation of hypotheses about the prevalence, treatment, and prognostic significance of psychiatric disorders in children in the United States. In B. P. Dohrenwend, B. S. Dohrenwend , M. S. Gould, B. Link, R. Neugebauer, & R. Winsch-Hitzig (Eds.), *Mental illness in the United States: Epidemiological estimates* (pp. 9–45). New York: Praeger.

Graham, P. J. (Ed.). (1977). *Epidemiological approaches in child psychiatry.* New York: Academic.

Graham, P., & Rutter, M. (1977). Adolescent disorders. In M. Rutter, & L. Hersov (Eds.), *Child psychiatry: Modern approaches.* Oxford: Scientific Publications.

Haggerty, R. J. (1983). Epidemiology of childhood disease. In D. Mechanic (Ed.), *Handbook of health, health care, and the health professions* (pp. 101–119). New York: New York Free Press.

Haggerty, R. J., Roghmann, K. J., & Pless, I. R. (1975). *Child health and the community.* New York: Wiley.

Hankin, J. R., & Shapiro, S. (1980). The demand for medical service by persons under psychiatric care. In P. Robins, P. Clayton, & J. Wing (Eds.), *Social consequences of psychiatric illness* (pp. 17–32). New York: Brunner/Mazel.

Hankin, J. R., Starfield, B. H., Steinwachs, D. M., Benson, P., Livingston, G., & Katz, H. P. (1984). The relationship between specialized mental health care and patterns of primary care use among children enrolled in a prepaid group practice. In J. R. Greenley (Ed.), *Research in community and mental health, 4,* (pp. 203–220). Greenwich, CT: Sage Publications.

Hankin, J. R., Steinwachs, D. M., Regier, D. A., Burns, B. J., Goldberg, I. D., & Hoeper, E. W. (1982, Feb.). Use of general medical services by persons with mental disorders. *Archives of General Psychiatry, 39,* 225–231.

Joint Commission on Mental Health of Children. (1970). *Crisis in child mental health: Challenge for the 1970's.* New York: Harper & Row.

Jacobson, A. M., Goldberg, I. D., Burns, B. J., Hoeper, E. W., Hankin, J. R., & Hewitt, K. (1980, May). Diagnosed mental disorder in children and use of health services in four organized heath care settings. *American Journal of Psychiatry, 137,* 559–565.

Kellam, S. G., Branch, J. D., Agrawal, C. K., & Ensminger, M. C. (1975). *Mental health and going to school.* Chicago: University of Chicago Press.

Kessler, L. G., Tessler, R. C., & Nycz, G. (1983). Co-occurrence of psychiatric and medical morbidity in primary care. *Journal of Family Practice, 16,* 319–324.

Lipkin, M., Jr., & Kupka, K. (Eds.). (1982). *Psychosocial factors affecting health.* New York: Praeger.

Mitchell, S., & Shepherd, M. (1966). A comparative study of children's behavior at home and at school. *British Journal of Educational Psychology, 37:* 32.

Orvaschel, H., Sholomaskas, D., & Weissman, M. M. (1979). The assessment of psychopathology and behavior problems in children. A review of scales suitable for epidemiological and clinical research, 1967–1979. Final Report. Contract No. ADM 42-74-83 (DBE). National Institute of Mental Health. Rockville, MD.

Radloff, L. S. (1984, Sept. 10). Personal Communication. National Institute of Mental Health. Rockville, MD.

Regier, D. A., Burke, J. D., Jr., Burns, B. J., Clare, A. W., Gulbinat, W., Lipkin, M., Jr., & Spitzer, R. L. (1982). A proposed classification of social problems and psychological symptoms for inclusion in a classification of health problems. In M. Lipkin, Jr. & K. Kupka (Eds.), *Psychosocial factors affecting health* (pp. 153–184). New York: Praeger.

Rice, D., & Danchick, K. (1979). *Changing needs of children: Disease, disability, and access to care.* Paper presented at the session on Child Health: Meeting Basic Needs, Institute of Medicine Annual Meeting. Washington, D.C.

Robins, L. N. (1983). Continuities and discontinuities in the psychiatric disorders of children. In D. Mechanic (Ed.), *Handbook of health, health care, and the health professions* (pp. 195–219). New York: Free Press.

Robins, L. N. (1978). *Mental disorders in children.* Background paper prepared for the President's Commission on Mental Health. Superintendent of Documents, Washington, DC: U.S. Government Printing Office.

Robins, L. N. (1974). *Deviant children grown up.* Huntington N.Y.: Krieger.

Roghmann, K. J., Babigian, H. M., Goldberg, I. D., & Zastowny, T. R. (1982, Nov.). The increasing number of children using psychiatric services: Analysis of a cumulative case register. *Pediatrics, 70,* 790–801.

Rosen, B. M. (1979). Distribution of child psychiatric services. In J. D. Nospitz (Ed.), *Basic handbook of child psychiatry, 70*, Vol. IV, Part C. New York: Basic Books.

Rutter, M. (1977). Surveys to answer questions: Some methodological considerations. In P. J. Graham (Ed.), *Epidemiological approaches in child psychiatry* (pp. 1–30). New York: Academic.

Rutter, M., Tizard, J., & Whitmore, K. (1970). *Education, health, and behavior.* London: Longmans.

Shapiro, S., Hankin, J. R. & Steinwachs, D. M. (1980). Columbia Medical Plan, Columbia, Maryland. In I. D. Goldberg, D. A. Regier, & B. J. Burns (Eds.), Utilization of health and mental health outpatient services in four organized health care settings, *NIMH Series DN, No. 1, DHHS Publication No. (ADM)* 80–859. Washington, D.C.

Shepherd, M., Oppenheim, B., & Mitchell, S. (1971). *Childhood behavior and mental health.* New York: Grune & Stratton.

Starfield, B. (1982, April). Behavioral pediatrics and primary health care. *Pediatrics Clinics of North America, 29*, 377–390.

Starfield, B. (1981). Stability and change: Another view. *American Journal of Public Health, 71*, 301–302.

Starfield, B., Gross, E., Wood, M., Pantell, R., Allen, C., Gordon, I. B., Moffatt, P., Drachman, R., & Katz, H. (1980). Psychosocial and psychosomatic diagnoses in primary care of children. *Pediatrics, 66*, 168–172.

Starfield, B., Hankin, J., Steinwachs, D., Horn, S., Benson, P., Katz, H., & Gabriel, A. (1985). Utilization and morbidity: Random or tandem? *Pediatrics, 75*, 241–247.

Starfield, B., Hoekelman, R., McCormick, M., Benson, P., Mendenhall, R., Moynihan, C., & Radecki, S. (1984, December). Who provides health care to children in the United States? *Pediatrics, 74.*

Starfield, B., Katz, H., Gabriel, A., Livingston, G., Benson, P., Hankin, J., Horn, S., & Steinwachs, D. (1984, March 29). Morbidity in childhood: A longitudinal view. *New England Journal of Medicine, 310*, 824–829.

Tuddenham, R., Brooks, J., & Milkovich, L. (1974). Mothers' reports of behavior in ten year olds: Relationships with sex, ethnicity, and mother's education. *Developmental Psychology, 10*, 959–995.

U.S. Department of Commerce. (1980, January). Social indicators, 1976. In L. LaResche (Ed.), *The epidemiology of learning and behavior problems in children and adolescents.* A report submitted to the Human Learning and Behavior Branch, National Institute for Child Health and Human Development. NIH, Washington, D.C.

U.S. Department of Health, Education, and Welfare. (1971, 1972, 1972, 1974, 1974). *Vital and health statistics, Series 11, Nos. 108, 113, 121, 137, 139.* National Center for Health Statistics, Rockville, MD.

Williams, J. B. W., & Spitzer, R. (1982). A proposed classification of mental disorders for inclusion in a multi-axial classification of health problems. In M. Lipkin, Jr., & K. Kupka (Eds), *Psychological factors affecting health* (pp. 209–218). New York: Praeger.

Williams S. J., Diehr, P., Drucker, W. L., & Richardson, W. C. (1979). Mental health services: Utilization by low income enrollment in a prepaid group practice and in an independent practice plan. *Medical Care, 17*, 139–150.

World Organization of National Colleges, Academies, and Academic Associations of General Practitioners/ Family Physicians. (1979). *International classification of health problems in primary care.* New York: Oxford University Press.

6

Biopsychosocial and Epidemiologic Perspectives on Adolescent Health

ANN F. BRUNSWICK AND CHERYL R. MERZEL

INTRODUCTION

Adolescence has too long been ignored as a life stage with distinct patterns of health problems and requisite modes for providing health services. Indeed awareness of adolescents as a group with separable health needs is a phenonmenon chiefly of the past two decades (Brunswick, 1969, 1976; Brunswick & Josephson, 1972; Coates, Petersen & Perry, 1982; Gallagher, Heald & Garell, 1976; Kovar, 1978; Rogers & Reese, 1964; Select Panel for the Promotion of Child Health, 1981). Recognition of a field called "behavioral medicine" is even more recent (Birk, 1973, cited in Gentry, 1982). It is apparent also that the adolescent life stage is a natural and opportune locus for applying concepts and practices of behavioral medicine.

94

The predominance of behavioral factors in adolescent health can render it paradigmatic for understanding behavioral and psychosocial factors in health and illness more generally.

We set out in this chapter to review what is known about the major health problems of adolescents and to raise issues in providing services appropriate to meeting them. The discussion will be set in the context of the major developmental parameters and challenges of adolescence. The approach we take is an ecological one which views adolescent health and health related behavior as subject to a variety of influences from without and within and, accordingly, emphasizes the integrity of biological, psychological, and social factors in health.

The onset of adolescence is marked by a sudden physical growth spurt and is biologically determined. When adolescence ends, however, is a social phenomenon—presumably with the assumption of "adult" roles and economic independence. Consequently the developmental period of adolescence is quite literally a biopsychosocial phenomenon. It follows that any reasonable approach to health care and to understanding the health needs of adolescents must take into account this biopsychosocial nature of health (Engel, 1977). In addition the age boundaries of adolescence cannot be firmly established for any one point in time (12 to 17? or 10 to 19?) and certainly not across different historical periods. Cross-cultural and cross-national variations in the timing of adolescence have been noted by the World Health Organization (1977).

In early formulations the adolescent life stage was characterized as a period of turbulence, the so-called "sturm and drang" approach to adolescence (Hall, 1904). That view subsequently fell into disfavor as having been erroneously imputed by clinicians who saw only disturbed adolescents. It was replaced by one that saw "normal adolescence" experienced without great emotional outbursts and symptoms of distress (Douvan & Adelson, 1966). It is more than likely that each of these views was properly reflecting the youth of its own era. For today, if societally disapproved adolescent behavior such as cigarette smoking, drinking, sexual relations, pregnancy, use of illicit drugs, school dropout, risk-taking, and violence are taken as the yardstick, the earlier outlook on adolescence as a turbulent and difficult transition might not seem inappropriate. Others have proposed that we examine more closely differences between early adolescence—that is, junior high school ages versus senior high school ages—with the former constituting perhaps the more formidable transition task (Hamburg, 1974).

By any measure adolescence is a period of dilemmas and shifting boundaries. It is marked by rapid growth, change, and discontinuities in varied realms of experience—physical development, self image, cognitive and learning styles, family roles and relationships, peer relations, vocational plans and preparation. The rate of physical growth in adolescence is second only to that in the neonatal stage of development. But in adolescence it is complicated by increasing self awareness:

All important aspects of the individual are affected: accelerated physical development and, most distinctively, sexual maturation; expansion in emotional range of response (reflected in the wide mood swings that adolescents evidence); expanded cognitive or intellectual development when, as Piaget has noted, formal operational or abstract thinking and the ability to look at one's own ideas makes its first appearance; expanded range of interpersonal relations, with the same and the opposite sex. In turn, the adolescent's perceptions and expectations of those around him, as theirs of him, are changing and sometimes unpredictable, thereby intensifying and confusing the issues of identity search—at the very time adolescents are to prepare themselves for occupation and career and to individuate and separate themselves from their families of origin. (Brunswick, 1978, p. 3)

Thus the questions, Who am I? Where am I going? are the unifying themes of adolescence, and autonomy and self-esteem its crucibles. For adolescence by its very name, is a time of learning, acquisition, and maturing into adult roles. Even what adults frequently characterize as risk-taking in adolescence might be understood within the rubric of exploring the limits of identity and competence. Adolescent behaviors can be viewed as attempts at resolving conflicting demands stemming from status and experience in childhood and from expectations of adulthood: dependency and compliance versus autonomy and independent decision making; orientation toward family versus peers; competence in social, cognitive, and career-oriented skills; and developing personal controls required in handling new psychological, physical, and social situations. Inadequate opportunities for meeting these challenges contribute to feelings of powerlessness, anxiety, and stress which mark the young person who is vulnerable to increased physical and emotional problems and to the maladaptive behaviors of adolescence which have their health consequences for the individual adolescent and for society. Moreover, the challenges of the life stage, rooted in the sudden growth and discontinuities which mark it, pose stresses and strains that predispose to the onset of health problems which can surface at later ages.

More broadly, therefore, adolescent behaviors—prosocial or antisocial, adaptive or maladaptive—are best considered a function of how a society views its youth and provides opportunities for their growth and development. As Dragastin (1975) notes: "Not only is the term 'adolescence' a social definition, but what society perceives as an adolescent problem is also socially defined." Similarly, the locus for prevention—in encouraging values, motivations, and controls that foster healthy development and deter the onset of undesirable behaviors which have direct health consequences—lies with those opportunities and resources (medical, educational, occupational, and recreational) which a society makes available for its youth.

ADOLESCENTS AT SPECIAL RISK

As suggested above, rapid rates of change and resultant developmental discontinuities which are inherent in adolescence (Eichorn, 1975) are elements of potential risk for all adolescents. Further differentials often exist in rates of development over various spheres of cognitive, interpersonal, emotional, and/or physical development even within the same adolescent:

> Biological age, chronological age and psychosocial functioning are not always synchronized. We need to develop better indicators of physical, psychological, and social growth in order to have some idea about what the baselines are during the different periods of adolescent development. (Dragastin, 1975, p. 298)

Social variations in risk also exist. Certain characteristics predispose particular adolescents to different and/or more severe health problems. Some of these are considered here:

1.   Age.   Recently three subdivisions with different parameters and challenges have been suggested for use in appraising development in adolescence: early adolescence, covering ages 10 to 14; middle adolescence, ages 15 to 16; and late adolescence, ages 17 to 20. At the same time maturational age based on pubertal development (Tanner, 1974; Petersen & Taylor, 1980), rather than chronological age, is now being used to evaluate biobehavioral development during adolescence. For example, sleep and daytime patterns of sleepiness in adolescence have been found to correlate more closely with endocrine changes and secondary sex characteristics than with chronological age (Litt, 1982). Similarly recent research findings provide evidence that in girls the rate of pubertal development (early, on-time, late), is linked to differences in self-esteem and attitudes toward parents and peers (Brooks-Gunn & Petersen, 1983; Rierdon & Koff, 1980).

2.   Gender.   Not only are the "normal" or average timetables of development and change different for adolescent boys and girls, the relative importance of certain developmental issues and challenges may differ. On the basis of their research in the late 1950s, Douvan & Adelson (1966) observed that adolescent girls evidenced greater concern for interpersonal relations and intimacy and adolescent boys for asserting mastery and independence. Maccoby (1977) suggested that differences such as these have their origin in childhood: different role models that boys and girls have; varied adult responses to boys' and girls' behaviors; and innate biological differences. Block (1976) and Maccoby & Jacklin (1974) observed that girls evidence less self-confidence in their ability to handle a new task than boys do, have less of a sense of control over what happens to them, have greater susceptibility to anxiety, seek more help and reassurance, have greater proximity to friends, and are more concerned with what is socially desirable. Such differences may well be diminishing and can be expected to continue doing so as the social roles and expectations of males and females become more similar. But for now gender distinctions remain, and they continue to have an impact on the experience and problems of adolescence and what are considered appropriate responses to them.

3.   **Poverty, Ethnicity, and Race.**   Sixteen percent of all 16-to-21-year-olds were living below the poverty level in 1981. They accounted for 12 percent of the total poverty population. Among white youth, ages 16 to 21 , 12 percent were classified as below poverty level, compared to 37 percent for black and 28 percent for Hispanic. Although most 16-24-year-olds were either in school or working, fully 10 percent were not engaged in either activity. Almost one of every eight 16 to 24 year olds was a high school dropout (U.S. Bureau of the Census, 1982).

Several sources contribute to special impact from these conditions on adolescent health. One is the adolescent's heightened sense of differences—whether in material possession or in biological endowment. Another results from the effects of reduced access to career opportunities at a stage of life when expanded opportunities are needed for assertion and mastery as well as preparation for economic independence. It should come as no surprise that low income and minority group adolescents are at greater risk on every adolescent health indicator—mortality, acute morbidity, chronic impairments, disabilities and handicaps, and health related behaviors.

4.   **Changing Cohorts.**   Often overlooked, especially by those whose primary concern is with developmental issues, is the fact that the nature and prevalence of adolescent health problems and behaviors constantly change over time. The very definition of adolescence (for example its ages and expected roles) and even its biologic markers (for example, reduction in age at menarche over this century) are variable.

Certain periods of history may in fact be kinder to adolescents than others; that is, more adaptable to their needs in providing an environment conducive to physical growth and development, opportunities in occupational, cognitive, and social arenas and, most importantly, opportunities for meaningful and respected contributions to the community (Elder, 1980). Changing rates of adolescent problem behaviors (violence, truancy, substance abuse) may well be markers of these societal attitudes. It is important to recognize the state of flux within the social fabric as the backdrop for generational differences in the experience of adolescence and the health problems and behaviors that are manifestations of this experience.

HEALTH RISKS: MORTALITY AND MORBIDITY IN ADOLESCENCE

Epidemiological data describing what is currently known about health problems in adolescence will be reviewed here. Large gaps exist in the information which is available; for example, national mortality statistics are collected regularly but population based studies of the nature and extent of adolescent health problems reported by adolescents themselves are limited indeed.

Behavioral and psychosocial factors are in evidence in almost all indicators of adolescent mortality and morbidity. Three possible processes are at work. First, behavioral and psychosocial factors may predispose individual adolescents to illness; for example, the links between poverty and illness which come about through reduced stamina, poor health practices, and/or reduced access to the medical care system. Second, behavioral and psychosocial factors may modify the course and severity of an illness, for example, through poorer adherence to medical regimens. Third, they may extend the effects of a given illness across multiple domains of experience which are critical in adolescence—for example, dermatological disorders (even at mild levels), musculoskeletal deformities (even relatively minor ones), and other physical anomalies that have cosmetic effects which have an impact on the adolescent's self-image and self-confidence over and above their direct physical and functional implications. They may affect the adolescent's feelings of acceptance by peer group and significant adults. In similar fashion periodic acute episodes of chronic illness (for example, asthma) and physical handicaps may inhibit an adolescent's participation in peer-group activities and thereby close this critical avenue toward expanding his or her interpersonal skills and relationships and feelings of worth.

Mortality.   Overall mortality and death rates for most *diseases* ("natural" causes) are lower for adolescents than for other age groups. But statistics for mortality from "natural causes" present a limited view of the adolescent situation. Accidents are the single leading cause of adolescent mortality nationwide and account for more deaths in the 12 to 17 age range than all other causes combined, with motor vehicle accidents being most prominent. In 1976,[1] 36 percent of all adolescent deaths were due to motor vehicle accidents, and 6 percent to drowning (Table 6.1). A recent literature review on unintentional injuries among adolescents and young adults suggests that male gender and substance abuse are important risk factors in accidents (Halperin et al., 1983).Violence (homicide and suicide) accounted for 12 percent of all adolescent deaths in 1976 (Table 6.1). When such fatali-

[1]Mortality data are reported for different time periods, for example, 1976, 1979, or 1981, depending on when the most recent data were available for the age, gender, and/or race groupings of interest.

TABLE 6.1.   MORTALITY IN ADOLESCENCE, UNITED STATES, 1976

| | | Ages | |
Cause	Total (100%)	12–15 (100%)	16–17 (100%)
All accidents & violence	69.9	62.5	76.8
Accidents	56.5	52.5	60.4
Motor vehicle	36.0	28.3	43.2
Fire & flames	1.6	2.2	1.0
Drowning	6.3	7.5	5.3
Suicide	5.4	4.0	6.7
Homicide	6.5	4.5	8.3
All diseases & conditions	30.1	37.5	23.2
Neoplasms	8.9	11.2	6.8
Malignant neoplasms	8.4	10.5	6.5
Leukemia	3.2	4.3	2.1
Congenital anomalies	2.5	3.4	1.6
Heart	1.3	1.7	0.8
Nervous system	3.3	4.1	2.6
Respiratory system	2.9	3.8	2.1
Pneumonia	1.8	2.3	1.3
Circulatory system	4.5	5.4	3.7
Infective & parasitic	1.4	1.9	0.9

Source: Original table published in Kovar, M.G. (1979). Some indicators of health-related behavior among adolescents in the United States. *Public Health Reports, 94*, p. 117.

ties are combined with mortality figures for accidents the total climbs to 70 percent, as compared to 30 percent for deaths due to all diseases and conditions (neoplasms, congenital anomalies, circulatory problems, etc.).

Within the adolescent period, the nature and rate of mortality undergo marked change. Mortality rates climb from 44 per 100,000 earlier in adolescence (ages 12 to 15) to 91 at ages 16 to 17. The major sources of increase are violent and accidental deaths, which rise from 27 per 100,000 adolescents ages 12 to 15 to 70 among 16 to 17 year olds (Kovar, 1979).

More detailed information concerning mortality rates is provided in somewhat different age groupings: 5 to 14, 15 to 24, and so on in Table 6.2. The remaining discussion of trends in adolescent deaths, therefore, will be based on reports for the 15 to 24 year age group and, consequently, reflects experiences of older adolescents. Deaths from natural causes in the 15 to 24 age group declined through 1979, more so for females than for males. But motor vehicle mortality, homicide, and suicide, which, in that order, are the three leading causes of death in the age group, have increased substantially over recent decades. Furthermore, these increases in violent deaths

TABLE 6.2. MORTALITY RATES BY AGE AND SELECTED CAUSES, UNITED STATES, 1981 (NUMBER OF DEATHS PER 100,000 POPULATION)

Age	All Causes	Heart Disease	Malignant Neoplasms	Motor Vehicle Accidents	Homicide and Legal Intervention	Suicide
Under 1 yr.	1,207.3	21.3	2.5	6.1	6.1	—
1–4	60.2	2.5	4.9	7.8	2.6	—
5–14	29.4	0.9	4.1	7.5	1.3	.5
15–24	107.1	2.6	5.7	41.2	14.7	12.3
25–34	132.1	8.4	13.0	28.6	18.5	16.3
35–44	221.3	43.2	47.2	20.2	14.4	15.9
45–54	573.5	177.7	178.1	17.8	11.3	16.1
55–64	1,322.1	481.5	434.8	17.3	7.1	16.4
65–74	2,922.3	1,175.8	814.8	19.4	4.8	16.2
75–84	6,429.9	2,850.3	1,221.8	27.3	5.3	18.6
85+	15,379.7	7,458.8	1,575.3	25.8	5.3	17.7

Source: Compiled from National Center for Health Statistics. (1984). Advance report, final mortality statistics, 1981. *Monthly Vital Statistics Report, 33* (No. 3, Suppl.).

explain why 15 to 24 year olds are the *only* age group to have shown an *increase* in mortality since 1950 (National Center for Health Statistics [NCHS], 1982a). In fact the mortality rate from motor vehicle accidents is higher at ages 15 to 24 than at any other age. Homicide rates for these ages are second only to the rates for ages 25 to 34 (Table 6.2).

Important differences appear by race. Motor vehicle accidents account for upwards of 40 percent of the white deaths at these ages. But homicides are the leading cause of deaths among young black men and women, accounting for approximately 40 percent of black male deaths, nationwide, at these ages. These differences, as well as those in deaths from natural causes where the death rate for the black population also exceeds the white, are acknowledged to reflect socioeconomic disparities between racial groups (NCHS, 1982a). Racial differences in rates of mortality from external causes have been narrowing. While motor vehicle accident deaths among whites, especially females, and also white male homicides have increased (the latter nearly doubled between 1970 and 1979), black homicide and nonmotor vehicle accident mortality decreased. Still, the black male homicide rate is far higher than the white. Gender differences in mortality from accidents and violence far outweigh racial differences (NCHS, 1982a).

Morbidity.   Information about adolescent chronic and acute illness, disabilities and handicaps affecting normal growth, development or function must be pieced together from different sources. National data based on physical examinations of normal samples of adolescents will be presented first, followed by other national data and then community based data.

In the 1960s and 1970s, physical examinations were included as part of national health surveys (Health Examination Survey [HES] and Health and Nutrition Examination Survey [HANES]) which documented the prevalence of the following adolescent disorders: skin, dental and periodontal, vision, nutritional, neuromuscular and musculoskeletal, blood pressure and other cardiovascular, and neurologic disorders. Over half of the examined 12 to 17 year olds had one or more decayed teeth and periodontal disease was found among one-third. Thirty-six percent of this age group had significant skin pathology (Klerman, Kovar & Brown, 1981). Elevated blood pressure[2] was noted in 4 percent, 9 out of 10 cases of which had not been previously diagnosed (NCHS, 1982b). Regarding vision, among the 34 percent who used corrective lenses, almost a third (31 percent) did not meet the 20/20 testing level with correction. At least 15 percent of the age group had abnormalities of the ear, with hearing problems diagnosed in one percent of all adolescents (NCHS, 1973).

Documenting nutritional deficiencies, 12 to 17-year-old-males' caloric intake averaged 15 percent below the daily recommended allowance. Among females, caloric intake deficiency averaged at least 30 percent in the older 15 to 17 year group and approximately 25 percent among those 12 to 14 years old. Female adolescents, on average, registered at least 30 percent below recommended daily levels in iron intake (NCHS, 1977).

Abnormalities affecting normal growth, development, and/or functioning were reported for more than one of five 12 to 17 year olds. Thirty-four percent of the diagnosed abnormalities were neuromuscular; 34 percent were musculoskeletal; 21 percent cardiovascular; 8 percent neurological; and 5 percent involved renal problems.

For reasons not yet well understood, certain health conditions which begin in childhood may become more prominent during adolescence, for example, diabetes and chronic inflammatory bowel disease. Hormonal influences and medical regimen compliance difficulties have been suggested as etiological factors (Litt, 1982).

National prevalence of physical, cognitive, and emotional disability is reported from different sources. It is estimated to include 7 to 11 percent of all children and youth under age 21 (Gliedman & Roth, 1980; Kakalik, Brewer, Dougharty, Fleischauer, & Genensky, 1973). The rate of disability is higher among 14 to 17 year olds than among younger children (Ireys, 1981). Medically significant disabilities have been estimated to occur one and a half to two times more often among poor children than among the more affluent (Gliedman & Roth, 1980). In classifying the most common types of childhood impairment, over a third involved mental retarda-

[2]Criteria were systolic pressure of at least 140 mm Hg and/or diastolic pressure of at least 90 mm Hg.

tion; 30 percent were cases of crippling and/or other physical health impairment, almost one-fifth were speech impairments; emotional disturbance, learning disabilities, and multiple handicaps were each estimated at five percent of the impaired population (Gliedman & Roth, 1980; see Brunswick, 1985, for a discussion of disability in adolescence).

Community studies, mainly of poor and minority adolescents, provide additional information about morbidity in adolescence. Medical examinations of a random sample of black adolescents from Harlem (Brunswick & Josephson, 1972) revealed that sizeable proportions of young adolescents aged 12 to 15 had the following health problems: vision, upper respiratory, cardiac and blood pressure, skin, nervous-emotional, nutritional, neuromuscular or musculoskeletal, lung and bronchial, blood problems (chiefly anemia), urinary tract, and speech. Examining physicians in the Harlem study found that 61 percent of 12-to 15-year-old boys and 74 percent of the girls had at least one significant medical problem. Furthermore, evidence that adolescents were not receiving medical attention they needed was reflected in the fact that for each condition already under treatment, there were eight that needed referral to care (Brunswick & Josephson, 1972). A different study in a predominantly black, male, urban high school in New York City (Schonberg & Cohen, 1979) also revealed a wide range of acute and chronic conditions in that presumably healthy sample of teenagers.

Self-reports are an important source of information about adolescents' health (Brunswick, 1976). In the Harlem study of black adolescents, consistent with their medical examination findings, the 10 most frequently self-reported problems among all males and females aged 12 to 17 were: dental, weight (both obesity and, especially among boys, underweight), vision, frequent colds, repeated headaches, nervous-emotional problems, skin, stomach pains, speech, and menstrual problems. Health problems increased over the adolescent years and did so about two years earlier among girls than boys (Brunswick, 1980a).

While health problems observed in young people using health services cannot be taken as a measure of the full range of health problems in the population at large, they add to the knowledge base concerning adolescent health risks. Hospitalization at ages 12 to 17 is relatively infrequent compared to older age groups and is occasioned chiefly by injuries and pregnancy-delivery. Hospitalization rates for injury are almost three times greater among adolescent males, especially older ones, than females. Hospitalization for illness is higher among females than males (Kovar, 1979). Eighteen percent of all female hospital days are accounted for by delivery. Major illnesses leading to hospitalization are respiratory, digestive, and psychiatric (Brunswick, Hamburg, & Kovar, 1978).

In a hospital in New York City (Schonberg & Cohen, 1979), adolescent in-hospitalization was occasioned by gastrointestinal illnesses (1 in 10 admissions); trauma, due mainly to automobile and athletic injuries (7 percent of admissions); neurological, cardiac, orthopedic, asthma, Ob-Gyn, and endocrine disorders (each of which comprised another 6 percent). Leading reasons for visits to the hospital *outpatient* clinic were: venereal disease, contraception, health maintenance and assessment, infections, dermatologic, pregnancy, depression and anxiety (Schonberg & Cohen, 1979).

As can be seen from the above, emotional disorders were identified as a major health risk in almost every data source. Furthermore in the mid-1970s, mental disorders were the fourth ranking reason for hospitalization of 12 to 17 year olds, accounting for 11 percent of all hospital days. The most frequent diagnoses were schizophrenia, adjustment reactions, and depressive disorders (Klerman et al, 1981). The risk rises sharply with age in adolescence, evidenced in admission rates to inpatient psychiatric facilities: 127 per 100,000 of 10 to 14 year olds compared to 433 among older 15 to 17 year olds (Select Panel for the Promotion of Chilld Health, 1981).

Health Behaviors.   Included here are both health-compromising practices and health-promoting activities. Among adolescents, health-risk practices include cigarette, alcohol, and illicit substance use; careless sexual practices; and careless risk-taking resulting in accidents and injuries. Of these, systematic epidemiologic data are available only for reproductive and substance-use behaviors.

Trends in adolescent sexual activity have been reported by the Alan Guttmacher Institute (1981): "In the course of the 1970s, sexual activity among unmarried women ages 15-19 living in metropolitan areas rose by two-thirds." Approximately 7 in 10 females and 8 in 10 males had intercourse by the end of their teens.

Rates of contraceptive use are rising among teenagers. Still, according to a recent national survey, only about one-third (34 percent) of sexually active women between ages 15 and 19 use contraception regularly. Chief methods are the pill, condom, and withdrawal. About a quarter (27 percent) never practiced contraception, their chief reason being that they did not believe they were at risk of pregnancy. Evidence suggests that teen-aged women alternate their contraceptive methods rather than staying with a single preferred one. Furthermore the proportion of adolescent women using the most effective forms of birth control, the pill and IUD, decreased between 1976 and 1979 while the percentage using less effective methods such as withdrawal, condom, foam, and diaphragm increased during this period (Alan Guttmacher Institute, 1981).

Reports on pregnancy outcomes indicate that in 1978 about half of all pregnancies among women under age 20 were terminated either by abortion or miscarriage. Almost one quarter (22 percent) of the pregnancies resulted in births to unmarried women, and a quarter (27 percent) of pregnancies were conceived and/or delivered after marriage (Alan Guttmacher Institute, 1981). While abortions increased through the 1970s, among all age groups, the proportion of abortions relative to live births has been consistently highest among women under age 15 (NCHS, 1983). These practices have important implications for the health care of sexually active adolescents.

Trends in substance use are reported in two national surveys (Johnston, O'Malley, & Bachman, 1984; Miller et al., 1983).[3] Cigarettes, alcohol, and marijuana are the substances most commonly used by adolescents. Although trending up in the 1970s, the prevalence of use of all substances, except cocaine, is now declining among 12 to 17 year olds. Current[4] rates of use (Table 6.3) show that in 1982 better than a quarter of 12 to 17 year olds were drinking alcohol, about one in seven were smoking cigarettes, one in nine were smoking marijuana, 2 percent were using cocaine, and one percent were using hallucinogens (PCP or angel dust, LSD or acid, mescaline, etc.).

These figures cover the full range of 12 to 17 years and may mask the substantial increase observed during adolescence.[5] During the same time period, high school seniors reported much higher current rates of use: alcohol, 70 percent; cigarettes, 30 percent; marijuana, 28.5 percent; cocaine, 5 percent; hallucinogens, 4 percent; and nonprescribed stimulants, 10 percent (Table 6.3).

Importantly, note that not only did rates of use increase during adolescence, but that the adolescent years are the chief period of risk for recruitment into substance use (Brunswick & Boyle, 1979; Johnston, et al., 1984; Kandel, Murphy & Karus, 1984). In other words, most users of recreational substances, licit and illicit, begin use in adolescence. Finally, national data have been discussed here because they are useful for describing general trends. Their very aggregate nature, however, conceals important variations to be found among population subgroups. Rates of illicit drug use generally are higher among males than females, higher in the Northern and Western states than the South, higher in urban areas than rural. Race and economic level have influenced rates in the past (Brunswick, 1980b) but convergence across these boundaries is appearing (O'Donnell, Voss, Clayton, Slatin, & Room, 1976).

While the epidemiological and medical literature has generally viewed adolescent health as the absence of health-compromising behaviors and the proper use of diet, rest, exercise, and timely seeking of medical care, a newer concept of *positive* health is emerging, as illustrated in the work of Jessor (1984) and Perry and Jessor (1985). Positive health is perceived as encompassing four interrelated domains: physical health (adequate func-

[3]One, the National Survey on Drug Abuse (Miller et al., 1982), is conducted through personal interviews in a representative sample of households. The other, Monitoring the Future (Johnston et al., 1982), is conducted annually with a national sample of high school *seniors* by self-completed questionnaire.

[4]In both studies, "current" use is defined as within the 30 days prior to survey.

[5]These are acknowledged to underestimate true prevalence, since high school dropouts and absentees are omitted and they have higher rates of drug use.

TABLE 6.3 LIFE TIME PREVALENCE AND CURRENT USE OF SELECTED SUBSTANCES, UNITED STATES, 1982[a] (IN PERCENTS)

	Household Survey[b] (12–17 Year Olds)		High School Seniors[c]	
	Lifetime Prevalence (N = 1581)	Current Use (N = 1581)	Lifetime Prevalence (N = 17,500)	Current Use (N = 17,500)
Cigarettes	49	15	70	30
Alcohol	65	27	93	70
Marijuana	27	11	59	29
Hallucinogens[d]	5	1	15	4
Cocaine	7	2	16	5
Heroin	*	*	1	*

*Less than .5%

[a]Lifetime prevalence includes use one or more times in lifetime. Current use refers to use within past month (30 days).

[b]Compiled from Miller, J., et al. (1983). *National survey on drug abuse: Main findings 1982* (DHHS Publication No. ADM 83-1263). Washington, DC: U.S. Government Printing Office.

[c]Compiled from Johnston, L., O'Malley, P. & Bachman, J. (1984). *Drugs and American high school students 1975–1983* (DHHS Publication No. ADM 85-1374). Washington, DC: U.S. Government Printing Office.

[d]Includes LSD and other hallucinogens such as PCP (angel dust), mescaline, peyote, psilocybin, and/or DMT.

tioning of the major body systems), psychological health (subjective sense of well-being), social health (effectiveness in fulfilling tasks within the social setting), and personal health (integrative capacity for personal self actualization). In this context, health promotion activities are directed toward changing the adolescent's behavior, personality, and environment in order to weaken health compromising behavior and strengthen health-enhancing behavior.

MEETING THE HEALTH NEEDS OF ADOLESCENTS

Biopsychosocial markers and challenges of adolescence were examined in the first part of this chapter. These are useful guidelines both for understanding the health problems in that life period and for approaches to caring for them.

The prominence of so-called stress-related symptoms and behaviors among the predominant health risks of adolescents is particularly noteworthy in a volume focussed on psychosocial and behavioral determinants, manifestations, and interventions in illness. These behaviors are reflected in adolescent mortality, which derives largely from risk taking (accidents), violence (homicides), and self-destruction, and in the dramatic rise in psychiatric hospitalization in later adolescence. The fact that these conditions are so prevalent calls into question how well we are attending or even defining mental health risks in adolescence. We have identified the following psychosocial states as major adolescent emotional risks: depression, anxiety, poor self-esteem, diminished sense of competency and control, attention problems, agression/poor impulse control, denial, sociopathy, alienation, and anhedonia (Brunswick & Merzel, 1983). These states should be taken as early-warning signals of potentially serious emotional disorders ahead.

Another set of symptoms, so-called "neurological soft-signs," also merit comment. These recognized symptoms of stress figure prominently in adolescents' reports of their own health problems. In the Harlem study, for example, 19 percent reported that they had repeated headaches, 17 percent frequent stomach pains, and 12 percent often had chest pains (Brunswick, 1980a). Lacking "hard" signs that can be detected by the physician, these "soft" signs do not appear often enough in the rosters of observed adolescent medical problems. Such physical complaints among adolescents may actually reflect a pattern of illness behavior developed in childhood in response to illness episodes and stress situations (Mechanic, 1980).

The biopsychosocial perspective on adolescents' health needs which is the focus of this paper is depicted in Figure 6.1. This ecological or contextual model of influences on health and behavior has been modified from Bronfenbrenner's (1979) generalized model (see also Brunswick, 1985; Kurdek, 1981). In it, health influences are arrayed according to four domains of varying complexity and distance from the individual. Essentially, the model reminds us that the adolescent lives in a variety of settings, any or all of which may interact with his/her own biological and psychological predispositions in affecting health outcomes.

1.   At the broadest macrosocial level, gender, ethnicity, socioeconomic status, and historic time are some of the sources of influence on health outcomes.

2.   At the next level of complexity are structural factors, including availability of health services and/or allocation of other societal and institutional resources, for example, health insurance, housing conditions, and neighborhood quality. Included in this situational domain also are availability of illicit substances and other environmental hazards, or, on the positive side, availability of recreational facilities and jobs.

3.   The third level, called the "microsystem," covers the important area of interpersonal relations: the adolescent's relations with family, peers,

Macrosystem ⟶ Exosystem ⟶ Microsystem ⟶ Ontosystem

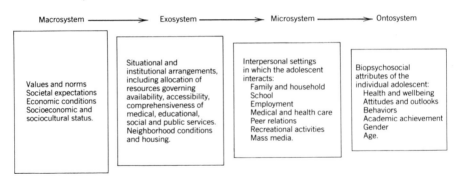

Values and norms Societal expectations Economic conditions Socioeconomic and sociocultural status.	Situational and institutional arrangements, including allocation of resources governing availability, accessibility, comprehensiveness of medical, educational, social and public services. Neighborhood conditions and housing.	Interpersonal settings in which the adolescent interacts: Family and household School Employment Medical and health care Peer relations Recreational activities Mass media.	Biopsychosocial attributes of the individual adolescent: Health and wellbeing Attitudes and outlooks Behaviors Academic achievement Gender Age.

FIGURE 6.1.   Ecological paradigm: influences on adolescent health.

teachers, physicians, and others. This domain, particularly, has important feedback effects with intraindividual characteristics.

4.   The individual level subsumes the full range of intraindividual qualities—physical, cognitive, and emotional—which enter into assessing the adolescent's needs for care.

It is useful to keep the above broad model of influences on health in mind in conceptualizing suitable settings, services, and delivery styles for meeting adolescents' health care needs. As a starting point some specific observations and recommendations are raised below.

1.   Education and information on matters that concern adolescents are an important part of the process of their health care. These matters include: nutrition, exercise, body systems (structure and function), sexual responses and reproduction, emotions, cigarette smoking, alcohol, drug use (licit and illict); resources for medical care and how to use the health care system; how to deal with health information and use it in decision making; and handling responsibility for one's own health and assisting others in managing their health care.

2.   Heightened concern about the body and how it works (brought about by rapid changes in physical appearance and function) provides the motivational base for adolescents to develop good health maintenance practices which can extend through the life span.

3.   A number of services adolescents need have not been available through their usual source of care (if they have one). As an example, widespread need for gynecologic and contraceptive services and for mental-health services by adolescents is in evidence, but access to those services usually requires resort to a separate clinic or provider. Note that some of the more successful models for adolescent health care, to date, have been multiservice centers (including traditional medical care and also career guidance, family planning, nutrition and dietary guidance, drug "rap" groups, etc.).

4. The adolescent's access to medical care has in the past been conditional on adults (consent to care and ability to pay for it). Different arrangements may be needed to bypass these barriers and also to provide as much confidentiality in the doctor-patient relationship as the adolescent desires.

5. It is important to make adolescents active participants in the process of their health care, so that the provider is doing things *with* not *to* them.

6. Youthful age in the health counselor and provider of adolescent medical services probably is less important than his or her attitude and outlook. Adolescents have not infrequently been characterized as threatening, mischievous, and/or unreliable, given to exaggerating their health problems. There is little objective basis for these attitudes. It is critical for the individual practitioner to recognize his or her feelings about adolescents before entering into a relationship to treat them. Practitioners who have worked with adolescents are generally impressed by young people's responsiveness to genuine respect and concern.

It is very appropriate that issues in adolescents' health and health care be addressed in a volume concerned with behavioral pediatrics. As noted throughout this chapter, such a discussion is also suggestive of what remains to be done in meeting the biopsychosocial health needs of adolescents. Certainly adolescence can be recognized as a life-stage in its own right, with distinct patterns of health problems, which in turn, demand distinct programs of health services.

REFERENCES

Alan Guttmacher Institute. (1981). *Teenage pregnancy: The problem that hasn't gone away*. New York: Author.

Block J. (1976). Issues, problems, and pitfalls in assessing sex differences: A critical review of the psychology of sex differences. *Merrill-Palmer Quarterly, 22*, (4).

Bronfenbrenner, U. (1979). *The ecology of human development*. Cambridge, MA: Harvard University Press.

Brooks-Gunn, J., & Petersen A. (Eds.). (1983). *Girls at puberty: Biological and psychosocial perspectives*. New York: Plenum

Brunswick, A.F. (1969). Health needs of adolescents: How the adolescent sees them. *American Journal of Public Health, 59*, 1730–1745.

Brunswick, A.F. (1976). Indicators of health status in adolescence. *International Journal of Health Services, 6*,475–492.

Brunswick, A.F. (1978, April). *Adolescent health needs: A developmental and psychosocial perspective*. Paper presented at the meeting of Southern Region, Maternal and Child Health Professionals. Chapel Hill, NC.

Brunswick, A.F. (1980a). Health stability and change: A study of urban Black youth. *American Journal of Public Health, 70*, 504–513.

Brunswick, A.F. (1980b). Social meanings and developmental needs: Perspectives on Black youth's drug abuse. *Youth & Society, 11*, 449–473.

Brunswick, A.F. (1985). Health services for adolescents with impairment, disability, and/or handicap: An ecological paradigm. *Journal of Adolescent Health Care, 6* (in press).

Brunswick, A.F., & Boyle, J. (1979). Patterns of drug involvement: Developmental and secular influences on age at initiation. *Youth & Society, 11,* 139–162.

Brunswick, A.F., Hamburg, B., & Kovar, M.G. (1978, November). *Adolescent health indicators.* Paper presented at 106th Annual Meeting of the American Public Health Association, Los Angeles, CA.

Brunswick, A.F., & Josephson, E. (1972). Adolescent health in Harlem. *American Journal of Public Health,* (October Supp.), 1–62.

Brunswick, A.F., & Merzel, C. (1983) *The development of a classification scheme for identifying high risk adolescents.* Unpublished manuscript.

Coates, T.J., Petersen, A.C., & Perry, C. (Eds.). (1982). *Promoting adolescent health: A dialog on research and practice.* New York: Academic.

Douvan, E., & Adelson, J. (1966). *The adolescent experience.* New York: Wiley.

Dragastin, S. (1975). Research themes and priorities. In S. Dragastin & G. Elder, Jr. (Eds.), *Adolescence in the life cycle* (Epilogue). Washington, DC: Hemisphere Publishing Corporation.

Eichorn, D. (1975). Asynchronizations in adolescent development. In S. Dragastin & G. Elder, Jr. (Eds.), *Adolescence in the life cycle.* Washington, DC: Hemisphere Publishing Corporation.

Elder, G. (1980). Adolescence in historical perspective. In J. Adelson (Ed.), *Handbook of adolescent psychology* (pp. 3–465). New York: Wiley.

Engel, G.L. (1977). The need for a new medical model: A challenge to biomedicine. *Science, 196,* 129–136.

Gallagher, J., Heald, F., & Garell, D. (1976). *Medical care of the adolescent* (3rd ed.). New York: Appleton-Century-Crofts.

Gentry, W.D. (1982). What is behavioral medicine? In J.R. Eiser (Ed.), *Social psychology and behavioral medicine* (pp. 3–13). New York: Wiley.

Gliedman, J., & Roth, W. (1980). *The unexpected minority: Handicapped children in America.* New York: Harcourt Brace Jovanovich.

Hall, G.S. (1904). *Adolescence: Its psychology and its relation to physiology, anthropology, sociology, sex, crime, religion and education* (Vol. 1). New York: Appleton.

Halperin, S., Bass, J., Mehta, K., & Betts, K. (1983). Unintentional injuries among adolescents and young adults: A review and analysis. *Journal of Adolescent Health Care, 4,* 275–281.

Hamburg, B.C. (1974). Early adolescence: A specific and stressful stage of the life cycle. In G. Coelho, D. Hamburg, & J. Adams (Eds.), *Coping and adaptation.* New York: Basic Books.

Ireys, H. (1981). Health care for chronically disabled children and their families. In Select Panel for the Promotion of Child Health, *Better health for our children: A National strategy: Vol. 4, Background papers* (pp. 321–353). (DHHS Publication No. PHS 79-55071). Washington, DC: U.S. Government Printing Office.

Jessor, R. (1984). Adolescent development and behavioral health. In J.D. Matarazzo, S.M. Weiss, J.A. Herd, N.E. Miller, & S.M. Weiss (Eds.), *Behavioral health: A handbook of health enhancement and disease prevention* (pp. 69–90). New York: Wiley.

Johnston, L., Bachman, J., & O'Malley, P. (1982). *Student drug use, attitudes and beliefs, national trends 1975-1982.* (DHHS Publication No. ADM 83-1260). Washington, DC: U.S. Government Printing Office.

Johnston, L., O'Malley, P., & Bachman, J. (1984). *Drugs and American high school students 1975–1983.* (DHHS Publication No. ADM 85-1374). Washington, DC: U.S. Government Printing Office.

Kakalik, J., Brewer, G., Dougherty, L., Fleischauer, P., & Genensky, S. (1973). *Services for handicapped youth: A program overview.* Santa Monica, CA: The Rand Corporation.

Kandel, D., Murphy, D., & Karus, D. (1984). Cocaine use in young adulthood: Patterns of use and psychosocial correlates. In N. Kozel & E. Adams (Eds.), *Cocaine technical review*. Rockville, MD: National Institute on Drug Abuse.

Klerman, L., Kovar, M.G., & Brown, S. (1981). Adolescents: Health status and needed services. In Select Panel for the Promotion of Child Health, *Better health for our children: A national strategy: Vol. 4, Background papers* (pp. 285–319). (DHHS Publication No. PHS 79-55071). Washington, DC: U.S. Government Printing Office.

Kovar, M.G. (1978). Adolescent health status and health-related behavior (Summary). *Institute of medicine conference on adolescent behavior and health* (pp. 29–38). Washington, DC: National Academy of Sciences.

Kovar, M.G. (1979). Some indicators of health related behavior among adolescents in the United States. *Public Health Reports, 94*, 109–118.

Kurdek, L. (1981). An integrative perspective on children's divorce adjustment. *American Psychologist, 36*, 856–866.

Litt, I. (1982). Adolescent health in the U.S. as we enter the 1980's. In T.J. Coates, A.C. Petersen, & C. Perry (Eds.), *Promoting adolescent health: A dialog on research and practice* (pp. 45–60). New York: Academic Press.

Maccoby, E. (1977). Sex differentiation during childhood development. *Master lectures on developmental psychology*. Washington, DC: American Psychological Association.

Maccoby, E., & Jacklin, C. (1974). *The psychology of sex differences*. Stanford, CA: Stanford University Press.

Mechanic, D. (1980). The expense and reporting of common physical complaints. *Journal of Health and Social Behavior, 11*, 146–155.

Miller, J., Cisin, I., Gardner-Keaton, H., Harrell, A., Wirtz, P., Abelson, H., & Fisburne, P. (1983). *National survey on drug abuse: Main findings 1982* (DHHS Publication No. ADM 83-1263). Washington, DC: U.S. Government Printing Office.

National Center for Health Statistics. (1973). Examination and health history findings among children and youths, 6–17 years, United States. *Vital and Health Statistics* (Series 11, No. 129). (DHEW Publication No. HRA 74-1611). Washington, DC: U.S. Government Printing Office.

National Center for Health Statistics. (1977). Dietary intake of persons 1-74 years of age in the United States. *Advance data* (No. 6). Rockville, MD: Health Resources Administration. (DHEW Publication No. HRA 77-1250).

National Center for Health Statistics. (1982a). *Health, United States, 1982*. (DHHS Publication No. PHS 83-1232). Washington, DC: U.S. Government Printing Office.

National Center for Health Statistics. (1982b). Blood pressure levels and hypertension in persons ages 6-74 years: United States, 1976-80. *Advance data* (No. 84). Hyattsville, MD: National Center for Health Statistics. (DHHS Publication No. PHS 82-1250).

National Center for Health Statistics. (1983). *Health, United States, 1983*. (DHHS Publication No. PHS 84-1232). Washington, DC: U.S. Government Printing Office.

O'Donnell, J., Voss, H., Clayton, R., Slatin, G., & Room, R. (1976). *Young men and drugs—A nationwide survey* (Research Monograph No. 5). Rockville, MD: National Institute on Drug Abuse.

Perry, C., & Jessor, R. (1985). The concept of health promotion and the prevention of adolescent drug abuse. *Health Education Quarterly, 12*, 169–184.

Petersen, A.C., & Taylor, B. (1980). The biological approach to adolescence; biological change and psychological adaptation. In J. Adelson (Ed.), *Handbook of adolescent psychology* (pp. 97–155). New York: Wiley.

Rierdon, J., & Koff, E. (1980). The psychological impact of menarche: Integrative versus disruptive changes. *Journal of Youth and Adolescence, 9*, 49–58.

Rogers, K., & Reese, G. (1964). Health studies—presumably normal high school students, Pt. 1, physical appraisal. *American Journal of Diseases of Children, 108,* 572–600.

Schonberg, S.K. & Cohen, M.I. (1979). Health needs of the adolescent. *Paediatrician, 8* (Suppl. 1), 131–140.

Select Panel for the Promotion of Child Health. (1981). *Better health for our children: A national strategy: Vol. 3. A statistical profile.* (DHHS Publication No. PHS 79-55071). Washington, DC: U.S. Government Printing Office.

Tanner, J.M. (1974). Sequence and tempo in the somatic changes in puberty. In M.M. Grunbach, G.D. Grave, & F.E. Meyer (Eds.), *Control of the onset of puberty.* New York: Wiley.

U.S. Bureau of the Census. (1982). *Statistical abstract of the United States, 1982-83* (103rd ed.), Washington, DC: U.S. Government Printing Office.

World Health Organization, (1977). *Health needs of adolescents.* (Technical Report Series No. 609). Geneva: Author.

PART **III**

DETERMINANTS

7

Psychoneuroimmunology: Developmental Perspecitves

ROBERT ADER

"Behavioral medicine is the interdisciplinary field concerned with the development and integration of behavioral and biomedical science knowledge and techniques relevant to the understanding of health and illness and the application of this knowledge and these techniques to prevention, diagnosis, treatment, and rehabilitation." (Schwartz & Weiss, 1978).

I presume that behavioral pediatrics similarly involves an integration of the behavioral and biomedical sciences as these apply to an understanding of developmental processes related to health and disease. As such, behavioral pediatrics must be concerned with basic research on normal growth and development in behavior and physiology as well as in the application of this knowledge in the treatment and prevention of disease. My purpose in this chapter is to focus on an integration of behavior and immunology,

Preparation of this paper was supported by a Research Scientist Award (K5 MH06318) from the National Institute of Mental Health, USPHS.

two "disciplines" that, until recently, have remained almost totally independent.

Immunologists know little about behavior, and behaviorists know little about the immune system. If we behaviorists had any course work in immunology at all, we were taught that the immune system is an autonomous agency of defense, a self-regulating system devoted to the recognition of what is "self" and what is "not self." Indeed, immunology has been defined as that agency of defense that is independent of the central nervous system (Snell, 1972). However, the situation seems to be changing. Converging data from a variety of disciplines suggest that there is a "dynamic flow of information" (Besedovsky, del Ray, & Sorkin, 1983) between the immune system and the central nervous system, and that the immune system is integrated with all other physiological systems that operate to maintain the integrity of the individual and the species in its adaptation to prevailing environmental circumstances. As such, the immune system is sensitive to behavioral processes and may, in turn, influence behavioral processes of adaptation.

Recently the Developmental Immunology Program of the Genetics and Teratology Section of the National Institute of Child Health and Human Development elaborated upon its interests in a developmental perspective in immunologic research by enumerating areas that were of particular concern. The areas identified reflected a practical concern with development, aging, and health and disease from the perspective of the immunologist. There was no explicit consideration of the potential role of behavioral processes. It seems appropriate then to reexamine these interest areas from the integrative perspective of behavioral pediatrics to determine the possible impact of behavior on these very same priority areas. A strong case, based on a great deal of direct experimental evidence, can not be made. However, something of a case based on a limited number of provocative studies can be made, and in my view, is sufficient to warrant new research initiatives that adopt a developmental strategy with respect to studies of the interactions between behavior and immune function.

Specific interests in developmental immunology research relate to observations that (1) abnormal immunologic development leads to immunodeficiency disease; (2) deficits in bodily defenses can result in intrauterine and postnatal infections that are known to be teratogenic; and (3) immunologic interactions between mother and fetus are possible causes of intrauterine growth retardation, abortion, premature births, and congenital malformations.

There is an extensive literature on the effects of prenatal maternal stress, early postnatal experiences, and pre- and postnatal endocrine interventions on the development of behavioral and physiological processes. It would not be unreasonable, therefore, to suppose that (1) environmental stimulation or direct neuroendocrine interventions during early (postnatal) life are capable of altering immune development (thereby influencing the likelihood of developing immunodeficiency diseases); (2) "stressful" stimulation experienced by pregnant females can influence bodily defenses including immunocompetence (and thereby alter susceptibility to intrauterine and postnatal infections); and (3) prenatal maternal "stress" plus a variety of other postnatal circumstances are capable of influencing behavioral interactions between mother and young (thus influencing a variety of psychobiologic processes). Conversely, there is evidence to indicate that early infectious disease has behavioral consequences and that these differ from those that follow from infectious disease in the older individual. Let me then expand upon each of these possible behavioral determinants of immunocompetence.

EFFECTS OF INTERVENTIONS DURING EARLY (POSTNATAL) LIFE

There is extensive literature on the effects of psychosocial factors (including "stress") on infectious, parasitic, and autoimmune diseases (Plaut & Friedman, 1981; Solomon, 1981). Of particular interest to behavioral pediatrics, for example, are the studies indicating that "stress" is related to an increased susceptibility to streptococcal disease in families (Meyer & Haggerty, 1962) and that the duration of respiratory illness is prolonged in children that score high on a scale of life-event changes (Boyce et al., 1977). Events that occur during early life have been shown capable of modifying behavioral and physiological development and influencing susceptibility to a variety of spontaneously occurring or experimentally induced disease processes in a variety of species (Ader, 1980, 1981). Only a few studies (Amkraut, Solomon, & Kraemer, 1971; Friedman, Glasgow, & Ader, 1969; Levine & Cohen, 1959), however, have examined the effects of early life experiences on disease processes that may involve immunologic defense mechanisms. Although it is not entirely clear to what extent different kinds of cancer have a viral etiology or involve immune surveillance, I might at least note that several studies have documented the effects of different early life experiences on the development and/or the course of different neoplastic processes (LaBarba, 1970; Sklar & Anisman, 1981).

There are few generalizations that can be gleaned from this literature on the effects of psychosocial factors (including early life experiences) on disease susceptibility except to indicate that environmental manipulations are capable of altering the susceptibility or response to pathophysiologic processes. The effects obtained are a function of the nature of both the environmental intervention and the pathogenic stimulus, several biological characteristics of the host (for example, species, strain, age, gender), and the psychophysiological state of the organism upon which the environmental and pathogenic stimuli are superimposed. The same interacting variables also determine the effects of psychosocial factors on immune function (Ader, 1980, 1983; Monjan, 1981).

With respect to the direct measurement of immune function, Solomon, Levine, and Kraft (1968) subjected infant rats to daily handling from birth until weaning at 21 days of age. At nine weeks of age the handled animals and an unmanipulated control group were immunized with flagellin, a bacterial antigen. Both the overall primary and secondary response to antigenic stimulation was greater in the handled animals. Handling during infancy did not, however, alter the course of an adjuvant-induced arthritic condition in rats (Amkraut et al., 1971). In terms of interventions during early life, most of what could be described as developmental psychoneuroimmunologic research has concerned endocrine manipulations. Several papers have dealt with the parallel development of endocrine and immune function (Pierpaoli, 1981). Part of the evidence for interactions between the endocrine and immune systems comes from observations that endocrine manipulations influence immune process and immune responses elicit endocrine changes. Such findings are reinforced by the results of developmental studies. Dieter and Breitenbach (1970), for example, manipulated the endocrine status of immature (3-week-old) white Leghorn cockerels. There is a high corticosterone response to ACTH and "stress" at one month of age, which is also about the time of lymphoid organ growth and development in the cockerel. Different doses of corticosterone or testosterone proprionate injected daily for two weeks resulted in a dose-related involution of the bursa of Fabricius, the thymus, and the spleen. Two weeks later, the lymphoid organs of the cockerels treated with corticosterone did not differ from those in control birds; the effects of testosterone, however, were still evident. Histological evidence indicated that the effects of testosterone were permanent, particularly with respect to the bursa of Fabricius.

In birds, the bursa of Fabricius is a primary lymphoid organ critical to the development of humoral immunity. It is the origin of B cells and is active during embryonic life and in young chickens. Data obtained by Pedernera, Romano, Besedovsky, and Aguilar (1980) suggest that the bursa of Fabricius may also be required for normal endocrine development. In the search for a bidirectional link between endocrine and immune function, chick embryos were bursectomized after 68 hours of incubation. A second group of bursectomized chicks received a graft of bursal tissue. Relative to values obtained from sham-operated controls, bursectomy diminished the *in vitro* production of corticosterone by the adrenals and increased the *in vitro* production of testosterone by the testes. Bursal grafting obviated these endocrine alterations. Such results suggest that the bursa of Fabricius produces factors that can modify endocrine function during development of the chick embryo.

Hormonal differences between males and females appear to be related to the gender differences in immunologic reactivity. Skin allografts, for example, are rejected more rapidly by females than males, and allograft rejection is accelerated by castration in males but is only minimally affected by castration in females (Castro & Hamilton, 1972; Graff, Lappe, & Snell,

1969). In humans as well as in lower animals, females tend to be more reactive and, with age, are more liable to autoimmune disease (Dubois, 1974). Sex differences in behavior are dependent upon differences in neural organization laid down during early development (Gorski, 1979). Neonatal exposure to androgens masculinizes the sexual behavior of females and alters the ability of the hypothalamus to regulate cyclic gonadotrophin secretion by the pituitary. Ovarian hormones, however, do not exert an analagous influence on the development of the brain. A sexual dimorphism has also been confirmed morphologically with respect to singing in birds (Arnold, 1981). Is there a sexual dimorphism in the brain that governs immunologic reactivity? That is, one could ask if the differences in immunologic reactivity between males and females are also related to differences in neural organization, if the neonatal administration of testosterone would permanently "masculinize" the immunologic reactivity of females, and where in the brain steroid might exert such an effect on immune function.

There are sex differences in the development of immunologic reactivity (Krzych, Thurman, Goldstein, Bressler, & Strausser, 1979) and there are other experiments suggesting that manipulation of gender-related hormonal levels during early life has long-term consequences. Female SJL/J mice, for example, display a high incidence of spontaneous neoplasms and are particularly vulnerable to the development of lymphosarcomas in response to oral administration of dimethylbenzanthracene (DMBA). Pierpaoli, Haran-Ghera, and Kopp (1977) masculinized SJL/J female mice with a single injection of 1 mg of testosterone at either two or three days of age. Mice were treated with DMBA at 60 days of age. Early testosterone treatment decreased the incidence of lymphosarcomas from 82 percent to 23 percent and prolonged the latency to develop tumors. It remains to be determined, however, if the results of this alteration in hormonal state actually represents an "early" experience effect. Provocative results were also obtained by Tartakovsky and Klimenko (1981), who injected rats with testosterone on days 2 and 16 of life. At 60 days of age half the testosterone-treated group and untreated controls were immunized with sheep erythrocytes. Testosterone treatment decreased complement level and the phagocytic activity of leukocytes (two measures of nonspecific defense mechanisms) and, in response to the antigenic stimulation, reduced humoral and cell-mediated immunity. Unfortunately the abstract of this report (in Russian) did not specify the gender of the animals that were used and, again, it was not determined if these long-term effects of testosterone actually represent "early" experience effects.

The development of autoimmune disease in New Zealand hybrid mice represents another model within which to relate sex hormones and immune function. The female (NZBxNZW)F_1 mouse eventually develops a lethal glomerulonephritis and several studies (Roubinian, Talal, Greenspan, Goodman, & Siiteri, 1978; Steinberg et al., 1979) have shown that the immunologic defect that results in manifest disease is sensitive to the manipulation of sex hormones. Castration and/or testosterone treatment of females prolongs survival and castration and/or estradiol treatment of males accelerates mortality relative to sham-treated controls. Steinberg et al. (1979) have shown that the effects of such hormonal interventions are a function of age. Castration of males markedly accelerates the development of autoimmune disease only if performed at two or three weeks of age. Castration has only a minor effect if performed at five weeks and has no effect if it is delayed until 15 weeks of age. It appears, then, that hormone production early in life or, perhaps, the balance or pattern of hormones that affect other endocrine or lymphoid tissue are critical to the development or maintenance of immunocompetence.

PRENATAL INFLUENCES

There is now abundant evidence concerning the deleterious effects of chemical contamination of the environment, and there are data indicating that the immature organism is particularly sensitive to such adverse environmental circumstances. It has also been shown that the effects of environmental pollutants may be detected in behavioral changes before physical symptoms become evident. As a matter of fact prenatal exposure to environmental toxins may not cause detectable defects at birth but still result in behavioral impairments later in life as behavioral processes of adaptation emerge. Presumably the developing brain is especially vulnerable to chemical insult, and alterations in brain development are sensitively indexed by alterations in behavior. More recent data indicate that neuroanatomic and neurochemical alterations in the developing brain resulting from exposure to a variety of environmental contaminants are also reflected in compromised immune defense mechanisms (Koller, 1979). Like the alterations in behavior, immune function is modified by levels of contamination that do not necessarily produce clinical signs of toxicity; and like the alterations in behavior, long-term effects on immunologic reactivity may be greater when exposure occurs during infancy.

Spyker (1975), for example, described the behavioral changes that eventually occurred in mice that were exposed to methyl mercury prenatally but were "normal" at birth. During the course of this study, she observed an increased incidence of bacterial infection with advancing age in the mice exposed to methyl mercury *in utero*. In another sample of differentially treated animals, a specific antigenic challenge was used to assess immunocompetence and revealed an impairment of immune function in the elderly group of prenatally exposed mice.

Another illustration is provided by the immunomodulating effects of alcohol. There have been several studies of the growth, development, and behavioral effects of pernatal exposure to alcohol (Abel, 1980; Randal & Riley, 1981). Clinical evidence indicates that alcohol abuse is toxic to the immune system, and Monjan and Mandell (1980) examined the effects of *in utero* exposure to alcohol on the immunologic reactivity of rat offspring. Females were intubated daily with different doses of ethyl alcohol or sucrose beginning two weeks before mating and continuing until parturition. Mitogenic stimulation of splenic lymphocytes was introduced when the offspring were 7, 11, and 18 months of age. There were no differences in B-cell function, but T-cell function, as measured by the response to conconavalin A (Con A), was depressed at 7 and 11 months of age in the offspring of females that received a high dose of alcohol. Exposure to alcohol *in utero* has some transient and some relatively long lasting effects on the steady-state levels, metabolism, or release of neurotransmitter substances (Druse, 1981) that have been implicated in the modulation of immune responses (Hall & Goldstein, 1981). Whether the patterning of these neurotransmitter changes or direct effects on the developing thymus could account for the immunosuppressive effects of prenatal exposure to alcohol remains to be examined. These data nevertheless suggest that the teratogenic effects of alcohol intoxication extend to the immune system. A variety of other psychoactive drugs are also capable of influencing immune function in adult organisms (Ferguson, Schmidtke, & Simmons, 1978; Saunders & Muchmore, 1964). It might be important, therefore, to determine if the abuse of such agents is also teratogenic for the immune system.

In summarizing the effects of prenatal exposure to methyl mercury (which may be generalized to other environmental and, perhaps, pharmacologic stimuli), Spyker (1975) speculates that the "apparent dysfunction of the immune system may also be an example of how impairment of a system other than the nervous system can affect behavior. On the other hand, decreased immunological competence may be altering nervous system function and thus indirectly affecting behavior." (p. 1843). One could also hypothesize that the effects of prenatal stimulation on immune function result directly from the neuroanatomical and/or neurochemical changes induced by environmental contaminants, pharmacologic agents, and experiential events.

MOTHER-YOUNG INTERACTIONS

The development of immunocompetence, which is critical to the survival of the organism, is accomplished in part through the transfer of cells and antibodies from mother to young (Stini, 1981). The intimate contact of mother and young during suckling, for example, provides warmth and nurturance and, in addition, exposes mother and young to pathogenic stimuli. When animal pups are licked, pathogens present on the neonate enter the mother's respiratory and gastrointestinal tracts. The lymphatic circulation of the gastrointestinal tract (in humans, at least) also supplies the mammaries. Thus any immunologic changes elicited by antigens derived from the infant are contained in breast milk and immunity can be transmitted to the infant in this manner. In seeking the stimuli responsible for the increase in maternal behavior that lactating rats display toward their experimentally stimulated pups, one might therefore ask if such behavior serves to protect the infant from the environmental pathogens to which it may be exposed when it is taken away from the nest. One might even ask if the recognition (i.e., acceptance and/or rejection) of young is mediated by the major histocompatibility complex which has already been implicated in mate selection in mice (Andrews & Boyse, 1978; Yamaguchi, Yamazaki, & Boyse, 1978; Yamazaki, Yamaguchi, Andrews, Peake, & Boyse, 1978) and might be hypothesized to mediate the early social interactions among gerbils that depend upon the transfer of saliva (Block, Volpe, & Hayes, 1981).

There are also potential hazards in mother-young relationships. Since the bloodbrain barrier in the rat and the human is not fully developed at birth, maternal specific antibodies are present in the cerebrospinal fluid (CSF) of infants (Thorley, Holmes, Kaplan, McCracken, & Sanford, 1975). When labelled IgG antibodies against brain antigens are injected into adult and infant rats, transfer into the CSF is observed only in the infants (Adinolfi & Dodd, 1981). These authors have postulated that abnormal endocrine states or immune perturbations in the mother (e.g., the presence of antibrain antibodies) might cause changes in the brain during fetal or early life that ultimately result in specific neurologically mediated behavioral disorders. Related to these speculations, perhaps, are some observations on Snell-Bagg (dwarf) mice. These animals have a pituitary defect and are deficient in somatotrophic hormone and thyroxine. They are also immunologically compromised. A similar wasting disease can be induced by immunologic blockade of hypothalamic-pituitary function, but only when such intervention occurs during the first few weeks of life; there is no impairment of cellular immunity when antipituitary serum is given to adult animals (Pierpaoli, Fabris, & Sorkin, 1970). It is of related interest that there are striking behavioral differences between dwarf mice and heterozygous controls and their sensitivity to rearing in a perceptually "enriched" environment (Bouchon & Will, 1982).

Although there are relatively few studies on alterations in immunocompetence as a function of behavioral interactions between mother and young, the importance and potential of such studies are being recognized. The data available illustrate, again, the dependence of immunologic development and, perhaps, subsequent immune function on extraimmune factors. Reite, Harbeck, and Hoffman (1981) recently reported that peer separation in pigtailed monkeys results in an impairment of cellular immunity that was evidently unrelated to the changes in hormone levels that were measured at the same time. In a second experiment, Laudenslager, Reite, and Harbeck (1982) examined the effects of mother-young separation in bonnet monkeys. In two mother-infant pairs, mothers were removed to another room for two weeks and then returned to their young. Relative to a two-week baseline, both infants displayed a depressed lymphocyte response to mitogenic stimulation with Con A and phytohemagglutinin (but not to pokeweed) during the period of separation. The two mothers also showed a depression of cellular immunity during separation. Both infants and one of the two mothers recovered normal immune responses within two weeks of reunion. As these authors point out, any generalization may be tenuous at this point, but maternal separation in rhesus monkeys is not accompanied by any consistent change in adrenocortical steroids (Gunnar, Gonzalez, Goodlin, & Levine, 1981).

Michaut et al. (1981) examined the immunologic effects of maternal deprivation in mice. Lactating females were removed from their litters for four hours each day during the first postpartum week and for eight hours each day during the second week and the litters were weaned at 15 days postpartum. Control litters were unmanipulated and remained with the lactating female until 21 days of age. Between seven and eight weeks of age, all mice were immunized with sheep red blood cells. There were no differences in body weight or adrenal weight, but maternally deprived animals showed a depressed antibody response to the antigenic stimulation.

Preliminary data on the effects of premature weaning in the rat have been reported by Keller et al. (1983). Half the rats were weaned at 15 days of age and half the animals were weaned at the customary age of 21 days. At 40 days of age there was a significant suppression of the lymphocyte response to phytohemagglutinin stimulation in the samples of whole blood obtained from the prematurely weaned group. There was also a significant lymphopenia in these animals. Using a fixed number of lymphocytes in an isolated lymphocyte stimulation assay, however, confirmed the decreased responsivity in the prematurely weaned animals. Adult determinations were obviated by a respiratory infection in the laboratory which resulted in the death of 8 of 22 prematurely weaned animals and none of 22 controls, a serendipitous observation that is obviously worth pursuing. As the authors note, it will be important to determine if and how nutritional deficits, temperature regulation, and/or changes in hormone or neurotransmitter levels may have contributed to these alterations in immunologic reactivity.

In contrast to the above, extending maternal influences can also have immunologic consequences. As mentioned above, Snell-Bagg mice have immunologic deficiencies. The prolonged nursing of dwarf mice by foster mothers, however, attenuates the deleterious effects of their pituitary deficiency on lymphoid tissue and partially restores their response to antigenic stimulation. Whether the restoration of immune function is attributable to some maternal milk factor, other nutritional influences, or some maternally mediated modification of endocrine status (Pierpaoli et al., 1970) needs to be examined.

As previously noted, one may not always be able to specify the direction of the effects, but there is considerable literature indicating that experiential events influence susceptibility or responses to infectious disease. There are also data indicating that infectious disease can influence behavior. Furthermore, the effects of viral infection on behavior may be a function of the age at which the infection is experienced and may be modified by mother-young interactions. Hotchin, Benson, and Gardner (1970) inoculated mice with lymphocytic choreomeningitis (LCM) virus when they were two days old. At nine days of age, a mother not previously exposed to LCM virus was substituted for the litter's natural mother. This intervention caused a 20 percent decrease in mortality. Introducing two "normal" mothers reduced mortality by 32 percent. Conversely, if a mother from LCM-infected mice was substituted for the natural mother of uninfected animals, there was a 15 percent increase in mortality. The daily rotation of lactating females within each group increased mortality among infected mice but had no effect on control litters. The mothers' health clearly influenced survival of the pups, but it is not clear how this influence was exerted. Mothers of infected mice did receive contact infection that resulted in mild illness six days after their pups were inoculated, and pup survival might have been influenced by illness-induced behavioral changes in the mother rather than or in addition to any changes in milk secretion, for example. In this connection it is interesting that rotating the mothers (which the authors describe as "mildly stressful") had little effect on normal mice but acted synergistically to potentiate the lethal effects of the viral infection. This interpretation is consistent with other data on the interaction between "stress" and viral infection (Friedman, Ader, & Glasgow, 1965).

More recently McFarland, Sikora, and Hotchin (1981) inoculated weanling mice and 8-week old mice with herpes simplex type 1 virus. When tested in an open-field two weeks later, mice inoculated at weaning were hypoactive and mice inoculated at eight weeks of age were hyperactive compared to uninfected controls. Although housing conditions were changed following infection and may have differentially affected the mice (Edwards, Rahe, Stephens, & Henry, 1980), these results are consistent with the hypothesis that the effects of infectious disease on behavior, like the effects of behavior on infectious disease, are influenced by an interaction between the host (for example, stage of development) and the infectious agent.

DISCUSSION

It is not necessary to detail here the extent to which hormones influence behavior, or the extent to which behavior and early life experiences influence endocrine function. Also it is beyond the scope of this paper to present all the evidence for hormonal modulation of immune responses; several very complete reviews are available (Ahlqvist, 1981; Comsa, Leonhardt, & Wekerle, 1982). I think that we will now begin to see more research that focuses on the role of hormones in the *development* of immuno-competence. As Comsa et al. (1982) point out, the vast majority of the research relating endocrine and immune function has concentrated on the thymus. Because of its central role in the ontogeny of immune function, the endocrine functions of the thymus have not received the attention they deserve. Conversely, hormones other than those of the thymus have not received sufficient attention as modulators of immune responses.

Lymphocytes bear receptors for neurotransmitter substances as well as hormones, and the influence of neurotransmitters on immunologic reactivity (Hall & Goldstein, 1981) is a rapidly growing field of research. Modulators of neurotransmitter level also influence behavior, perhaps especially when their effects are exerted early in the development of the central nervous system (Cuomo et al., 1981; Shaywitz, Yager, & Klopper, 1976). It will be interesting and important to determine if there are parallel effects on the development of immunocompetence. Based on the literature from developmental psychobiology, it is plausible to hypothesize that some of the effects of behavior in modifying immunologic reactivity are mediated by neuroendocrine changes. It would be premature, however, to specify the multiple pathways through which behavioral processes might influence immune processes—and vice versa. There are data to show that behavioral processes, including conditioning (Ader & Cohen, 1981), can influence immune responses. There is also a growing literature showing that neuroendocrine changes influence immune function, and there are now data documenting the innervation of lymphoid tissue.

In view of the available data, it would not be surprising to find that behavioral factors, particularly those that occur during early development, are capable of influencing those immune processes that have been identified as important to health. Based on the available data, the relationship between behavior and immune function would appear to be a promising new field of interdisciplinary research. If I have expanded upon the concerns of developmental immunology, then, it is in the belief that a developmental perspective to the study of psychoneuroimmunology will add a very meaningful dimension to such an integrative venture and that the data obtained will have important clinical implications in behavioral pediatrics.

REFERENCES

Abel,E.L. (1980). The fetal alcohol syndrome: Behavioral teratology. *Psychological Bulletin, 87,* 29–50.

Ader, R. (1980). Psychosomatic and psychoimmunologic research. *Psychosomatic Medicine, 42,* 307–321.

Ader, R. (1981). Animal models in the study of brain, behavior and bodily disease. In H. Weiner, M. A. Hofer, & A. J. Stunkard (Eds), *Brain, behavior, and bodily disease* (pp. 11–26). New York: Raven.

Ader, R. (1983). Developmental psychoneuroimmunology. *Developmental Psychobiology, 16,* 251–267.

Ader, R., & Cohen, N. (1981). Conditioned immunopharmacologic effects. In R. Ader (Ed.), *Psychoneuroimmunology* (pp. 281–319). New York: Academic.

Adinolfi, M., & Dodd, S. (1981). Immunologic aspects of central nervous system maturation. In K.J. Connolly & H.R. Prechtl (Eds.), *Maturation and development: Biological and psychological perspectives. Clinics in developmental medicine. 77/78* (pp. 162–185). Suffolk, England: Spastics International.

Ahlqvist, J. (1981). Hormonal influences on immunological and related phenomena. In R. Ader (Ed.), *Psychoneuroimmunology* (pp. 335–403). New York: Academic.

Amkraut, A.A., Solomon, G.F., & Kraemer, H.C. (1971). Stress, early experience and adjuvant-induced arthritis in the rat. *Psychosomatic Medicine, 33,*203–214.

Andrews, P.W., and Boyse, E.A. (1978). Mapping of an H-2-linked gene that influences mating preference in mice. *Immunogenetics, 6,* 265–268.

Arnold, A.P. (1981). Model systems for the study of sexual differentation of the nervous system. *Trends in Pharmacological Sciences, 3,* 148–149.

Besedovsky, H.O., del Ray, A., & Sorkin, E. (1983). Neuroendocrine immunoregulation. In H. Fabris, E. Garaci, J. Hadden, & N.A. Mitchison (Eds.), *Immunoregulation* (pp. 315–339). New York: Plenum.

Block, M.L., Volpe, L.C., & Hayes, M.J. (1981). Saliva as a chemical cue in the development of social behavior. *Science, 211,* 1062–1064.

Bouchon, R., & Will, B. (1982). Effects of early enriched and restricted environments on the exploratory and locomotor activity of dwarf mice. *Behavioral and Neural Biology, 35,* 174–186.

Boyce, W.T., Cassel, J.C., Collier, A.M., Jensen, E.W., Ramey, C.T., & Smith, A.H. (1977). Influence of life events and family routines on childhood respiratory tract illness. *Pediatrics, 60,* 609–615.

Castro, J.E., & Hamilton, D.N.H. (1972). Adrenalectomy and orchidectomy as immunopotentiating procedures. *Transplantation, 13,* 614–616.

Comsa, J., Leonhardt, H., & Wekerle, H. (1982). Hormonal coordination of the immune response. *Reviews of Physiology Biochemistry and Pharmacology, 92,* 115–189.

Cuomo, V., Cagiano, R., Coen, E., Mocchetti, I., Cattabeni, F., & Racagni, G. (1981). Enduring behavioral and biochemical effects in the adult rat after prolonged postnatal administration of haloperidol. *Psychopharmacology, 74,* 166–169.

Dieter, M.P., & Breitenbach, R.P. (1970). A comparison of the lymphocytic effects of corticosterone and testosterone proprionate in immature cockerels. *Proceedings of the Society for Experimental Biology and Medicine, 133,* 357–364.

Druse, M.J. (1981). Effects of maternal ethanol consumption on neurotransmitters and lipids in offspring. *Neurobehavioral Toxicology and Teratology, 3,* 81–87.

Dubois, E.L. (Ed.) (1974). *Lupus erythematosus.* Los Angeles: University of California Press.

Edwards, E.A., Rahe, R.H., Stephens, P.M. & Henry, J.P. (1980). Antibody response to bovine serum albumin in mice: The effects of psychosocial environmental change. *Proceedings of the Society for Experimental Biological Medicine, 164,* 478–481.

Ferguson, R.M., Schmidtke, J.R., & Simmons, R.L. (1978). Effects of psychoactive drugs on *in vitro* lymphocyte activation. *Birth Defects, 14,* 379–405.

Friedman, S.B., Ader, R., & Glasgow, L.A. (1965). Effects of psychological stress in adult mice inoculated with Coxsackie B viruses. *Psychosomatic Medicine, 27,* 361–368.

Friedman, S.B., Ader, R., & Glasgow, L.A. (1965). Effects of psychological stress in adult mice inoculated with Coxsackie B viruses. *Psychosomatic Medicine, 27,* 361–368.

Friedman, S.B., Glasgow, L.A., & Ader, R. (1969). Psychosocial factors modifying host resistance to experimental infections. *Annals of the New York Academy of Sciences, 164,* 381–392.

Gorski, R. (1979). The neuroendocrinology of reproduction: An overview. *Biology of Reproduction, 20,* 111–127.

Graff, R.J., Lappe, M., & Snell, G.D. (1969). Influence of gonads and adrenals on tissue response to skin grafts. *Transplantation, 7,* 105–111.

Gunnar, M.R., Gonzalez, G.A., Goodlin, B.L., & Levine, S. (1981). Behavioral and pituitary-adrenal response during a separation period in infant Rhesus Macaques. *Psychoneuroendocrinology, 6,* 66–75.

Hall, N.R., & Goldstein, A.L. (1981). Neurotransmitters and the immune system. In R. Ader (Ed.), *Psychoneuroimmunology* (pp. 521–543). New York: Academic.

Hotchin, J., Benson, L. & Gardner, J. (1970). Mother-infant interaction in lymphocytic choriomeningitis virus infection of the newborn mouse: The effect of maternal health on mortality of offspring. *Pediatric Research, 4,* 194–200.

Keller, S.E., Ackerman, S.H., Schleifer, S.J., Schindledecker, R.D., Camerino, M.S., Hofer, M.A., Weiner, H., & Stein, M. (1983). Effect of premature weaning on lymphocyte stimulation in the rat. *Psychosomatic Medicine 45,* 75.

Koller, L.D. (1979). Effects of environmental contaminants on the immune system. *Advances in Veterinary Science and Comparative Medicine, 23,* 267–295.

Krzych, U., Thurman, G.B., Goldstein, A.L., Bressler, J.P., & Strausser, H.R. (1979). Sex-related immunocompetence of BALB/C mice. I. study of immunologic responsiveness of neonatal, weanling, and young adult mice. *Journal of Immunology, 123,* 2568–2574.

LaBarba, R.C. (1970). Experiential and environmental factors in cancer. *Psychosomatic Medicine, 32,* 259–276.

Laudenslager, M., Reite, M., & Harbeck, R.J. (1982). Suppressed immune response in infant monkeys associated with maternal separation. *Behavioral and Neural Biology, 36,* 40–48.

Levine, S., & Cohen, C. (1959). Differential survival to leukemia as a function of infantile stimulation in DBA/2 mice. *Proceedings of the Society for Experimental Biology and Medicine, 102,* 53–54.

McFarland, D.J., Sikora, E., & Hotchin, J. (1981). Age at infection as a determinant of the behavioral effects of herpes encephalitis in mice. *Physiological Psychology, 9,* 87–89.

Meyer, R.J., and Haggerty, R.J. (1962). Streptococcal infection in families: Factors altering individual susceptibility. *Pediatrics, 29,* 539–549.

Michaut, R-J., Dechambre, R-P., Doumerc, S., Lesourd, B., Devillechabrolle, A., & Moulias, R. (1981). Influence of early maternal deprivation on adult humoral immune response in mice. *Physiology and Behavior, 26,* 189–191.

Monjan, A. (1981). Stress and immunologic competence: Studies in animals. In R. Ader (Ed.), *Psychoneuroimmunology* (pp. 185–227). New York: Academic.

Monjan, A.A., & Mandell, W. (1980). Fetal alcohol and immunity: Depression of mitogen-induced lymphocyte blastogenesis. *Neurobehavioral Toxicology and Teratology, 2,* 213–215.

Pedernera, E.A., Romano, M., Besedovsky, H.O., & Aguilar, M. (1980). The bursa of Fabricius is required for normal endocrine development in chicken. *General and Comparative Endocrinology, 42,* 413–419.

Pierpaoli, W. (1981). Integrated phylogenetic and ontogentic evolution of neuroendocrine and identity-defense, immune functions. In R. Ader (Ed.), *Psychoneuroimmunology* (pp. 575–606). New York: Academic.

Pierpaoli, W., Fabris, N., & Sorkin, E. (1970). Developmental hormones and immunological maturation. In G.E.W. Wolstenholme & J. Knight (Eds.), *Hormones and Immune Response* (pp. 126–153). London: Churchill.

Pierpaoli, W., Haran-Ghera, N., & Kopp, H.G. (1977). Role of host endocrine status in murine leukaemogenesis. *British Journal of Cancer, 35,* 621–629.

Plaut, S.M., & Friedman, S.B. (1981). Psychosocial factors, stress, and disease processes. In R. Ader (Ed.), *Psychoneuroimmunology* (pp. 3–29). New York: Academic.

Randall, C.L., & Riley, E.P. (1981). Prenatal alcohol exposure: Current issues and the status of animal research. *Neurobehavioral Toxicology and Teratology, 3,* 111–115.

Reite, M., Harbeck, R., & Hoffman, A. (1981). Altered cellular immune response following peer separation. *Life Sciences, 29,* 1133–1136.

Roubinian, J.R., Talal, N., Greenspan, J.S., Goodman, J.R., & Siiteri, P.K. (1978). Effect of castration and sex hormone treatment on survival, antinucleic acid antibodies, and glomerulonephritis in NZB/NZW F_1 mice. *Journal of Experimental Medicine, 147,* 1568–1583.

Saunders, J.C., & Muchmore, E. (1964). Phenothiazine effect on human antibody synthesis. *British Journal of Psychiatry, 110,* 84–89.

Schwartz, G.E., & Weiss, S.M. (1978). Behavioral medicine revisited: An amended definition. *Journal of Behavioral Medicine, 1,* 249–251.

Shaywitz, B.A., Yager, R.D., & Klopper, J.H. (1976). Selective brain dopamine depletion in developing rats: An experimental model of minimal brain dysfunction. *Science, 191,* 305–308.

Sklar, L.S., & Anisman, H. (1981). Stress and cancer. *Psychological Bulletin, 89,* 369–406.

Snell, G. (1972). *Immunology, immunopathology and immunity.* Hagestown: Harper.

Solomon, G.F. (1981). Emotional and personality factors in the onset and course of autoimmune disease, particularly rheumatoid arthritis. In R. Ader (Ed.), *Psychoneuroimmunology* (pp. 159–182). New York: Academic.

Solomon, G.F., Levine, S., & Kraft, J.K. (1968). Early experience and immunity. *Nature, 220,* 821–822.

Spyker, J.M. (1975). Assessing the impact of low level chemicals on development: Behavioral latent effects. *Federation Proceedings, 34,* 1835–1844.

Steinberg, A.D., Melez, K.A., Raveche, E.S., Reeves, J.P., Boegel, W.A., Smathers, P.A., Taurog, J.D., Weinlein, L., & Duvic, M. (1979). Approach to the study of the role of sex hormones in autoimmunity. *Arthritis and Rheumatism, 22,* 1170–1176.

Stini, W.A. (1981). Body composition and nutrient reserves in evolutionary perspective. *World Review of Nutrition and Dietetics, 37,* 55–83.

Tartakovsky, W.L. & Klimenko, O.A. (1981). The influence of testosterone on immune reactivity of new born rats. In E. Korneva (Ed.), *The regulation of immune homeostasis* (pp. 98–99). Leningrad.

Thorley, J.D., Holmes, R.K., Kaplan, J.M., McCracken, G.H., & Stanford, J.P. (1975). Passive transfer of antibodies of maternal origin from blood to cerebrospinal fluid in infants. *Lancet, i,* 561–653.

Yamaguchi, M., Yamazaki, K., & Boyse, E.A. (1978). Mating preference tests with the recombinant congenic strain BALB.HTG. *Immunogenetics, 6,* 261–264.

Yamazaki, K., Yamaguchi, M., Andrews, P.W., Peake, B., & Boyse, E.A. (1978). Mating preferences of F_2 segregants of crosses between MHC-congenic mouse strains. *Immunogenetics, 6,* 253–259.

8

Developmental Determinants and Child Health Behavior: Research Priorities

FRANCES DEGEN HOROWITZ AND MARION O'BRIEN

Our knowledge about the course of normal development is relatively recent. Despite 19th century interest in the topic by Darwin and others, systematic empirical observation and recording of early development were not begun until Gesell and his colleagues worked to map the young child's motor development in the 1920s and 1930s. At about that time Piaget first described sequences of cognitive development in his own three children, although it was some decades later before Piagetian constructs made their way into the mainstream of American developmental psychology and education. Both of these pioneer developmentalists had their early training in biology—Gesell as a physician and Piaget as a specialist in mollusks. Their approaches, guided by their biological training and orientation, have undoubtedly influenced the long-standing debate concerning the degree to which biological versus environmental factors control the course and quality of behavioral development in young children.

Our task in this chapter is to consider developmental determinants of behavioral development. There is a sense that this might be thought of as a recursive assignment in that behavioral development and developmental determinants could be considered iterations of the same basic concept. However, as we have become increasingly sophisticated in our understanding of behavioral development we have come to apppreciate the pervasive influence of constraining parameters that guide its course. These undoubtedly result from eons of evolutionary history in which the human behavioral repertoire has been biologically and genetically honed to a hardy course not easily deflected by the ordinary fluctuations of environmental experience. The sequences and general topography of human behavioral development are well tuned as the basic theme upon which the variations of individual differences appear to build. Some of the individual differences are also likely to be genetically and biologically determined; others may be environmentally determined.

The heredity-environment or nature-nurture controversy cannot be ignored in trying to understand the degree to which one can assign to the environment the responsibility for developmental outcome. However, the issue is most likely going to be resolved in the context of an interactional focus, whereby biologically and genetically controlled developmental determinants set the general course of development and the organism's predisposition to respond to environmental stimulation. But without environmental stimulation and stimulus input, behavioral development will not occur. We know this from some of the unfortunate "experiments in nature" in which abandoned and isolated children, left without natural sources of environmental stimulation, show quite aberrant behavioral development. The significant scientific questions now revolve around understanding how environmental stimulation interacts with biological and genetic predispositions to determine the individual differences and variations in behavioral developmental outcome.

We will look first at what we know about the normal developmental course of children and we will describe the limitations of our knowledge base. We will also consider the role of the physician who understands this knowledge base as we review each period of development. We will discuss how environmental factors may affect behavioral development; we will suggest a model of organism-environment interaction to account for behavioral development; and we will make a distinction between the role of behavioral management and the role of developmental determinants as contributors to developmental outcome. Finally, we will suggest the agenda for programmatic research most likely to advance our ability to help children and to foster optimal development in children.

THE KNOWLEDGE BASE AND ITS LIMITATIONS

Infancy

The logical beginning for this discussion is with infancy. At the moment of birth the normal human infant has the capability of responding to visual, auditory, tactile, olfactory, and kinesthetic stimulation. The infant's direct response to stimulation is brief and variable, but the rudiments of behavioral organization and attention are intact and functioning. Newborns also engage in short bursts of interactive behavior, and these increase in duration and frequency with each passing day. Under controlled laboratory conditions, newborns have been shown to form simple associations and exhibit response decrement to repeated presentations of the same stimulus (Lipsitt, 1977, 1982; Lipsitt & Wenner, 1981).

Yet not all newborns are alike. Some crying infants are easy to console, others difficult, and still others may soothe themselves. Some newborns move smoothly and gradually between states whereas others change states rapidly and frequently. These early individual differences are thought to contribute to the nature of interaction between parent and child, but it is also likely that the nature of interaction influences the infant's temperamental characteristics (Horowitz, Linn & Buddin, in press). There is evidence that infants who are strong in attending to and tracking sounds and objects and who are low in irritability in the first few days of life also elicit positive interaction from mothers over their early months. Furthermore, we have found that newborn infants can be categorized by whether their behavior is consistent or variable during two successive administrations of the Brazelton neonatal behavioral assessment scale, one day apart. Interestingly those babies who show variable response on the assessment also have mothers who are *more* responsive to them. Perhaps behavioral variability is inherently more interesting to mothers or is a sign of a wider repertoire of available behaviors and thus a biologically better-organized infant (Linn & Horowitz, in press).

Developmental change over the period of infancy is rapid and relatively regular. We will briefly review what is known and not known in the major areas of development.

1. Physical Development. The course of motor development was charted by Gesell and tends to follow a regular progression from rolling over to sitting alone to crawling or scooting and finally to the first step sometime around the end of the first year. There are factors, both biological and environmental, that influence the rate, if not the progression, of motor development. For example, American black infants tend to show more rapid motor development than caucasians; height-weight ratios influence motor development; and the opportunity for free exploration also appears to affect motor development.

Only recently has another aspect of physical development been investi- gated—that is, physical appearance or attractiveness. Babies who are seen as attractive—and there is reasonably high agreement across judges on these categorizations—receive more positive attention from adults. The potential importance of physical appearance is suggested by a recent dem- onstration in Israel, where surgical techniques developed in Germany have been used to normalize the appearance of Down's Syndrome children. In simply looking at the "before-and-after" photographs, one finds oneself "expecting" different kinds of behavior from the child.

2. Cognitive Development.   In the area of cognitive development, or the tracking of the infant's ability to understand relationships and respond to them, we are really attempting to describe the infant's increasing ability to make use of learning opportunities and to participate more actively in social interchanges (Brainerd, 1978).

Piaget termed infancy the "sensori-motor period" because it is during these months that a child initially learns to regulate and coordinate motor activity in response to (or pursuit of) a sensory stimulus. For example, when a new parent hangs a mobile over an infant's crib, the infant's initial response will be visual: the baby will watch the mobile as it moves in re- sponse to air currents, another person's movements, or even a wind-up motor. But soon—by 10 to 12 weeks of age—the baby will begin to per- ceive that the mobile is more likely to move if the baby is also moving. If the infant can touch the mobile, random movements of the infant will rap- idly be replaced by directed arm movements aimed at making the mobile move. These interactions are evidence that the infant's motor behavior is coming under control of the external stimulus of the mobile. By 4 or 5 months the infant will reach, grasp, and pull on the mobile—at which point the wise parent will raise the mobile out of baby's reach and the learning process will begin again (Langer, 1980).

Similarly early cognitive development is intimately involved in the in- fant's social relationships. In the first year a baby learns to recognize par- ents and other familiar adults and children and to respond emotionally when mother and other caregivers leave and return.

At times in the infant's acquisition of understanding of relationships, the parent may find the experience frustrating. In the course of learning how the world and its objects fit together, the infant must practice. But when practice means dropping the spoon from the high chair over and over and over and over and over most parents become weary. The inability of infants to "turn off" a newly acquired behavior can also be exasperating to parents. Sometimes babies will persist in a behavior, such as batting a mobile, almost in an obligatory fashion and eventually begin to cry out of frustration. Parents are sometimes mystified at this behavior, but a pedia- trician can help parents be sensitive to their baby's lack of control and can help them learn the "tricks" of redirection and distraction that ease the frustration of both parent and child.

As with motor development, the fact that cognitive development occurs rapidly and with regularity in most infants does not mean that the process is automatic and preprogrammed. The normal environment of most infants is replete with learning opportunities and experiences that promote the infant's awareness of relationships. When these opportunities and experiences are absent, there is evidence that cognitive development does not proceed normally (Hunt, Paraskevopoulis, Schickendanz & Uzgiris 1975). It is likely that many aspects of later intellectual performance build on a cognitive base formed in infancy.

3. Language.   The acquisition and creative use of language is what makes us humans unique in the biological world. Like other aspects of development in infancy, language acquisition follows a normal course from production of sounds to imitation of sounds, from comprehension of others' speech to single word utterances to two or more word strings of consistent structure (Brown, 1973). Developmental psycholinguists have differed over the years on their interpretations of the impetus for language—biological, environmental, or, of course, both. The data make clear by now that the quality of the environment has an important influence on the rate of sound production in early infancy and the rate of vocabulary acquisition in the second and third years.

"Motherese," or the simpler form of language typically used by mothers in talking to infants, in combination with facial expressions and gestures, likely teaches babies a great deal about the communication medium of the culture. Similarly contingent responsiveness appears to be an important factor in encouraging language production. Language acquisition also appears to be affected generally by the socioeconomic status of the family as well as cultural, racial, and ethnic factors. The reasons for these influences are not entirely known. It is clear however, that consistent and meaningful interaction with adults is necessary if the infant's language development is to be fostered (Horowitz, 1980).

It is perhaps obvious that language development and cognitive development are interdependent. Language fosters cognitive processes and cognition promotes speech. Each appears to depend heavily on the environment for impetus and direction. Individual differences in cognitive and language development are evident where there is somatic disorder; many deficits or differences may be associated with organic constraints that we have not yet learned to detect or even to look for.

4. Social, Personality, and Emotional Development.   Our knowledge of the normal course of social and emotional development lags far behind that of the areas previously discussed. Major interactive events—the social smile, the first laugh, "stranger anxiety"—are well known, and their relationship to the infant's cognitive, motor, and language competencies is not hard to discern.

There is little doubt that the emotional bonding between parents and child is a big factor in the socialization of children. Some have pinpointed bonding as occurring most readily immediately after birth, but evidence increasingly accumulates to show that the process of emotional attachment is gradual, occurring steadily over at least the first year of life (Leiderman, 1978).

Extensive studies have been carried out to describe infant distress on separation from the mother and the mixture of positive and negative emotions that often accompany reunion. Controversy continues among developmental psychologists over the interpretation of these events, although infant psychiatry leans heavily on the use of attachment disorders as symptomatic of trouble between mother and infant.

Recent studies on infants' recognition of emotional signals from adults and use of these signals in guiding their actions strongly suggest that the human infant is a more sophisticated interpersonal being than we had previously thought. Within the first few months of life, the emotional expressions of infants show that they are not merely imitating, but processing and responding to their mother's expressions. Furthermore within the first year infants whose mothers react with expressions of fear to a "visual cliff" situation refuse to cross the clear glass "cliff," whereas those whose mothers show happy expressions cross without apparent concern (Sorce, Emde, Campos & Klinnert, 1981).

The field of emotional development has only just begun to be tapped, and it is becoming clear that there is much to be learned about the children's development in this domain (Emde, 1980).

Preschool and Middle Childhood

Moving beyond infancy, we find that the patterns in our knowledge of development are much the same. Motor development has been described, and amounts generally to a smoothing out of skills rather than the acquisition of new skills. Some children are clearly more agile and graceful than others, and the reasons for these differences—whether they are due more to genetic factors or to practice and the importance of physical activity within the family and the culture—are not known.

Our understanding of cognitive development follows directly from Piaget's work. Preschool children are termed "preoperational" in that their thinking and problem solving strategies are largely intuitive and almost magical. The period of concrete operational thinking, beginning at about the time children enter school and lasting to adolescence, is characterized by the child's ability to think logically, understand the constancy of matter in the face of seeming transformations, and grasp more complex relationships among objects and events. The mechanisms by which children advance in cognitive development have not been thoroughly described. Language clearly facilitates cognitive development, and most preschool and early-school-age children actively use language in fostering their own development. Some have estimated that a typical 4-year-old asks upwards of 400 questions a day. While not all of the answers they receive convey information, still, the process of inquiry undoubtedly leads to growth in understanding (Flavell, 1977).

An appreciation for the level of cognitive development a child has achieved may be particularly helpful to parents and physicians who attempt to communicate effectively with children. The type of explanation offered for illness or treatment should be consistent with the child's ability to understand, and should neither underestimate nor overrate the child's capacities. Although little research has been done to describe the processes of successful parenting, it is likely that the ability to adjust communication level so that it is appropriate to the child as he or she grows older may be an important aspect in promoting harmonious relationships (Broen, 1972; Snow & Ferguson, 1977).

Whereas motor development seems to slow down in the preschool period, language development becomes particularly rapid. Normally developing children imitate just about all the sounds they hear, including those parents would rather not have repeated, and seem to delight in their newfound ability to converse. Many children talk so quickly that they cannot always be understood; most children lose the tendency toward nonfluent speech, but a few continue to stutter, sometimes severely. Language appears to be promoted by patient adults who listen to the child, respond appropriately, and encourage elaboration of language.

Social-emotional development during the early school years becomes more and more involved with peer relationships as the child develops a self-concept and a sex role identity. Parent concerns often arise from school problems or conflict over child compliance or sibling relationships. It is not always easy for the pediatrician to determine whether a particular parental concern is a true indicator of trouble, and it is often difficult to get any information from a preteenager; still, sometimes a few questions about the child's and family's wider experiences can suggest whether a concern requires attention or the parent should be reassured that the situation is normal.

Adolescence

This most troublesome time for parents has been perhaps least studied by developmental psychologists. The physical changes that occur at puberty are obviously reflected in emotional upheaval. For some adolescents these changes are extremely dramatic and difficult, whereas for others the transition into adulthood seems less intense and altogether less upsetting. The reasons for these individual differences are not known.

Along with the more obvious changes, children reaching adolescence also move into a new cognitive stage—that of "formal operations." At this point, the child gains the ability to handle abstractions, demonstrate logical flexibility, and mentally test alternative hypotheses. These developing abilities undoubtedly influence other aspects of the child's life. The newly acquired ability to play intellectual games, in the form of experimenting with ideas, may lead to parental conflict when parents fail to recognize the game and take the child's expressions as being in earnest, as of course the adolescent momentarily believes they are. It is common for parents to overreact to adolescent statements and actions, and confrontation is almost inevitably the result. Difficulties in communication contribute to the level of conflict. Parents who see the need for isolating disagreements to the particular event involved and not let them take over the relationship contribute to communication by not making every interaction contentious. Parents also need to work at seeing the adolescent's drive for independence as a necessary and important aspect of development and not as a threat.

According to the psychoanalytic literature, adolescence is particularly difficult for parents partly because the issues that arise are those that most adults have not fully resolved: sexuality, independence-dependence, identity. When these issues must be confronted with a child, the adult's own ambivalences also emerge, creating more of a conflict than the situation deserves. If given the opportunity, pediatricians can help parents see the need for balance and for avoiding continual confrontation, and can also exploit the adolescent's cognitive competencies by suggesting alternative views.

Although it seems obvious that biology plays a major role in the turmoil of adolescence, it is also clear that environmental influences are strong. Cultural expectations, peer influences, and imitation of admired adults all play a part in adolescent behavior. How these factors interact with biological events and constitutional predispositions to produce developmental change is simply not known. The increase in adolescent suicide and widespread drug abuse lend urgency to the study of development in this period.

AN INTERACTIONAL MODEL

Throughout our brief look at development, it has been clear that the theoretical orientation adopted involves consideration of both organismic characteristics and environmental experience as important in behavioral development. During the evolutionary history of the human organism, particular characteristics, propensities, and high-probability events have come to determine universal developmental phenomena which act as con-

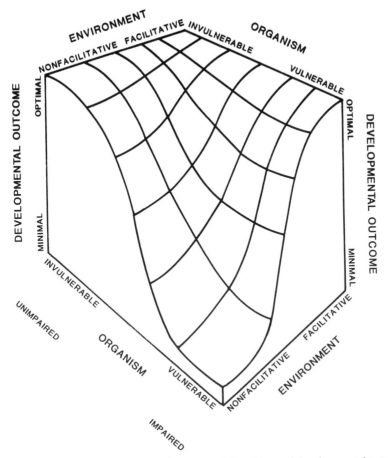

FIGURE 8.1.   Model of organism-environment relationships and developmental outcome.

straints to environmental influences. These constraints are likely lodged in the genetic code and are extremely powerful, particularly in early development. From the moment of conception, however, environmentally introduced elements must be considered as contributing some of the determinants of development (Horowitz, 1980, 1982).

An interactional model that may serve to guide the kind of research agenda needed to more fully understand developmental determinants is shown in Figure 8.1. In this model characteristics of the organism—whether impaired or unimpaired, vulnerable or invulnerable, or somewhere in between—interact with characteristics of the environment to produce a developmental outcome that lies on the continuum between minimal and optimal. According to this model environmental determinants play differing roles depending on the vulnerability of the organism. Furthermore at different stages of development and in different domains of development, a child may be more or less vulnerable, more or less impaired, and the overall outcome will be accordingly affected.

What does this model suggest in relation to child-health behavior? First of all, if it is accepted that certain aspects of behavioral development are determinants either of medical conditions or of the ability to pursue and respond to treatment, then it is clear that an understanding of behavioral development is necessary. According to an interactional model, this involves a knowledge of the nature of the organism plus a knowledge of the nature of the organism's interaction with the environment and the processes by which the interaction occurs. For this reason, as will be discussed below, it is important to foster good basic research aimed at illuminating the nature of behavior, at mapping individual differences, at describing functional environmental stimulation, and at trying to understand the interactive equation responsible for developmental outcome in normal and at-risk children.

An interactional model is essentially a common-sense model, though increasingly supported by the data base related to developmental outcome. We know that prediction of developmental outcome from a single event—such as prematurity or perinatal insult (unless inflicting mass physiological damage to the organism)—is not possible. Further, early to later correlations grow weaker the longer the intervening time span. Some behavioral scientists have taken the evidence of weak prediction from early to later periods of development as an indication of essential discontinuity in development and/or as suggesting preeminence of a genetic unfolding of preprogrammed development that is independent of environmental experience. Such pronouncement is premature and also ignores the proper focus of the scientific understanding of behavioral development.

A simple analogy will advance the argument being developed here. If one is interested in the etiology and treatment of cancer, it is generally assumed that we must understand the normal processes of cell division as well as the processes of abnormal cell division. The fact that a cell is normal at one point in time and cancerous at a later point in time is not taken as an indication that there is discontinuity, but rather that significant changes have occurred in the basic processes that control and inhibit cell division. It is agreed that the ultimate understanding and prevention of cancer will come as a result of a basic understanding of these processes. This analogy presents a model for scientific strategy in the study of cancer that is no less valid for the study of behavioral development, though it is likely that behavioral development is far more complex than cell division and inhibition.

The interactional model involves an appreciation of the fact that the developmental course of human behavior may be highly overdetermined in the sense that a variety of environmental circumstances provide equally effective stimulus conditions for development to occur. Thus environments that differ significantly may equally foster normal motor development. To make this observation is not equivalent to asserting that environmental stimulation is irrelevant to motor development. Rather given the variety of conditions under which normal motor development occurs, the best hypothesis is that each of the variations contains the necessary and sufficient conditions to foster normal motor development. The scientific challenge is to identify these necessary and sufficient conditions.

Yet defining the conditions that insure normal development may not fully explain the variation in developmental outcome. For example, we know that most children whose hearing is unimpaired will develop language. And we know that the necessary and sufficient conditions for language development involve some linguistic input from the environment. We also know, however, that there are enormous variations in the quality of language development in children. Some of these variations do correlate with gross environmental conditions. Middle and upper-middle class children are likely to have larger vocabularies and use language in a more sophisticated manner than children of lower class backgrounds. Additionally we know that some children from lower class backgrounds develop language abilities similar to middle and upper-middle class children. How much of this variation is due to differences in environmental stimulation and individual reinforcement histories, how much to individual differences in propensity to learn or not learn from environmental experience, and how much to genetic or biological constraints we do not now know. According to the model shown in Figure 8.1, a child highly vulnerable to the specific character of environmental stimulation may be disadvantaged by a given set of experiences that have little influence on the development of another child who is less vulnerable, and more developmentally "insured," as it were. Concretely in an environment where linguistic input is simple and minimal, one child may develop language abilities barely appropriate for his or her age whereas another child may develop language abilities above the norm. One child would be classified as "vulnerable" to environmental conditions; the second child as "invulnerable"—that is, not easily affected by adverse circumstances. For the vulnerable child a highly functional environmental experience is necessary for optimal development; for the invulnerable child functional environmental experience may be less important.

Complicating the picture is the probable fact that vulnerability is specific to a particular behavioral domain. For example, a child may require an enriched environment for optimal language development but not for optimal social or emotional development. Additionally relative vulnerability to environmental stimulation may change from one developmental period to another, leading to seeming discontinuities in development. The fact that a child does well in language development during the preschool period and poorly during the middle years of childhood may reflect a change in adequacy of environmental factors and/or an organismic shift in relative dependence upon environmental input. The shifts will be understandable when we understand the basic processes involved and can measure the relevant variables. When low correlations across two periods of time are found, the proper reaction is not to assert an inherent "discontinuity" in development but to attempt to formulate a theoretical blueprint of the basic processes involved and to proceed to investigate various hypotheses that can be derived from that blueprint (Horowitz, in press).

The model shown in Figure 8.1 is an attempt to draw the basic dimensions of a fruitful theoretical blueprint. It recognizes that the general course of behavioral development is likely highly overdetermined. This is not the same as claiming that behavioral development occurs independently of the necessary and sufficient conditions of environmental stimulation. Given the ethical and moral considerations in human experimentation, we would never countenance experiments to prove this position. However, Kuo (1967) did demonstrate that it was possible to reverse even seemingly instinctual behavior in dogs if the conditions were properly arranged. Thus while one takes as a given the highly probable developmental course—particularly in the area of sequences of development—that course is not without its determining processes and variables.

There is, from the point of view described here, a practical distinction to be made between behavioral development and behavioral management. Concomitantly, the implication, alluded to in examples given throughout this chapter, is that behavioral management is likely to be more successful if it takes into account facts of behavioral development than if those facts are ignored. An obvious example is available with respect to achieving verbal control over a child's behavior. That control is more likely to occur if the verbal stimulation involves a vocabulary the child understands and a grammatical construction compatible with the child's level of cognitive development. Similarly a training program is more likely to be successful if it utilizes a natural sequence of developmental progression than if it does not

The principles that determine the success of behavioral management may or may not be the same principles that underlie behavioral development. One of the overgeneralizations common to neophyte behavior modifiers is assuming that the principles demonstrated to achieve behavior modification are the same ones that are responsible for behavioral development in the natural environment. There may well be overlap but this is not a necessary conclusion from the exercise of successful behavior modification. Additionally the conditions necessary to the laboratory demonstration of behavioral control may not be those obtained in the natural environment. It has been suggested, for example, that conditioning phenomena in the natural environment may occur under a wider variation of circumstances than appear to be permissible in the laboratory environment (Horowitz, 1968).

PRIORITIES FOR A RESEARCH AGENDA

The field of behavioral pediatrics will be most well served by an increased understanding of basic developmental phenomena, of the processes that are responsible for behavioral development, and of the techniques that can be employed to intervene to avert or remediate poor development. Behavioral pediatrics will also be well served by more broadly educating physicians with respect to an understanding of behavioral development and of the role of properly timed intervention in ameliorating developmental problems. As has been indicated, it is likely that development follows an inexorable course in the normal child, with wide individual variations—some of which are trivial, others significant indicators of problems. Unfortunately there is a tendency to let the normal wide individual variability among children cloud the need for assessment and diagnosis of developmental delay and deficit. Parents are often the first to observe signs of abnormality and deviation but too often physicians pass off parental concerns about developmental problems by reassuring the parents, telling them that there is a wide range of individual differences in children. It would be useful for physicians to have enough knowledge of basic developmental phenomena and of brief screening assessments that can be done in the office to carry out an independent check, often casual and informal, of problems noted by parents. There is increasing evidence that early detection followed by some intervention program of early stimulation constitute an effective strategy for preventing developmental retardation—especially in high-risk children (Ramey & Campbell, 1977).

Though there has been a steady increase in our knowledge base in the area of behavioral development, especially with respect to infant behavior and development, much remains to be understood. Continued descriptive data of infant capabilities, of the range of individual differences and of the relevant variables in environmental stimulation during infancy and childhood are high priority for any programmatic research agenda. There is a danger that the very productive era of research on infants and of the increasingly obvious relative paucity of information concerning, for example, the adolescent period will encourage a deemphasis on infant development in order to emphasize research on adolescents. This would be unfortunate because the opportunities to study basic processes may be better with younger organisms and it is still meaningful to entertain the hypothesis that early experience lays a considerable part of the foundation for later development. Additionally with the increased survival rate among high-risk infants, focus upon comparative studies of normal and high-risk populations could be extremely informative.

The substantive research agenda for the infancy period and for other periods of development must contain a priority for understanding the functional elements of environmental stimulation. This is a particularly troubling area because we do not yet know the proper level of measurement necessary in order to understand basic processes. For example, is functional maternal stimulation best understood by a microanalytic level of measurement—of conditional probabilities and tracking interactions response by response? Or will the basic processes be just as easily illuminated by a more macroanalytical strategy involving gross ratings of maternal warmth or responsiveness? In the absence of clear indicators for strategy choices it is important that the research horizon contain a variety of research strategies.

Because individual differences are likely a major source of relevant variables controlling basic processes, systematic efforts to understand the important ranges of individual differences in children will be fruitful. Studies of temperament, emotionality, cognitive style, sensitivity to different kinds of stimulation, patterns of response acquisition, and modality differences and preferences ought to provide important information. These individual difference variables need to be studied at different periods of development and no *a priori* assumptions should be made that they are necessarily stable across time. The interaction of individual differences and environmental variables in a process of mutual "shaping" also needs attention.

Our understanding of emotional and social development during infancy and during the preschool, middle-school and adolescent years is minimal. We need to identify the most useful system of descriptors and to gather descriptive data. Additionally we need to understand how behavioral development in these domains affects and interacts with cognitive factors and to describe the functional environmental variables involved.

One of the major problems encountered in developing a meaningful agenda of research priorities is the fact that some problems will require following samples of children over time. Because of funding patterns of two- and three-year grants such systematic efforts are difficult to mount and maintain. Attention needs to be given to mechanisms whereby the programmatic research essential to advancing our knowledge base in a significant manner can be supported. Further, in the behavioral sciences there has been much less of a tendency to develop core research teams that work together over a period of years in laboratory or field setting groups. Encouragement of such a pattern of research is needed if systematic and programmatic efforts are to be undertaken. Again, funding patterns militate against such efforts. This has been particularly true in the area of infancy where core support necessary to an ongoing program of research is an absolute necessity. It has been suggested that consideration should be given to identifying a key group of senior investigators who have maintained ongoing programmatic research, often with great difficulty, who would be eligible for core support to keep a laboratory functioning, to keep trained technicians on staff and to keep the skeletal staff necessary to recruiting subjects, insuring quality control.

Special emphasis on the need for a better understanding of adolescent behavior and development is warranted given the major social problems encountered in our society during adolescence. It is interesting to note that our most solid base of knowledge concerning adolescence is in the area of physical development. During this period of development there is a culmination of physical developmental processes and socialization processes that often catapult the young person into public and semipublic settings involving significant pressures. We understand very little of how all the factors work to determine differential developmental and behavioral patterns. Additionally in a pluralistic society that is also socioeconomically heterogeneous the importance of variables related to racial, ethnic and social-class membership cannot be underestimated. There is also the likelihood that the larger variable of history—the social milieu of our time compared to that of other periods—must be considered as well (Elder, 1974). It is during adolescence that the self-destructive behaviors such as drug and alcohol abuse and sexual promiscuity that bedevil our society become most obvious. Adolescent suicide is the most dramatic of self-destructive behaviors and is a serious problem in the United States. It is not known to what extent precursors of these behavioral patterns are to be found in earlier periods of development, represent shifts along the continuum of vulnerability at the point of adolescence, or are influenced by powerful factors associated with contemporaneous neighborhood influences and social pressures.

There is a temptation to recommend research priorities closest to one's own theoretical and research-strategy approaches, not to mention one's own area of particular interest and expertise. Certainly one makes the most convincing case when one can discuss in some depth one's own area of speciality—be it neonatal assessment, infant habituation, or preschool cognitive development. However, every argument for good information is valid no matter the special topic identified, especially as our need to understand is so pervasive when it comes to behavioral development. In recognition of this we have chosen to conclude this chapter with a more generic plea: The greatest single need with respect to increasing our understanding of behavioral development is for stable programmatic research aimed at illuminating the basic processes that control behavioral development. Such a program is most likely, ultimately, to contribute to advancing the efficacy of the practice of behavioral pediatrics because understanding of basic processes will lead, eventually, to practical applications in prevention and treatment, and will permit more effective and useful research on successful techniques for prevention and treatment. While one may quibble over whether it is really necessary to understand the mechanisms of a phenomenon in order to prevent or treat its deviant expressions, it is clear that such understanding makes successful and enduring prevention and treatment much more likely.

REFERENCES

Brainerd, C. (1978). *Piaget's theory of intelligence.* Englewood Cliffs, NJ: Prentice-Hall.

Broen, P. A. (1972). The verbal environment of the language learning child. *American Speech & Hearing Association Monograph,* No. 17.

Brown, R. (1973). *A first language—The early stages.* Cambridge, MA: Harvard University Press.

Elder, G. H. (1974). *Children of the great depression.* Chicago: University of Chicago Press.

Emde, R. (1980). Emotional availability: A reciprocal reward system for infants and parents with implications for prevention of psychosocial disorders. In P. M. Taylor (Ed.), *Parent-infant relationships* (pp. 87–115). New York: Grune-Stratton.

Flavell, J. (1977). *Cognitive development.* Englewood Cliffs, NJ: Prentice-Hall.

Gelman, R., & Shatz, M. (1977). Appropriate speech adjustments; The operation of conversational constraints on talk to two-year-olds. In M. Lewis, & L. A. Rosenblum (Eds.), *Interaction, conversation, & the development of language* (pp. 27–61). New York: Wiley.

Horowitz, F. D. (1982). Child development for the pediatrician. *Pediatric Clinics of North America,* (April), *29,* 359–375.

Horowitz, F. D. (1968). Infant learning and development: Retrospect & prospect. *Merrill-Palmer Quarterly, 14,* 101–120.

Horowitz, F. D. (1980). Intervention and its effects on early development: What model of development is appropriate? In R. Turner, & H.W. Reese (Eds.), *Life span developmental psychology: Intervention* (pp. 235–248). New York: Academic.

Horowitz, F. D. (1978). Normal & abnormal child development. In K. E. Allen, V. A. Holm, & R. L. Schiefelbusch (Eds.), *Early intervention—A team approach* (pp. 3–25). Baltimore: University Park Press.

Horowitz, F. D. (in press). The psychobiology of parent-offspring relations in high-risk situations. In L. P. Lipsitt (Ed.), *Advances in infancy research.* New York: Ablex.

Horowitz, F. D. (1980). Receptive language in the first year of life. In J. Gallagher (Ed.), *New directions for exceptional children. Young exceptional children* (pp. 1–20). San Francisco: Jossey-Bass.

Horowitz, F. D., Linn, P. L., & Buddin, B. J. (in press). Neonatal assessment: evaluating the potential for plasticity. In T. B. Brazelton, & B. Lester (Eds.), *New approaches to developmental screening of infants.* New York: Elsevier Science.

Hunt, J. McV., Paraskevopoulos, J., Schickendanz, D., & Uzgiris, I. (1975). Variations in mean ages of achieving object permanence under diverse conditions of rearing. In B. Friedlander, G. Sterritt, & G. Kirk (Eds.), *Exceptional infant, Vol. 3.* (pp. 247–262). New York: Brunner/Mazel.

Kuo, Z. Y. (1967). *The dynamics of behavioral development.* New York: Random House.

Langer, J. (1980). *The origins of logic.* New York: Academic Press.

Leiderman, H. (1978). The critical period hypothesis revisited: Mother to infant social bonding in the neonatal period. In F. D. Horowitz (Ed.), *Early developmental hazards: Predictors & precautions.* Boulder, CO: Westview Press.

Linn, P. L., & Horowitz. F. D. (in press). The relationship between infant individual differences and mother-infant interaction during the neonatal period. *Infant Behavior & Development.*

Lipsitt, L. P. (1982). Infant learning. In T. M. Field, A. Huston, H. C. Quay, L. Troll, & G. E. Finley, (Eds.), *Review of human development* (pp. 62–78). New York: Wiley.

Lipsitt, L. P. (1977). The study of sensory & learning processes of the newborn. *Clinics in Perinatology,* Vol. 4, No. 1, March, 163–186.

Lipsitt, L. P., & Werner, J. (1981). The infancy of human learning processes. In E. Gollen (Ed.), *Developmental plasticity.* New York: Academic.

Ramey, C., & Campbell, F. (1977). Prevention of developmental retardation in high-risk children. In P. Mittler (Ed.), *Research to practice in mental retardation: Care & intervention. Vol. 1.* Baltimore: University Park Press.

Snow, C. E., & Ferguson, C. A. (1977). *Talking to children*. Cambridge: Cambridge University Press.

Sorce, J. F., Emde, R. N., Campos, J. J., & Klinnert, M. D. (1981). Maternal emotional signaling: Its effect on the visual cliff behavior of one-year-olds. Paper presented at the meeting of the Society of Research in Child Development, Boston, MA.

9

A Behavioral Systems Perspective in Childhood Psychopathology: Expanding the Three-Term Operant Contingency

ROBERT G. WAHLER AND DELLA M. HANN

Child development can basically be seen as a process of surviving and adapting to the increasing demands of the environment. As such the developing child is continuously interacting with and being influenced by those objects and agents which compose the environment. In this light child behavior can be viewed as a product of the physically developing child interacting with the surrounding environment. Of particular importance to this adaptational process are the behaviors and characteristics of the direct caregivers, parents. Parental behavior provides a main avenue through which socially acceptable ways of behaving can be introduced to and incorporated by the child. Thus the surrounding environment, which the parents partially provide, can have a major impact on the successful adaptation and development of the child.

Exactly how the environment comes to influence the development of the child has become a concern of much psychological inquiry and theory. One approach widely applied in the past two decades is known as the behavioral approach. This orientation focuses directly on the present behavior of the child and the events (stimuli) surrounding behavioral responding. Environmental stimuli are of concern in that these events are seen to determine and control the emission of behavior. Hence it is the interaction between the child and the environmental stimuli which leads to the acquisition and maintenance of behavior, that is, the learning of behavior. Within this framework the classification of behavior as normal or abnormal is a societal decision, for all forms of behavior are learned and under the control of one's surrounding environment.

As the above arguments would suggest, learning processes provide a conceptual framework for the behavioral explanation and treatment of childhood disorders. Within the traditional behavioral model, three major learning paradigms have been utilized: (1) classical conditioning, (2) operant conditioning, and (3) observational learning. Although all three learning paradigms are of applicational value in the behavioral framework, the present chapter is concerned primarily with the operant conditioning paradigm. As such only this model will be more fully presented[1].

Operant conditioning centers on observable responses which are emitted by an individual, yet are capable of being influenced by the environmental events which follow. Any behavior which operates on the environment primarily by generating consequences is called an operant response (Skinner, 1953). With this definition the conditioning of behavior involves the manipulation of events that directly follow behavior. Those consequent events that increase the probability of subsequent similar behavior are said to reinforce behavior. With operant conditioning, learning then involves changes in response frequency and/or intensity via the alteration of consequent environmental events. Thus the process of learning and the performance of behavior are determined and controlled by environmental events which directly follow behavior.

Although consequent events are of primary concern in the operant paradigm, the effect of antecedent events is not neglected. Situations which reliably precede reinforced episodes may come to act as cues or signals for reinforcement. In this sense antecedent events serve as discriminative stimuli which "set the stage" for the occurrence of previously reinforced behaviors; discriminative stimuli tend to increase the likelihood of responding without demanding (eliciting) the behavior (Kazdin, 1980).

With the inclusion of the discriminative stimulus, the operant paradigm provides a three-component framework from which to approach and describe behavior: Antecedent-Response-Consequence. Since behavior is un-

---

[1]For extended coverage of classical conditioning and observational learning, see Agras, 1978; Craighead, Kazdin, and Mahoney, 1981; Kazdin, 1980.

der the direct control of the environmental events which precede and follow responding, describing and changing existing behaviors becomes a task of identifying the environmental events which surround the response.

Such a conceptual base forms the orientation of behavioral assessment and treatment. Assessment of behavioral pathology is concerned with two key elements: (1) the present problem behavior, and (2) the surrounding environment of the behavior. Keeping in reference developmental norms and trends, the presenting problem-behavior (target behavior) is examined as to the extent of the problem and degree of change desired. In conjunction with this evaluation of the target behavior, the environment in which the behavior occurs is also assessed. The examination of the environment focuses primarily on those events that immediately precede and follow the occurrence of the target behavior. The behavioral therapist gains information as to what events may be serving to elicit and/or reinforce the target response—that is, what is controlling the inappropriate behavior. Although a variety of techniques are available for the assessment of target behavior and environmental conditions (Mash & Terdal, 1982), traditional behavioral assessment has primarily employed various forms of naturalistic observation. By using this mode for assessment, one can obtain a fairly clear description of the natural events which precede and follow the target behavior.

Having described the target reponse and identified the immediate environmental events, strategies for behavioral intervention may be devised and implemented. The major theme of behavioral treatment is that changes in the environment will lead to changes in behavior. Thus treatment involves the manipulation of those antecedent and consequent events which immediately surround the target behavior. Since the focus of behavioral interventions is on the events which surround behavior, treatment is typically conducted in the setting natural to the behavior. To aid the process of in-the-field treatment, the cooperation of natural agents (for example, parents) may be enlisted. By having natural contact with the child, these individuals also have the greatest opportunity to regulate and monitor antecedent and consequent events. Inclusion of natural agents may be particularly important in cases where their own behavior may be contributing to and/or supporting the target behaviors; behaviors of the natural agents may be serving as disciminative stimuli and/or reinforcement for the problem behavior (Patterson & Reid, 1970; Wahler, 1976).

Overall the behavioral approach to the assessment and treatment of psychopathology focuses on natural environmental events and circumstances which immediately surround present problem behavior. The behaviors of natural agents in the environment may be most important in that they serve to cue, reinforce, and thereby control the occurrence of problem behavior. Thus by altering these aspects of the environment, one will alter the target behavior. In essence then the traditional behavioral model understands current behavior from a dyadic exchange viewpoint. Naturally occurring events (a parental refusal) may serve as discriminative stimuli for a problem behavior (a temper tantrum). The emitted response then acts on the environment by producing a consequence (parental yielding) which then affects the probability of subsequent similar responding. Hence dyadic interchanges between antecedent-response and response-consequent comprise the conceptual roots of the traditional behavioral approach.

The treatment and explanation of psychopathology from this orientation has been quite extensive. In the case of child psychopathology behavioral strategies which focus on the alteration of antecedent-response and/or response-consequent dyads have been applied successfully in the treatment of social skills deficits (Bonney, 1971), asthma (Miklich, 1973), obesity (Lansky & Brownell, 1982), and a host of other childhood disorders. In addition to treatment, this behavioral orientation has been helpful in explaining the intricacies of childhood behavior pathology. In working with families of children with conduct disorders, Patterson (1976, 1979) has utilized this behavioral framework in describing the occurrence of child oppositional behavior. Accordingly children displaying oppositional behavior typically do not heed parental requests and commands. Instead a scenerio such as the following often occurs. A mother asks her child to pick up toys. The child makes no attempt to comply and continues to watch T.V. The child's noncompliance is then followed by a more forceful command from the mother. Again the child does not comply. This mother-child interaction continues with increasing anger and frustration on the mother's part and increasing stubborness on the child's part until one of the members (usually the mother) stops the interaction by exiting the situation.

Behavioral interpretation of this scenario first focuses on the role of the mother. The first maternal request can be viewed as a discriminative stimulus which sets the stage for the target response of noncompliance. In turn, child noncompliance serves as a consequence for the mother's initial request and also as a disciminative stimulus for the mother's next command. The next command serves as a consequence for the child's opposition and functions also as a discriminative stimulus for further noncompliance. Such reciprocal dyadic interchanges continue in a serial fashion until the terminating escape-behavior occurs. The escape behavior not only acts to reinforce the prior responses (due to the cessation of an aversive interchange), but also increases the probability of subsequent similar dyadic episodes.

Overall this behavioral interpretation of a coercive interchange stresses that the behavior of a parent may be extremely important in the initiation and continuance of child problem-behavior. As such familial behavior has become a focal point in the clinical treatment of children. Behavioral methods which maintain this family focus by changing parental behavior in the direction of reinforcing desirable child behavior while ignoring or punishing undesirable behavior are collectively known as parent-training (O'Dell, 1974). By training parents to alter the stimulus consequences for their children's behavior, Herbert et al. (1976), Wahler (1969a), and Zeilberger, Sampen, and Sloane (1968) have shown that such changes may serve to control and reduce episodes of undesirable child behavior.

In the dyadic scheme just presented operant influences represent a bi-directional process. Parents and siblings set stimulus contingencies that govern the troubled child's behavior, and the child, in turn, exerts a recip-rocal influence on these family members. Accordingly the behavior of each family member becomes understandable as a direct function of dyadic ex-changes with other people in that natural group. In following this logic, the previously discussed parent training method makes good sense as an inter-vention strategy. The parent presents reinforcers and discriminative stim-uli for child problem behavior *because* the child reinforces the parent for this unfortunate caretaking style. Therefore if a clinical mediator can then teach the parent to alter the presentation of these stimuli, two processes ought to be set in motion: (1) the child's behavior will change in accordance with the new stimulus contingencies, and (2) the modified patterns of child behav-ior will serve to reinforce the parent's new caretaking style. In effect the therapeutically planned dyad becomes a self-perpetuating unit within the family. Since parents usually constitute a significant segment of the young child's environment, these therapeutic contingency changes could be ex-pected to yield important lifestyle shifts for the troubled youngster. To the extent that other dyads involving this child (for example, teacher-child; peer-child) can likewise be studied and, if necessary, subjected to contin-gency management, lifestyle shifts of even greater generality should be possible.

GENERALIZATION PROBLEMS WITH THE OPERANT MODEL

While the notion of a self perpetuating dyad is a useful guideline in the understanding and treatment of troubled children, proponents of the oper-ant model have long recognized that each dyad operates in a multitude of different environmental contexts (Bijou and Baer, 1961). This being the case, the issue of stimulus control for each member of the dyad is actually broader than we have portrayed it. A mother's response to her crying child might entail pleading with the child in a grocery store and shouting at the child in the privacy of her home. Presumably these situational differences in stimulus control are due to the fact that the social context also provides antecedents and consequents for the mother's child-care responses. This situational complexity would then mean that the study of a parent-child dyad, in order to reflect a complete picture of stimulus control, would have to entail a representative sampling of environmental contexts in which that dyad is embedded. A similar sampling process would be required to pro-duce generalized changes in the parent-child dyad. In line with the gen-eralization strategy outlined by Stokes and Baer (1977), the contingency shifts within a dyad must be accomplished in multiple environmental contexts—to the point that stimulus context becomes irrelevant to the dyadic contingencies.

The situational view of interpersonal behavior has a lengthy and controversial history in the child development field (Bowers, 1974). Early empirical work on the view tended to emphasize self-report and global judgement measures of behavior, and the findings suggested that child interpersonal behavior is consistent across situations (Alport, 1966; Mann, 1959). However when direct observational strategies came into popular use, findings on interpersonal consistencies were the exception rather than the rule (Mischel, 1968). Given molecular measures of child interpersonal behavior, these behaviors seem closely tied to the stimulus context in which the observations are made (Gewirtz, 1956; Sears, 1963; Wahler, 1969b), thus supporting an operant model of behavior influence.

In recent years the situational conception of child behavior has again been questioned, this time through refinements in direct observational procedure. Two avenues of procedural inquiry have been pursued: (1) consideration of the response unit as a *class* of covarying molecular measures instead of the molecular measures in isolation; for example, instead of studying the stimulus control of a child's hitting, yelling, and noncompliance as separate responses, one could study the measures as a single response unit by tracking their intercorrelations, and (2) instead of choosing stimulus contexts (situations) arbitrarily, one might search for functionally similar situations. Once again the procedural shift would entail a unit expansion, in this case the analysis of stimulus *class* rather than a focus on individual stimulus situations. Results of these new inquiries, while limited to a handful of studies, provide an intriguing new look at the situational quality of child behavior.

Harris and Reid (1981) examined the aggressive responses of normal children in two situations, a school classroom and a school playground. Aggressive behavior was analyzed as a class of eight molecular responses in which a rank order correlation coefficient expressed the classroom-playground consistency of each child's output of the responses. Of the 53 boys studied, 37 displayed statistically significant correlations between their classroom and playground responses, thus reflecting a cross-situational constistency in these latter children's rank order use of the various aggressive behaviors. In a group study of the same phenomenon, Harris (1979) discovered that a sample of 10 normal boys produced rates of aggressive responses that yielded a significant rank order across children in the two settings. Surprisingly a second sample of 10 boys designated by teachers as moderate problem-aggressors, displayed no rank order consistency between classroom and playground. But then on an individual level (Harris, 1979) found that one extremely aggressive youngster was highly consistent in his across-setting output of the eight coercive responses. Similarly Patterson and Maerov (1976) found high response class correlations (.90s) in the home-school deviant behaviors of two clinic-referred boys. All in all then these response class studies of child behavior demonstrate a remarkable across-situational consistency in social interchanges. The conceptual problem posed by these findings is of no small magnitude: if child behavior is primarily a function of its *short term* environmental contingencies, how do we account for one child's similar interpersonal style in different environments?

Studies exploring functional connections between environmental situations lend further documentation to the permeability of environmental boundaries. Fowler and Baer (1981) observed seven preschool children in two free-play periods separated by intervals of 15 to 45 minutes. Observers recorded the children's sharing behaviors as well as social attention from peers and teachers. After a baseline phase, the children were told they would receive points for sharing. During this reinforcement phase, the children were given feedback immediately after the first (early) play period. If a child met criteria of increased sharing in this early period, a point reward was assigned. Sharing increments in the late period were never followed by points. Observational records then showed exactly what one would expect: The children increased their rate of sharing in the early period but remained at baseline sharing rates in the late period. Next, the feedback reinforcement session was delayed until the end of each school day, but still based only on sharing increments in the early period. Following this simple operation, the children now increased their sharing in the late period. The authors' further analyses of late period associations between sharing and points plus social attention were crucial to the explanation of increased sharing in this later free-play period. That is could increases in the late period sharing be due to changes in teacher and/or peer social attention contingencies? Or equally possible, could the increased sharing be caused by a systematic association between late period sharing and the points? Results showed answers to both questions to be negative: late period sharing was no more likely to be followed by social attention; associations between sharing in the late period and points were purely random. Why then did sharing increase during the late period when the feedback and reinforcement sessions were delayed to day's end? At the beginning of each school day, the children were reminded that increased sharing would lead to points. Thus when point deliveries were delayed to day's end it appears that these morning instructions now set the occasion for late period sharing, even though the point consequences for this behavior were noncontingent.

Fowler and Baer (1981) demonstrated that morning instructions along with delayed point deliveries could serve an across-situation "bridge" function for preschool children's sharing. Moreover the behavioral control power of this "bridge" was *not* due to its discriminative function. During the late period, the children behaved as if the morning instructions were discriminative for reinforcement. In fact no such contingencies existed in the late period. Another example of this "as if" discriminative function is provided by Simon, Ayllon, and Milan (in press). In this study the math performance of seven middle-school children was observed in three class-room settings, each manned by a different teacher. Rate of correct math responses was computed each day by dividing the number of problems correctly completed by number of minutes taken to complete the work. In a baseline phase, only teacher attention followed correct responses. Then a token reinforcement phase was initiated in which one token could be earned for each correct response in all three settings. Results, as expected, showed clear rate increases in each of the three settings. Next, baseline conditions were reinstated in two of the settings while token reinforcement continued in the third setting. Following this step correct response rate dropped predictably in the first two settings, but almost doubled in the third setting. Finally, a return to token reinforcement in all settings was followed by a reduced rate in the third setting and higher rates in the first two settings.

The authors interpreted their results as similar to those "behavioral contrast" phenomena already well documented in the animal literature (Reynolds, 1961). That is animals have been shown to alter their response rates on unchanged reinforcement schedules when the availability of reinforcement is manipulated in other settings frequented by the animals. Thus when the children in Simon et al. (in press) were subjected to extinction conditions in two of the settings, they behaved in the third setting (their response rates doubled) as if the reinforcement schedule had changed. In terms of stimulus control, it is apparent that the extinction operations served an across situation function similar to that shown in Fowler and Baer (1981).

The perplexing demonstrations of stimulus control described above were also reported in a correlational study by Wahler (1980). In this case the aggressive child care behaviors of troubled mothers were shown to covary with events outside the home setting. On days outside the home in which the mothers reported a high proportion of coercive exchanges between themselves and kinfolk or helping agency representatives, objective observers were likely to see higher rates of mother-child punitive exchanges later in the day at home. In other words the adult-mother arguments appeared to serve an across situation influence on the mothers' tendencies to be aversive with their children. As in Fowler and Baer (1981) and Simon et al. (in press) it is difficult to conceptualize these influences as discriminative stimuli.

SETTING EVENTS IN OPERANT STIMULUS CONTROL

The studies of Simon et al. (in press), Fowler and Baer (1981), and Wahler (1980) suggest a behavioral influence which is not subsumed under the concept of discriminative stimulus control. Rather than a discrete and temporally proximate condition serving to set the stage for reinforced behavior, an environmentally complex and temporally distant phenomenon appears to be affecting observed behavioral patterns. Consequently these "setting factors" require closer examination so that the impact of the environment on behavior may be more fully understood.

Although relatively new to the applied field of clinical psychology, the setting event concept has existed for several decades in the "interbehavioral psychology" proposed by J.R. Kantor. In his writings, setting factors referred to those circumstances which influence the occurrence of various stimulus-response relationships already built up through past organism-environment interactions (Kantor, 1959). More specifically setting factors were conceived as complex behavioral-environmental conditions (for example, food or sleep deprivation) which temporally preceded or overlapped with the occurrence of behavior and affected this occurrence in either a complementary or inhibitory manner. Thus setting factors can be differentiated from the previously described discriminative stimuli along three major dimensions: (1) the complexity of the behavioral-environmental event, (2) the temporal proximity of the event to the occurrence of behavior, and (3) the effect of the event on behavioral performance.

Having defined and described setting factors, an example of this form of environmental control may be taken from the basic operant conditioning literature conducted with laboratory animals. Powell (1973) used operant conditioning in the training of pigeons to respond discriminatively to several stimuli. Following this discrimination learning, several hours of food deprivation were included in the design. Results of this investigation indicated that when food deprivation was introduced, the accuracy of discriminative responding decreased. Basically then a condition which had little direct reference to the discriminative stimulus-response-consequence triad influenced performance by inhibiting the accuracy of responding; food deprivation functioned as a setting factor for later discriminative behavior.

The Powell study provides a working example of the original Kantorian concept of setting factors. However, complex conditions such as food deprivation need not be the only type of events which function in this manner. In a writing concerned with the child's developing psychological environment, Bijou and Baer (1961) expanded the setting factor by referring to this phenomenon as ". . . a stimulus-response interaction, which simply because it has occurred will affect other stimulus-response relationships which follow it" (p. 21). The inclusion of stimulus-response relationships then allows reference to a more elaborate conception of the setting event, that is, complex environmental conditions and/or behavioral interactions which precede or overlap with the occurrence of behavior, yet influence this later behavioral performance.

With this definition of setting events, the at first puzzling across-situation influences noted by Wahler (1980) may be more logically explained. Recalling his comments, days which were marked with higher than average mother-child coercive interchanges were directly correlated with negatively valenced adult-mother interactions. These adult-mother episodes could occur hours prior to the mother-child exchanges, therefore being too temporally removed, environmentally complex, and nonreinforcement linked to be classified as discriminative stimuli. However, with use of the setting event concept, these preceding adult-mother interactions may be viewed basically as complex stimulus-response events. Because this type of event occurred, the later interchanges of the mother-child dyad were affected. Thus the across-situation influence of aversive adult-mother interactions on coercive mother-child behavior may be described via the setting event concept.

Overall the studies of Powell (1973) and Wahler (1980) have served to demonstrate that temporally distant events, which do not function as discriminative stimuli, may still exert a form of environmental control over proximal behavior. The setting event, however, does not appear to fit conceptually within the well-known operant boundaries. Hence the question of incorporating setting events into the operant paradigm has become one of theoretical importance.

Skinnerian Behaviorism Revisited

The original formulations of operant theory were presented by B.F. Skinner. In his first major writing Skinner (1938) outlined the fundamental assumptions, objectives, and goals which constituted the then "new" psychology. One such fundamental was the assumption that behavior is lawful—it can be predicted and controlled by identifying and manipulating those events of which behavior is a function. Behavior then is systematically related to, a function of, or "caused" by the external variables which surround its occurrence. "The external variables of which behavior is a function provide for what may be called a causal or functional analysis. We undertake to predict and control the behavior of the individual organism. This is our 'dependent variable'—the effect for which we aim to find the cause. Our 'independent variables'—the causes of behavior—are the external conditions of which behavior is a function. Relations between the two—the 'cause-and-effect relationships' in behavior—are the laws of science" (Skinner, 1953, p. 35).

In alliance with this position, the primary aim of Skinnerian behaviorism lies in the identification and description of systematic behavioral-environmental covariations. As noted this goal states nothing about the complexity or temporal span of events involved in the functional relationship. One may then surmise that the measurement unit used to reflect the behavioral-environmental relationship is not an issue of much concern. Instead of striving to remain on molecular levels, one should deal conceptually with these covariations on levels which will further elucidate their systematic nature. Thus, discrete as well as complex behavioral-environmental events can constitute the functional relationships with which operant theory is concerned.

In light of this Skinnerian behaviorism, the concept of setting events has always been included but not specifically named as part and parcel of a behavioral psychology. Setting events refer to complex behavioral-environmental interactions which can occur separate in time from other behavioral-environmental interactions, yet still influence these latter interactions. Basically the setting event describes a systematic relationship between two temporally separate behavioral events. The complexity and temporal span between the two events is not an issue, since the concern of this behaviorism rests solely in the *reliable covariation* of the two interactions.

SETTING EVENT INFLUENCES IN CHILDHOOD PSYCHOPATHOLOGY: A BEHAVIORAL SYSTEMS VIEWPOINT

If the setting event is considered an integral part of operant processes, the previously reviewed generalization phenomena become understandable. In addition a number of developmental findings on childhood problem behaviors can be viewed usefully from this expanded stimulus control model. As we now intend to argue, the expanded model not only makes reasonable sense out of perplexing generalization phenomena; a treatment or intervention plan for troubled children can also be derived by viewing childhood psychopathology from this perspective. Both contributions to the understanding and treatment of childhood problems center on the expanded model's conceptualization of *indirect* as well as *direct* stimulus influences on human behavior. As we outline the impact of these influences, our illustrations will focus on one very prevalent childhood disorder— conduct problems. Although other forms of childhood psychopathology seem equally understandable from this viewpoint, the bulk of research has been aimed at troubled children who "conduct" themselves in a manner best described as oppositional and/or aggressive.

As stated in the previous section the setting event addition to operant processes means that our basic unit in the analysis of interpersonal behavior becomes triadic instead of dyadic. Thus instead of an exclusive look at mother-child interchanges (the direct stimulus influences), we would also want to examine, for example, father-mother and father-child interchanges. The latter two sets of interchanges, while they too represent direct stimulus influences, will contribute indirectly to the mother-child exchanges. In other words we can account for more variance in any dyadic interaction if we know about each member's contact patterns with other people.

Figure 9.1 represents our schematic analysis of a social system based on the triad as a fundamental unit of system function. According to the

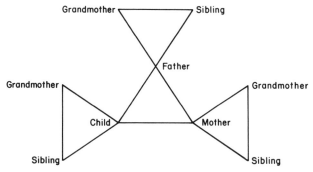

FIGURE 9.1.   A behavioral systems scheme depicting the operating characteristics of family. The five members in this group are shown interacting in a pattern of triangles representing direct and indirect social influences. For example, consider the child-mother dyad shown in the center of Figure 9.1: while these individuals respond directly to one another, each person's response will be indirectly determined by three other people.

scheme a community of people should be studied as a pattern of social triangles. Each member of this sytem will react directly to the behavior of other members, but the nature of each direct reaction will be determined, partially, by other exchanges making up the behavioral context of the system. For purposes of communication clarity we will now refer to the Figure 9.1 scheme as a *behavioral systems* viewpoint.

When children are classified as emotionally troubled because of oppositional and/or aggressive behavior, direct observations are apt to portray their dyadic interactions as "coercive" (after Patterson, 1976). When these children are compared to nontroubled children, the former are shown to make more use of aversive social behaviors such as nagging, noncompliance, crying and hitting. In turn the coercive child is more likely to receive aversive input from other people. Thus, the typical dyadic pattern presented by these problem children is one of matching aversive interchanges (Patterson, 1976). Presumably aversive stimuli are the relevant discriminative and reinforcing events in the maintenance of child conduct problems—at least at the dyadic level of our behavioral system. The more complete triadic picture of maintenance will again implicate the function of aversive social stimuli, but this time a setting event interpretation will prove useful. Since there are longitudinal data on the development of conduct problems in children, the triadic maintenance picture can best be painted by starting with a look at coercion processes during infancy.

Mother-infant relationships have been studied extensively by observers interested in the phenomenon of social attachment (Ainsworth, 1979). These investigators have suggested a bipolar relationship category called "secure-insecure" which appears to have a bearing on the formation of coercive infant behavior. Insecurely attached infants are marked by a high likelihood of aversive response to their mothers, in the form of crying and noncompliance with maternal prompts (Stayton, Hogan, & Ainsworth, 1971). However, contrary to what is known about coercive dyads involving older children, the mothers of insecurely attached infants typically do not provide matching aversive responses for their "difficult" babies. Instead this maternal caretaking style is best described as insensitive or noncontingent; the mothers' response to infant behavior appears determined less by what the infants do and more by the mothers' prevailing moods. Interestingly enough the longitudinal analyses by Bell and Ainsworth (1972) indicate that maternal insensitivity in the first three months of infant life predicts the infant's *later* development (next three months) of aversive behavior. As this developmental lag in the infant's behavior suggests, the mother's noncontingent caretaking style is predictive of her infant's crying and noncompliance rather than the other way around. If this interpretation is correct, one might argue some sort of causal connection between noncontingent caretaking and the emergence of infant coercive behavior. Perhaps as we will argue in a later section of this chapter, an unpredictable stimulus context has an aversive function; if the infant discovers that crying will generate a temporary state of contingent or predictable maternal response, then crying has, by definition, been negatively reinforced.

In our present quest for understanding triadic influences in mother-child coercive relationships, the issue at hand centers on *why* a mother would initiate her caretaking role with a noncontingent interpersonal style. Once again the social attachment researchers have provided some intriguing answers. Crockenberg (1981) observed a sample of 48 nonproblem mother-infant dyads when the infants were 3 months of age. Mothers were then classified as responsive or nonresponsive based on the latency of their attending to infant distress. Then when the infants reached 12 months of age, the mother-infant dyads were again observed for purposes of classifying the infants as securely or insecurely attached. Finally, the triadic picture of this caretaking system was completed through use of two additional measures: (1) The quality of maternal social contact with adults ("social support") was assessed by interview with mothers when the infants were at the 3 month age period; (2) Infant temperament (high or low irritability) was assessed at the fifth and tenth days following birth. Results showed the expected correlation between maternal insensitivity at 3 months and infant insecure attachment at 12 months, but the *indirect* influences of maternal social support and infant temperament also contributed significant variance to this dyadic relationship. The most difficult year-old infants were those who were classified as highly irritable at birth and whose mothers reported low social support. In addition the mothers of such babies were quite likely to be unresponsive caretakers in the early months. Thus although a mother's insensitive or noncontingent caretaking appears to be a direct influence on infant coercive behavior, these mother-infant transactions appear indirectly determined by infant temperament and quality of the mother's adult social relationships. The role of both factors as indirect contributors to maternal insensitivity was supported in several prior studies of infant attachment (Waters, Vaughn & Egeland, 1980; Vaughn, Egeland, Sroufe & Waters, 1979).

The above described developmental patterns suggest that a continuation of insensitive maternal care might ultimately lead to mother-child "coercive entrapment." In other words the noncontingent, insensitive mother could be expected eventually to respond in kind to her child's coercive behavior and, thus, the repetitive, spiraling aversive exchanges commonly observed in childhood conduct disorders would be established. While this developmental linkage between insecure attachment and later conduct problems has yet to be documented, there are indications of the linkage. Several studies suggest that abusive mother-child episodes are associated with infancy attachment problems as well as childhood conduct problems. Egeland and Sroufe (1981) compared two samples of mother-infant dyads in which the mothers were known to either mistreat their babies or to provide excellent care. When the infants were 12 months of age, only 25 percent of babies in the excellent care group were classed as insecurely attached, but 62 percent of the maltreatment group were so classified. George and Main (1979) continued the developmental linkage hypothesis in their finding that abused toddlers (1 to 3 years of age) were much more likely to assault or threaten their caregivers than were children in a control sample. Likewise, Wolfe and Mosk (1983) found that parent-report measures on child behavior problems showed these to be more severe in an abuse sample than in a nonproblem sample.

From our behavioral systems viewpoint, the most interesting facet of the attachment-abuse-conduct linkage concerns the commonality of mother insensitivity. This maternal characteristic is not only a prevailing part of insecure infant attachments; mothers who abuse their children and who rear conduct-problem children also demonstrate this indiscriminate mode of response to their youngsters (Crittenden, 1981; Patterson, 1976). While mothers of the latter children are also likely to consequate child aversive response (for example, hit) with their own aversive action (for example, slap), these parents will often respond aversively to their children's prosocial behaviors as well. In this respect it is interesting to review the Dumas and Wahler (in press) group comparison of moderate and severely disturbed families with conduct problem children. Degree of disturbance was defined by the number of social and socioeconomic stressors reported by the mothers in each family. Home observations revealed mother-child dyads in the severely disturbed families exchanged significantly more aversives than did those in the moderately disturbed families. In addition the former mothers were found to dispense their aversives (for example, yelling and screaming) more indiscriminately following their children's aversive and prosocial behavior.

Consistent with the functioning of a behavioral system, maternal insensitivity appears to be a keystone index of indirect stimulus influences in the previously reviewed studies of insecure infant attachment (Crockenberg, 1981). That is this mode of maternal caretaking response was associated with the setting factors of mother social support and infant temperament. As one might suspect the covariation between such setting events and maternal insensitivity continues to be evident in families marked by abuse and conduct problems. Thus in the earlier cited study by Egeland and Sroufe (1981), the troubled relationships between abusive mothers and their infants (observed when the infants were 12 months of age) had a striking association with environmental stressors in the mothers' day-to-day lives. Six months after these mother-infant dyads were observed to be insecurely attached, many of the mothers happened to experience improvements in the quality of their family environments. When observers then repeated assessments of the dyads (at 18 months of infant age), the mother-infant attachments were now classified as secure. Evidently stressful environmental context may have served an indirect stimulus function with respect to the mothers' infant care routines. A more specific source of indirect stimulus control was suggested in the Reid, Taplin and Loeber (1981) comparison study of abusive and normal families. In this case, mother-father aversive exchanges were observed to occur at higher rates in families referred for child abuse. To complete the setting event picture along this hypothesized attachment-abuse-conduct linkage, Wahler (1980) presented correlational evidence of indirect stimulus influences on the mother-child interchanges of conduct problem children. On a day to day basis, maternal reports of adult friendship contacts in the community bore inverse associations with the mothers' aversive response to their problem children. Observers found the mother-child relationships to be significantly less coercive on days in which the mothers reported high proportions of friendship contacts earlier in the day.

A summary of suspected developmental progressions in coercive child interactions would highlight the formation of a pathology-inducing triangle. If a mother rears her infant within an environment marked by aversive exchanges, her caretaking style is apt to reach a quality described as insensitive, indiscriminate or noncontingent. Given this style, the infant is likely to respond to the mother in a coercive manner described as insecure attachment. Once this sort of dyadic relationship has formed, an escalation in coercive response can be expected for both members of the dyad. Such escalation might then increase the chances of maternal abuse of the child and/or the child's formation of conduct problems. However each step of the hypothesized progression appears to depend on the complete social triangle. Should the mother's aversive environmental context lose its stressful function, she is likely to become more sensitive and less aversive in her manner of child care. The child, in turn, would be expected to become less coercive and more prosocial. While the treatment or prevention-intervention implications of this developmental model are compelling, our focus in this chapter is on further comprehension of this developmental process.

Thus the following and final section offers an explanatory look at how the pathology-inducing triangle might be formed.

RESPONSE GENERATED PREDICTABILITY: A SUSPECTED PRINCIPLE OF SETTING EVENT STIMULUS CONTROL

Thus far in our discussion of deviance supporting social systems, we have primarily offered descriptions of system operations. On the side of *explanation* we alluded to reinforcement principles as a useful means of accounting for the dyadic parts of a social system. However, when triadic exchanges became our focal point of discussion, we remained at a purely descriptive level in outlining the Kantorian setting event as a needed addition to the operant view of system functions. For example, we presented evidence to show that a troubled mother's indiscriminate and aversive response to her difficult child is influenced by stressful encounters in other spheres of her environment. While the encounters fit a setting event definition, the definition says nothing about *why* these contextual stimuli should affect the mother's child care routine. Certainly, the triadic process will make intuitive sense to the lay public (You're apt to kick the dog if you're in a bad mood). Likewise researchers and theorists who postulate structures or forces within the organism are likely to achieve explanatory closure (for example, adult-adult conflict affects one's "perception" of what is later said and done; a child's smile might be "perceived" as sarcastic provocation following the adult conflict). From a behavioral viewpoint, explanation must entail observable processes, and it is this criterion that makes indirect stimulus control so difficult to comprehend for the behaviorist. However, since the behavioral viewpoint of system functioning has proven valuable thus far, we see little reason to deviate from its strategic aims. Therefore our following efforts to comprehend setting events will stay within the behavioral framework, but we must warn the reader not to expect a complete conceptual picture.

Like much of the progress in behavioral psychology, explanatory notions of indirect stimulus control started within the confines of laboratory experimentation. The animal studies by Herrnstein (1966) and Reynolds (1961) indicated that one can create unusual forms of stimulus control by manipulating the organism's history of reinforcement. As Herrnstein demonstrated, it is possible to produce an analogue of the previously described maladaptive mothering phenomenon through gradually fading an animal's reinforcement schedule from intermittent to random presentations; pigeons, for example, will eventually display "superstitious" responding to stimuli after the cues have long ceased to serve a discriminative function for reinforcement. D'Amato (1974) and, more recently, Imada and Najeishi (1982) argued that these reinforcement schedule outcomes could be expected via an "uncertainty" principle of reinforcement. In essence, the principle states that the reinforcement function of a stimulus lies in its relationship with the surrounding stimulus setting. The aversive or positive quality of the stimulus event is immaterial to its potential reinforcement function; it is the *relational* quality of that stimulus vis-a-vis the stimulus context that determines its reinforcement value. Thus the common operant notion of cataloging stimuli in terms of their demonstrable aversive, positive and neutral functions would not be applicable to the uncertainty principle. If the stimulus context becomes uncertain or noncontingent, that context will serve an aversive function for the organism. Then if the organism living within this context produces a response that is followed or consequated by an increase in the predictability of stimulus events, that consequence will prove to be reinforcing. The critical feature of this consequence is its predictability compared to the surrounding stimulus context: as long as the consequence exceeds its context in predictability, that consequence will serve a reinforcement function. The bizarre quality of animal behavior produced under these conditions is highlighted by Morse and Kellher (1977). These investigators showed that squirrel monkeys will perform behaviors that are reinforced solely by painful electric shock. As long as the animals' environments were kept unpredictable, they continued to behave in this "masochistic" fashion.

If animals can be made to behave in these unusual, sometimes maladaptive ways, it seems plausible to argue that humans might create social networks that also serve as an uncertainty function. If so the mothers we described in the previous section of this chapter could be viewed as behaving in ways that are likely to produce order in their chaotic lives. Their infants, confronted with a similar pattern of uncertain or insensitive maternal care, would be expected to likewise act in a manner designed to induce predictability in their more limited environments. With respect to childhood conduct problems, aggressive and oppositional behaviors are unfortunate but powerful ways of creating certainty—even though that certainty is composed of aversive reactions by the child's mother. It is not surprising, then, to find observational documentation showing that conduct problem children live in families marked both by inconsistent parental discipline and prolonged episodes of consistent parent-child exchanges of aversive behavior (Patterson, 1976; Snyder, 1977; Wahler, Hughey & Gordon, 1981).

According to the uncertainty principle, triadic stimulus control requires an environmental context that flows over time in an unpredictable fashion. An individual who lives in that environment (for example, mother) will, by definition, respond to the context as an aversive stimulus field. A respite from this aversive context would be achieved if the individual could engage another person in some form of comparatively predictable interchange (such as coercion). We suspect that mother-child dyads who are on the road to pathological conduct-problem relationships do interact in ways that generate a figure-context sort of predictability. Consider, for example, the recent observation findings on chronic conduct problem children described by Wahler and Dumas (in press). The mothers in this study were shown to increase their likelihoods of aversive child-care responding following daily incidents of coercive interchanges with adults. Conditional probabilities of mother-child aversive exchanges were found to be unaffected by these coercive setting events, thus demonstrating the nondiscriminative function of the adult-adult pole of the triangle. However, since both mother and child produced higher rates of aversive responding during these days, it can be said that the "bad" days of mother-child interchange were predictably different from the other days at home. Presumably the mothers' aversive child-care behaviors on the "bad" days generated behavioral episodes that exceeded their daily context in predictability.

The indiscriminate infant-care responding of troubled mothers also makes a certain degree of sense from the uncertainty principle. Perhaps these mothers are responding to their stressful contextual encounters as pseudo discriminative stimuli for the child-care routines described by observers as "insensitive" or "noncontingent." Given that the mothers offer this sort of uncertain stimulus context for their babies, the babies ought to behave in ways that generate greater certainty, that is, crying and other coercive responses. The comparatively greater predictability generated by the babies' coercive behavior will then reinforce the mothers' participation in such coercive exchanges. What appears to be a "pseudo" discriminative stimulus from a strict operant viewpoint might actually function to predict a dependable consequence, if one is willing to consider the consequence as a figure-ground pattern. Without doubt these speculations are only a start at explaining triadic or indirect stimulus control of child behavior. Our point in presenting this section on "response generated predictability" is heuristic: We hope that other researchers and clinicians concerned with childhood psychopathology might consider our arguments as a springboard for further research and discussion.

IMPLICATIONS OF A BEHAVIORAL SYSTEMS VIEWPOINT FOR PEDIATRICS

Other chapters in this book present some clearly outlined pictures of how psychological processess impinge on the medical problems of children. Although this behavioral systems perspective is more general in its application to the pediatric field, there is a focal point that intersects perspective and field. Parent and child compliance with the medical regimen is critical to the success of any prescriptive intervention. In our reading of the pediatric literature we were struck by the sometimes extraordinary instructional requirements placed on both child and parent in the course of certain medical treatments. Because of these instruction-compliance issues, the behavioral systems perspective could constitute an important set of guidelines in pediatric intervention. In some families, the principal caregiver may understand and agree with the needed medical regimen, but may not pursue its completion because of reinforcement and setting event factors operating within family and community. Thus a mother who is prepared to institute regimen adherence with her diabetic child could be involved in a variety of inhibiting systems factors. Not only might she be faced with a number of directly presented aversive contingencies in the form of her child's noncompliance, nagging and temper outbursts; she might also encounter the critiques of spouse and extended family, as well as a reduction in her usually available positive interchanges with these people. The cumulative effects of both direct and indirect stimulus experiences could reduce the regimen to a haphazard series of events.

In a related issue of medical compliance, the pediatrician is also faced with "lifestyle" problems sometime presented by older (adolescent) children. Drug, alcohol and dietary abuse have become increasingly more common referral problems in pediatric practice, again leading to the question of how one institutes appropriate changes in the troubled youth's lifestyle. Undoubtedly these maladaptive behavior patterns are maintained by direct reinforcement contingencies in the youth's peer- and adult-governed environments *and* through indirect sources represented by setting event stimulus control. For example, an anorectic girl's refusal to eat will bear a contingent relationship to peer approval and parent disapproval, but the indirect influences in her dietary problem will not be so obvious. That is this youth's dependency interactions with her mother might be shown to influence her sparse eating pattern as well as her frequently voiced worries about how plump she seems to be. While the girl's dependency manipulation with mother may have no direct connection to the dietary problem, the former exchanges could serve as setting events for the latter behavior. As we argued in the earlier section describing this sort of triadic stimulus control, the setting event may function to predict states of "certainty." In our case example the dependency striving between girl and mother could create contextual uncertainty within the family; the girl's eating regimen, although it creates unpleasant parental response, may also reduce uncertainty.

There is little doubt that a behavioral systems perspective has been a useful conceptual tool in child clinical psychology. Since the pediatric profession has become increasingly involved in the psychological processes of families, it seems reasonable to anticipate similar benefits when pediatric workers employ these guidelines. Whether the issue be medical regimen adherence or maladaptive lifestyle, an appreciation for the principles of triadic stimulus control might lead to some new formulations of these complex problems.

REFERENCES

Agras, W.S. (Ed.). (1978). *Behavior modification: Principles and clinical applications* (2nd ed.). Boston: Little, Brown.

Ainsworth, M.D.S. (1979). Attachment as related to mother-infant interaction. In J.S. Rosenblatt, R.S. Hinde, C. Beer, & M. Busnel (Eds.), *Advances in the study of behavior* (Vol. 9; pp. 2–51). New York: Academic Press.

Allport, G.W. (1966). Traits revisisted. *American Psychologist, 21*, 1–10.

Bell, S.M., & Ainsworth M.D.S. (1972). Infant crying and maternal responsiveness. *Child Development, 43*, 1171–1190.

Bijou, S.W., & Baer, D.M. (1961). *Child development I: A systematic and empirical theory.* Englewood Cliffs, NJ: Prentice-Hall.

Bonney, M.E. (1971). Assessment of effort to aid socially isolated elementary school pupils. *Journal of Educational Research, 64*, 359–364.

Bowers, K.S. (1974). Situationism in psychology: An analysis. *Psychological Review, 81*, 506–520.

Craighead, W.E., Kazdin, A.E., & Mahoney, M.J. (1981). *Behavior Modification: Principles, Issues, and Applications* (2nd ed.). Boston: Houghton Mifflin.

Crittenden, P.M. (1981). Abusing, neglecting, problematic, and adequate dyads: Differentiating by pattern of interaction. *Merrill-Palmer Quarterly, 27*, 201–218.

Crockenberg, S.B. (1981). Infant irritability, mother responsiveness, and social support influences on the security of infant-mother attachment. *Child Development, 52*, 857–865.

D'Amato, M.R. (1974). Derived motives. *Annual Review of Psychology, 25*, 83–106.

Dumas, J., & Wahler, R.G. (in press). Indiscriminate mothering as a contextual factor in aggressive-oppositional child behavior. *Journal of Abnormal Child Psychology.*

Egeland, B. & Sroufe, L.A. (1981). Attachment and early maltreatment. *Child Development, 52*, 44–52.

Fowler, S.A., & Baer, D.M. (1981). Do I have to be good all day? The timing of delayed reinforcement as a factor in generalization. *Journal of Applied Behavior Analyses, 14*, 14–24.

George, C., & Main, M. (1979). Social interactions of young abused children: Approach, avoidance, & aggression. *Child Development, 50*, 306–318.

Gewirtz, J.L. (1956). A factor analysis of some attention-seeking behaviors of young children. *Child Development, 27*, 17–366.

Harris, A. (1979). An empirical test of the situation specificity/consistency of aggressive behavior. *Child Behavior Therapy, 1*, 257–270.

Harris, A., & Reid, J.B. (1981). The consistency of a class of coercive child behaviors across school settings for individual subjects. *Journal of Abnormal Child Psychology, 9*, 219–227.

Herbert, E.W. Pinkston, E.M., Hayden, M.L., Sajewaj, T.E., Pinkston, S., Cordura, G., & Jackson, C. (1976). Adverse effects of parental attention. *Journal of Abnormal Psychology, 6*, 15–30.

Herrnstein, R.J. (1966). Superstition: A corollary of the principles of operant conditioning. In W.K. Honig, (Ed.), *Operant behavior: Areas of research and application* New York: Appleton-Century-Crofts.

Imada, H., & Najeishi, Y. (1982). The concept of uncertainty in animal experiments using aversive stimulation. *Psychological Bulletin, 91*, 573–588.

Kantor, J.R. (1959). *Interbehavioral Psychology.* Granville, OH: Principia Press.

Kazdin, A.E. (1980). *Behavior Modification in Applied Settings.* Homewood IL: Dorsey.

Lansky, D., & Brownell, K.D. (1982). Comparison of school-based treatments for adolescent obesity. *Journal of School Health, 52*, 384–387.

Mann, R.D. (1959). A review of the relationships between personality and performance in small groups. *Psychological Bulletin, 56*, 241–270.

Mash, E.S., & Terdal, L.G. (Eds.). (1982). *Behavioral assessment of childhood dissorders.* New York: Guilford.

Miklich, D.R. (1973). Operant conditioning procedures with systematic desensitization in hyperkinetic asthmatic boy. *Journal of Behavior Therapy and Experimental Psychiatry, 4,* 177–182.

Mischel, W. (1968). *Personality and assessment.* New York: Wiley.

Morse, W.H., & Kellher, R.T. (1977). Determinants of reinforcement and punishment. In W.K. Honig, & J.E.R. Staddon (Eds.), *Handbook of operant behavior* (pp. 174–200). Englewood Cliffs, NJ: Prentice-Hall.

O'Dell, S. (1974). Training parents in behavior modification: A review. *Psychological Bulletin, 81,* 418–433.

Patterson, G.R. (1976). The aggressive child: Victim and architect of a coercive system. In L.A. Hannerlynck, L.C. Handy, & E.J. Mash (Eds.), *Behavior modification and families I. Theory and research* (pp. 267–316). New York: Brunner/Mazel.

Patterson, G.R. (1979). A performance theory for coercive family interaction. In L.G. Cairns (Ed.), *Social interaction: Methods, analysis, and illustration.* Chicago: University of Chicago Press.

Patterson, G.R., & Maerov, S. (1976, December). A functional analysis of controlling stimuli in two settings. Paper presented at meeting of the Association for the Advancement of Behavior Therapy, New York.

Patterson, G.R., and Reid, J.B. (1970). Reciprocity and coercion: Two facts of social systems. In C. Neuringer, & J.L. Michael (Eds.), *Behavior modification in clinical psychology* (pp. 133–177).

Powell, R.W. (1973). Effects of stimulus control and deprivation upon discriminative responding. *Journal of the Experimental Analysis of Behvior, 19,* 351–360.

Reid, J.B., Taplin, P.S. ,& Loeber, R. (1981). A social interactional approach to the treatment of abusive families. In R. Stuart (Ed.), *Violent behavior: Social learning approaches to prediction, management and treatment.* New York: Brunner/Mazel.

Reynolds, G.S. (1961). Behavioral contrast. *Journal of the Experimental Analysis of Behavior, 4,* 57–71.

Sears, R.R. (1963). Dependency motivation. In M.R. Jones (Ed.), *Nebraska symposium on motivation* (pp. 25–64).

Simon, S.J., Ayllon, T., & Milan, M.A. (in press). Behavioral compensation: Contrast-like effects in the classroom, *Behavior Modification.*

Skinner, B.F. (1938). *The behavior of organisms.* New York: Appleton-Century-Crofts.

Skinner, B.F. (1953). *Science and human behavior.* New York: Free Press.

Snyder, J.J. (1977). A reinforcement analysis of intervention in problem and nonproblem children. *Journal of Abnormal Psychology, 86,* 5, 528–535.

Stayton, D.J. Hogan, R., & Ainsworth, M.D.S. (1971). Infant obedience and maternal behavior: The origin of socialization reconsidered. *Child Development, 42,* 1057–1069.

Stokes, T.F., & Baer, D.M. (1977). An implicit technology of generalization. *Journal of Applied Behavior Analysis, 10* 349–367.

Vaugh, B., Egeland, B., Sroufe, A., & Waters, E. (1979). Individual differences in infant-mother attachment at twelve and eighteen moths: Stability and change in families under stress. *Child Development, 50,* 971–975.

Wahler, R.G. (1969a). Oppositional children: A quest for parental reinforcement control. *Journal of Applied Behavior Analysis, 2,* 239–246.

Wahler, R.G. (1969b). Setting generality: Some specific and general effects of child behavior therapy. *Journal of Applied Behavior Analysis, 2,* 239–246.

Wahler, R.G. (1976). Deviant child behavior within the family: Developmental speculations and behavior change strategies. In H. Leitenbert (Ed.) *Handbook of behavior modification and behavior therapy* (pp. 516–543). Englewood Cliffs, NJ: Prentice-Hall.

Wahler, R.G. (1980). The insular mother: Her problems in parent-child treatment. *Journal of Applied Behavior Analysis, 13*, 207–219.

Wahler, R.G., & Dumas, J.E. (in press). Stimulus class determinants of mother-child coercive interchanges in multidistressed families: Assessment and intervention. In J. Buchard (Ed.), *Vermont Conference on the Primary Prevention on Psychopathology.*

Wahler, R.G., Hughey, J.B., & Gordon, J.S. (1981). Chronic patterns of mother-child coercive interchanges in multidistressed families: Assessment and intervention. In J. Buchard (Ed.), *Analysis and intervention in developmental disabilities, 1, 2,* 145–156.

Waters, E., Vaughn, B.E., & Egeland, B.R. (1980). Individual differences in infant-mother attachment relationships at age one: Antecedents in neonatal behavior in an urban, economically disadvantaged sample. *Child Development, 51,* 208–216.

Wolfe, D.A., & Mosk, M.D. (1983). Behavioral comparisons of children from abusive and distressed families. *Journal of Consulting & Clinical Psychology, 51,* 702–708.

Zeilberger, J., Sampen, S.E., & Sloane, H.N. Jr. (1968). Modification of a child's problem behaviors in the home with the mother as therapist. *Journal of Applied Behavior Analysis, 1,* 47–53.

PREVENTION

10

Appropriate Functions of Health Education in Schools: Improving Health and Cognitive Performance

LLOYD J. KOLBE, LAWRENCE GREEN, JOHN FOREYT,
LINDA DARNELL, KEN GOODRICK, HARRIET WILLIAMS,
DIANNE WARD, A.S. KORTON, ISMET KARACAN,
ROGER WIDMEYER, AND GENE STAINBROOK

INTRODUCTION

The disappointment of some professionals who have studied the performance of health education in schools (Knowles, 1977; U.S. Department of Health, Education and Welfare, 1973) attests to a gap between outcomes and expectations. The disappointment appears to stem largely from expectations in the health sector that school health education should have given us more spectacular gains in health outcomes. In contrast to the high

171

expectations, the 15 to 24 age group is the only age group in the United States to have experienced an increased death rate in recent decades. Teenage pregnancies and sexually transmitted diseases have increased, and the rate of injuries from automobile crashes and violence is higher in this age range than in any other.

This chapter asks whether the high expectations of some health professionals are based on a valid interpretation of the function of education in general and of health education in or out of schools, and, if not, whether health education in schools can be justified and supported on some other basis.

ASSUMPTIONS AND IMPLICIT MODELS OF CAUSATION

Biomedical and Public Health Models

When medical and public health workers speak of function, they refer generally to the assumed or expected relationship between an intervention and a health outcome. It is assumed that the effectiveness and efficiency of an intervention, which may be a technique, strategy, program or institution, are to be judged on the basis of the intervention's causal relationship to the "saving" of lives (usually meaning the deferring of death), the improvement of health (usually meaning the removal or control of symptoms), or the prevention of disease or injury. For any given intervention, this relationship is more or less supported by "hard" evidence, meaning controlled trials in which randomized subjects who received the intervention showed significantly better health outcomes than their randomized controls. Most interventions, except FDA-approved drugs, immunizing agents and medical appliances, have not been submitted to this test of evidence. Instead, they are defended on the basis of an implicit model of indirect or mediated causation. Thus, the simple medical and public health models,

(a) medical intervention→individual health outcome
(b) public health intervention→population health outcome,

are elaborated with assumptions and evidence concerning the primary impact of the intervention on some immediate outcome or series of effects. These in turn are assumed or known from other studies to be directly related to the intended health outcome:

(c) intervention→impact→outcome.

Biobehavioral Models

The "impact" variables range from specific, physiologically documented risk factors, such as blood pressure control, to theoretical constructs, based solely on subjective, self-reported statements, such as attitudes or beliefs. The latter are typically imbedded in more elaborate hybrids of behavioral science and biomedical science models, in which the number of intermediate impact variables multiply into complex chains of causation with some strong links and some weak. For example,

$$(d) \quad \text{intervention} \rightarrow \text{impact} \rightarrow \text{impact}$$
$$\searrow \quad \downarrow \quad \quad \downarrow$$
$$\text{impact} \rightarrow \text{impact} \rightarrow \text{outcome,}$$

is a generic form of model in which the intervention is assumed or expected from diverse data and experience to set into motion a series of actions and reactions, direct and indirect effects, as well as interaction effects, leading ultimately to the desired health outcome.

Public Health Education Models

In a world of such models, medicine has had a distinct advantage because its interventions are subject to more immediate and controlled testing for health outcomes than those of public health. In the area of public health, health education has required more complex and difficult-to-test models because of the linkages of cognitive, environmental and behavioral variables, each of which is variously and sometimes tenuously related to the others and to health outcomes. A generic health education model is one that contains, by definition, a "combination of interventions designed to predispose, enable, and reinforce voluntary adaptations of behavior conducive to health" (Green, Kreutor, Deeds & Partridge, 1980):

$$(e) \quad \text{educational} \xrightarrow{\nearrow \text{predisposing factors} \searrow} \text{behavior} \rightarrow \text{health} \rightarrow \text{quality of life}$$
$$\text{interventions} \xrightarrow{\searrow \text{reinforcing factors} \nearrow}$$

School Health Education Models

Within health education, school health education has had an even more arduous path to define between its interventions and the expected health outcomes. Although schools independently can increase predispositions to healthy behavior (by increasing health knowledge, fostering healthful attitudes, and teaching health skills), they frequently depend on community health promotion interventions to enable and reinforce those behaviors depicted in model (e). Documenting with experimental or even nonexperimental prospective data the relationship between classroom interventions and health outcomes has been a rare feature in even the best evaluations of school health education (Coates, Perry, & Petersen, 1982; Green & Iverson, 1982; Kreuter & Christenson 1981; Mechanic, 1979). Nevertheless, an impressive record of impact on health behavior has accumulated in the past few years, as documented in a number of recent meta-evaluations and reviews (Evans & Raines, 1982; Evans, Hill, Raines, & Henderson, 1981; Green, Heit, Iverson, Kolbe & Kreuter, 1980; Iammarino, Weinberg & Holcomb, 1980; Levy, Iverson & Wahlberg, 1980; Olsen, Redican, & Krus, 1980; Schaps, DiBartolo, Moskowitz, Polly, & Churgin, 1981; Thompson, 1978), though the more impressive record is with improvements in knowledge, attitudes and skills assumed to be important in the subsequent development of health behavior. In this hierarchy and temporal sequencing of effects lies an implicit model imposed upon, rather than inherent in school health education:

$$(f)\ \text{School health education} \rightarrow \begin{array}{c} \nearrow \text{cognitive development} \searrow \\ \text{affective development} \\ \searrow \text{skill development} \nearrow \end{array} \rightarrow \text{behavior} \rightarrow \text{health}$$

This model, derivative of the public health education model (e), places ultimate importance on health outcomes and the behavior necessary to achieve them. The problem is that schools are not medical institutions nor public health agencies and have never adopted the same mission and goals. School health educators have worked valiantly to live up to the expectations of their public health education colleagues, but they have been fighting an uphill battle within the education sector in recent years because of the "back to basics" movement, and public health agencies have not always worked with the schools to enable and reinforce the targeted behavior. In any case the schools simply cannot be held accountable for solutions to all the ills of society (Green, 1980b; Kolbe, 1979; Kolbe, 1982), and the line is now being drawn more clearly between the primary educational mission of the schools and the functions other agencies would like for them to perform.

The Comprehensive School Health Program Model

One result of this recognition that the classroom could not be expected to accomplish behavioral and health outcomes by itself was a return to a basic model of school health programs which was not derivative of public health education, but rather of education in general. This generic model of school health programs combines health teaching with school and community health services, as well as with interventions in the school and community environment to produce that level of health necessary to ensure that students can perform optimally in school. The two significant departures of this model from the preceding models are the combination of education with school and community services and environmental interventions to promote health, and the emphasis on health as an instrumental as well as a terminal objective.

The comprehensive school health program model would look something like the following:

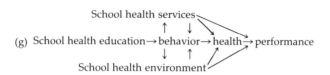

It is important to emphasize that in this model (g) the school health program is intended to increase educational performance directly (through preventive health services and the environment) as well as indirectly through the mediating influence of behavior and health.

The Community Health Promotion Model

The comprehensive school health program model shown in (g) approximates in two ways at the school level what has come to be associated with health promotion at the community and national level. First, the combining of health education with organizational and environmental services and resources in support of health behavior in both the school health program model and in the health promotion model (Green, 1980a; Green, 1981; Green, Wilson, & Bauer, 1982) mitigates the unrealistic expectations that health education and the school alone can accomplish desirable behavioral and health outcomes. Second, the recognition that health is not necessarily an end in itself but may serve other values and social goals or quality-of-life concerns is in keeping with the positive concepts of health as "physical, mental and social well-being" inherent in the earliest approaches to health education in the World Health Organization (1954) and in more recent formulations of policy in health promotion (U.S. Dept. of Health and Human Services, 1979).

This instrumentality of health is reflected in the resolution of the World Health Assembly of 1977: "The main social target of Governments and WHO in the coming decades should be the attainment by all the citizens of the world, by the year 2000, of a level of health that will permit them to lead a socially and economically productive life." Whereas the World Health Organization, the U.S. Surgeon General and private industries initiating worksite health promotion programs speak of productivity, the schools speak of performance and academic achievement. Whereas the school health model speaks of combining education with school health services and interventions on the school environment, WHO defines "primary health care" as consisting of these three elements, and the Surgeon

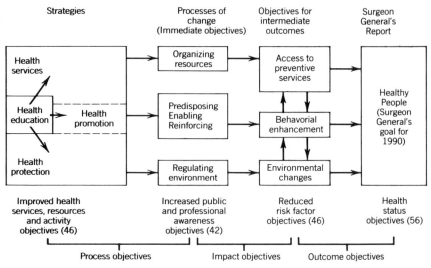

FIGURE 10.1. Structure and logical relationships of the objectives for the nation in disease prevention and health promotion. (From Green, L.W., Wilson, R.W. and Bauer, K.G. *American Journal of Public Health*, Volume 73, 1982.)

General's initiative in disease prevention and health promotion consists of parallel elements in preventive health services, health promotion directed at behavior and health protection directed at the environment. (See Figure 10.1.)

One other revelation that the health promotion "movement" has forced upon us is that there are immediate benefits to be gained from lifestyle modification that most health professionals and scientists would normally not count as health outcomes. Some would not be counted because they are too subjective, such as "feeling good," "feeling alert," and "feeling more energetic." Others would not be counted because they are considered to have more to do with cosmetics, economics, or social norms than with objectively defined health. These include outcomes of healthier lifestyles such as weight control, agility, endurance, concentration, efficiency of movement, good muscle tone, and improved performance of daily living activities.

Together these benefits and related "intangibles" make up a large part of the quality of life or social concerns which were considered a consequence of health in the public health education model. They were given prominence there because public health education begins "where the people are" as a matter of principle or philosophy, and because educational and health research, especially on adult populations, has demonstrated that commitment of people to the goals of a program increases the probability of their participation in or behavioral response to a program. Recognizing that the priority concerns of a population are seldom expressed in terms of health, public health education has typically worked to show people how health can contribute to their quality of life or social concerns.

Schools are not obliged to justify their attention to performance and achievement in terms of their contribution to health. Yet, they cannot escape the need to assure that time and resources allocated to the school health program are working for rather than against educational objectives. Schools, therefore, share several interests with public health, public health education and health promotion. How can these common interests be merged in a model of school health promotion that uses the capacity of the school to contribute to health while recognizing that such capacity will not be used to full advantage unless school administrators can be convinced that the outcomes will include improved academic achievement?

A RATIONALE FOR AN INTEGRATED SCHOOL HEALTH PROMOTION MODEL

As portrayed in the foregoing review of models and assumptions, the major difference between those derived from the heatlh fields (biomedical, public health, biobehavioral and public health education) and those derived from education (for example, the comprehensive school health model) is their respective placement of health as an ultimate outcome or an instrumental outcome. Part of the disagreement here lies in the missions of the two sectors, health and education. With the increasing complexity of etiologies and causal pathways for specific diseases and health problems (Stallones, 1980), the health establishment seems ready to entertain more complex and time-lapsed models of intervention for health outcomes. The growing interest in disease prevention and health promotion attests to this. At the same time the schools and their constituencies are demanding more "time on task" and improved achievement of their students. The convergence of these trends suggests a new rationale for health promotion in the schools in which the variables targeted for the short-term outcomes are lifestyle and performance variables:

$$(h) \; intervention \rightarrow lifestyle \rightarrow performance \rightarrow achievement$$

Persuasion of the education establishment to adopt this model will depend largely on evidence documenting the association between lifestyle and performance as measured in educational terms. The remainder of this review will assess that evidence in four lifestlye areas: diet, exercise, sleep and stress. The corresponding evidence for alcohol and drug abuse has been thoroughly reviewed in recent publications (McAlister, 1982) and its influence on performance in school is hardly in question.

To obtain the support of the health establishment, this model needs to be extended to show its potential contribution to health outcomes. The main argument and body of evidence affirming the relevance of this model to health is the pervasive and inescapable correlation between educational attainment and health (Bachman, O'Malley, & Johnston, 1978; Mechanic, 1979). The connection between educational attainment and health is most logically explained in behavioral terms, although genetic and economic factors undeniably enter into both the educational attainment and the health behavior of children and parents. The empirical evidence supporting the causal link between educational attainment and health behavior is consistent but tenuous in that it is not experimental (Bachman et. al., 1978; Mechanic, 1979). Similarly, the link between health behavior and long-term health outcomes is widely documented and accepted (Breslow & Enstrom, 1980), but nearly impossible to establish experimentally.

With these caveats in mind, we propose the following integrated model for health promotion in schools:

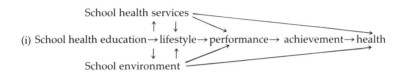

This model is of course highly simplified, leaving out the "exogenous" influences of other aspects of the curriculum on performance, factors other than performance on achievement, and factors outside the school, including coordinated community health promotion efforts, on all of the outcomes. Our purpose is simply to specify the essential elements linking school health promotion interventions with health outcomes in a causal chain that gives primacy to the educational outcomes that are the main, if not the sole concern of the schools.

In the following section, we review the literature linking each of four aspects of lifestyle—diet, exercise, sleep, and stress—to cognitive performance and related variables in school achievement.

DIET*

Evidence is accumulating about the effects of nutrition and social environments on attention, memory, cognitive performance, emotional affect, and social functioning (Popkin & Lim-Ybnanez, 1982; Pollitt & Thompson, 1977; Ricciuti, 1981; Scrimshaw, 1974). These factors directly influence the academic achievement of students. The reported effects of malnutrition, iron deficiency anemia, food additives, caffeine, sugar, fasting, overeating, and obesity briefly are reviewed below.

*Material on Diet written by John Foreyt, Linda Darnell, and Ken Goodrick.

Chronic Food Deprivation and Cognitive Function

Studies of malnourished populations in Latin America (Cravioto, DeLicardie, & Birch, 1966), India, Japan, Europe, Italy, and Britain (Birch, 1972) consistently found that undernourished children performed more poorly than their well-nourished counterparts on global measures of short-term cognitive performance (Popkin & Lim-Ybnanez, 1982). In these studies, cognitive abilities were assessed by measuring the child's recognition of geometric forms and problem solving skills. These measures (Birch, 1972; Popkin & Lim-Ybnanez, 1982) were designed to circumvent the cross-cultural validity problems that are incurred by using culture-sensitive tests developed in more industrialized societies.

Chronic Food Deprivation and Intellect

Pollitt and Thomson (1977) reviewed 21 studies and concluded that mental functioning, as measured by long-term intellectual and developmental quotients, was vulnerable to severe undernutrition during the first year of life. Intellectual function was found to be reduced by as much as one to two standard deviations below the average developmental quotient among malnourished one-year-olds. Severe undernutrition during the second and subsequent years of life, however, did not seem permanently to impair intellectual abilities.

Environmental Stimulation and Intellect

In a series of experiments with rats, Levitsky and Barnes (1972) examined the effects of undernutrition on emotional responses to stress (that is, open field locomotion, fighting, and fear responses). Permanent exaggerated responses to stress were produced by early malnutrition experiences. In subsequent studies, these exaggerated responses were increased further by combining early social isolation with early malnutrition experiences (Levitsky & Barnes, 1972). Further studies found that by handling the rats and allowing them time to "play" with other rats, the effects of early nutritional trauma could be eliminated. If the rats were kept under standard cage conditions (not handled), early nutritional trauma continued to influence adult behavior by exaggerating responses to stress.

Monckeberg, Tiser, Toro, Guttas & Vega (1972) reported similar effects of malnutrition and social environment on mental development in a human population. Preschoolers from a lower socioeconomic group were found to have lower growth rates and to have lower developmental quotient scores than their counterparts in a well-fed, higher socioeconomic group, thus implicating either social or nutritional factors (or both) with intellectual development. Richardson (1976) controlled for both of these variables and found social background to be a better predictor of IQ than nutrition in a chronically malnourished population.

McKay, Sinisterra, McKay, Gomez, and Lloreda (1978) took the nutrition/social background issue one step further and compared children of contrasting economic environments before and after a nutritional and academic intervention. Cognitive functioning of previously malnourished school children from deprived environments was increased to the levels of well-fed children from favorable environments. These data should be of particular interest to school administrators in economically depressed areas in the United States.

Iron-Deficiency Anemia

Estimates of iron-deficiency anemia in the school age population in the United States range from less than one percent among younger children (Foxman, Lohr, & Brook, 1983), to 20 percent among adolescents (Pollitt, Greenfield, & Leibel, 1979). Iron deficiency may impair attention, arousal, memory, and learning. One of the proposed mechanisms by which iron deficiency may alter cognitive processes is through the enzyme monoamine oxidase (MAO). The enzyme is particularly sensitive to body iron stores and has been observed to fluctuate in less time than required to observe development of frank anemia. Some behavioral changes have been noted upon administration of monoamine oxidase inhibitors (Oski & Honig, 1978; Pollitt & Leibel, 1976).

Webb and Oski (1973) found iron-deficient black children in an economically deprived area who had hemoglobin values of 10.1 to 11.4 gm/dl to score significantly lower on Iowa Tests of Basic Skills than children with hemoglobins of 14.0 to 14.9 gm/dl. The iron-deficient group also scored lower on scales of personality disturbance, conduct problems, and inadequacy-immaturity. The authors point out that it is unclear whether these data are confounded by ethnic and social variables. If children who were more economically deprived comprised the iron-deficient group, then either social-economic or extraneous nutritional variables could have been measured rather than iron status. Additionally black children are known to have normal hemoglobin concentrations anywhere from 0.5 to 1.0 gm/dl lower than white children. The anemic group thus may have been more undernourished than iron deficient.

In a blind trial carried out in Indonesia (Pollitt, 1984), 9-to-12-year-old children initially were treated for parasites, classified as iron-deficient-anemic or nonanemic, and administered a battery of psychological tests (including the Raven Progressive Matrices IQ test, a concentration task, and achievement tests on educational materials). The anemic children scored lower on the concentration and achievement tests, but not on the IQ test. Both groups then randomly were assigned to either iron treatment or placebo supplements. After 3 months the anemic group had recovered hemoglobin and transferrin saturation to the level of the control children, and had significantly increased their concentration and scholastic achievement scores. The nonanemic students did not increase their scores upon iron supplementation, and neither the nonanemic group nor the anemic group who received placebos increased their scores.

In another study (Ricciuti, 1979) iron-deficient children in the United States were shown to perform less well than noniron-deficient children on measures of selective attention, use of memory strategies, and ability to respond to salient stimuli. These deficits were eliminated when iron was restored to normal.

A nationwide food consumption survey (U.S. Department of Agriculture, 1980) revealed that iron intake among school-aged children in the United States is far below recommended levels. However, few educational programs emphasize the need for adolescents to select foods that will assure they have adequate iron.

Food and Hyperactivity

It is often asserted that hyperactivity among children is caused by salicylates, artificial food colors and flavors, preservatives, sugar, and caffeine. These beliefs have been fostered by the reported clinical experience of Feingold (Rumsey & Rapoport, 1983), and by anecdotal, nonblind studies (Kolata, 1982; Wender, 1981). Of particular concern to investigators attempting to study hyperactivity is the difficulty of classifying individuals with a syndrome that may be defined more subjectively than objectively. One classification scheme defines those children who respond to amphetamines by decreased activity as hyperkinetic; yet approximately 25 percent of symptomatically hyperactive children do not respond to amphetamines. In addition, hyperactivity and minimal brain damage frequently are considered synonymous. One hypothesized connection between hyperactivity and minimal brain damage is suggested by the neurotoxic effects of additives such as erythosin (FD&C 3) among animals (Rumsey & Rapoport, 1983).

The validity of hypotheses about additive neurotoxicity is difficult to establish by using retrospective clinical trials of human populations that must rely on imprecise and possibly multiple diagnoses. Nonetheless, there currently is little acceptable evidence to support the assertion that food substances cause hyperactivity (Kolata, 1983; Rumsey & Rapoport, 1983; Wender, 1981). There may be some subset of hyperactive children who can benefit from severe elimination diets; but methodological and diagnostic problems make it difficult to discover who they are or to discover how helpful the diets may be.

Caffeine

The Food and Drug Administration (FDA) recently has recommended that pregnant women not consume caffeine because of the possibility it might cause birth defects. The FDA also has expressed concerns about possible neurobehavioral effects of caffeine on children (Rumsey & Rapoport, 1983). Perhaps the most prevalent source of caffeine for children is soft drinks. Soft-drink consumption among children has increased dramatically over the last few decades (Mayer & Mayell, 1981). The percentage of children who consume soft drinks increases with age, with 11 percent of infants, 40 percent of 1-to-2-year-olds, 50 percent of 3-to-8-year-olds, and 60 percent of 15-to-18-year-olds consuming soft drinks. Some soft drinks contain from 31 to 46 milligrams of caffeine. For smaller children this is equivalent to one cup of coffee. Little is known about the effects of caffeine on the cognitive functions of children.

Sugar

Sugar has been suspected as an agent of various health problems and diseases; yet whether it causes problems other than dental caries among children remains unknown. Consumption of simple sugars can cause a rapid rise in blood sugar, followed by a larger reduction. This overcompensating reduction may cause lowered energy and poorer cognitive performance. Despite claims that children suffer behavioral disturbances after ingestion of sugar, there is no evidence that sugar causes such behavioral problems (Rarick, 1976; Shephard, 1983).

Breakfast and Fasting

Dickie and Bender (1982) recently studied children who habitually ate or did not eat breakfast. They also looked at children who normally ate breakfast but skipped it for the study. On tests of attentional detection, memory search, addition, and sentence verification, no differences were found in association with habitual or deliberate omission of breakfast. The authors acknowledged that children who were aware of being deprived of breakfast may have aroused themselves in compensation to perform normally during the relatively short experimental period.

Studies of breakfast-skipping comprise one subset of more general studies of food deprivation and its relation to available energy for brain metabolism and cognitive performance. Pollitt and his colleagues (1981), notable for their work in this area, report that the brains of children use 50 percent of the body's oxygen supply. During periods of fasting, the liver provides glucose to the blood. Children have a higher ratio of brain weight to liver weight, and a 50 percent greater metabolic rate per unit of brain weight compared to adults. Thus, fasting places a greater demand on the child's glycogen stores than on the adult's.

To test whether this greater metabolic stress has behavioral or cognitive consequences, Pollitt (1981) had 9-to-11-year-old children skip breakfast. Testing occurred at noon. The fasting condition produced significantly higher levels of betahydroxybutyrate, lactate anf free fatty acids, indicating that the fast was physiologically stressful. Such fasting had an adverse effect on accuracy in problem solving, but a beneficial effect on immediate short-term memory recall. Ability to discriminate between relevant and irrelevant features of visual stimuli also was impaired. Thus, it seems that hungry children are more vigilant but less reflective and analytical.

Obesity

The most prevalent form of childhood malnutrition in the U.S. population is obesity. Prevalence estimates vary with criteria used to define obesity (for example, skinfold thickness or weight for height) and with the standards used. Thus estimates have large ranges. LeBow (1984) estimated that 20 to 40 percent of lower socioeconomic children, and 3 to 25 percent of higher socioeconomic children, may be obese. Concerns about the academic achievement of the obese center around low self-esteem derived from societal and peer condemnation of the obese and the short-term effects of fasting for many obese students who diet frequently.

LeBow (1984) summarized several studies in which societal condemnation of the obese was assessed. Children repeatedly rated silhouettes of endomorphic characters as stupid, lazy, and cheaters; while mesomorphs were rated as smart, clean and brave, regardless of the phenotype of the rater. The direct effects of the negative self-image of obese children on their scholastic achievement, however, have not been measured. LeBow hypothesized that emotional turmoil might be accentuated by the double message communicated throughout our society that associates food with splendor, but fat with ugly and that associates eating with friendship, but depicts obese persons as unworthy of friends.

Although the adage that fat babies become fat adults is losing credibility, 80 to 85 percent of obese teenagers do become obese adults (Collipp, 1980). In lower ranges of excess body fat or in temporary caloric increase, hypertrophy only of existing fat cells occurs. In advanced obesity of adolescence and adulthood, however, fat cells proliferate, producing a hyperplastic as well as hypertrophic form of obesity (Sjostrom, 1980). The refractoriness of obesity reflects the inability of an individual to lose fat cells once they are developed. Adherents of the fat-cell theory maintain that once individuals become obese they may reduce the size of their fat cells and appear thinner through diet or exercise, but the number of cells remain, waiting to refill to their accustomed, if not ahove average, size. Childhood, therefore, is the crucial period for intervention to prevent obesity-related diseases such as heart disease, diabetes, and hypertension and to prevent the negative effects of obesity on a child's social development.

It is important that appropriate messages about obesity be communicated sensitively to children. Information about obesity and motivation to prevent it can be provided in the school setting, as can support for the weight-control efforts of obese schoolmates. Brownell and Stunkard (1980), for example, have designed a weight control program that can be implemented in schools.

In addition, short-term overeating needs to be examined more thoroughly. Many children may experience somnolence after overeating. Indeed this is a natural response that has been observed in animals. There may be optimal feeding patterns for school children to maintain energy and attention levels with a range for best learning. Furthermore, the short-term cognitive effects of fasting and malnutrition may be regulated to ensure that persons who are dieting or restricting calories can perform at optimal levels.

EXERCISE*

There is little doubt that physical activity contributes to health and well-being among children and adults. A growing body of evidence is developing that more and more strongly ties physical activity to a healthy, optimally functioning brain and thus potentially to improved cognitive performance in young and old alike.

Perceptual-Motor Development and Cognitive Performance

Developmental psychologists (particularly in France) and experts in the field of perceptual-motor development have for a long time pointed to significant relationships between early psychomotor and neuromuscular development and cognitive growth in young children of elementary school age. Early development of optimal neuromuscular control and psychomotor function seem to help the early stages of academic learning (Shephard, 1983). An important part of early education is the organization and refinement of crude movement responses into finely tuned, coordinated movement patterns. (Rarick, 1976). Barker and Wright (1958) suggest that in a single 24-hour period, a child may perform as many as 2000 movement responses which involve over 660 behavioral objects in a variety of cognitive activities. Children who are "slowly developing" in school achievement tend to show less well-developed neuromuscular and psychomotor skills than do children of comparable chronological ages who do not have similar academic difficulties (Williams, Temple & Bateman, 1978).

Perceptual-motor development theory and research suggest that early motor development (physical activity) experiences and cognitive growth go hand in hand. Although limited in scope and design, most research in this area indicates that basic neuromuscular skills (for example, gross object and body projection skills and fine eye-hand coordination skills involved in writing, drawing, and object manipulation) provide an important

*Material on Exercise written by Harriet Williams and Dianne Ward.

foundation for the development of more sophisticated perceptual and cognitive behaviors (Belka & Williams, 1978; Chissom, Thomas, & Biasiotto, 1972). Such relationships clearly are stronger in children younger than seven years of age than they are in children who are older. In essence, evidence suggests that to function efficiently in a cognitive mode, the young child must develop at least a minimal set of neuromuscular and psychomotor skills (Belka & Williams, 1978). Belka and Williams (1979) and Williams (1983) also have shown that cognitive performances of kindergarten-age children can be predicted from observation of a child's perceptual-motor development at prekindergarten level. In the Trois-Rivieres study in Quebec, both mathematics and language ability (reading and writing) were enhanced by the introduction of additional physical activity in the primary school curriculum (Shephard, 1982).

These findings are consistent with Piaget's theory that the development of adequate psychomotor abilities is a vital part of the total cycle of the child's cognitive growth and is particularly important in the early years of development (Piaget, 1963).

Level of Arousal and Exercise

Both physical and mental performance are affected by the degree of arousal of the individual. An important condition for learning and for cognitive performance, therefore, is an appropriate level of arousal. Physical activity has a strong and immediate effect on the individual's level of arousal. Shephard (1983) suggests that the physiological basis for the arousal effects of exercise is an increase in the activity of reverberating neuronal circuits in the reticular formation of the brainstem produced by the stimulation of muscle, tendon and joint proprioceptors which project via central pathways to these reticular neuronal loops. Release of both norepinephrine and epinephrine during vigorous physical activity may also contribute to the heightened level of alertness or arousal. Whatever the mechanism, it appears that exercise does positively influence arousal. Although some arousal may be advantageous to both physical and mental performance, intense arousal, which often accompanies highly competitive, organized sports programs for young children, may have some immediate deleterious effects on behavior (Blinkie et al., 1977; Skubic, 1955). These effects, however, do not appear to be of long duration (Rivard et al., 1977).

Self-esteem and Exercise

Adequate self-esteem is important to mental health and can indirectly affect cognitive functioning. Physical activity may have some lasting effect on one's sense of self-worth and thereby indirectly influence the cognitive performance of children. Self-efficacy, or a person's estimate of his ability to perform specific actions within highly specific circumstances, is effectively enhanced through performance and experience (Coates, Peterson, & Perry, 1982). Increasing the child's capacity to undertake physical and mental work increases the child's confidence in his or her ability to perform. In addition, participation in physical activity tends to enhance body-image and thus create a positive effect upon the child's attitude toward work and his or her potential for goal achievement (Shephard, 1983).

There also is considerable evidence to suggest that physically active individuals tend to respond less intensely to emotionally laden stimuli (Cox, Evans, & Jameson, 1979; Raab & Krzywanek, 1966). Those who exercise seem to exhibit greater emotional stability and greater ability to cope with stress. Such comparisons, however, are mostly from nonrandomized studies and self-selection bias must be taken into account.

Mechanisms Linking Physical Activity to Cognitive Performance

Animal studies indicate that an important element in early brain growth and development is sensory stimulation. Brains of sensory-enriched (stimulated) animals demonstrate significant changes in anatomical and biochemical parameters that are believed to be indicative of a more efficiently functioning nervous system (Dobbing & Sands, 1973; Goldman, 1972; Greenough, Fass, & Devoogd, 1976; Purpura, 1977; Rosenzweig & Bennett, 1972; Rosenzweig, Bennett, & Diamond, 1972). If cognitive performance is in any way a reflection of optimal brain growth and development, then sersory stimulation through physical exercise must be considered an important factor in at least the early development of the child's cognitive abilities.

From another perspective, individuals with cardiac insufficiency are slower in psychomotor and cognitive functions than those without such health problems (Birren, Carden & Phillips, 1963; Light, 1975; Wilke, Eisdorfer, & Nowlin, 1976). Memory and intelligence also deteriorate more in hypertensive individuals than in normal individuals (Hamsher & Benton, 1978; Hertzog, Schaie, & Gribben, 1978). Even individuals who are predisposed to cardiovascular disease (regardless of age) but who do not show clinical symptoms of such are slower in psychomotor and cognitive responses than controls (Abraham & Birren, 1973). Again, untangling the genetic, environmental and behavioral web of causation is the major barrier to drawing definitive policy guidelines for schools from such relationships.

Deterioration of the respiratory and cardiovascular system reduces cerebral blood flow (CBF). There is little doubt that brain activity is affected by cerebral circulation. In addition the relationship between EEG activity, oxidative metabolism of brain tissue and CBF is well documented (Ingvar, 1967; Ingvar & Lassen, 1975; Ingvar, Sjolund, & Ardo, 1976). It is known that total CBF tends to remain constant regardless of the level of physical work being performed (Fixler, Atkins, Mitchell, & Horowitz, 1976), but CBF shifts according to metabolic demands of different regions of the brain (Halsey, Blauenstein, Wilson, & Willis, 1979; Lassen, Ingvar, Shinhoj, 1978). Specific areas of the brain performing an active task receive increased blood flow to support the work; other less active areas received reduced blood flow. Increased CBF has been shown to occur following gross physical activity (for example, treadmill running), manual activity and arousal reactions. Physical activity in particular has been shown to increase regional CBF in prefrontal somatosensory, and primary motor cortices (Lassen, Ingvar, & Shinhaj, 1978; Orgogoza & Larsen, 1979) in some cases by as much as 30 percent. Such evidence suggests a potentially important link among cardiovascular fitness, exercise and psychomotor and cognitive performance. These data, however, do not provide an unequivocal case for causal links among these variables.

Glucose uptake and metabolism in the brain also is affected by exercise. Glucose is important in brain function because it serves as the main fuel for energy metabolism in the mammalian brain. The rate of glucose utilization has been found to be closely related to functional brain activity. Reduction in glucose utilization ultimately impairs local functional activity of the brain (Adelman, 1970; Chen, Warshaw, & Sanadi, 1972). Charp (1976) clearly has demonstrated that there are differences in glucose consumption in the brains of exercising versus resting animals. If during physical activity different areas of the brain are regularly and systematically activated and, as a result, blood flow to these areas is increased or maintained for long periods of time, exercise could act to develop and maintain optimum vascularization of the brain for glucose production and utilization. If these processes are maintained at a high level, then the energy required to support optimal neural functioning is more likely to be available. Thus exercise could contribute in significant ways to the neurophysiological substrate that underlies cognitive performance.

Level of Physical Activity Among the Young

For children, sufficient physical activity was thought to occur naturally during play, so that little concern was expressed about lack of activity in the lives of children. Although this might have been a safe assumption in the past, times have changed and with these changes have come associated health concerns. As many as 40 percent of children aged 11–14 are estimated to have one or more risk factors associated with heart disease, including overweight, high blood pressure, elevated blood cholesterol, smoking, lack of exercise, and diabetes (U.S. Dept. of Health and Human Services, 1979). The American Academy of Pediatrics has recognized that substantial numbers of children are not getting adequate physical activity during the growing years, even though research has shown that physical activity can decrease degree of overweight (Goldbloom, 1979), improve physical work capacity (Goode, 1979; Lindner & DuRant, 1982), and contribute to intellectual development (Shephard, 1983).

Current research indicates a change in the pattern of children's use of leisure time (Lindrer & Durant, 1982; Sherif & Rattany, 1976; Sutton-Smith & Rosenberg, 1961). Increased time watching television, adult intrusion in organizing children's play (for example, Little League), development of video games, and the role model presented by sedentary adults are speculated reasons for this change in children's exercise behavior (Ryan, 1976). These changes in children's physical activity patterns have resulted in decreases in energy expenditure when compared to children of several years ago (Griffiths & Payne, 1976); this has been accompanied by a concomitant decline in cardiovascular fitness (Shephard, 1982). Reversing the decline in the cardiovascular condition of children may be more difficult than maintaining it (Hertzog et al., 1978).

In 1964 a UNESCO Council recommended a balance of intellectual, physical, moral and aesthetic development, with 1/6 to 1/3 of the total waking time of the child being devoted to physical activity (Bailey, 1976). As with Plato's philosophy of combining a healthy body and a healthy mind, the UNESCO position represents a plea for balance. The Canadian Medical Association (Bailey, 1979) and the U.S. Public Health Service (Green & Horton, 1982) both have stressed the need for increased time for and participation in physical education. Volpe (1979) encouraged more time for physical activity in order to develop the adaptive potential for students. Adaptive behavior, as he defines it, constitutes a fundamental process needed by children and adults to operate effectively as agents in their own development, including cognitive performance.

The Trois Rivieres study clearly indicated that five additional hours of physical activity per week positively affected school performances of public school primary level students. In addition to showing expected gains in maximal oxygen uptake, muscle strength, and physical performance measures, these children also had consistently higher marks in classroom activities than did control students who did not participate in the additional physical activity (Shephard, 1983). This improvement occurred in spite of the reduction in classroom time by 13 to 14 percent. Similarly a ten-year study (1951 to 1960) in Vanves, France showed that increasing the time devoted to physical activity (7 to 8 hours per week) for elementary school children resulted not only in improved health, fitness and motor development, but also in enhanced academic performance, in increased independence of students, and in decreased susceptibility to stress (Bailey, 1976).

Bailey (1973), in a similar school-based study in Saskatoon, also found that students who engaged in additional physical activity increased concentration ability and showed less disruptive behavior than did control students.

Implications for School Health Promotion

Physical education has been a standard component of elementary and secondary education over the past few decades, and, until recently, an increasing number of states required it in education codes. A worsening economy however, resulted in deteriorating physical education facilities in the schools and declining support for physical education. This has been justified on the grounds that greater emphasis needed to be placed on academic subjects in curriculum, and that physical education was not contributing to cognitive performance. The evidence, however, suggests otherwise. The contribution of physical education to academic performance could possibly be made more efficient by integrating the physical education component of the curriculum with components addressing health and lifestyle, rather than tying it to sports, but that is another subject.

The Houston Independent School District hired only 250 new teachers for the 1983–84 academic year. Normally they hire approximately 700. The difference is made up in large part by physical education teachers not being replaced. Physical educators and other professionals concerned with the exercise component of health and development would do well to familiarize themselves with the rationale for its place in the curriculum or at least in the school environment. The evidence reviewed here provides such a rationale, and the objectives of the program could be recast in line with the model proposed earlier in this chapter for school health promotion.

SLEEP*

Sleep is generally defined in such a way that it is tautologically related to cognitive performance. The Sleep Disorders and Research Center at Baylor College of Medicine defines sleep as a state of rest so that vigilance may be maintained during working hours. This definition does not deal with the several neurochemical theories about sleep and wakefulness, nor does it really define what sleep in all its complexity is. It does, however, underscore the need for a restful night's sleep for a school child. It is impossible for the sleep disorders clinician or researcher to imagine a chronically sleep-disturbed child performing well in school.

Normal Sleep

The normal sleep of children is quite a different physiological phenomenon than that of adults, as seen in Figures 10.2 and 10.3. Adults tend to need about seven hours of sleep per night, whereas school-age children re-

*Material on Sleep written by A.S. Korton, Ismet Karacan, and Roger Widmeyer.

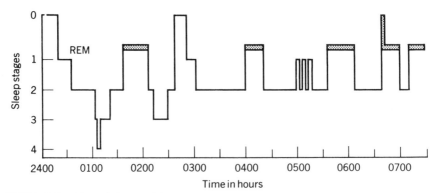

FIGURE 10.2. Normal sleep, adult 40 years. Histogram of all-night sleep recording of normal adult male. Note the relatively short sleep latency and the minimal amount of wakefulness during the night. The early night shows the characteristic progression through the sleep stages into the intial REM period one and one-half hours after sleep onset. The REM periods total 23% of sleep time, Stages 3 and 4 combine for 8%.

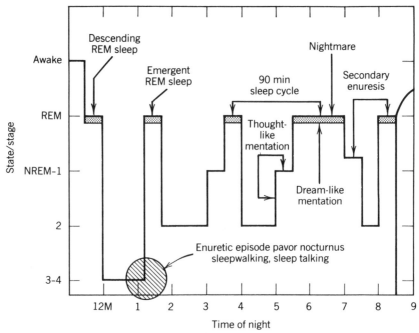

FIGURE 10.3. Idealized histogram, child 8 years. As compared to the adult histogram, note the child's shorter initial REM latency and the larger percentage of REM. Note, too, the much larger percentage of Stages 3 and 4 sleep. (From Guilleminault, C. and Anders, T. Sleep Disorders in Children. *Advances in Pediatrics*, Vol. 22, Chicago, 1976.)

190

quire about nine or ten. As seen in Figure 10.4, adults typically present about 20 percent of their sleep as REM (rapid-eye movement or "dream" sleep), whereas children up to age 10 present about 30 percent REM. Deep sleep, stages three and four, are absent in many adults past the age of 50, and accounts for only about 10 percent of the total night's sleep in 30-year-olds. Deep sleep is crucial for children and makes up about 25 percent of a ten-year-old's sleep.

These three parameters—total sleep time, REM sleep, and stages three and four deep sleep—are the foci of much of the research in childhood sleep. The Baylor clinic has found that much of the daytime impairment a child may experience can be traced to an abnormality within one or more of these parameters.

As Figure 10.4 illustrates, a number of changes occur in sleep patterns as one progresses from infancy into adulthood (Williams, Karacan, & Hursch, 1974). Total sleep time gradually decreases from 700 minutes per day shortly after birth, to 600 minutes per day at one year of age, and continues to decline—somewhat rapidly during the first decade of life. A child

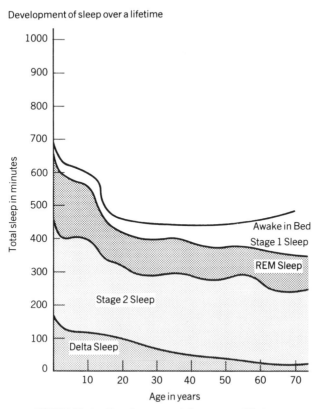

FIGURE 10.4.   Development of sleep over a lifetime.

of five or six will usually protest being told to take a nap—a further indication of the declining physiological need for sleep.

REM sleep dramatically decreases over age also. The most common
question about infant REM is, What could a newborn baby be dreaming
about? We do not know; we only know the compelling urge for infants to
have REM sleep, including REM-onset sleep (the single most most important sign of narcolepsy in the adult).

Deep sleep is the time when the human growth hormone is secreted.
The need for children to have a large percentage of this sleep is obvious.
But as the common name for stages three and four indicates, this sleep is
deep and restful; the appropriate sleep for an organism that has spent
much of its time growing, trying new muscle tissue, continually moving
while awake. Paradoxically it is also the sleep when most pathological
sleep-related conditions are presented in children: night terrors, sleep-
talking, sleep-walking, and enuresis. These are not disorders of REM
sleep, as commonly thought.

The quality and quantity of sleep are essentially the same for both boys
and girls (Williams et al., 1974). One of the few differences is that boys 10
to 12 years of age show a larger number of sleep stages during the night
than do girls of the same ages. During puberty—even during the menstrual cycle—the sleep polysomnograms of both sexes are virtually indis-
tinguishable.

The Sleep Disorders

In order to explore sleep and sleep disorders in children, and the effect
sleep can have on cognitive ability in children and adolescents, we will
summarize the prevalent child-related syndromes as enumerated in the
Association of Sleep Disorders Centers' Classification of Sleep and Arousal
Disorders (Rollwarg, 1979).

1.   Disorders of Initiating and Maintaining Sleep (The Insomnias).   Insomnia is rare in children. One typically thinks of the insomniac lying
awake for hours on end, tossing and turning, waiting for the blissful moment of sleep onset. Although not so rare in the anxiety-ridden adult, the
disorder of *initiating* sleep with difficulty is not often seen in children. It is
not necessarily that stresses and worries are less acute in children—their
concerns are every bit as real to them—only that their need for sleep may
be more physiologically pressing. Certain parasomnias (to be discussed
shortly) may cause difficulty *maintaining* sleep (certainly a type of insomnia), and so they may secondarily be labeled as insomnia complaints.

It should be noted that very few systematic studies involving sleep deprivation in children exist: no reputable university or research center's human subjects committee would allow the same protocols for children and
adults. Much of the literature, then, is built on case histories and common-

sensical approaches to presented complaints. The conclusions of the clinicians, however, seem viable to almost all sleep experts.

The definitive study to date on sleep loss in children (Carskadon et al., 1980) showed there was daytime sleepiness when the volunteers in the study were involved with their performance tasks (as there would well be at school work); however, during physical activity periods, vigilance was maintained quite easily by all the children. The twelve children in the study (age range 11.7 to 14.6) were not totally sleep deprived, but were allowed 20-minute nap periods across the thirty-six-hours covered by the study. If the subjects did not go to sleep during the performance test batteries (also administered, as were the naps, at two-hour intervals), results of their tests showed no significant decrement. If sleep, or "microsleeps," occurred during the test periods, significant decrements were seen on the test performances. The study was limited to the thirty-six hour period, plus the adaptation night and the return-to-baseline night.

Carskadon's results show that disturbed nighttime sleep can cause impaired daytime intellectual functioning (Williams et al., 1974). As mentioned earlier, insomnia is extremely rare in children. Hauri and Olmstead (1980) found the largest number of insomniac children to be depressed, the next largest segment to have attention-deficit problems, and a third group to have conduct disorders.

The issue of whether insomnia is a primary disorder or a secondary symptom still remains unresolved. The sleep disorders discussed in this chapter are presented four times more often to child psychiatrists than to pediatricians and family practitioners (Bixler, Kales, & Soldatos, 1979).

Drug-dependency insomnia in adults is frequently seen in sleep disorders clinics. Kales describes a case of severe insomnia that developed in a child kept too long on increasing doses of trimeprazine syrup originally prescribed by a pediatrician in response to complaints of moderate "hyperactivity" in the late afternoons (Kales, Soldatos, & Kales, 1980). In the occasional case in which a hypnotic or benzodiazepine must be prescribed for a child, weekly evaluations must also be done; long-term prescriptions for sleep medications for children are never advisable.

2.   Disorders of Excessive Somnolence (The Hypersomnias).   Children presenting fatigue, irritability, and lowered mental functioning during the day may be showing symptoms of insomnia, but more probably these children are exhibiting one of the hypersomnias.

Sleep apnea—caused either by a central nervous system inhibition of respiratory effort or a chronic upper-airway obstruction—is most often seen in males over the age of 40; the symptoms, however, are the same in children. This cessation of breathing during sleep causes the victim to awaken every 30 to 60 seconds (marked by an EEG arousal on the sleeprecording) gasping for breath. The oxygen saturation in the blood falls drastically. There is gross thoracic and body movement. The child, however, is not aware of the arousals. Sleep is fragmented, with a substantial decrease in deep sleep. Daytime fatigue is the most common complaint.

Guilleminault's (1976) study of nine children with apnea included results worthy of attention by school personnel. Although disrupted sleep accounted for excessive daytime sleepiness, 35 percent of the children were diagnosed as "borderline retarded;" the sleep apnea/hypersomnia had a greater impact on intellectual functioning than narcolepsy (to be discussed presently). To appreciate the severity of the syndrome, consider the mean of 319 apnea episodes per night in Guilleminault's population. In sleep apnea, proper diagnosis and treatment always result in significantly improved daytime functioning and increased IQ scores.

Narcolepsy is another disorder of excessive somnolence increasingly seen in children and adolescents. Previous studies have indicated that the usual age of onset is between the ages of 15 and 25, but 20 percent of adult narcoleptics recite a history of daytime fatigue and one or more of the "narcoleptic tetrad" (cataplexy, sleep paralysis, hypnogogic hallucinations, and sleep attacks) before the age of 11. Although full blown cases of narcolepsy which present all of the narcoleptic tetrad are rare, school personnel need to be aware of the warning signs of the disease. A family history usually reveals a strong familial link in narcolepsy. It is treatable with methylphenidate and a regimen of short, carefully scheduled naps.

A child presenting hypersomnolent symptoms during school should be evaluated by a sleep disorders center to differentiate the several possible disorders—sleep apnea, narcolepsy, or psychophysiological excessive somnolence. Especially with children, an accurate assessment of the dysfunction requires information from several sources, including parents, teachers and child. Commonly, parent and child reports differ.

3. Disorders of the Sleep-wake Schedule. This ASDC third group of disorders is extremely rare in children. Certainly, there are children who suffer along with their parents from "jet lag," but there are few children who experience "work shift" or chronically changing sleep-wake schedules.

4. Dysfunctions Associated with Sleep, Sleep Stages, or Partial Arousals (The Parasomnias). This group of disorders represent the most common complaints presented to pediatricians, child psychiatrists, and school health officials (Anders, Carskadon, & Dement, 1980; Anders, Carskadon, Dement, & Harvey, 1978; Busby, Firestone, & Pivik, 1981; Simonds & Humbarto, 1982). Sleep-talking, sleep-walking, and night-terrors, though worrisome to parents, will usually in time disappear from the child's sleep. Sleep-talking is seldom more than mumbling and incoherencies, and it does not disturb a child's sleep architecture. As do the other parasomnias discussed here, sleep-talking originates in stage four sleep and should not be confused with nightmares ("dream anxiety attacks" as the ASDC terms them). Sleep-terrors are remarkable for several reasons: the child's scream, the immediate lapse back into sleep if awakened, and the total absence of recall after the event. Nightmares occur in REM sleep, and the memory of a particularly bad dream may linger for days and weeks. Only 1 to 6 percent of children present night-terrors, and most children will outgrow this parasomnia by the age of five.

Sleep-walking (somnambulism) also occurs in stage four, is not recalled afterwards, and is also usually outgrown by school age. If frequent attacks of sleep-walking occur, the child's sleeping quarters should be made accident proof.

All of the above disorders have been treated with imipramine, but drug therapy is not recommended unless the disorder is severe enough to disrupt home life and affect the child's daytime wakefulness.

Enuresis (bed-wetting) is unsettling for the child and the parents. Of course occasional enuretic attacks are common and to be expected up to the age of three, and not uncommon to the age of five. After that, a differential diagnosis must be made and some therapy attempted. Impairment of daytime functioning is generally slight. Many adolescents who present enuresis do not have confirmed psychopathology. Nevertheless supportive therapy is usually helpful. There is a correlation between transient daytime stress and accompanying attacks in the evening.

Dream anxiety attacks (REM sleep dysfunctions) can occasionally severely disturb a child's sleep and consequently impair his or her cognitive abilities the following day.

A sometimes troubling occurrence for the adolescent male is frequency of nocturnal emissions ("wet dreams"), but nocturnal erections and emissions are normal phenomena during REM sleep in males through most of their lifetime (Karacan, Hursch, Williams & Littell, 1972; Williams, Karacan, Hursch & Davis, 1972).

Sleep Hygiene; Implications for School Health Promotion

Karacan and associates (1975) thoroughly studied the sleep patterns of two adolescent age groups: those 13–15, and those 16–19 years old. The patterns of these early adolescent groups showed quite a number of significant differences from those of 10–12 years-olds. Normal childhood sleep gradually changed to early adulthood sleep patterns—notably decreased time in bed and total sleep time. Time in bed and total sleeptime continued to decrease in the later adolescent group also.

From the standpoint of the earlier definition of night time sleep as a period of rest which promotes daytime vigilance, 10 to 12 years of age appears to be the ideal age for sleep: children in that range typically sleep soundly and long enough to be fully alert all day. They go to sleep easily and wake refreshed without the aid of "zeitgebars"—clocks, meals, and other indicators of time. Their circadian rhythm is well-established in that they go to bed and awake about the same time each day. The adolescent period, on the other hand, is marked by irregularities: a changing endocrine system, a quickening of social life and inherent pressures, an increased work schedule, and so on. Picture the stereotypical teenager arising in the morning, protesting, grouchy, sleepy-eyed, stumbling about trying to get his or her work day begun.

Even though many sleep experts believe most of us could get by comfortably on a little less sleep each day, there is certainly some question about whether adolescents get enough sleep (Carskadon et al., 1981). Teenagers, for example, are wont to make up for their "sleep deprivation" on the weekends, and most sleep quite long in the mornings, albeit they often have later bedtimes on the weekends. This see-saw schedule in a teen's sleep is far from ideal (Bonnet, 1982). A regular bedtime and arising time strengthens circadian cycling; a more natural wake/activity time and a distinct sleep/rest time emerge, with much less dependence on "zeitgebars." The somewhat sleep-deprived adolescent (studying late during the weekdays, socializing late on weekends, occasionally trying to "catch up" by sleeping late Saturday and Sunday and napping) is, in truth, creating a perpetual hypersomnolence (Salzarulo & Chevalier, 1983). (Studying before bed is probably beneficial: deep sleep stages three and four occur more regularly and sooner in the night.)

Interaction of Sleep and Other Lifestyle Factors

The typical high schooler's diet is not conducive to heathful sleep patterns. Caffeine is well known for the disturbing effect it has on sleep; yet it remains a pervasive additive in most people's daily food and drink intake, and especially in that of teenagers. As little as one cola or one cup of cocoa or coffee in the evening can prolong sleep onset.

Caloric intake also affects sleep. Chronic dieters (as many teenagers are) appear to sleep poorly; overeaters generally sleep soundly. Naturally, a median should be struck and the appropriate caloric intake for age and size should be considered in sleep problems. Some investigators recommend a light dairy product as a bedtime snack, cheese or milk for example, because of the natural tryptophans involved. The ritual itself may promote short sleep latency.

Nicotine is a central nervous system stimulant; smokers generally sleep more poorly than nonsmokers. Sleep is significantly improved in smokers who quit.

Although a light cocktail or glass of wine may relax some insomniacs, alcohol generally destroys sleep architecture by suppressing both deep sleep and REM sleep. Additionally, over indulgers may awake for prolonged periods in the middle of the night.

Few systematic studies have been done on the effects of street drugs on sleep. Marijuana has essentially the effect on sleep that alcohol does. A plethora of studies clearly show that hypnotics and stimulants eventually destroy the natural sleep architecture and circadian rhythms; it is safe to assume that street drugs do likewise.

Several studies have shown that exercise deepens sleep. Professional athletes have a significantly high percentage of stages three and four sleep. Regularity, however, is important. A sudden increase of exercise has little affect on sleep overall. Morning exercise appears to have less affect on sleep onset and stages three and four than does afternoon or early evening exercise. Ideally early evening exercise could aid in diminishing the amount of psychological stress in an adolescent as well as aid in initiating sleep.

Finally a sleeper should sleep in a room that is environmentally conducive to sleep. A hot room adversely affects sleep; but a room that is too cold does also. Bright lights and noises disturb sleep, even if the sleeper is seemingly unaware of them. Studies have indicated that women are more sensitive to noise than men; that noise during REM is incorporated into the dream and is thus less likely to arouse the sleeper; and that noise arousals from sleep largely depend on the sleep stage—that is, it is more difficult to be aroused from stage four than from stage two. Nevertheless, noises such as those to which adolescents often expose themselves during sleep— radios, stereos, television—usually cause an EEG arousal.

A harmonious blend of diet, exercise and sleep will certainly benefit the child or adolescent in daytime vigilance and therefore in cognitive performance. The schools, therefore, can justify allocations of at least enough time and resources in the school health program to promote adjustments of behavior in these three areas, although more research is needed to define what the optimal adjustments are for specific ages and socioeconomic groups.

STRESS*

Interaction of Stress, Social Behavior and Academic Performance

In considering the relationship between stress and school performance, the question is whether stress, as reflected in reports and measures of test or performance anxiety and negative ratings of school and classroom environments, has an important influence on behavioral adjustment and academic performance. Behavioral adjustment, social competency, and school performance are highly interactive and are often impossible to separate satisfactorily.

Biologic potential or basic aptitude is extremely hard to isolate because most standard tests, such as IQ assessments, are subject to considerable

*Material on Stress written by Gene Stainbrook.

negative biasing. Negative biasing leading to performance deficits both on achievement and aptitude tests can derive from two general types of factors. A short-term situational anxiety about performance is generally termed "test" or "performance" anxiety. In this, the individual may be highly motivated to perform, but because of constitutional factors such as a tendency toward CNS hyperarousal and physiologic overreactivity, compounded by pressures to excel from parents or teachers, often fails to perform well on competitive examinations. A second factor that can contribute to poor performance on aptitude tests is lassitude or low motivation. This lassitude can occur infrequently or chronically. A prior history of failures leading to low self-esteem, a feeling of pessimism and hopelessness and lack of positive reinforcement will have a negative influence on motivation and performance. In short, stress in home and school settings is an important factor in the motivation and performance of children.

Assessment of Test Anxiety

The effects of anxiety or arousal on acute-situational performance has been studied for many years (Barrios, Hartmann, & Shigetouri, 1971; Becker, 1982; Tryon, 1980). In general, performance on tasks, especially more complex cognitive tasks, tends to follow the form of the inverted U-shaped curve (Yerkes & Dodson, 1908; Broadhurst, 1959; Welford, 1976). At low levels, performance is low; it reaches an asymptote at some intermediate level, and at high levels of stress performance drops off markedly. This relationship has been replicated numerous times in a wide variety of learning and performance situations. Factors that commonly increase stress are time pressure, lack of control over the conditions of testing and actual or perceived threat regarding the outcomes.

Experimental Studies of Arousal and Performance

In a number of investigations, experimentally increased stress has been found to improve efficiency on simple tasks but to decrease performance on complex tasks (Krohne & Laux, 1982). This is comparable to the finding on sleep deprivation reported in the previous section. Studies also have been carried out to examine the effects of experimentally induced fear of failure on performance (Child, 1954; Mandler & Sarason, 1952; Sarason, Davidson, Lighthall, Waite & Ruebush, 1952). It has been observed that anxiety generated by expectation of failure was related to responses that were defensive and not relevant to the task.

Stress induced by fear of failure also has been related to poorer performance on learning and recall of nonsense syllables, digit symbol substitution, arithmetic, sentence formation, digit span, card sorting, and reaction time (Friedman, Das, & O'Conner, 1981).

The effects of stress generated by time pressure and task complexity has frequently been examined with simultaneous variations in the two components of stress to measure their effects on physiologic responses and performance (Doerr & Hokanson, 1965; Fiske & Maddi, 1961). Typically a linear relationship has been found between the level of stress and physiologic response, and an inverted U-shaped relationship between stress and task performance.

A number of studies suggest that minority children tend to react to examiners and test situations with greater suspicion and fear and consequently to perform below their potentials (Katz, 1963; Stattler, 1970; Riegler & Butterfield, 1968; Ziegler, Abelson, Trickett, & Seitz, 1982).

Preexamination arousal has been found to correlate with level of aspiration, estimates of exam difficulty, and ratings of personal competency (Becker, 1982). Success-oriented students had anxiety levels that rose early and dropped before examinations, but failure-oriented students had anxiety levels that also rose early but continued to remain high before examinations.

The literature on test anxiety has been reviewed recently by Tryon (1980). He concluded that high test anxiety consistently has been negatively associated with scores on aptitude and achievement tests and with grade-point averages.

Environmental Stress

1. **Schools and Classroom Settings.**   From William James' *Talks to Teachers* in 1899 (1962) to B.F. Skinner's 1965 essay, "Why Teachers Fail," psychologists have offered advice on how best to structure learning environments. Both James and Skinner advocated nonaversive learning environments. The negative effects of threat and fear on motivation and performance are well documented (Krohne & Laux, 1982). Determining the aversiveness and stress in school environments, however, requires getting honest feedback from students, which often threatens administrators and teachers.

For many young adolescents the transition from elementary school to junior high school is very stressful. If potential emotional adjustment problems are not anticipated and reduced shortly after their onset, they can seriously compromise academic performance.

In a study by Armstrong (1964), 45 percent of the boys and girls with high elementary-school grades performed only at a fair or poor level in junior high school. Finger and Silverman (1966) supported the earlier findings with their study and noted as well that many students whose performance initially dropped did not subsequently recover in performance. These observations suggest that the stress of coping with pervasive social and environmental changes and challenges divert attention from course work and lower motivation for academic performance. Hamburg (1974) has discussed this issue both from the point of view of motivation and of differences in cognitive functioning between early and late adolescence.

Perry (1982) recently conducted a survey of school environments, basing her classification of "healthy" environments on four measures: student absenteeism, illegal absenteeism, suspension rates, and referral rates. Academic performance was not measured. Phillips (1978) examined the relationships between student ratings of the stressfulness of school environments and their academic performance in public schools. He found that school procedural differences influenced the reported number of stressors and overall perceived levels of stress at the schools. Stress levels were negatively correlated both with achievement and intelligence test scores. Children in minority groups and those from low SES families tended to rate school as more stressful and perform more poorly.

Size of schools has been found to correlate negatively with the number of activities that students participate in (Barker & Gump, 1964) and with expressed attitudes of belonging (Williams, 1967).

Classroom environments have been assessed by direct observation and by student ratings on standardized scales. Stallings (1975) rated first to third grade classrooms with a detailed observational system. Systematic relationships were found between qualities of the classrooms and the behavior and academic performance of children. The structure of the classroom was a better predictor of reading and math achievement than the aptitude scores at school entry. Students in structured classes had higher achievement scores than those in flexible classes. Yet students in flexible classes had higher nonverbal reasoning scores, worked longer on their own, and were absent less often.

Moos (1974, 1979) has developed and standardized scales to rate environments, including school classrooms. Three social climate domains consistently have been found to be important: relationship, personal development, and system maintenance and change. These relate significantly to ratings of mood, satisfaction and behavior.

Trickett and Moos (1979) used the Classroom Environment Scale (CES) with high school students. Students from classes that rated high in competition reported that they learned more than did those from classes rated lower in competition. However, students from classes rated high in teacher support and student involvement felt more satisfied and had fewer absences.

While studies comparing the average characteristics of classrooms to group behavior are important, it is also useful to know how a particular individual adapts to and performs in different settings, or what the person environment fit (PEF) is. Several authors have investigated this issue (Grimes & Allinsmith, 1961; Kelly, 1979; Reiss & Martell, 1974). A consistent finding has been that more creative children learn better and report higher self esteem in more open and flexible clasrooms. On the other hand children who tended to be more distractable and show poorer concentration learned more in structured classrooms.

The assessment of positive and negative stress-producing aspects of school and classroom environment both by expert observers and by student ratings appears to be a promising area of research. For a better understanding of the reasons for good and poor student social behavior and academic performance school environments warrant more systematic analysis. At present, the relationships between specific school and classroom characteristics and student social behavior and academic performance are highly suggestive but have not been examined systematically enough to provide explicit guidelines for structural and process changes.

2. Stress in Homes and Family Settings. Families or home settings influence the social-behavioral adjustment and academic motivation of children. When home events are physically or emotionally damaging they can have short-term and sometimes long-lasting effects on behavioral adjustment and school performance. More minor events or daily hassles, if perceived to be aversive, can also be sources of stress that burden physical and emotional reserves and create a mental/emotional load which, through decreased attention and motivation, impair learning and school performance. Adults in the lowest income levels report more life changes and a significantly larger number of aversive or socially undesirable events than those in middle and upper income levels (Dohrenwend, 1973; Gersten, Langer, Eisenberg, & Orzeck, 1974). Consistent with this observation, children from low income families also experience more negative life changes than those from higher income families (Coddington, 1972; Grad & Johnson, 1980; Sandler & Ramsey, 1980).

Situational stresses within families have been examined in relationship to child abuse by Justice and Duncan (1976). They found that abusive parents reported more recent life changes than control parents. It was suggested that parents who undergo a life crisis often become exhausted, have a decreased ability to adjust, and are at increased risk of losing control.

Life change scores were found related to a number of psychological problems by Gesten et al. (1977). An index of total life changes and in particular a subgroup of negative life changes were both correlated with measures of anxiety, conflict with parents, fighting, delinquency, self-destructive tendencies, and learning problems. Hotaling et al. (1978) observed that level of life change was positively related to high scores on a psychological problem index.

Sandler and Block (1979) compared children judged to have adjustment problems by teachers and parents to normals on an index of life stress which included only items over which the child had no apparent control.

Children exhibiting a high rate of behavioral problems experienced more life changes, had higher life change unit scores, and a greater number of undesirable events. In another study, Sandler and Ramsay (1980) observed that family troubles, financial setbacks, legal problems, and entrance events (for example, addition of a new person to the family) were associated with poorer child adjustment on the basis of parent ratings. Furthermore, Grad and Johnson (1980) found measures of negative life change to correlate with several indicies of adjustment. These included reported visits to a school counselor, reports of personal problems, and self-rated ability to cope with personal problems. Johnson and McCutcheon (1980) found negative life changes to correlate significantly with measures of anxiety, depression, and a measure of general maladjustment. High levels of negative change were also associated with an external locus of control orientation. Thus the higher the level of negative change the less subjects perceived themselves as having control over environmental events.

Findings are also available that directly address the effects of stress on intelligence as measured by standardized intelligence (IQ) or aptitude tests. In the NINCDS Collaborative Study the impact of biological and social factors on intelligence was studied (Broman, Nichols, & Kennedy, 1975). Relationships were found between IQ and the family characteristics of income, parental education, parental employment, mother's marital status, and father presence in the home. Further analysis of these data has examined the relationship of IQ to stress, measured with a composite index of family characteristics and negative life events (Brown & Rosenbaum, 1983). A strong association was found between scores on the stress index and IQ, with high stress inversely related to IQ. In general stress levels were higher in low income families. The results of these studies strongly suggest that the frequency of life change events in families, particularly when they are viewed to be negative or stressful, are often associated with behavioral adjustment problems, decremented school performance, and lowered intelligence test scores in children. Therefore interventions that aim at improving sociobehavioral competence and academic achievement must give careful and systematic attention to stress in families.

Stress Management and Social and Academic Performance

Several types of interventions have been conducted in school settings that can be considered to be conducive to stress management or stress-resistance. These approaches have been used widely with children who have exhibited behavioral adjustment problems and associated school performance deficits.

During the past 10 years, some of the most popular and successful methods of treating psychological and emotional problems in adults have been variants of a procedure termed Rational-Emotive Therapy (RET) which was developed by Ellis (1961). A rationale emotive education (REE) curriculum based on the RET model has been developed and used with students. A number of reports of outcomes on the use of the REE curriculum have been published (Knaus, 1977). Albert (1971) found that REE reduced anxiety and increased positive classroom behaviors in fifth-grade students. Short-term decreases in test anxiety and improvements in self-esteem in children were observed by Knaus and Bokor (1975). Finally, participation in a six-month REE program by 17- and 18-year-old, inner city students was found to increase self-concept and school attendance and decrease drop-out rates (Knaus & Bloch, 1976). Most of these studies report only short-term pre-post program outcomes and did not use comparable enough control groups to rule out general positive demand effects. Nevertheless, the short-term outcomes suggest that more work should be done with this program.

Two other curricula that can be considered stress resistance building programs have been developed and tested. One is the Social Problem-Solving (SPS) Curriculum developed by Spivak and Shure (1976). A second is the Social Problem-Solving Program developed by Cowen and his colleagues (Weissberg, Gesten, Liebenstein, Schmid, & Hutton, 1980). Both of these programs are designed to help young children learn to solve interpersonal problems through a competency building approach. Parents, teachers, and other professionals or volunteers working in schools have been trained to use these curricula.

Successful results using the SPS program have been reported for students ranging from young children to early adolescents. In comparison studies, students trained with the SPS program were observed to display greater gains than controls in level of social problem-solving skills and behavioral adjustment (Shure & Spivak, 1980; Spivak, Platt, and Shure, 1976). Children who achieved higher levels of SPS skills also showed less impatience, hyperemotionality, and aggresive behavior both in school and at home.

The Rochester Social Problem-Solving Program (RSPS) has evolved out of the Primary Mental Health Project (PMHP) (Cowen, 1975). Through teacher referral and systematic screening, children with behavioral problems that interfere with social adjustment and academic performance are referred to the program. Children referred for assistance get help from nonprofessional child aides who have been trained in the use of curriculum materials and procedures and work under close professional supervision. At present, the PMHP is located in more than 20 Rochester-area schools and comparable programs have been initiated in more than 300 schools in 80 different school districts in the U.S. (Cowen, Spinelli, Wrighty & Weissberg, 1983). Outcomes of this program have been carefully documented and summarized in several reports (Cowen, 1975; Cowen, Gesten, & Wilson, 1979; Weissberg, Cowen, Lotyzawski, & Gesten, 1983). Weissberg et al. (1983) have provided a recent summary of the program outcomes. The children were assessed prior to and after program completion on measures of social-emotional adjustment, achievement motivation, and level of learning problems. Ratings were made by teachers, aides, and supervising mental health professionals. The intervention consisted of 20 to 25 individual contacts of 30–45 minutes' duration with a child aide. Training sessions occurred once or twice weekly.

The main findings were that the program reduced shy-anxious and acting-out behavior, and increased competency in frustration tolerance, adaptive assertiveness and peer sociability. These outcomes were consistent with earlier reports of PMHP outcomes (Cowen, 1975; Cowen, Gesten, & Wilson, 1979). It was also noted that the program was generally more effective in reducing shy-anxious behavior than in decreasing acting-out, aggressive behaviors. This is an important finding in light of the outcomes of longitudinal studies by Kellam (1975) who has found that poor behavioral adjustment, in particular acting-out and aggressive behavior, was related to learning problems and later substance use.

Screening for early behavioral adjustment problems and social skill deficits, since they are frequently related to learning problems and poor academic performance, seems highly advisable. Moreover, the wisdom of implementing low-cost intervention services to remedy or reduce problems as soon as detected in schools or even preschool settings rests on sound logic and an increasingly firm empirical base.

Relaxation and Biofeedback Training

In addition to the curricula and training methods for developing and strengthening behavioral and social skill competencies, other methods that show considerable promise for reducing stress and improving learning performance are relaxation and biofeedback interventions.

Stress management programs, in which relaxation training and biofeedback methods are important components, are being used increasingly in the treatment of physical and emotional disorders. Relaxation and biofeedback training programs have been found useful and cost-effective in the treatment of mild to moderate affective disorders, most notably anxiety, and in psychosomatic disorders such as insomnia and headaches (Butler, 1978; Fotopaulos & Sunderland, 1978; Rosenbaum, 1981). As noted previously, anxiety, if severe and prolonged, can be a serious block to social competency and scholastic performance. In addition recurrent headaches and insomnia, which are both often sensitive indicators of stress overload, can also interfere with social and academic capabilities. Furthermore, biofeedback has been found useful in the management of hyperactivity, a common early childhood behavioral problem which interferes with learning and performance (Linn & Hodge, 1980; Sandvick, 1981).

Relaxation and biofeedback training also have been found to enhance academic performance more directly. Biofeedback has been shown to improve examination performance of test-anxious college students (Collatz &

Gordon, 1980). Finally, Carter (1981, 1983), in a large study, has observed that stress management, using electromyographic (EMG) biofeedback training and providing relaxation tapes, significantly improved a number of academic skills in children with learning problems. Compared to matched controls, children who received training showed significant gains in IQ, math, reading, spelling, auditory memory and penmanship. Combined biofeedback training and listening to tapes was the most effective intervention. Children in the treatment groups received three 20-minute sessions each week for six weeks. The sessions were conducted by teachers in school settings. Most of the improvements at the end of the intervention were found to have been retained at a 10-month follow-up. Treatment results from over 400 children suggest that a combination of biofeedback/relaxation procedures implemented by teachers in public schools effectively helps children achieve and maintain relaxed attentiveness and improve academic performance in a number of important areas.

The impressive results of this program and the relative ease and low cost of implementing the relaxation-training component suggest that much wider utilization of relaxation training for children, both with and without identified learning problems, would be highly advisable.

SUMMARY AND CONCLUSIONS

Those responsible for appropriating health and educational resources are interested in the extent to which such appropriations will result in attaining important health and educational outcomes. School health education programs have focused largely on improving health outcomes by modifying behaviors associated with diseases frequently not manifested until mid- to late-adulthood (for example, cardiovascular disease, cancer). Especially given increasing interest in designing educational reforms to improve the educational achievement of American students, those responsible for appropriating educational resources (including curriculum time) may legitimately be more interested in improving educational outcomes by modifying health-related behaviors. Indeed reviewed in this chapter is considerable evidence that dietary, exercise, sleep, and stress-related behaviors directly influence the cognitive performance of students.

For example, although severe undernutrition experienced during the first year of life may impair intellectual functioning permanently, the intellectual effects of undernutrition during the second and subsequent years seem reversible. Several studies have shown that undernourished children perform less well than their well-nourished couterparts on global measures of short-term cognitive performance. Dietary habits influence short-term attention, memory, emotional affect, and social functioning, which may exacerbate or be exacerbated by deprived social environments. Iron consumption among school-aged children in the U.S. is far below recommended levels, and about 20 percent of adolescents suffer iron-deficiency anemia. Iron-deficiency has been shown to reduce attention, concentration, memory, and achievement.

Although the excitatory effects of caffeine among adults is well-documented, we know little about the effects of caffeine on the concentration and cognitive performance of children. Similarly, although the rapid rise and fall of blood-sugar in response to concentrated sugar consumption is well documented, we know little about the effects of sugar on the cognitive performance of children. Relatedly, despite the fact that consumption of caffeinated and highly sugared soft drinks among children has increased dramatically during the last few decades, little is known about the combined effects of these substances on children's cognitive performance. Research conducted to date, however, does not support the hypothesis that sugar consumption contibutes to behavioral problems among children, or that food additives contibute to childhood hyperactivity.

Fasting (for example, skipping breakfast or lunch) causes greater physiological consequences among children than among adults. While fasting may increase vigilance, it reduces reflective and analytical abilities. Little is known about the short-term effects of the opposite behavior, overeating. Although many children experience somnolence after eating, the short-term effects of eating or overeating on cognitive performance are unknown. The long-term consequence of overeating, obesity, is particularly prevalent in the United States. Anywhere from 20 to 40 percent of lower socioeconomic children, and 3 to 25 percent of higher socio-economic children are thought to be obese. Among these children, poor self-esteem and frequent fasting may diminish cognitive performance.

A growing body of evidence suggests that physical activity improves brain function, and, consequently, may improve cognitive performance among young and old alike. Exericse increases cerebral blood flow, as well as glucose uptake and metabolism; and the brains of sensory-enriched animals exhibit significant anatomical and biochemical differences that seem indicative of a more efficient nervous system. Among young children, the establishment of neuromuscular and psychomotor skills provides an important foundation for the development of more sophisticated perceptual and cognitive behaviors. Exercise also may improve cognitive performance among young and old alike by heightening levels of alertness, increasing capacities to undertake physical and mental work, increasing perceptions of self-efficacy and self-esteem, and reducing the intensity of responses to emotionally laden stimuli. Indeed, several controlled studies have indicated that specific school-based physical activity programs not only increased maximal oxygen uptake and other physical performance measures, but also improved concentration, mathematics, reading, and writing abilities, and reduced disruptive behaviors and susceptibility to stress.

The evidence is quite clear that quantity and quality of sleep also are important determinants of cognitive performance, yet sleep is a topic much neglected by educational researchers and health educators alike. Many adolescents experience a see-saw pattern in their sleep schedules: frequently studying late on weekdays or socializing late on week-ends, and trying to "catch-up" by sleeping late on Saturdays and Sundays. This pattern may reduce both the quantity and quality of sleep by disrupting the establishment of circadian rhythms; and consequently may result in a state of insidious, chronic hypersomnolence. Chronic dieting and substances frequently used by adolescents, including caffeine, alcohol, tobacco, and marijuana, may also significantly diminish the quality of sleep. On the other hand, regular exercise and a sleeping environment protected from temperature extremes, bright lights, and noise markedly improve the quality of sleep.

Finally, the amount and nature of stress experienced by young people at home and in school, and their capacities to cope with stress, are important determinants of cognitive performance. Although some stress may be needed to stimulate performance, excessive or inappropriate stress can reduce the motivation as well as the actual ability to perform. Stressful events in the home or family can cause short-term as well as long-lasting impairments in behavioral adjustment and cognitive performance. Major family life changes experienced by young people (for example, parental discord or divorce, moving, etc.), as well as more minor daily problems (if excessively numerous and adverse) may decrease school attention, motivation, and performance. Few studies have attempted to determine the extent to which the quality of family or peer relationships (that is, social support networks) influence cognitive performance.

The psychological climates created in the school and in the clasroom are also powerful determinants of cognitive performance. For many, the transition from elementary to junior high school is especially stressful, and the need to cope with pervasive environmental and social changes may divert attention away from schoolwork, as well as reduce motivation for academic performance. In addition, certain individuals may be well motivated and well prepared to perform on "tests," but may not perform to their potential because of "performance anxiety." The extent to which such anxiety may reduce test performance depends upon the individual's tendency to experience hyperarousal, the degree to which the individual perceives performance expectations to be achievable, and the individual's skills in coping with performance anxiety. Several school-based programs specifically designed to address various sources of stress have reduced general and test anxiety, impatience, hyperemotionality, and aggressive behavior. They have also increased social problem-solving skills and peer sociability and have improved scores on tests of auditory memory, mathematics, reading, and intelligence.

The greatest potential for improving the cognitive performance of students probably lies in school-based interventions designed to achieve synergistic effects by modifying relevant dietary, exercise, sleep, and stress-related behaviors simultaneously. In addition students may be more inclined to practice health-enhancing behaviors if they are taught to perceive short-term cognitive effects, rather than if they are taught only to anticipate adverse physical effects that may (or may not) result in the somewhat distant future. Similarly educational administrators might be more inclined to allocate school resources to achieve improvements in immediate cognitive performance of their students than only to assure their students' future health.

REFERENCES

Abraham, J.P., & Birren, J.E. (1973). Reaction time as a function of age and behavioral predisposition to coronary heart disease. *Journal of Gerontology, 28,* 471–478.

Adelman, R.C. (1970). An age-dependent modification of enzyme regulation. *Journal of Biological Chemistry, 245,* 1032–1035.

Albert, S. (1971). A study to determine the effectiveness of affective education with fifth grade students. Unpublished master's thesis, New York, Queens College.

American Academy of Pediatrics. (1976). Fitness in the preschool child. *Pediatrics, 58,* 88.

Anders, T., Carskadon, M., & Dement, W. (1980). Sleep and sleepiness in children and adolescents. *Pediatric Clinics of North America, 27,* 29–43.

Anders, T., Carskadon, M., Dement, W., & Harvey, K. (1978). Sleep habits of children and the identification of pathologically sleepy children. *Child Psychiatry and Human Development, 9,* 56–63.

Armstrong, C. (1964). Patterns of achievement in selected New York State schools. Albany: New York State Educational Department.

Bachman, J.G., O'Malley, P.M., & Johnston, J. (1978). *Change and stability in the lives of young men: Adolescence to adulthood* (Vol. 6). Ann Arbor, MI: Institute for Social Research.

Bailey, D. (1979). Inactivity and the Canadian child. In R.G. Goode & R. Volpe (Eds.), *The child and physical activity, Proceedings of a workshop for educational leaders.* Toronto.

Bailey, D.A. (1973). Exercise, fitness and physical education for the growing child. In W.A.R. Orban (Ed.), *Proceedings of The National Conference on Fitness and Health* (pp 13–22). Department of National Health and Welfare, Ottawa.

Bailey, D.A. (1976). The growing child and the need for physical activity. In J.G. Albinson & G.M. Andrews (Eds.), *Child in sport and physical activity* (pp 81–96). Baltimore: University Park Press.

Barker, R.G., & Gump, P.V. (1964). *Big school, small school.* Stanford, CA: Stanford University Press.

Barker, R.G., & Wright, H.F. (1958). *Midwest and Its Children.* Evanston, IL: Row Peterson.

Barrios, B.A., Hartmann, D.P., & Shigetouri C. (1971). Fears and anxieties in children. in E.J. Mash & L.G. Terdal (Eds.), *Behavioral assessment of childhood disorders.* New York: Guilford.

Becker, P. (1982). Fear reactions and achievement behavior of students approaching an examination. In H.W. Krohne & L. Laux (Eds.), *Achievement, stress, and anxiety.* Washington: Hemisphere.

Belka, D., & Williams, H.G. (1978). Canonical relationships among perceptual-motor, perceptual and cognitive behaviors in young, normal children. Unpublished paper. The University of Toledo.

Belka, D., & Williams, H.G. (1979). Prediction of later cognitive behavior from early school perceptual-motor, perceptual and cognitive performances. *Perceptual and Motor Skills, 49,* 131–141.

Birch, H.G. (1972). Malnutrition, learning and intelligence. *American Journal of Public Health, 62*, 773–784.

Birren, J.E., Carden, P.V., & Phillips, S.L. (1963). Reaction time as a function of the cardiac cycle in young adults. *Science, 140*, 195–196.

Bixler, E., Kales, A., & Soldatos, C. (1979). Sleep disorders encountered in medical practice: A national survey of physicians. *Behavioral Medicine, 1*, 1–6.

Blimkie, C.J., Cunningham, D.A., & Leung F.Y. (1977). Urinary catecholamine excretion and lactate concentration in competitive hockey players aged 11 to 23 years. In H. Lavelle & R.J. Shephard (Eds.), *Frontiers of activity and child health* (pp. 313–321). Quebec: Pelican.

Bonnet, M. (1982). Effects of irregular versus regular sleep schedules on performance, and body temperature. *Biological Psychiatry, 14*, 287–296.

Breslow, L., & Enstrom, J.E. (1980). Persistence of health habits and their relationship to mortality. *Preventive Medicine, 9*, 469–483.

Broadhurst, P.L. (1959). The interaction of task difficulty and motivation: The Yerkes-Dodson law revived. *Acta Psychologica, 16*, 321–338.

Broman, S.H., Nichols, P.L., & Kennedy, W.A. (1975). *Preschool IQ: Prenatal and early correlates.* Hillsdale, NJ: Erlbaum.

Brown, B., & Rosenbaum, L. (1983). Stress effects on IQ. Unpublished manuscript.

Brownell, K.D. (1980). Behavioral treatment for obese children and adolescents. In A.J. Stunkard (Ed.), *Obesity.* Philadelphia: W.B. Saunders.

Busby, K., Firestone P., & Pivik, R.T. (1981). Sleep patterns in hyperkinetic and normal children. *Sleep,* 4:366–383.

Butler, F. (1978) *Biofeedback: A survey of the literature.* New York: IFI/Plenum.

Carskadon, M., Harvey, K., & Dement, W. (1981). Sleep loss in young adolescents. *Sleep,* 4(3), 299–312.

Carskadon, M., Harvey, K. Duke, P., Anders, T., Litt, I, & Dement, W. (1980). Pubertal changes in daytime sleepiness. *Sleep, 2*, 453–460.

Carter, J.L. (1983). Application of biofeedback/relaxation procedures to handicapped children: Second Year Report to the U.S. Office of Education. Proj #443CH00207.

Carter, J.L., & Russell, H.L. (1981). Application of biofeedback/relaxation procedures to handicapped children. Report to the U.S. Office of Education. Project #443CH00207.

Charp, F.R. (1976). Relative cerebral glucose uptake of neuronal perikarya and neuropil determined with 2-deoxyglucose in resting and swimming rat. *Brain Research, 110*, 127–139.

Chen, J.C., Warshaw, J.B., & Sanadi D.R. (1972). Regulation of mitochondrial respiration in senescence. *Journal of Cellular Physiology, 80*, 141–148.

Child, I.L. (1954). Personality. In C.P. Stone & Q. McNemar (Eds.), *Annual Review of Psychology,* (pp. 149–70). Stanford, CA: Annual Reviews.

Chissom, B.S., Thomas, J.F., & Biasiotto, J. (1972). Canonical validity of perceptual-motor skills for predicting an academic criterion. *Educational & Psychological Measurement, 32*, 1095–1098.

Coates, T.J., Peterson, A.C., & Perry, C. (1982). Crossing the barriers. In T.J. Coates, et al., *Promoting adolescent health: A dialog on research and practice.* New York: Academic.

Coates, T.J., Perry, C., & Peterson, A.C. (Eds.). (1982). *Promoting adolescent health: A dialog on research and practice.* New York: Academic.

Coddington, R.D. (1972). The significance of life events as etiologic factors in diseases of children, II. A study of a normal population. *Journal of Psychosomatic Research, 16*, 205–213.

Collatz, F.A. & Gordon, K. (1982). Efficacy of EMG biofeedback training in improving examination performance of test-anxious college students (pp. 62–65). *Consolidation and new dimensions: Proceedings of the biofeedback society of America,* Eleventh Annual Meeting.

Collipp, P.J. (1980). Obesity in childhood. In A.J. Stunkard (Ed). *Obesity*. Philadelphia: W.B. Saunders.

Cowen, E.L. (1925). *New ways in school mental health: Early detection and prevention of school maladjustment*. New York: Human Sciences.

Cowen, E.L., Gesten, E.L., & Wilson, A.B. (1979). The primary mental health project (PMHP): Evaluation of current program effectiveness. *American Journal of Community Psychology, 7*, 293–303.

Cowen, E.L., Spinelli, A., Wright, S., & Weissberg, R.P. (1983). Continuing dissemination of a school-based mental health program. *Professional Psychiatry, 13*, 118–127.

Cox, J.P., Evans, J. & Jameson, J. (1979). Aerobic power and tonic heart rate response to psychological stressors. *Personality & Social Psychology Bulletin, 5*, 160–165.

Cravioto, T., DeLicardie, E.R., & Birch, H.G. (1966). Nutrition, growth and neurointegrative development. An experimental and ecological study. *Pediatrics, 38*, 319–372.

Dickie, N., & Bender, A. (1982). Breakfast and performance in school children. *British Journal of Nutrition, 48*, 483–496.

Dobbing, J., & Sands, J. (1973). Quantitative growth and development of human brain. *Archives of Disease in Childhood, 48*, 757–767.

Doerr, H.O., & Hokanson, J.E. (1985). A relation between heart rate and performance in children. *Journal of Personality and Social Psychology, 2*, 70–76.

Dohrenwend, B.S. (1973). Life events as stressors: A methodological inquiry. *Journal of Health and Social Behavior, 14*, 167–175.

Ellis, A., & Harper, R. (1961). *A Guide to Rationale Living*. New York: Prentice-Hall.

Evans, R.I., Hill, P.C., Raines, B.E., & Henderson, A.H. (1981). Current behavioral, social and educational programs in control of smoking: A selective, critical review. In S. Weiss, A. Herd, & B. Fox (Eds.), *Perspectives on Behavioral Medicine*. New York: Academic.

Evans, R., & Raines, B. (1982). Control and prevention of smoking in adolescents: A psychosocial perspective. In T. Coates, A. Peterson, & C. Perry (Eds.), *Promoting adolescent health: A dialog on research and practice*. New York: Academic.

Finger, J., & Silverman, M. (1966). Changes in academic performance in the junior high school. *Personnel Guidance Journal, 45*, 157–164.

Fiske, D.W., & Maddi, S.R. (1961). *Functions of varied experience*. Homewood, IL.: Dorsey.

Fixler, D.E., Atkins, J.M., Mitchell, J.H., & Horowitz L.D. (1976). Blood flow to respiratory, cardiac and limb muscles in dogs during graded exercise. *American Journal of Physiology, 231*, 1515–1519.

Fotopoulos, S.S., & Sunderland, W.P. (1978). Biofeedback in the treatment of psychophysiological disorders. *Biofeedback and Self-Regulation, 3*, 331–361.

Foxman, B., Lohr, K.N., & Brook, R.H. (1983). *Measurement of physiologic health for children, Vol. 5: Anemia*. Santa Monica, CA,: Rand.

Friedman, M., Das, J.P., & O'Conner, N. (Eds.) (1981). *Intelligence and learning*. New York: Plenum.

Gesten, J.C., Langer, T.S., Eisenberg, J.G., & Orzeck, L. (1974). Child behavior and life events: Undesirable change or change per se. In B.S. Dohrenwend & B.P. Dohrenwend (Eds.), *Stressful life events: Their nature and effects*. New York: Wiley.

Gesten, J.C., Langer, T.S., Eisenberg, J.G., & Simcha-Fagan, O. (1977). An evaluation of the etiological role of stressful life-change events in psychological disorders. *Journal of Health and Social Behavior, 18*, 228–244.

Goldbloom, R.B. (1979). Obesity in childhood. In R.G. Goode & R. Volpe (Eds.), *The child and physical activity, Proceedings of a workshop for educational leaders*. Toronto.

Goldman, P.S. (1972). Developmental determinants of cortical plasticity. *Acta Neurobiologaiae Experimentia, 32*, 495–511.

Goode, R.C. (1979). The child and physical activity. In R.G. Goode & R. Volpe (Eds.), *The child and physical activity, Proceedings of a workshop for educational leaders*. Toronto.

Grad, M.T., & Johnson, J.H. (1980). Correlates of adolescent life stress as related to race, SES, and levels of perceived social support. *Journal of Clinical Child Psychology, 9*, 13–16.

Green, L.W. (1980a.) Healthy people: The surgeon general's report and the prospects. In W.J. McNerny (Ed.), *Working for a healthier America*. Cambridge, MA: Ballinger.

Green, L.W. (1980b). To educate or not to educate. Is that the question? *American Journal of Public Health, 70*, 625–626.

Green, L.W. (1981). National policy in the promotion of health. In M.D. Hiller (Ed.), *Medical ethics and the law: Implications for public policy*. Cambridge, MA: Ballinger.

Green, L.W., Heit, P., Iverson, D.C., Kolbe, L.J., & Kreuter, M.W. (1980). The school health curriculum project: Its theory, practice, and measurement experience. *Health Education Quarterly, 7*, 14–34.

Green, L.W., & Horton D. (1982). Adolescent health: Issues and challenges. In T.J. Coates, A.C. Peterson, & C. Perry (Eds.), *Promoting adolescent health: A dialog on research and practice*. New York: Academic.

Green, L.W., & Iverson, D.C. (1982). School health education. *Annual Review of Public Health, 3*, 321–338.

Green, L.W., Kreuter, M.W., Deeds, S.G., & Partridge, K.P. (1980). *Health education planning: A diagnostic approach*. Palo Alto, CA: Mayfield.

Green, L.W., Wilson, R.W., & Bauer, K.G. (1982). Data requirements to measure our progress on the Objectives for the Nation in health promotion and disease prevention. *American Journal of Public Health, 73*, 18–24.

Griffiths, M., & Payne, P. (1976). Energy expenditure in small children of obese and non-obese parents. *Nature, 260*, 698–700.

Greenough, W., Fass, B., & Devoogd, T. (1976). The influence of experience on recovery following brain damage in rodents: Hypothesis based on developmental research. In Walsh & W. Greenough, *Environments as therapy for brain dysfunction* (pp. 10–50). New York: Plenum.

Grimes, J.W., & Allinsmith, W. (1961). Compulsivity, anxiety, and school achievement. *Merrill-Palmer Quarterly, 7*, 247–271.

Guilleminault, C., Eldridge, F., Simmons B., & Dement, W. (1976). Sleep apnea in eight children. *Pediatrics, 58*, 23–30.

Halsey, J.J., Blauenstein, U.W., Wilson, E.M., & Willis, E.H. (1979). Regional cerebral blood flow comparison of right and left hand movement. *Neurology, 29*, 21.

Hamburg, B.A. (1974). Early adolescence: A specific stressful stage of the life cycle. In G.V. Coehlo, D.A. Hamburg, & J.E. Adams, *Coping and adaptation* (pp. 101–124). New York: Basic Books.

Hamsher, K. des, & Benton, A.L. (1978). Interactive effects of age and cerebral disease on cognitive performances. *Journal of Neurology, 217*, 195–200.

Hauri, P., & Olmstead, E. (1980). Childhood-onset insomnia. *Sleep, 3*, 59–65.

Hertzog, D., Schaie, W., & Gribben K. (1978). Cardiovascular disease and changes in intellectual functioning from middle to old age. *Journal of Gerontology, 33*, 872–883.

Hotaling, G.T., Atwell, S.G., & Linsky, A.S. (1978). Adolescent life changes and illness: A comparison of three models. *Journal of Youth and Adolescence, 7*, 393–403.

Iammarino, W., Weinberg A., & Holcomb J. (1980). The state of school heart health education: A review of the literature. *Health Education Quarterly, 7*, 320.

Ingvar, D.H. (1967). Cerebral metabolism, cerebral blood flow and EEG. In L Widen (Ed.), *Recent advances in clinical neurophysiology, electroencephalography and clinical neurophysiology*, Supplement 25 (pp. 102–106).

Ingvar, D.H., & Lassen, N.A. (Eds.) (1975). *Brainwork.* Munksqaard. Copenhagen: Alfred Benzon Sympsium VIII.

Ingvar, D.H., Sjolund, B., & Ardo A. (1976). Correlation between dominant EEG frequency, cerebral oxygen uptake and blood flow. *Encephale Clinical Neurophysiology, 41,* 268–276.

James, W. (1962). *Talks to teachers on psychology.* New York: Dover.

Johnson, J.H., & McCutcheon, S.M. (1980). Assessing life stress in older children and adolescents: Preliminary findings with the life events checklist. In I.G. Sarason & C.D. Spielberger (Eds.), *Stress and anxiety* (Vol. 7). Washington, D.C.: Hemisphere.

Justice, B., & Duncan, D.F. (1976). Life crisis as a precursor to child abuse. *Public Health Reports, 91,* 110–115.

Kales, J., Soldatos, C., & Kales, A. (1980). Childhood sleep disorders. In S. Gellis & B. Kagan (Eds.), *Current pediatric therapy.* Philadelphia: W.B. Saunders.

Karacan, I., Anch, M., Thornby, J.I., Okawa, M., & Williams, R.L. (1975). Longitudinal sleep patterns during pubertal growth: Four-year follow-up. *Pediatric Research, 9,* 842–846.

Karacan, I., Hursch, C.J., Williams, R.L., & Littell, R.C., (1972). Some characteristics of nocturnal penile tumescence during puberty. *Pediatric Research, 6,* 529–537.

Katz, I. (1963). Factors influencing Negro performance in the desegregated school. In M. Deutsch, I. Katz, & A.R. Jensen (Eds.), *Social class, race, and psychological development.* New York: Holt, Rinehart & Winston.

Kellam, S.G., Branch, J.D., Agrawal, K.C., & Ensmingen, M.E. (1975). *Mental health and going to school: The Woodlawn program of assessment, early intervention, and evaluation.* Chicago: University of Chicago Press.

Kelly, J.G. (Ed.). (1979). *Adolescent boys in high school: A psychological study of coping and adaptation.* New York: Wiley.

Kolata, G. (1982). Consensus on diets and hyperactivity. *Science, 215,* 958.

Kolbe, L.J. (1979). Evaluating effectiveness: The problems of behavioral criteria. *Health Education monographs, 10,* 12–16.

Kolbe, L.J. (1982). What can we expect from school health education? *Journal of School Health, 52,* 145–150.

Knaus, W. (1977). Rational emotive education. In A. Ellis & R. Grieger (Eds.), *Handbook of rational emotive therapy.* New York: Springer.

Knaus, W., & Bloch, J. (1976). Rational emotive education with economically disadvantaged inner city high-school students: A demonstration study. Unpublished manuscript.

Knaus, W., & Bokor, S. (1975). The effect of rational-emotive education lessons on anxiety and self-concept in sixth grade students. *Rational Living, 11,* 7–10.

Knowles, J.H. (Ed.). (1977). *Doing better and feeling worse: Health in the United States.* New York: Norton.

Kreuter, M.W., & Christenson, G.M. (1981). School health education: Does it cause an effect? *Health Education Quarterly, 8,* 43–56.

Krohne, H.W., & Laux, L. (1982). *Achievement, stress and anxiety.* Washington, DC: Hemisphere.

Lassen, N.A., Ingvar, D.H., & Shinhoj, E. (1978). Brain function and blood flow. *Scientific American, 10,* 62–71.

LeBow, M. (1984). *Child obesity: A new frontier of behavior therapy.* New York: Springer.

Levitsky, D.A., & Barnes, R.H. (1972). Nutritional and environmental interactions in the behavioral development of the rat: Long term effects. *Science, 176,* 68–71.

Levy, S., Iverson, B., & Wahlberg, H. (1980). Nutrition-education research: An interdisciplinary evaluation and review. *Health Education Quarterly, 7,* 107–126.

Light, K.C. (1975). Slowing of response time in young and middle aged hypertensive patients. *Experimental Aging Research, 1*, 209–227.

Lindner, C.W., & DuRant, R.H. (1982). Exercise, serum lipids, and cardiovascular disease risk factors in children. *Pediatric clinics of North America, 6*, 1341–1355.

Linn, R.T., & Hodge, J.K. (1980). Use of EMG biofeedback training in increasing attention span and internalizing locus of control in hyperactive children. In *Consolidation and new dimensions: Proceedings of the biofeedback society of America* (pp 81–84). Eleventh Annual Meeting.

Mandler, G., & Sarason, S.B., (1952). A study of anxiety and learning. *Journal of Abnormal Social Psychology, 47*, 166–173.

Mechanic, D. (1979). The stability of health and illness behavior: Results from a 16-year follow-up. *American Journal of Public Health, 69*, 1142–45.

McAlister, A. (1982). The development and prevention of substance abuse: an introduction to research and policy. In T.J. Coates, A.C. Peterson, & C. Perry (Eds.), *Promoting adolescent health: A dialog on research and practice.* New York: Academic.

McKay, H., Sinisterra, L., McKay A., Gomez H., & Lloreda, P. (1978). Improving cognitive ability in chronically deprived children. *Science, 200* (No. 4339), 270–278.

Monckeberg, F., Tisler, S., Toro, S., Guttas, V., & Vega, L. (1972). Malnutrition and mental development. *American Journal of Clinical Nutrition, 25*, 766–772.

Moos, R. (1974). *The social climate scales: An overview.* Palo Alto, Ca.: Consulting Psychologists Press.

Moos, R. (1979). *Evaluating educational environments: procedures, measures, findings, and policy implications.* San Francisco: Josey-Bass.

Moyer, G., & Mayell, M. (1981). The soft drink explosion. *Nutrition Action, 8*(8), 8–10.

Olsen, L., Redican, K., & Krus P. (1980). The school health curriculum project: A review of research studies. *Health Education Monographs, 11*, 16–21.

Orgogoza, J.M., & Larsen, B. (1979). Activation of the supplementary motor area during voluntary movement in man suggests that it works as a supramotor area. *Science, 206*, 847–850.

Oski, F.A., & Honig, A.S. (1978). The effects of therapy on the developmental scores of iron-deficient infants. *Journal of Pediatrics, 92*, 21–25.

Perry, C. (1982). Adolescent health: An educational-ecological perspective. In T.J. Coates, A.C. Peterson, & C. Perry (Eds.), *Promoting adolescent health: A dialog on research and practice.* New York: Academic.

Phillips, B. (1978). *School stress and anxiety: Theory, research, and intervention.* New York: Human Sciences.

Piaget, J. (1963). *The origins of intelligence.* New York: Norton.

Pollitt, E. (1984). *Nutrition and educational achievement* (Nutrition Education Series, Issue 9). Paris, United Nations Educational, Scientific and Cultural Organization.

Pollitt, E., Greenfield, D., & Leibel, R. (1979). U.S. needs and priorities on behavioral effects of nutritional deficiencies. In J. Prozek (Ed.), *Behavioral effects of energy and protein deficits.* Washington, DC: U.S. Government Printing Office (NIH Pub. No. 79-1906).

Pollitt, E., & Leibel R.L. (1976). Iron deficiency and behavior. *Journal of Pediatrics, 88*, 373–381.

Pollitt, E., Leibel, R., & Greenfield, D. (1981). Brief fasting, stress, and cognition in children. *American Journal of Clinical Nutrition, 34*, 1526–1533.

Pollitt, E., & Thomson, C. (1977). Protein-calorie malnutrition and behavior: A view from psychology. In R.J. Wurtman & J.J. Wurtman (Eds.), *Nutrition and the brain* (Vol 2). New York: Raven.

Popkin, B., & Lim-Ybnanez, M. (1982). Nutrition and school achievement. *Social Science and Medicine, 16*, 53–61.

Purpura, D. (1977). Factors contributing to abnormal neuronal development in cerebral cortex of human infant. In Berenberg, *Brain fetal and infant development* (pp. 54–78). The Hague: Martinus Nijhoff Medical Division.

Raab W., & Krzywanek A. (1966). Cardiac sympathetic tone and stress response to personality patterns and exercise habits. In W. Raab (Ed.), *Prevention of ischemic heart disease* (pp. 121–134). Springfield, IL, Charles C Thomas.

Rarick, G.L. (1976). Concepts of motor learning: Implications for skill development in children. In J.G. Albinson & G.M. Andrew, *Child in sport and physical activity* (pp. 203–218). Baltimore: University Park Press.

Reiss, S., & Martell, R. (1974). Educational and psychological effects of open space education in Oak Park, IL. *Final report to board of education*, District 97, Oak Park, IL.

Ricciuti, H. (1979). Malnutrition and cognitive development: Research issues and priorities. In J. Prozek (Ed.), *Behavioral effects of energy and protein deficits*. Washington, DC: U.S. Government Printing Office (NIH Pub. No. 76-1906).

Ricciuti, H. (1981). Adverse environmental and nutritional influences on mental development: A perspective. *Journal of the American Dietic Association, 79*, 115–120.

Richardson, S.A. (1976). The relation of severe malnutrition in infancy to the intelligence of school children with differing life histories. *Pediatric Research, 10*, 57–61.

Rivard, G., Lavellee, H., Rajic, M., Shephard, R.J., Thinaudeau, P., Davignon, A., & Beaucage, C. (1977). Influence of competitive hockey on physical condition and psychological behavior of children. In H. Lavallee & R.J. Shephard (Eds.), *Frontiers of activity and child health* (pp. 335–354). Quebec: Pelican.

Rollwarg, H. (1979). Diagnostic classification of sleep and arousal disorders. *Sleep, 2*, 1–137.

Rosenbaum, L. (1981). Ongoing assessment: Experience of a university biofeedback clinic. *Biofeedback and Self-Regulation, 6*, 103–112.

Rosenzweig, M.R., & Bennett, E.L. (1972). Cerebral changes in rats exposed individually to an enriched environment. *Journal of Comparative and Physiological Psychology, 80*, 304–313.

Roenzweig, M., Bennett E., & Diamond M. (1972). Brain changes in response to experience. *Scientific American, 226*, 22–29.

Rumsey, J.M., & Rapoport, J.L. (1983). Assessing behavioral and cognitive effects of diet in pediatric populations. In R.J. Wurtman & J.J. Wurtman (Eds.), *Nutrition and the brain* (Vol. 6). New York: Raven.

Ryan, T.J. (1976). Psychosocial developments and activity in middle childhood—Comments and extensions. In J.G. Albinson & G.M. Andrews (Eds.), *Child in sport and physical activity*. Baltimore: University Park Press.

Salzarulo, P., & Chevalier, A. (1983). Sleep problems and their relationship with early disturbances of the waking-sleeping rhythms. *Sleep, 6*(1), 47–51.

Sandler, I.N., & Block, M. (1979). Life stress and maladaptation of children. *Journal of Community psychology, 7*, 425–439.

Sandler, I.N., & Ramsey, T.B. (1980). Dimensional analysis of childrens' stressful life events. *American Journal of Community Psychology, 8*, 285–301.

Sandvick, R.W. (1981). Some differential effects of biofeedback-assisted relaxation training in reducing hyperactive behavior in children. In *The integration of biofeedback with other therapy: Proceedings of the biofeedback society of America* (p. 43). Twelfth Annual Meeting.

Sarason, S.B., Davidson, K.S., Lighthall, F.F., Waite, R.R., & Ruebush, B.K. (1960). *Anxiety in elementary school children*. New York: Wiley.

Schaps, E., DiBartolo, R., Moskowitz, J., Polly C., & Churgin, S. (1981). A review of 127 drug abuse prevention program evaluations. *Journal of Drug Issues, 11*, 17–43.

Scrimshaw, N. (1974). Myths and realities in international health planning. *American Journal of Public Health, 64*, 792–798.

Shephard, R.J. (1982). *Physical activity and growth.* Chicago: Year Book Medical Publishers.

Shephard, R.J. (1983). Physical activity and the healthy mind. *Canadian Medical Association/Journal, 128*, 525–530.

Sherif, C.W., & Rattary, G.D. (1976). Psychosocial development and activity in middle childhood (5-12 years). In J.G. Albinson & G.M. Andrews (Eds.), *Child in sport and physical activity.* Baltimore: University Park Press.

Shure, M.B., & Spivak, G. (1980). Interpersonal problem-solving as a mediator of behavioral adjustment among disadvantaged school children. *Child Development, 42*, 1791–1803.

Simonds, F., & Humbarto, P. (1982). Prevalance of sleep disorders and sleep behaviors in children and adolescents. *Journal of the American Academy of Child Psychiatry, 21*, 383–388.

Sjostrom, L. (1980). Fat cells and body weight. In A.J. Stunkard (Ed.), *Obesity.* Philadelphia: W.B. Saunders.

Skinner, B.F. (1965). Why teachers fail. *Saturday Review,* October 16, 1965.

Skubic, E. (1955). Emotional responses of boys to little league and middle league competitive baseball. *Research Quarterly, 26*, 342–352.

Spivak, G., Platt J.J., & Shure, M.B. (1976). *The problem-solving approach to adjustment.* San Francisco: Jossey-Bass.

Stallings, J. (1975). Implementation and child effects of teaching practices in follow-through classrooms. *Monographs of The Society for Research in Child Development* 40 (Serial #163).

Stallones, R.A. (1980). To advance epidemiology. *Annual Review of Public Health, 1*, 69–82.

Stattler, J.M. (1970). Racial "experimenter effects" in experimentation, testing interviewing, and psychotherapy. *Psychological Bulletin, 73*, 137–160.

Sutton-Smith, G., & Rosenberg, B. (1961). Sixty years of historical change in the game preference of American children. *Journal of American Folklore, 74*, 17–46.

Thompson, E.L. (1978). Smoking education programs 1960–1976. *American Journal of Public Health, 68*, 250–57.

Trickett, E.J., & Moos, R.H. (1979). Personal correlates of contrasting environments: Student satisfaction in high school classrooms. *Journal of Community Psychology, 7*, 279–291.

Tryon, G.S. (1980). The measurement and treatment of test anxiety. *Review of Educational Research, 50*, 343–372.

U.S. Department of Agriculture. (1980, September). *Nationwide food consumption survey 1977–78: Food and nutrient intakes of individuals in one day in the United States* (Spring 1977). U.S. Department of Agriculture, Science and Education Administration.

U.S. Department of Health and Human Services. (1979). *Healthy people: The surgeon general's report on health promotion and disease prevention.* Washington, DC: Government Printing Office.

U.S. Department of Health, Education and Welfare. (1973). *Report of the president's committee on health education.* Washington, DC.

Volpe, R. (1979). Physical activity, intellectual and emotional development. In R.G. Goode & R. Volpe (Eds.), *The child and physical activity, Proceedings of a workshop for educational leaders.* Toronto.

Webb, T.E., & Oski, F.A. (1973). Iron deficiency anemia and scholastic achievement in young adolescents. *Journal of Pediatrics, 82*, 827–830.

Weissberg, R.P., Cowen, E.L., Lotyzcewski, B.S., & Gesten, E.L. (1983). The primary mental health project: Seven consecutive years of program outcome research. *Journal of Consulting & Clinical Psychology, 51,* 100–107.

Weissberg, R.P., Gesten, E.L., Liebenstein, N.L., Schmid, K.D., & Hutton H.P. (1980). *The Rochester social problem-solving program.* Rochester, NY: Primary Mental Health Project.

Welford, A.T. (1976). *Skilled performance in perceptual and motor skills.* Glenview, IL: Scott Foresman.

Wender, E. (1981). Diet and hyperkinesis. In L. Ellenbogen (Ed.), *Controversies in nutrition.* New York: Churchill Livingstone.

Wilke, F.L., Eisdorfer, C., & Nowlin, J.B. (1976). Memory and blood pressure in the aged. *Experimental Aging Research, 2,* 2–16.

Williams, E.P. (1967). Sense of obligation to high school activities as related to school size and marginality of student. *Child Development, 38,* 1247–1260.

Williams, H.G. (1983). *Perceptual and motor development.* Englewood Cliffs, NJ: Prentice-Hall.

Williams, H, Temple, I, & Bateman, J. (1978). Perceptual-motor and cognitive learning in the young child. *Psychology of motor behavior and sport II.* Champaign, IL: Human Kinetics Press.

Williams, R.L., Karacan, I., & Hursch, C.J. (1974). *Electroencephalography (EEG) of human sleep: Clinical applications.* New York: Wiley.

Williams, R.L., Karacan, I, Hursch, C.J., & Davis, C.E. (1972). Sleep patterns of pubertal males. *Pediatric Research, 6,* 643–648.

World Health Organization. (1954). *Expert committee on health education of the public.* Geneva, WHO Technical Report Series, No. 89.

Yerkes, R.M., & Dodson, J.D. (1908). The relation of strength of stimulus to rapidity of habit formation. *Journal of Comparative Neurology and Psychology, 18,* 459–482.

Ziegler, E., Abelson, W.D., Trickett, P.K., & Seitz, V. (1982). Is an intervention program necessary in order to improve economically disadvantaged children's IQ scores? *Child Development, 53,* 340–348.

Ziegler, E., & Butterfield, E.C. (1968). Motivational changes in IQ test performance of culturally deprived nursery school children. *Child Development, 39,* 1–14.

11

Childhood Injury
Control

MICHAEL F. CATALDO, ROBERT A. DERSHEWITZ,
MODENA WILSON, EDWARD R. CHRISTOPHERSEN,
JACK W. FINNEY, STEPHEN B. FAWCETT, AND
THOMAS SEEKINS

The technology and affluence of our modern society have produced a new public health hazard for this nation's children: Death and
damage from injury constitute the most important health problem children
as a population face.

This chapter will discuss (1) the epidemoiology of childhood injuries, (2)
conceptual frameworks for considering injury control, (3) research on injury control to date, (4) an example of instituting child-passenger safety
legislation, and (5) research priorities for the future.

EPIDEMIOLOGY OF CHILDHOOD INJURIES

Injuries are the cause of more deaths in children than the six next frequent causes combined (cancer, congenital anomalies, pneumonia, heart

TABLE 11.1. LEADING CAUSES OF DEATH IN CHILDREN LESS THAN 1 YEAR OLD

Cause of Death	N
1. Problems Related to the Perinatal Period	22,745
2. Congenital Anomalies	9,220
3. SIDS	5,510
4. Injuries	1,166
Ingestion of food/object	271
Motor vehicle	249
Mechanical suffocation	168
Fires, burns	161
Drowning	92
The total number of deaths from all causes is 45,526.	

Source: From National Center of Health Statistics, Public Health Service. U.S. Department HHS. These are the latest (1980, unpublished) official statistics.

disease, homicide, and stroke) (Mofenson & Greensher, 1978). About half of all deaths in young children result from injuries. This rate increases to more than 50 percent in preadolescents and to almost 80 percent in the 15 to 24 age group (Insurance Institute for Highway Safety, 1984).

Injuries are the leading cause of death in all children except those less than one year old, for whom injuries are the fourth leading cause of death (see Table 11.1). In all age groups, motor-vehicle-related injuries are the leading causes of accidental death, except in children under one year of age, for whom it is ingestion of food or objects. As shown in Table 11.2, the leading causes of fatal injuries for the 1 to 4 and 5 to 14 age groups are parallel, with the exception that "firearm-related deaths" replaces "ingestion of food/objects" as the fourth leading cause.

Even though most minor injuries are not reported and official injury rates are usually underreported (Barancik, Chatterjee, Greene, Michenzi, & Fife, 1983), the published morbidity statistics due to injuries are nevertheless grimly overwhelming. Each year, 19 million children less than 15 years of age obtain medical care for an injury. In the toddler age group alone, 1 in 10 are treated in hospital emergency rooms for injuries and poisonings (Rivara, 1982a). Injuries incapacitate about two million children for two weeks or longer, and at least 100,000 suffer permanent disabilities (Garfield, 1983).

In multinational comparisons of historical trends and types of injuries, patterns are remarkably similar, even though actual rates vary (Pless & Stulginskas, 1982; Westfelt, 1982). In 1920, injuries accounted for only 1 out of every 20 deaths in children compared with 1 out of 3 in 1980, largely due to the precipitous decline in the number of deaths due to infectious disease, while the number of deaths due to injuries declined much less dra-

TABLE 11.2. LEADING CAUSES OF INJURY-RELATED
DEATHS IN CHILDREN

Age	N
1–4 Years	
Motor vehicle	1,179
Drowning	711
Fires, burns	685
Ingestion of food/objects	136
Falls	111
Deaths from all injuries	3,313
Total number of deaths	8,187
5–14 years	
Motor vehicles	2,747
Drowning	856
Fires, burns	478
Firearms	271
Falls	89
Deaths from all injuries	5,224
Total number of deaths	10,689

Source: Latest official (1980, unpublished) data from the National
Center of Health Statistics, Public Health Service, U.S. Dept. of
HHS.

matically. The decline that did occur for injury-related deaths resulted primarily from a 60 percent decrease in the death rate from unintentional injuries not related to motor vehicle crashes. Greatest declines were in deaths related to falls, nonfarm machinery, and burns other than house fires. Death rates from motor vehicle injuries and poisonings have changed little, while mortality from house fires has increased (Baker, O'Neill, & Karpf, 1984; Mofenson & Greensher, 1978).

The emotional expense to injured children and their families is incalculable. Furthermore, the comprehensive costs to society, which could be calculated, have not been. However, annual costs incurred from motor vehicle injuries alone have been estimated at more than 25 billion dollars, a sum that is second only to the costs associated with cancer (Baker et al., 1984).

As a cause of death, injuries can be categorized as: homicide, suicide, and unintentional. Child abuse is classified in the homicide category, as are a multitude of other causes that reflect violence in society, such as gang warfare. Most injury deaths (66 percent) are unintentional, and this group of injuries is the subject of this chapter.

Epidemiological Framework

The formal study of injuries is derived from classic epidemiology, in which consideration of host, agent, environment, and vectors is paramount. Because injuries, like diseases, are usually not randomly distributed among the population, the interplay of these factors determines the probability and nature of the injury. An understanding of susceptibility is necessary to formulate effective preventive countermeasures. For example, by first ascertaining that infants are at greatest risk of death from vehicular injuries, falls, and asphyxiation, and then examining why, one can implement a more targeted, and hence more effective, strategy to reduce the death rate from these causes.

Host (the child).   To be sure, not all susceptible children sustain injuries, and many children not considered at increased risk become seriously injured. However, certain developmental disabilities (for example, mental retardation), personality traits (for example, impulsiveness, engaging in rough-and-tumble play), and sensorineural deficits (for example, poor coordination, poor vision, impaired depth perception) make some children more susceptible to injury (Angle, 1975; Berger, 1981; Rivara, 1982a; Rivara, 1982b).

Agent.   The agent producing injury is energy—mechanical, thermal, electrical, chemical, or radiation (see Table 11.3). Injury occurs when exposure to energy exceeds the body's tolerance. The vast majority of injuries (an estimated 95 percent) are due to mechanical energy. Themal energy causes burns, and chemical energy causes poisonings; both are more likely to injure younger children (Baker et al., 1984; Rivara, 1982a).

Environment.   Hazards are present in the environment. Weather and road conditions are important environmental variables in motor vehicle injuries (Feldman, 1980). Most accidental deaths of children younger than 5 years of age occur at home (Westfelt, 1982). Each year, approximately 3,000 children under 14 years of age die of home injuries, with the three leading causes being fires and burns, suffocation from an ingested object, and drownings. In terms of location in the home, more minor injuries occur in the kitchen (18 percent) than in any other room (Dershewitz & Christophersen, 1984). The psychological environment is also important; higher rates of injury occur in families at times of stress (for example, during moves) and in stressed families (Rivara, 1982a).

Vector or Vehicle.   The agent is transmitted to the body by means of an inanimate object (a vehicle) or a living thing (a vector). For example, cars are, in the literal sense, a vehicle for mechanical energy; poisons are a vehicle for chemical energy; a hot iron is a vehicle for thermal energy; and a bit-

TABLE 11.3. INJURIES AS TRANSFERS OF ENERGY

Form of Energy	Examples of Injuries
Mechanical	Fractures
	Lacerations
	Subdurals
Thermal	Heat stroke
	Scald burns
Electrical	Asystole
	Burns
Chemical	Lead encephalopathy
	Methemoglobinemia from nitrates
	Corneal scars from corrosives
Radiation	Radiation sickness
	Postirradiation cancers

Reproduced with permission from Berger, L.R.: Childhood injuries: recognition and prevention. In Gluck, L., et al. (Eds.): *Current problems in pediatrics.* Copyright © 1981 by Year Book Medical Publishers, Inc., Chicago.

ing dog is a vector for mechanical energy. The 10 most dangerous vehicles (in order of severity and frequency) are bicycles, stairs, doors, cleaning agents, tables, beds, footballs, swings, liquid fuels, and glass (Haddon, 1980; Rivara, 1982a; United States Consumer Product Safety Commission, 1980).

Causative Variables

Risk factors account for the nonrandom distribution of injuries to children, of which the following are considered to be the most important.

Age.   There is a bimodal age-distribution pattern of childhood injuries in that the rate rises rapidly in the first year of life and again peaks in adolescents (Haddon & Baker, 1981; McCormick, Shapiro, & Starfield, 1981; Rivara, 1982a). However, age-fatality rates in all injury categories vary widely (Baker et al., 1984).

Sex.   Injury rates vary greatly by sex. A male predominance is evident by one year of age (McCormick et al., 1981). Lacerations, contusions, abrasions, concussions, drowning, bicycling, and pedestrian deaths in traffic are markedly more common in males. In contrast, there are no sex differences in the rates of foreign-body ingestions, poisonings, and burns (Rivara, Bergman, & LoGerfo, 1982).

Race and Socioeconomic Status (SES).   There are higher injury rates among blacks than whites, with a clustering of homicides and house-fire fatalities among the urban poor (Baker & Dietz, 1979). Much of the racial difference disappears when per capita income is controlled (Insurance Institute for Highway Safety, 1984; Wise, Mills, & Wilson, 1983). Moreover certain categories of injuries are related to income. For example, children have considerably greater likelihood of drowning if their home has a swimming pool.

Location.   Death rates are generally highest in rural areas, due, in part, to farm accidents and lack of sophisticated trauma services. Home accident rates have been noted to be highest in depressed urban areas even though there are considerable regional variations in urban-rural injury rates and patterns (Westfelt, 1982).

Temporal Variation.   Many types of injuries have seasonal fluctuations. In the summer there is a rise in deaths from motorcycles, bicycles, motor vehicles, drowning, and electrocution. The November peak in unintentional shootings is attributable to the hunting season. Fatal house fires are highest in the winter months, as are carbon monoxide poisonings. Deaths from falls increase slightly during the winter months. Deaths from injuries occur more commonly during weekends. In contrast, most poisonings have little monthly variation (Baker & Dietz, 1979; Baker et al., 1984).

Body Parts.   Certain body parts are injured more frequently than others, and some injuries occur most commonly in certain areas of the body. Forty percent of all injuries to infants involve the head, but this rate drops to 19 percent in preschool children. Young children also have a higher frequency of injuries to the face, mouth, and eyes, whereas extremities are the usual site of injuries to adolescents (Rivara, 1982a). Injuries to the eyes are disproportionately more serious than those elsewhere on the body. Of the 500,000 eye injuries that occur each year, many result in permanent loss of vision (Mofenson & Greensher, 1978).

Types of Injuries

Descriptive and epidemiological data on the major childhood injuries have been extensively reported and allow a quite detailed breakdown as follows, especially with regard to morbidity and mortality (Baker & Dietz, 1979; Baker et al., 1984; Berger, 1981; Christoffel & Tanz, 1983; Feldman, 1980; Garfield, 1983; Harris, Baker, Smith & Harris, 1984; Hongladarom, Allard, & Miller, 1978; Karwacki & Baker, 1979; McCormick et al., 1981; McIntire, 1980; Mofenson & Greensher, 1978; O'Shea, Collins, & Butler, 1982; Paulson, 1979; Rivara, 1982a; Williams, 1976).

Motor Vehicle.   The categories of mortality from motor vehicle injuries are occupant, motorcyclist, pedestrian, and bicyclist. Each has its own age-

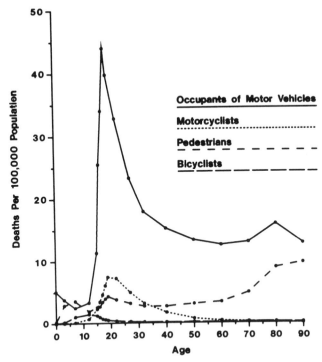

FIGURE 11.1. The effect of age on vehicle-related fatalities. Reprinted by permission of the publisher, from THE INJURY FACT BOOK by Susan P. Baker, Brian O'Neill, and Ronald S. Karpf, Lexington, Mass.: Lexington Books, D. C. Heath and Company, Copyright 1984, D. C. Heath and Company.)

related pattern (see Figure 11.1). The type and severity of injury are related to the size of the child. Younger children have relatively larger heads than older children, thereby giving them higher centers of gravity. This fact explains, in part, why so many young children (about one-third) that are thrown from a vehicle have a tendency to land head first. Their likelihood of being killed is thus increased.

Motor vehicle injuries are the leading cause of death in children in the United States. Approximately 1 out of 20 infants born in the U.S. will become seriously injured in a motor vehicle accident by young adulthood. Each year motor vehicle injuries claim the lives of approximately 4600 children, and for every one death 39 children become disabled. Childhood mortality rates from vehicular injuries have remained relatively constant over the past 50 years. With the adoption of child-passenger restraint laws in most states, this trend may be reversed.

Pedestrian injuries are usually more serious than occupant injuries because of the higher fatality rate. More children between 3 and 12 years of age die from pedestrian injuries than from passenger injuries. In the

United States there are more than 2000 child-pedestrian fatalities each year. Most of these deaths occur while the child is crossing a street. One-third of pedestrian deaths occur in rural areas, and one-half are at night.

Controlling for person-miles of travel, the death rate from motorcycles is 15 times the death rate from cars. For each year an adolescent rides a motorcycle, he or she has a 2 percent chance of being killed or seriously injured. States that have mandatory helmet requirements report up to a 30 percent reduction in motorcyle fatalities; and states in which that law has been subsequently repealed have experienced increases in motorcycle fatalities of up to 40 percent.

About 1000 bicyclists die each year, two thirds of whom are between 5 and 14 years of age. Most bicycle deaths involve a collision with an automobile. There are an estimated one million bicycle injuries each year, 370,000 of which are brought to hospital emergency rooms. Children who are seriously hurt most commonly have their heads injured; most injuries, however, consist of cuts and abrasions to the lower extremities. The age of the bicyclist is strongly correlated with responsibility for the injury. In 90 percent of the cases of injury to children less than 12 years old, the children are responsible. They usually dart into the street or fail to obey stop signs. After age 12 the responsibility steadily decreases in inverse relation to age.

Drowning.   One third of all drowning victims in the U.S. are children less than 15 years old. Drowning is the second leading cause of death in children between 5 and 14 years of age. Most drownings do not involve boats but rather occur among poorly supervised children who cannot swim. In the United States blacks have almost double the drowning rates as whites, and drowning rates are higher in rural rather than urban areas. The average age of a home swimming-pool victim is 3 years, with younger children drowning in less common ways around their homes (for example, in bathtubs and through pail immersion).

Burns and Fire Deaths.   House fires cause three-quarters of all deaths from fires and burns, and these rates are highest among the very young and the elderly. Other types of fatal burn and fire injuries include clothing ignition, hot substances (for example, coffee burns and electrical burns, including lightning), combustibles (for example, gas in space heaters), stoves, matches, and chemicals. Of the 1.75 million burn victims each year, 40 percent are children less than 15 years old. Three-quarters of all burns in children are scalds, and three-quarters of scalds occur in the kitchen, with coffee being the major vehicle. Tap-water scalds are an important category of burns in children both because of the large number of cases, and because they serve as a prototype of injuries that could virtually be eliminated by legislation (that is, by mandatory lowering of home water temperature). Most electrical burns result from children mouthing live extension cords, and most of these injuries produce third-degree burns. Even though the death rate from house fires has increased, there has been an 85 percent decline in burn deaths from other causes. Overall there has been a downward trend in burn mortality.

Asphyxiation.   Aspiration is the most common cause of household deaths in children less than 6 years old. Infants' oral tendencies and toddlers' penchant for running with food in their mouths predispose young children to aspiration. More than 90 percent of deaths from aspiration of food occur in children less than 5 years old; 65 percent in infants less than 2 years old. Asphyxiation by choking may be due to either food or nonfood products. The most frequent food causing asphyxial death is hot dogs; nuts and grapes are the second and third leading causes, respectively. In one study, 503 out of 703 asphyxial deaths in children were caused by nonfood products. The most common nonfood vectors in this category include safety pins, pacifiers, small balls, jacks, and balloons.

Mechanical suffocation is the fourth leading cause of death in males between 10 and 14 months of age. The circumstances vary by age, and injury can occur in a variety of unanticipated ways. For example, a heavy toy chest lid may fall against a child's neck and compress the airway. Victims of crib strangulation and injury as a result of wedging between crib mattress and frame are most commonly 6 to 8 months of age. Suffocation by fallen earth at construction sites most often occurs in children between 8 and 10 years old.

Firearms.   Roughly 75 percent of all homes in the United States have guns. Approximately one-fifth of those killed from firearm accidents are children less than 15 years old. Unintentional shootings are the third leading cause of accidental death in children aged 10 to 19. The peak occurs in males between 13 and 17 years of age; male death rate from firearms is sixfold greater than the rate for females. About 55 percent of accidental firearm deaths occur at home with children less than 15 years old as victims in approximately 30 percent of the cases.

Morbidity data from firearm injuries are scant. In 1972 there were an estimated 155,000 nonfatal shootings in all age groups. Many such shootings lead to severe disability such as spinal cord injury and blindness. Each year spring-operated guns marketed as toys produce many fatal and nonfatal injuries. The U.S. Consumer Product Safety Commission estimated that in 1973 11,000 injuries associated with gas, air, and spring-operated guns (including BB guns, pellet guns, and air rifles) were treated in emergency rooms.

Falls.   Falls are the fifth leading cause of accidental death in children. Each year about 500 children younger than 14 years old are killed from falls; 150 are under five years of age. Even though the death rate from falls is low, falls result in a great many injuries. As an example, 147,000 children

TABLE 11.4. FALLS OF SPECIAL CONCERN FOR CHILDREN

Type	Comment
Crib accidents	Most of these falls occur when infants climb out of cribs.
Bunk beds	Many of these falls occur at times of rough play.
Changing tables	Most of these falls are caused by lack of supervision.
High chairs	In 1974, 7,000 children were treated in emergency rooms for falls from high chairs.
Infant carriers	Children should never be left unattended in an infant carrier on an elevated surface.
Jumpers and walkers	Falls down stairs are common, leading to thousands of hospital emergency room visits each year.
Falls from windows	These falls accounted for 20% of all child accidental deaths in New York City in 1966.

Data from Mofenson, H. C., & Greensher, J. (1978). Childhood accidents. In R. A. Hoekelman (ed.), *Principles of pediatrics—Health care of the young* (pp. 1806–1807). New York: McGraw-Hill

in 1978 were injured by falling down stairs. In one study, 43 percent of all injury-related emergency room visits were due to falls. Most of the injuries resulted from playing, bicycling, roller-skating, walking, or falling from a bed. Because of development patterns and risk exposure, certain types of falls are either unique to, or predominate in, children (see Table 11.4).

Sports and Recreational Injuries. In 1978, 1.8 million children had injuries related to sports and recreational activities. Preadolescents have a lower injury rate than adolescents. Football is the leading cause of sports injuries. In one study 80 percent of high school football players and 75 percent of wrestlers were injured. Gymnasts have four times the spinal cord injury rate of football players. Table 11.5 lists the leading causes of morbidity and mortality from sports.

Several other recreational activities are particularly dangerous to children. Between 100,000 and 155,000 children are brought to emergency rooms each year because of injuries on playgrounds; about half these injuries occur on home playground equipment. An estimated 300 children were killed in 1968 from sledding accidents, and many more were seriously injured. Snowmobiles are even more dangerous than sleds. Of the esti-

TABLE 11.5.   SPORTS-RELATED INJURIES (1980) AND DEATHS (1973–1980)

Sport	Estimated Number of Injuries Treated in Hospital Emergency Rooms, 1980		Number of Deaths, 1973–1980	
	All Ages	Ages 5–14	All Ages	Ages 5–14
Football	463,800	173,100	260	19
Baseball	442,900	121,700	183	40
Basketball	421,000	92,800	37	6
Soccer	94,200	37,800	11	6
Racquet sports	74,700	5,400	3	1
Volleyball	73,700	13,900	4	0
Wrestling[a]	67,500	20,000	23	2
Gymnastics	61,400	38,200	8	0
Ice hockey	36,400	10,800	10	2
Track and field	31,600	8,800	10	2
Golf[b]	18,800	4,600	28	14
Trampoline	6,100	2,900	13	6

Source: G.W. Rutherford, R.B. Miles, V.R. Brown, and B. MacDonald, *Overview of Sports-Related Injuries to Persons 5–14 Years of Age*, Washington, DC: U.S. Consumer Product Safety Commission, 1981.

Note: Injuries were estimated from the Consumer Product Safety Commission's National Electronic Injury Surveillance System. Deaths were idetified from death certificates, newspaper clippings, consumer complaints, medical examiner reports, and NEISS data.

[a]Includes deaths from "rough-housing."

[b]Includes children playing with golf clubs, and spectators.

mated 100,000 annual skateboard injuries to children, thousands require medical attention.

Poisonings.   The peak age for poisoning in children is between 18 and 24 months of age. Children may be poisoned by drugs and medications, other solids and liquids, and gases and vapors. Over the past 25 years, the number of poisoning deaths among young children has dramatically declined. In 1960 the death rate from poisonings to children under 5 years old was 2.2 per 100,000; in 1980, the rate fell to 0.5. Most of this decrease is attributable to legislation banning lead in indoor paint and requiring safety caps for dangerous medications. Yet each year about 80 children under 5 years of age die from unintentional poisinings, and for every death, more than 1,000 ingestions are reported to poison control centers. Poisoning by antidepressants and cardiovascular drugs warrant special mention: Even though they represent only 1 percent of all ingestions of children under 5 years of age, they cause 13% of poisoning deaths in that age group.

Toys.   Each year approximately 700,000 children are injured by toys, resulting in 150,000 emergency room visits. A relatively small percentage of these injuries are serious. Only 1 percent of all fatal childhood injuries are toy-related. By virtue of the Child Prevention and Toy Safety Act of 1969, the Consumer Product Safety Commission has banned thousands of unsafe toys, thus preventing many injuries. Most toy injuries consist of minor cuts, abrasions, and falls.

Other Important Injuries.   Certain other lesser categories of injuries are particularly noteworthy:

> Fireworks—Of the 6,500 people injured by fireworks in 1973, 65 percent were children under 15 years of age. Every type of firework is able to produce serious injury. For example, a burning sparkler reaches temperatures of up to 2000° F, which can readily cause major burns and eye injuries.
>
> Minibikes—Sixty-five percent of the 20,000 minibike-related injuries treated each year in emergency rooms are to children under 15 years of age. These two-wheeled vehicles can travel up to 50 MPH. Collisions and falls often produce serious injuries.
>
> Wringer Injuries—Fortunately, the dangerous models of washing machine wringer attachments are no longer manufactured, but there are still millions in use. The mechanism of injury is by crushing soft tissue (usually an arm), which may then damage nerves, tendons, muscles, ligaments, and blood vessels. One-half of wringer injuries are to children under 5 years of age.
>
> Animal Bite Injuries—Children, who sustain 75 percent of all animal bites, receive between 450,000 and 750,000 bites annually. An estimated 60,000 of these bites result in serious injuries, such as facial disfigurement or psychological problems. Because of rabies prophylaxis, cases of human rabies are now extremely uncommon. The newer human diploid cell vaccine has largely replaced the duck embryo vaccine, and rabies immune globulin has similarly replaced antirabies serum, resulting in considerably fewer vaccine related side effects.

The descriptive, epdiemiological data amassed to date clearly indicate the magnitude of the problem of childhood injury. How then should we begin to consider and effect solutions? An important first step in problem solving is establishing a conceptualization of the problem that structures and results in successful solution strategies.

CONCEPTUAL FRAMEWORK

One conceptualization that has gained increased attention over the past two decades has been referred to as injury control. It has three aspects: (1)

preventing injury-producing events, many of which are the result of man-made hazards that can be eliminated, reduced, or modified; (2) reducing the likelihood of injury or the severity of injury if such events do occur; and (3) making the best emergency response, treatment, and rehabilitation available to injured children (Haddon, 1980; Haddon and Baker, 1981). The injury control conceptualization includes a careful look at the definition and description of the problem of injury in terms of epidemiological principles and a reorientation of interest toward a public health emphasis.

Defining the Problem

Calling the cause of injury an accident has confined much of the preventive effort to "accident prevention" or the prevention of injury-producing events. An accident is something occurring by chance or without intention. Injury-producing events are often accidents in the sense that no one intends for them to happen. They are, however, not random; the injury is quite predictable, given the event. Use of the term accident not only conveys a sense of helplessness or bad luck, it also tends to draw attention away from the fact that injury might be minimized or prevented even without preventing the event. Furthermore, attention to so-called accidents disguises the fact that the same preventive strategy may often reduce both deliberate and inadvertent injuries.

Injury has traditionally not been thought of as a disease. That it has not is based on two distinctions: (1) damage from injury is often clearly linked to some apparent injurious but nonpathogenic antecedent events, and (2) damage from injury appears quickly in relation to an energy exchange as opposed to biological process. As a result, injury has only recently been considered a proper concern by many nonsurgical health professions. Accordingly, childhood injury has not had the broadly based attention from health researchers that such a large problem deserves.

The difficulty of defining injury differently from disease is both subtle and important in identifying solutions. Indeed the same agent (heat energy from the sun) may cause a "disease" (skin cancer) or an "injury" (sunburn). Haddon (1980) proposes that injury be defined as damage to the body manifested within 48 hours of the energy exchange that produced it. Despite the conceptual distinction between injury and disease that can be drawn, methods of studying the problem and the solution to childhood injury may very well be similar to those employed for the prevention and treatment of disease.

Injury is damage to the body that results from the interaction of agent and host through some vehicle. This interaction takes place in an environment that permits it. Almost always one can describe the portion of the population that is at increased risk for sustaining a particular kind of injury in terms of age, sex, race, per capita income, geography, urbanization, occupation, and so on (Baker, O'Neill, & Karpf, 1984). These descriptors do

TABLE 11.6.   BASIC STRATEGIES FOR REDUCING INJURIES WITH EXAMPLES

Phase	Strategy	Examples of Countermeasures to Prevent Injury to Motor Vehicle Occupants
Preevent	Preventing the marshaling of potentially injurious agents or Reducing their amounts	Alternative travel modes; reduction in speed limits and speed capabilities
	Preventing inappropriate release of the agent	Vehicle and road designs that simplify driver's task
Event	Modifying release of the agent	Use of seat belts or infant restraint devices to decelerate occupant
	Separating in time or space or with physical barriers	Restricting transport of hazardous materials to certain times and places Highway medians
	Modifying surfaces and basic structures	Air bags to spread forces over wide area of body; removing projections in car
Post-event	Increasing resistance to injury	Therapy for osteoporosis
	Emergency response or medical care and rehabilitation	Systems that route patient to appropriately trained physicians

Source: Adapted from S. P. Baker and P. E. Dietz, Injury Prevention in Healthy People: The Surgeon General's Report on Health Promotion and Disease Prevention. *Background Papers.* Washington, D.C.: Department of Health, Education, and Welfare, 1979. From "Injuries and Injury Control" by M. H. Wilson. In C. De Angelis (Ed), *Pediatric Primary Care* (3rd ed.). Boston: Little, Brown, 1984, p. 537.

not necessarily have causal power but can suggest groups at particular risk. Clarifying the precise characteristics of the interaction of the agent and the susceptible host provides an important focus for conceptualizing injury. Realizing the parallels with infectious diseases directs attention toward control of the vehicle as a strategy for preventing injury. To maximize the possibilities for solutions, the conceptualization must consider the myriad of human and environmental factors that permit or promote the interaction. One tendency has been to focus on the behavior of the persons immediately involved in the energy exchange and to assign guilt or blame rather than focus on prior behavior of decision makers that may have contributed to the level of risk. Thus although some preventive efforts have been targeted toward behavior change in children and their caregivers, others have considered changes in outlook by policymakers and agency executives that relate to controllable or predictable aspects of the environment.

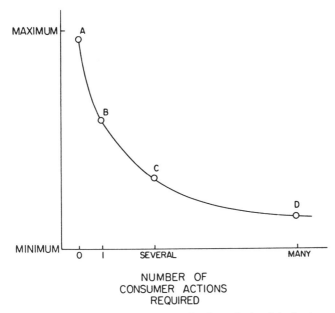

FIGURE 11.2. Effectiveness of preventive strategies for reducing injuries in a community. Hypothetical curve illustrates that automatic protection is far more effective than measures that require repeated actions on the part of individuals. (Modified from Baker, S.P. Childhood injuries: The community approach to prevention. *J. Public Health Policy*, 2:235, 1981. Reproduced with permission from Berger, L. R., "Childhood Injuries: Recognition and Prevention," in Gluck, L. et al. (Eds.), *Current Problems in Pediatrics*. Copyright © 1981 by Year Book Medical Publishers, Inc., Chicago).

Strategies for Injury Control

The objective of injury control is to reduce damage and death from injury. Haddon (1970) has listed 10 basic strategies for achieving this end; for a given injury-producing event, specific measures can be outlined that correspond to each of these strategies (see Table 11.6). However, for any given strategy to be effective, that is, to help achieve the goal of injury control, it must work if used and be used. Many strategies that would work if used are not used.

One current injury control effort is based on the supposition—an outgrowth of previous public health experience—that strategies are more likely to be effective if they do not depend on *frequent* actions of individuals. Thus, the more "passive" the strategy is on the continuum, the more likely the needed protection will result. This model is illustrated in Figure 11.2. An example of this kind of passive protection would be to limit the capability of water heaters to a maximum temperature that would not scald the skin. To extend this example, a measure that requires action only once

Injury matrix

Factors

	Human	Vehicles and equipment	Physical and socioeconimic environment
Pre-event	1	2	3
Event	4	5	6
Post-event	6	7	8

Phases

FIGURE 11.3. One example of a haddon matrix. Injury control measures can be classified according to three factors and three phases. (From: *To Prevent Harm*. Washington, D.C.: Insurance Institute for Highway Safety, 1978. Used by permission.)

(turning down the water heater) would be more effective than a measure that requires action every time proctection is needed (always supervising toddlers in rooms with hot-water taps).

Strategies can also be arranged in a two-dimensional matrix with the basic strategies—sometimes grouped into preevent, event, and postevent phases—along one axis, and enabling factors—divided into human, vehicle, and physical or sociocultural environmental factors—along the other axis (see Figure 11.3). Often called the Haddon matrix, it can be used for strategy identification and planning (Insurance Institute for Highway Safety, 1978). Such matrices can be used in program planning when strategies must be selected for implementation. For example, using the Haddon matrix to choose strategies might include the following considerations:

Emphasis should be placed on procedures that will most effectively control injury, even though they may not have an impact on the first or more important "cause" in the sequence of events.

The program should include several strategies, with strategies from each of the phases listed in Table 11.6.

Passive procedures should be given preference when they exist.

Economic resources should be allocated wisely to provide the largest possible impact on injury control.

The last two guidlines are familiar public health priorities only recently applied to the problem of injury.

When a strategy has been identified as worthy of implementation, there are a limited number of avenues open to achieve implementation: government action, voluntary action, litigation, or health education. Government action may take the form of regulation or legislation, along with appropriation of funds. Alternatively, responsible parties may be convinced to voluntarily make desirable modifications, that is, without government intervention. Often as a last resort, litigation has been used to motivate the implementation of strategies.

Overwhelmingly health education has been the means of attempting to modify the behavior of individuals. However, the success of health education efforts is dependent on several factors, including who delivers the message (the health professional, the teacher, the mass media) and the style of message. The aim of the health education message is usually some combination of increasing knowledge and changing attitudes. The hope is that these outcomes will lead to a behavior change and thus to the implementation of a strategy that will control injury. Unfortunately increased knowledge does not necessarily lead to behavior change, and the goal of decreased injury damage is often not reached.

Therefore other avenues to injury control (other than health education) are employed either (1) to encourage and motivate the individual to make the step from increased knowledge to behavior change (for example, car seat laws), or (2) to circumvent the need for individual action, that is, to implement passive strategies (for example, regulations controlling pacifier and crib designs, child-proof safety caps). Although behavior change may not reliably result from a single health education experience, serial and varying educational experiences over time may lead to the desired behavior change. For example, the decreasing percentage of smokers in the adult popuation may have resulted from many health messages from various sources delivered over many years. Certainly the problem of injury is so large that even small impacts may be important, especially if repeated exposure to messages about injury and injury control has a cumulative effect.

Ultimately, injury control must entail some degree of behavior change, requiring the establishment and maintenance of appropriate safety behavior—by parents, legislators, judges and juries, police, health educators, physicians, reporters, and the like. Thus even passive approaches, which do not require maintained responding to be effective, require an understanding of how to control human behavior to induce intital adoption of the passive procedure and to ensure that, once the procedure is adopted, people do not attempt to bypass or eliminate it.

Research on the principles of behavior change (operant conditioning, the experimental analysis of behavior, applied behavior analysis, etc.) has demonstrated the orderly relationship between behavior and its consequences. Many behavior change studies have addressed applied problems, including those related to injury. Thus this area of research can provide a conceptualization of the conditions under which behavior change can be expected to occur or not occur. For example, health education programs can be considered to be effective because the recipients have previously benefited (obtained positive reinforcement) from following similar health advice. Consequently, those who do not benefit as a result of health education—those whose behavior does not change—behave so because they lack the necessary positive learning history to follow such advice, even when it would ultimately be in their best interest.

This conceptualization of injury control should be differentiated from a logical or cognitive explanation. For example, logical, or cognitive, considerations would suggest that individuals, including children, find it hard not to engage in a pleasant or exciting activity (riding a motorbike at a dangerous speed, playing around a swimming pool, taking a chance that a bottle is filled with candy rather than medicine) just because the event may pose a health hazard. The learning-based approach would argue that such risk-taking behavior exists because the child has rarely, if ever, experienced an unpleasant result from such experiences and more frequently experiences a postive outcome.

Limitations of Conceptual Approaches

Despite any heuristic appeal these conceptualizations about injury control might have, they are not without their limitations. The passive approach to injury control indeed reduces the frequency with which individuals must rely on their own skills and vigilance to avoid dangerous situations; however this approach requires that each hazard be identified and appropriate action at a societal level be effected.

As noted above, the health education conceptualization very often does not result in behavior change. Thus while relatively inexpensive in terms of the cost per individual to dispense educational messages, this approach merely provides information that must compete with other motivational factors and must be consistent with an individual's learning history to result in desired behavior change.

With regard to approaches that attempt to provide differential consequences to increase safety behavior and thereby decrease injury, the advantage of the considerably greater power of these techniques is compromised by cost and practical problems. Application of operant principles to injury control requires that an individual's behavior be quantitatively noted, that reinforcing and/or punishing consequences be identified, and that these consequences be differentially contingent on certain aspects of behavior. Often risk-taking behavior is difficult to observe (it often occurs when a child is alone). Although identifying consequences that can be ethically controlled by others is decidedly easier for children than adults, this requirement for an operant approach becomes more difficult as the child grows older—thus injury control programs for adolescents using an operant approach would be much more difficult than those for younger children. Finally, while providing consequences contingent on desired behavior does not require a great deal of special training and is, in fact, informally and routinely carried out by parents and other caregivers, an injury control program would need to be consistently followed, and such consistency is often difficult for parents who have many and competing responsibilities.

How then are we to decide about approaches to injury control? The most reasonable answer is usually to consider a combination of approaches. However, the knowledge base on the use of these approaches to injury control is different and yields different outcomes for the health and safety of children. Assessment of this knowledge base requires a critical review of the intervention research literature.

RESEARCH ON INJURY CONTROL STRATEGIES

A variety of strategies for injury control have been the subject of research. A major thrust of this research has been the development of health education strategies that can be implemented in pediatric primary care (Finney & Christophersen, 1984) and delivered via mass media. Operant and learning-based approaches that manipulate consequences have been much less the focus of research but have demonstrated more precise and detailed measurement of behavior related to injury. Lastly, investigations have been made of the effects on injury prevalence as the result of city, state, and national legislation mandating safety-related measures (for example, Poisoning Prevention Packaging Act of 1970). This section will critically review research to date on the predominant approaches to injury control in terms of the conclusions that can be made about the efficacy of each approach and the gaps that exist in the research base. Although approaches with child populations will be of most interest, some studies on interventions for adult populations will also be discussed because of their methodological implications.

Health Education

Health education research is often focused on changes in knowledge and attitudes that lead to changes in behavior, but the gauge of effectiveness for health education is often, in addition to knowledge and attitude change, the resulting behavioral change that improves health (Green, Kreuter, Deeds, & Partridge, 1980). For injury control, behavioral changes that result in greater protection for infants and children must be the primary goal of health education. Research on health education in primary care has focused on numerous injuries and their prevention through active behavioral changes and passive environmental changes.

Educational Messages.   Studies of educational messages concerning injury control have been conducted with parents and children during the children's routine health care appointments. These studies have generally been well-designed investigations using objective, reliable data measures and between-group comparison designs. Early research reports suggested that educational messages delivered by pediatricians produced large and significant changes in parent safety behavior (Allen & Bergman, 1976; Kanthor, 1976). However, early studies used parent self-report as the outcome measure, now known to be a poor outcome measure for health education research (Pless, 1978). Unfortunately when observational measures of safety behavior are used, the research results for educational message interventions are often disappointing.

Educational messages about the importance of infant restraint seats, pamphlets on car safety, and the convenient purchase of a restraint seat in the hospital did not improve the percentage of parents who used infant seats at discharge (Reisinger & Williams, 1978). More extensive educational messages, incorporating safety messages during prenatal care, modeling of appropriate restraint seat use, free loan of a seat, and repeated safety messages during child health supervision have produced initial gains in the number of infants restrained properly (Christophersen & Sullivan, 1982; Greenberg & Coleman, 1982; Reisinger et al., 1981); however, these interventions have not produced restraint-seat usage durable beyond the first two or three months of the infant's life.

A similar lack of dramatic effects has been evident for poisoning-prevention counseling using "Mr. Yuk" materials (Fergusson, Horwood, Beautrais, & Shannon, 1982) and for messages regarding safe storage techniques (Sobel, 1969). Educational messages about the use of electrical outlet covers, installation of cabinet and drawer locks, and the reduction of fire hazards had limited success in changing parent behavior (Dershewitz, 1979; Dershewitz & Williamson, 1977).

Educational messages about installing smoke detectors and reducing water heater temperatures have produced more promising results. Pediatric counseling about the importance of smoke detectors and facilitating parents' convenient purchase of smoke detectors resulted in an increased number of correctly installed smoke detectors (Miller, Reisinger, Blatter, & Wucher, 1982). A later study did not find a significant increase from smoke detector counseling, but the sample included large percentages of experimental and control group parents who had smoke detectors before the study (Thomas, Hassanein, & Christophersen, 1984). The effectiveness for this counseling effort may be related to the fact that installing a smoke detector aproximates a passive strategy for injury control: once a smoke detector is installed, other behavior changes are not required. In addition, parents' use of a similar passive strategy recommended for burn control, reducing water heater temperatures (Feldman, Schaller, Feldman, & Mc-Millon, 1978), was significantly increased by pediatric counseling (Thomas et al., 1984).

Christophersen, Sosland-Edelman, and LeClaire (in press) reported on an evaluation of a comprehensive child passenger safety program that included health education by hospital pediatric and nursing staffs. Both the experimental and comparison programs were conducted in the State of Kansas, which had legislation mandating restraint seat usage with infants. Other components included an established loaner seat program and numerous public education campaigns regarding child passenger safety. Thus the major difference was the health education component. Both groups had more than 90 percent of parents using infant restraint seats at discharge from the hospital. One year later, after the transition from an infant seat to a toddler seat, both groups had more than 84 percent of parents using restraint seats. Thus the health education program, at least for the suburban, educated, middle-class population studied, did not produce higher compliance. Further research is necessary to conclude what components result in significant numbers of parents using safety precautions for their children.

For at least some injury control techniques, perhaps those that do not require repeated activities, educational messages delivered by primary care providers may be an effective means of increasing the safety of children. For other injury control techniques, educational messages may be insufficient or may need to be enhanced by comprehensive programs that include many components. Therefore, more intensive educational and motivational strategies may be needed.

Educational Programs.   The status of research on educational programs is illustrated by four educational programs designed to enhance parent and child knowledge about poisoning risks and emetics. The major limitation of current educational programs is a lack of assessment of the behavioral and health outcomes that are obtained from educational programs. For example, Dershewitz, Posner, and Paichel (1983) assessed the knowledge of the use of syrup of ipecac in a group of mothers counseled by their pediatricians. Mothers were able to describe the use of the emetic, but the relationship of this knowledge to the actual use of poison antidotes was not established. Braden (1979) taught preschoolers in a daycare center to discriminate poisons and poison warning labels ("NO!" "STOP") in verbal and performance tasks, but assessment of actual poison avoidance in the home or reduction in poison incidents was not established. A similar 10-lesson program for preschoolers using "Mr. Yuk" materials enhanced children's identification of poisons, but was not evaluated in terms of home behavior or poison outcome (Krenzelok & Garber, 1981).

Educational programs may ultimately provide much needed safety training for children and parents. However, the extensive training process required for successful injury control may not be feasible for pediatric primary care. However, they may represent a complementary injury control intervention for preschools, daycare centers, and elementary schools.

Mass Media. An obvious value of mass media is the ability to inform large numbers of people about safety hazards and injury control techniques. There have been few controlled studies of mass media campaigns for injury control, but one exemplary study on the effects of repeated messages on seat belt use found that no behavior change resulted from an expensive television advertising campaign (Robertson et al., 1974). A cable television system serving an urban area was split so that two groups of subscribers could be monitored. One group of subscribers received the repeated safety messages, while the other group received advertising messages. Seat belt use was not different for the families who were exposed to the safety message campaign.

Media presentations, such as the series produced by the Stanford Heart Disease Prevention Project (Farquhar et al., 1977), may produce knowledge increases without complementary behavior changes. Other media campaigns have been supplemented by social support groups; for example, a highly structured community support group that watched televised smoking-cessation programs had a larger percentage of persons who stopped smoking than a comparison group that watched the programs alone (McAlister, Puska, Koskela, Pallonen & Maccoby, 1980). A program in Sweden used groups of parents who functioned as "child-environment supervisors" combined with a media program to increase public awareness of hazards and the elimination of public injury hazards (Gustafsson et al., 1979). However, research on the effectiveness of mass media for injury control has been limited by poor research methodology and a limited number of studies. Future research on media injury-control programs may show that the incidence of injuries may be reduced by a combination of interventions that include detailed media programs that not only teach about environmental hazards but also demonstrate effective ways of eliminating hazards or protecting children from them.

Motivational Strategies

A recent and promising initiative for injury control research has been to include the programming of contingent consequences for safe behavior. Several published studies on injury control interventions based on motivational strategies illustrate this approach to injury control. Christophersen (1977) attempted to identify a positive reinforcing consequence for child car seat use and found that children who were placed in safety restraints were better behaved. A later study used an across-subjects experimental design to evaluate the effectiveness of using information about improved child behavior to encourage parents to use restraint seats (Christophersen & Gyulay, 1981). Restraint seat use increased after parents received the "improved child behavior" counseling. The hypothesis was that parents who used restraint seats consistently would experience better child behavior and that behavioral improvements would reinforce continued use of restraint seats; in fact, restraint use by parents who received this counseling was maintained across a one-year follow-up. Thus the motivation to use restraint seats was to improve child behavior rather than avoid the possibility of injury. A later study has shown that a counseling package containing information about improved child behavior and the possible injuries ("fear message") was more effective than either approach alone (Treiber, in press).

Contingent reinforcement has also resulted in increased use of seat belts (Geller, Johnson, & Pelton, 1982; Geller, Paterson, & Talbot, 1982). Controlled studies by these investigators have shown that receipt of incentives (coupons exchangeable for food, gift items, and dinners at local restaurants) contingent on seat belt use produced significant increases in seat belt use in the study setting. Promising behavioral solutions to the problem of adult seat belt use through motivational programs (contingent reinforcement) may have great generality for programs designed to protect children traveling in cars. The feasibility and cost effectiveness of such programs for application to the public at large must be established once effective programs are developed for children.

A recent study by Tertinger, Greene, and Lutzker (1984) evaluated a comprehensive home safety assessment and behavior change program. Within-subject experimental designs with in-home observational measures were used to evaluate the results of the safety program with six families. The comprehensive home safety checklist was completed by trained observers and was sensitive to changes in safety behavior of parents. Following educational feedback in the home, parents corrected specific targeted hazards, but corrections were not extended to untargeted but identified hazards in the homes. This study suggests that objective assessment and safety interventions can reduce the number of hazards in homes. However, the relationship of hazard reduction to reduced injuries in the home has not been established (Baltimore & Meyer, 1968), and the utility, benefits, and cost effectiveness of this approach have not been studied. Further research on motivational strategies is a clear direction for future injury control research. Because many injury control strategies depend on human behavior for their effectiveness, research on motivation variables for injury control programs can contribute to the development of effective programs.

Legislation

Legislation on injury control is a difficult area to study. Laws are not implemented in an experimental fashion and thus only quasiexperimental comparisons can usually be made for injury rates before and after the legislation is introduced. However, changes in injury rates are often substantial and are coincident with changes in the law so that the attribution of results to the laws are often quite believable.

A dramatic example of the beneficial effects that legislation can have on childhood injuries is the "Children Can't Fly" program developed by the New York City Department of Health to combat the high incidence of deaths due to window falls (Spiegel & Lindaman, 1977). The program included many components, including legislation, public education campaign, and a distribution system for free installation of window guards. Between 1973 and 1975, there was a 50 percent decline in reported falls, and no falls were reported from windows where guards had been installed. Thus a program based on legislation can dramatically reduce child injuries and deaths.

Childhood ingestions of poisons, especially medications such as aspirin, have been dramatically reduced through product safety legislation. Clarke and Walton (1979) analyzed data from poison control centers in the United States and showed that aspirin ingestions decreased from 12.4 per center in 1965 to 1.4 per center in 1974. During the same period, there was a corresponding decrease from a death rate of 3.4 per million in 1968 to only 1.5 per million in 1974. These decreases were attributed to the introduction of the Poison Prevention Packaging Act of 1970, which mandated child-resistant safety caps for medication bottles. A significant decrease in poisoning occurred following the introduction of child-resistant packaging in England and Wales (Craft & Jackson, 1977).

Comparisons of seat belt use in countries, states, and provinces with and without seat belt use laws have also been made (National Highway Traffic Safety Administration, 1979; Robertson & Williams, 1978). In countries with mandatory seat belt usage, such as Australia and New Zealand, more than 70 percent of drivers observed were correctly using seat belts. Other countries were even higher, with 92 percent of drivers in Belgium, 87 to 95 percent in Switzerland, and 80 percent in Israel. In contrast, in states in the U.S. in which there were no seat belt laws, usage rates were between 20 and 30 percent. Increases in the use of restraint seats for children have been observed following the introduction of legislation in Rhode Island, Tennessee, and Quebec (Stulginskas & Pless, 1983; Williams & Wells, 1981). Although comparisons such as these do not constitute experiments, such discrepant safety behavior suggests that legislation may play an important role in reducing childhood injuries.

In summary considerable differences can be found in the quantity, quality, and reported effectiveness of this research. Most studies employ health education procedures and measure knowledge change and other indirect indices of behavior change. Direct measures of behavior appear to be most precise and objective in the motivational studies, perhaps because the nature of the intervention depends so much on quantification of the target behavior(s). In contrast, a passive approach, including legislative or regulatory interventions, appears to result in the greatest demonstrated reductions in mortality and morbidity. Unfortunately, most studies include two or more approaches, even though one approach might be emphasized as an explanation for the results. For example, passive approaches employing legislative intervention also included media coverage. Combining approaches is a reasonable strategy for studies that attempt to demonstrate that injury rates can be reduced but makes determining the relative effectiveness of, and necessity for, particular components difficult.

A CASE STUDY ON IMPACTING POLITICAL DECISION MAKING: CHILD PASSENGER SAFETY LEGISLATION IN KANSAS

To date, the passive approach to injury control has produced the best results. The adoption and use of passive approaches (such as car safety seats) is more likely if antecedent events (such as educational and awareness campaigns) and consequent events (such as fines) are arranged. Such events are usually arranged by elected officials or agency policymakers in accordance with their legislative and regulatory responsibilities. Their prescriptions of safety laws and regulations can be targeted for change by researchers and advocates for child safety. Presented here are the details of a successful effort to use research information to affect the behavior of state legislators considering a specific piece of child safety legislation.

As noted earlier, motor vehicle injuries are the leading cause of death for children in the United States. The current consensus among medical professionals is that many deaths and injuries, and much related trauma, could be prevented through widespread use of child passenger safety devices (National Safety Council, 1981). In the past several years medical societies and highway safety groups have lobbied successfully for state legislation requiring that parents or guardians use approved safety devices for their young children. Child-passenger safety laws have been passed in all but one state, although they vary in the ages of children affected, locations in the vehicle covered, penalties for noncompliance, and other relevant dimensions.

In the course of original enactment and subsequent reconsideration of these laws, researchers are called on to provide expert testimony pertinent to the policy choices available for reducing risk to child passengers. Although public policy is not formulated or enacted on the basis of fact and rationality alone, timely presentations of research information can inform, and occasionally influence, political decision-makers. How behavioral scientists conducted policy research and presented it to legislators considering the original Kansas Child Passenger Safety Act represents a typology of information relevant to political decision making regarding child safety issues.

Conduct of Policy Research

James Coleman (1972) outlined five steps in conducting policy research designed to inform political decision making. These steps were applied in creating and communicating research information to legislators considering the original Kansas Child Passenger Safety Act (H.B. 2208) (for more detail, see Fawcett & Seekins, 1981). In this case, the behavioral scientists contacted the legislator and offered their assistance. Three weeks were available between the initial conversation between the sponsor of the bill and the behavioral scientists and the committee hearing in which research information could be communicated.

Step 1: Identify Interested Parties.   Interested parties are those for whom favorable action on proposed legislation might be expected to produce reinforcing consequences. In a structured interview, the behavioral scientists requested a complete list of such groups from the state representative interested in sponsoring a bill requiring use of approved child-passenger safety devices. She identifed other interested parties, including the Kansas Medical Society (a state lobbying group for physicians), the Kansas Women for Highway Safety (a public interest group), and a number of pediatricians, nurses, and specialists in behavioral pediatrics.

Step 2: Determine Interests of the Parties.   In the same interview, the behavioral scientists inquired about the types of responses that could be reinforcing for the sponsor and other parties. As passage of the bill was judged doubtful, the sponsor sought credible testimony from the researchers in a hearing before the House Committee on Public Health and Welfare.

Step 3: Determine Relevant Information Needs.   The behavioral scientists questioned the sponsor about the availability and relevance of several more specific types of information. She noted three important areas in which information was lacking: (1) the number of children at risk, (2) whether the issue was important enough to merit consideration by the legislature, and (3) whether constituents would support regulation in this area usually reserved for parental discretion.

Step 4: Obtain the Information.   The behavioral scientists agreed to examine these questions using methods of behavioral assessment and survey research. Using a response definition based on standards promulgated by the Physicians for Highway Safety, the behavioral scientists collected behavioral observations and calculated the percentages of children at risk in urban and rural areas. In addition, random digit dialing survey research methods were used to estimate the percentage of constituents who judged the issue to be important and who supported regulation in this area. The percentage of respondents who acknowledged specific reasons for not supporting regulation was also computed.

Step 5: Report the Results. The sponsor and lobbyist identified characteristics of effective expert testimony, including brevity, professional attire, avoidance of jargon, written testimony for media distribution, and oral summary of findings and unequivocal recommendations based on research. At a hearing of the House Committee, one of the behavioral scientists presented brief (five-minute) testimony consisting of introductory remarks, a description of the study, a reading of the three main findings, and a summary statement. This testimony was credited with influencing passage out of committee and eventually into law. (The original law that resulted was a weak one: it provided for an oral warning and limited coverage for children under two years riding in the front seat. A subsequent law provided for a fine and extended coverage.) Researchers can thus create and communicate knowledge relevant to policy choices for reducing accident risks for children.

Types of Information Useful in Political Decision Making

Researchers who would have their findings inform politicians and policymakers should themselves be knowledgeable about the kinds of information sought in expert testimony. A brief description of seven types of information, and their application in testimony regarding the Kansas Child Passenger Safety Act, follows.

Dimensions of an Issue. Policy analysts (Quade, 1975; Stokey & Zeckhauser, 1978) agree that the first step in developing research information is to define the problem. This step involves specifying and describing the behaviors and their antecedents and consequent events (Rein & Schon, 1977). For example, in testimony regarding the Kansas Child Passenger Safety Act, health officials presented epidemiological data indicating that automobile accidents are a leading cause of child injury and death. One of the behavioral scientists showed the film "Children in Crashes" to the legislative committee. Members of the Kansas Medical Society and Kansas Nurses Association provided anecdotes of the physical conditions of child victims they had treated. Displays of child car seats and demonstrations of their use were also provided.

Relative Standing on an Issue. Public officials are constrained to choose a limited number of issues to confront in any legislative session (Walker, 1977). Cobb and Elder (1972) and Walker (1977) suggested that information showing the relative standing of issues in the opinion of the general public and various groups may help establish decision priorities. For example, although not presented in this case study, data comparing the relative importance of child safety issues to other policy demands might have helped legislators determine the degree of effort they would invest in considering this proposed legislation. In the absence of these data, the legislative sponsor had to work exceptionally hard to keep the house speaker from placing the bill on the "bone pile" of those that would not be submitted for full consideration.

Number of People Affected.   Scale theories of policy formulation (Schattschneider, 1960) suggest that information concerning the number of people affected by an issue may serve to limit or resolve conflicts. For example, issues concerning child safety may command a great deal of attention from public officials, partly because they involve children, parents, grandparents, medical providers, law enforcement agencies, and commercial enterprises. The researchers presented data suggesting that 98 percent of the children in the state were at risk; thus, for example, 98 percent of parents with young children might potentially be affected.

Interests of Those Involved.   Coleman (1972) suggested that information about the various interests involved in regulation is important to public officials. The greater the intensity of conflict between competing groups, the greater the reinforcing value of its resolution. For example, the behavioral scientists presented survey data to legislators that those in opposition to child passenger safety legislation wanted to minimize government interference in their lives and maximize personal freedom. This information helped to clarify values implicit in complaints received by legislators regarding the proposed bill.

Controlling Variables.   Public officials typically employ educative, facilitative, and punitive strategies to solve problems (Balch, 1980). Information about the variables controlling the behavior of those involved in an issue conflict may suggest more effective policy methods. Such tactical research (Bulmer, 1981) may suggest how public officials might use such methods as media information, tax incentives, or fines to have some impact on the dependent variables of interest. For example, the Kansas Medical Society provided information about the use of fines in other state laws, and the Kansas Highway Patrol testified to the difficulty of enforcing such laws.

Technological Alternatives.   Bulmer (1981) described information about specific program arrangements and their effectiveness (consequences produced) as the most potent type of research information available to public officials. It is characterized by demonstrations of experimental control over dependent variables in the real world. Although no information of this type was presented, data on the effects of car seat loaner programs would have been useful.

Social Validity.   Wolf (1978) identified three dimensions of social validity for program alternatives, including the importance of goals, acceptability of procedures, and significance of the effects. In the Kansas testimony, behavioral scientists presented information that indicated most citizens believed child safety was important and found a law to mandate the use of child safety seats acceptable.

Limitations and Caveats

Using the steps outlined in the case study, relevant research knowledge can be produced and disseminated to elected officials when public policies regarding child risk to injury are formulated and when they are enacted. However, just as communication of relevant research is no guarantee of policy enactment, the passage of seemingly prudent legislation is no assurance of reduced risk for children. Indeed, an evaluation of laws in seven states (Seekins et al., 1982) suggests that the passage of state laws may not be sufficient to promote child safety. These observations suggest that, even with a large number of issued citations, use of safety seats rarely exceeds 50 percent observance. The passage of state legislation does not guarantee significant levels of implementation. Many states, such as Kansas, have "home rule" constitutions (Hahn & Levine, 1982), meaning that each city must adopt state legislation for local police to have the authority to implement the law. In general there are a large number of government agencies and autonomous groups that must be involved in any broad prevention effort and few mechanisms for coordinated implementation.

The finding that child passenger safety laws—when enforced at typical levels—do not produce clinically significant levels of compliance has important implications for government involvement in promoting safety. The assumption that passing a law will result in reduced risk is tempting, as in the U.S. Department of Transportation's decision to offer to postpone implementation of air bags if enough states pass laws requiring use of seat belts. As a more effective alternative the federal government might call for adoption of national safety goals, such as 80 percent use of approved safety restraints, and uniform measurement systems for detecting levels of attainment. A percentage of federal highway funds, perhaps 1 percent, might be awarded contingent on observed compliance with the national goal for child safety. This approach would leave to states and local communities the freedom to choose socially acceptable means for achieving national standards for child passenger safety and other legislation designed to reduce child injury.

Thus as successful as this positive approach may appear to be, it does have limitations. Clinicians, policymakers, parents, and scientists will need to continue to work on improving and extending this model for injury control, as well as to consider others. Science offers one possible decision-making strategy for identifying and choosing the best approaches, and appropriate priorities for research must be set.

RESEARCH PRIORITIES

The prevalence and costs of childhood injury argue well for making it a high priority for our problem-solving activities. Advances in health care practices during the past century have been increasingly based on the use of scientific method to better understand the underlying processes involved in health and illness and to assess the necessity for specific procedures. Although childhood injury may not be best reduced solely by a medical or public health approach, the methods of science as a problem-solving strategy offer some distinct and important advantages in that science provides a knowledge base that is objective (quantifiable), replicable, and cumulative. If then we are to look to science, in part, to identify solutions to the childhood injury problem, what should we do first, what should be our priorities?

Descriptive Studies of Changeable Factors

The majority of research to date has been correlational in nature; this type of research is appropriate to a new area of investigation as it allows for the identification of marker variables that are associated with and therefore may influence injury. However, to continue to maintain the same proportion of correlational to causal studies would not take advantage of the descriptive knowledge base so far accumulated and would likely result in interventions that are both less efficient and more expensive than necessary. Descriptive research should now be focused more on identifying factors associated with injury that can readily be altered through some combination of passive and active intervention strategies.

Proximal Indices of Injury-Related Mortality and Morbidity

The ultimate value of injury control approaches will be determined by the degree of reduction in mortality and morbidity. Although childhood injury is a major public health problem, the prevalence of serious injury is sufficiently low to require that large populations be studied. As a result, studies using mortality and morbidity as primary measures are costly, requiring large numbers of subjects; and long-term effects often require years of data collection to demonstrate an experimental effect. An alternative is to conduct studies that employ more frequently occurring and readily observable events, such as behaviors or environmental conditions presumed to be proximally related to injury (for example, children in car restraint seats, hot water heater temperatures). The advantages of this strategy are proportional to the degree of association between these proximal indices and eventual injury. Accordingly a critical area for research is the identification of proximal indices that are *highly* related to injury. Such measures would probably be prerequisites or conditions for injury, and their role in the occurrence of specific injury would appear intuitive rather than as a subject for measurement research. Yet such intuitive justifications for intervention programs are exactly the reason for the appeal and success during the past century of basing medical practice on experimental, quantitative evidence rather than solely on clinical experience. Childhood injury is too serious a problem to be approached in a manner similar to the clinical guesswork that has existed in medicine from the time of Hippocrates.

Basic Research on Risk-Taking and Safe Behavior

To date, almost all the intervention approaches to childhood injury have targeted one or, at most, a few causes of injury. Yet our descriptive data indicate that some children are likely to have multiple injuries, while others very few; that some children will be injured when very few risks are present in their environment, while others will suffer few or no injuries even when the environment contains many dangerous situations. Such data suggest that factors related to the child's behavior, mother-child interactions and learning, and possibly other family or social situations make some children more likely to be injured, independent of the overall number of hazards in their environment. For example, through early learning experiences some children may acquire response repertoires or classes of behavior that are either high-risk (result in frequent injuries) or safe (result in few injuries). Therefore, a potentially fruitful area for investigation would be the study of the environmental conditions and contingencies that promote hazardous versus safe behavior. Such research could precede both from the study of parents and children and from animal models, particularly those similar to studies on avoidance conditioning.

Observational studies are needed to identify and measure observable parent and child behaviors that lead to injury or safety (avoidance of injury) and environmental conditions that can be changed to reduce injury and promote safety. Such observational studies would lead to intervention research to determine effective strategies to reduce risk taking and injury and to determine specific educational procedures needed for special populations (e.g., strategies designed for infants, toddlers, and school-age children).

Multiple-Outcome Interventions

One of the limitations of the passive approach to injury control is its necessity for targeting only one risk or injury at a time. In this time of escalating health care costs, we must be sure not to effect prevention approaches that are as costly as the injuries themselves. Therefore we should expand our considerations to include possible interventions that target many types of injuries. For example, studying hazardous versus safe behavior could be such a multiple-outcome intervention, as could passive approaches that target a child-safe home where multiple hazards are eliminated (Tertinger et al., 1984).

Community-Based Interventions

Research should also focus on the development of methods for local communities to reach performance goals. One approach might be systematic manipulation of antecedent and consequent variables on a community-wide scale. For example, the effects of prompts and praise might be investigated by observing the effects of bank teller window operators suggesting the use of safety seats to those not using them (operators might say, "The city is encouraging the use of child safety seats by all drivers. Here's a brochure that explains it.") and praising those using them ("Those seats save lives."). In addition, consequent variables might be arranged through gift certificates exchangeable at local franchise restaurants.

State Legislation and Executive Agency Policy

State laws and executive agency policy represent another level at which injury control interventions can be designed, implemented, and evaluated. For example, the overwhelming majority of child passenger safety laws rely primarily on a regulatory strategy that requires citizens to comply with the law under threat of punishment and is implemented by state highway patrol and local law enforcement agencies. Conceivably, the effects of a police crackdown on public highways or city streets might coincide with statements of child safety promotion. The wisdom of using coercion to force compliance with important social goals such as reducing risks for children is a subject of debate. Some political scientists (Neiman, 1980) argue that such regulatory policies provide a basis for inflicting retribution on those who do not comply. In doing so, they contribute to a shared sense that a practice, such as not restraining a child in a safety device, is wrong. Others (Balch, 1980) caution that the punishment features of such regulations may result in side effects such as anger directed to supporters of the legislation, lowered self-esteem related to the stigma of punishment, or attempts to escape or avoid punishment by cheating or lobbying to repeal legislation. Attempts to repeal child passenger legislation have already occurred. If enforcement is increased, efforts by parents to subvert installation requirements, lie about childrens' ages, or otherwise attempt to avoid punishment may also be observed. Initiatives to repeal and revise existing child passenger laws may yield insights into more optimal legislative strategies for reducing this risk to child injury. Priority should be given to development of research knowledge that contributes to policy making. There are many points at which this could be achieved: agenda setting, policy formulation, enactment, implementation, evaluation, and reconsideration. Research investigating the effects of such public-private partnerships at the local level might be particularly productive.

CONCLUSION

Injury is the number one health problem of children and youth. Like the most prevalent health concerns of adults, childhood injury results from a combination of factors both biological and environmental in nature, related to life style as well as to social and personal characteristics. Solutions put forth to date have included the more traditional medical-health education approach, learning-based interventions, and political and legislative mandates.

Accordingly, the ultimate solution to this number one child health priority will come from the combined talents of biomedical and behavioral scientists, clinicians, politicians, and parents. As such this problem and its resolution represent an example of the fundamental necessity for an interdisciplinary approach to child health behavior.

ACKNOWLEDGEMENTS

The order of authorship does not represent the level of contribution but, rather, the order of sections that appear in the chapter: overall organization and coordination, research priorities—Cataldo and Finney; epidemiology—Dershewitz; conceptual framework—Wilson; research critique—Christophersen and Finney; Kansas case study—Fawcett and Seekins.

Preparation of this chapter was supported in part by grants 917 and MCJ-243270-01-0 from Maternal and Child Health. We wish to thank Ruth Cargo for her assistance, especially for the excellent editorial work that is so necessary on a multiple-author manuscript.

REFERENCES

Allen, D. B., & Bergman, A. B. (1976). Social learning approaches to health education: Utilization of infant auto restraint devices. *Pediatrics, 58*, 323–328.

Angle, C. R. (1975). Locomotor skills and school accidents. *Pediatrics, 56*, 819–822.

Baker, S. P., & Dietz, P. E. (1979). The epidemiology and prevention of injuries. In G. D. Zuidema, R. B. Rutherford, & W. F. Ballinger (Eds.), *The management of trauma* (3rd ed.; pp. 794–799). Philadelphia: W. B. Saunders.

Baker, S. P., O'Neill, B., & Karpf, R. S. (1984). *The injury fact book.* Lexington, MA: Heath.

Balch, G. I. (1980). The carrot, the stick, and other strategies: A theoretical analysis of governmental intervention. In J. Brigham & D. W. Brown (Eds.), *Policy implementation: Penalties or incentives?* (pp. 43–68). Beverly Hills, CA: Sage Publications.

Baltimore, C. L., & Meyer, R. J. (1968). A study of storage, child behavioral traits and mother's knowledge in 52 poisoned families and 52 comparison families. *Pediatrics, 42*, 312–317.

Barancik, J. I., Chatterjee, B. F., Greene, Y. C, Michenzi, E M., & Fife, D. (1983). Northeastern Ohio trauma study: 1. Magnitude of the problem. *American Journal of Public Health, 73*, 746– 751.

Berger, L. R. (1981). Childhood injuries: Recognition and prevention. *Current problems in pediatrics* (pp. 1–59). Chicago: Year Book Medical Publishers.

Braden, B. T. (1979). Validation of a poison prevention program. *American Journal of Public Health, 69*, 942–944.

Bulmer, M. (1981). Applied social research: A reformulation of "Applied" and "Enlightenment" models. *Knowledge: Creation, Diffusion, Utilization, 3*, 187–210.

Christoffel, K. K., & Tanz, R. (1983). Motor vehicle injury in childhood. *Pediatrics in Review, 4*, 247–254.

Christophersen, E. R. (1977). Children's behavior during automobile rides: Do car seats make a difference? *Pediatrics, 60*, 69–74.

Christophersen, E. R., & Gyulay, J. (1981). Parental compliance with car seat usage: A positive approach with long-term follow-up. *Journal of Pediatric Psychology, 6*, 301–312.

Christophersen, E. R., Sosland-Edelman, D., & LeClaire, S. (in press). An evaluation of a comprehensive infant car seat loaner program with one-year follow-up. *Pediatrics.*

Christophersen, E. R., & Sullivan, M. A. (1982). Increasing the protection of newborn infants in cars. *Pediatrics, 70*, 21–25.

Clarke, E. R., & Walton, W. W. (1979). Effect of safety packaging on aspirin ingestion by children. *Pediatrics, 63*, 687–693.

Cobb, R., & Elder, C. (1972). *Participation in American politics: The dynamics of agenda building.* Baltimore: Johns Hopkins University Press.

Coleman, J. S. (1972). *Policy research in the social sciences.* Morristown, NJ: General Learning Corporation.

Craft, A. W., & Jackson, R. H. (1977). Child-resistant packaging and accidental poisoning. *Lancet, 1*, 289–290.

Dershewitz, R. A. (1979). Will mothers use free household safety devices? *American Journal of Diseases of Children, 133*, 61–64.

Dershewitz, R. A., & Christophersen, E. R. (1984). Childhood household safety: An Overview. *American Journal of Diseases of Children, 138*, 85–88.

Dershewitz, R. A., Posner, M. K., & Paichel, W. (1983). The effectiveness of health education on home use of ipecac. *Clinical Pediatrics, 22*, 268–270.

Dershewitz, R. A., & Williamson, J. W. (1977). Prevention of childhood injuries: A controlled clinical trial. *American Journal of Public Health, 67*, 1148–1153.

Farquhar, J. W., Maccoby, N., Wood, P., Alexander, J., Breitrose, H., Brown, B., Haskell, W., McAlister, A., Meyer, A. Nash, J., & Stern, M. (1977). Community education for cardiovascular health. *Lancet, 1*, 1192–1195.

Fawcett, S. B., & Seekins, T. (1981). Policy research and child passenger safety: A case study. Unpublished manuscript available from the Center for Public Affairs, University of Kansas, Lawrence, KS 66045.

Feldman, K. W. (1980). Prevention of childhood accidents: Recent progress. *Pediatrics in Review, 2*, 75–82.

Feldman, K. W., Schaller, R. T., Feldman, J. A., & McMillon, M. (1978). Tap water scald burns in children. *Pediatrics, 62*, 1–7.

Fergusson, D. M., Horwood, L. J., Beautrais, A. L., & Shannon, F. T. (1982). A controlled field trial of a poisoning prevention method. *Pediatrics, 69*, 515–520.

Finney, J. W., & Christophersen, E. R. (1984). Behavioral pediatrics: Health education in pediatric primary care. In M. Hersen, R. M. Eisler, & P. M. Miller (Eds.), *Progress in behavior modification* (Vol. 16; pp. 185–229). New York: Academic.

Garfield, E. (1983, November 29). Child safety: Part 1. *Current Comments*, No. 48, 5–12.

Geller, E. S., Johnson, R. P., & Pelton, S. L. (1982). Community-based interventions for encouraging safety belt use. *American Journal of Community Psychology, 10*, 183–195.

Geller, E. S., Paterson, L., & Talbot, E. (1982). A behavioral analysis of incentive prompts for motivating seat belt use. *Journal of Applied Behavior Analysis, 15*, 403–415.

Green, L. W., Kreuter, M. W., Deeds, S. G., & Partridge, K. B. (1980). *Health education planning: A diagnostic approach.* Palo Alto, CA: Mayfield.

Greenberg, L. W., & Coleman, A. B. (1982). A prenatal and postpartum safety education program: Influence on parental use of infant car restraints. *Journal of Developmental and Behavioral Pediatrics, 3*, 32–34.

Gustafsson, L. H., Hammarstrom, A., Linder, K., Stjernberg, E., Sundelin, C., & Thulin, C. (1979). Child-environment supervisors: A new strategy for prevention of childhood accidents. *Acta Paediatrica Scandinavica, 275* (Suppl.), 102–107.

Haddon, W. (1970). On the escape of tigers: An ecologic note. *Technology Review* (Massachusetts Institute of Technology), *72*(May), 44–53.

Haddon, W. (1980). Landmarks in American epidemiology: Advances in the epidemiology of injuries as a basis for public policy. *Public Health Reports, 95*, 411–421.

Haddon, W., & Baker, S. P. (1981). Injury control. In D. Clark & B. MacMahon (Eds.), *Preventive medicine* (2nd ed.; pp. 109–140). Boston: Little, Brown.

Hahn, H., & Levine, C. (1980). Introduction: The politics of urban America and the study of urban politics. In H. Hahn & C. Levine (Eds.), *Urban politics: Past, present and future* (pp. 1–50). New York: Longman.

Harris, C.S., Baker, S. P., Smith, G. A., & Harris, R. M. (1984). Childhood asphyxiation by food. *Journal of the American Medical Association, 251*, 2231–2235.

Hongladarom, G. C., Allard, J., & Miller, W. F. (1978). Injuries due to falls—Washington. *Morbidity and Mortality Weekly Report, 27*, 192–198.

Insurance Institute for Highway Safety (1978). *To Prevent Harm.* Washington, DC: Author.

Insurance Institute for Highway Safety. (1984, April 27). *The highway loss reduction status report, 19*(7). Washington, DC: Author.

Kanthor, H. A. (1976). Car safety for infants: Effectiveness of prenatal counseling. *Pediatrics, 58*, 320–322.

Karwacki, J. J., & Baker, S. P. (1979). Children in motor vehicles. *Journal of the American Medical Association, 242*, 2848–2851.

Krenzelok, E. P., & Garber, R. J. (1981). Teaching poison prevention to preschool children, their parents, and professional educators through child care centers. *American Journal of Public Health, 71*, 750–752.

McAlister, A., Puska, P., Koskela, K., Pallonen, U., & Maccoby, N. (1980). Mass communication and community organization for public health education. *American Psychologist, 35*, 375–379.

McCormick, M. C., Shapiro, S., & Starfield, B. H. (1981). Injury and its correlates among 1-year-old children. *American Journal of Diseases of Children, 135*, 159–163.

McIntire, M. S. (Ed.) (1980). *Handbook on accident prevention.* Hagerstown: Harper and Row.

Miller, R. E., Reisinger, K. S., Blatter, M. M., & Wucher, F. (1982). Pediatric counseling and subsequent use of smoke detectors. *American Journal of Public Health, 72,* 392–393.

Mofenson, H. C., & Greensher, J. (1978). Childhood accidents. In R. A. Hoekelman (Ed.), *Principles of pediatrics—Health care of the young* (pp. 1791–1823). New York: Mc-Graw-Hill.

National Highway Traffic Safety Administration (1979). *Effects of safety belt usage laws around the world.* Washington, DC: U.S. Department of Transportation.

National Safety Council (1981). *Policy update.* Washington, DC: Author.

Neiman, M. (1980). The virtues of heavy-handedness in government. In J. Brigham & D. W. Brown (Eds.), *Policy implementation: Penalties or incentives?* (pp. 19–42). Beverly Hills, CA: Sage Publications.

O'Shea, J. S., Collins, E. W., & Butler, C. B. (1982). Pediatric accident prevention. *Clinical Pediatrics, 21,* 290–297.

Paulson, J. A. (1979). Accidents. In A. J. Moss (Ed.), *Pediatrics update: Review for physicians* (pp. 419–439). New York, Elsevier Science Publishing.

Pless, I. B. (1978). Accident prevention and health education: Back to the drawing board. *Pediatrics, 62,* 431–435.

Pless, I. B., & Stulginskas, J. (1982). Accidents and violence as a cause of morbidity and mortality in childhood. In L. A. Barness (Ed.), *Advances in Pediatrics* (Vol. 29; pp. 471–495). Chicago: Year Book Medical Publishers.

Quade, E. S. (1975). *Analysis for public decisions.* New York: American Elsevier.

Rein, M., & Schon, D. A. (1977) Problem setting in policy research. In C. H. Weiss (Ed.), *Using social research in public policy making* (pp. 235–251). Lexington, MA: Lexington.

Reisinger, K. S., & Williams, A. F. (1978). Evaluation of programs designed to increase the protection of infants in cars. *Pediatrics, 62,* 280–287.

Reisinger, K. S., Williams, A. F., Wells, J. K., John, C. E., Roberts, T. R., & Podgainy, H. J. (1981). Effect of pediatrician's counsleing on infant restraint use. *Pediatrics, 67,* 201–206.

Rivara, F. P. (1982a). Epidemiology of childhood injuries. In A. B. Bergman (Ed.), *Preventing childhood injuries* (pp. 13–17). Report of the Twelfth Ross Roundtable on Critical Approaches to Common Pediatric Problems, March 29-30, 1981, Seattle.

Rivara, F. P. (1982b). Epidemiology of childhood injuries: 1. Review of current research and presentation of conceptual framework. *American Journal of Diseases of Children, 136,* 399–405.

Rivara, F. P., Bergman, A. B., & LoGerfo, J. P. (1982). Epidemiology of childhood injuries: 2. Sex differences in injury rates. *American Journal of Diseases of Children, 136,* 502–506.

Robertson, L. S., Kelley, A. B., O'Neill, B., Wixom, C. W., Eiswirth, R. S., & Haddon, W., Jr. (1974). A controlled study of the effect of television messages on safety belt use. *American Journal of Public Health, 64,* 1071–1080.

Robertson, L. S., & Williams, A. F. (1978, May). *International comparisons of the effect of motor vehicle seat belt use and child restraint laws.* Presentation to the Child Passenger Safety Conference, Transportation Center, University of Tennessee, Nashville.

Schattschneider, E. E. (1960). *The semi-sovereign people: A realist's view of democracy in America.* New York: Holt, Rinehart & Winston.

Seekins, T., Fawcett, S. B., Cohen, S. H., Elder, J. P., Jason, L. A., Schnelle, F., & Winett, R. A. (1982). *Experimental analysis of child passenger safety legislation.* Washington, DC: American Psychological Association.

Sobel, R. (1969). Traditional safety measures and accidental poisoning in childhood. *Pediatrics, 44,* 811–816.

Speigel, C. N., & Lindaman, F. C. (1977). Children can't fly: A program to prevent childhood morbidity and mortality from window falls. *American Journal of Public Health, 67,* 1143–1147.

Stokey, E., & Zeckhauser, R. (1978). *A primer for policy analysis.* New York: Norton.

Stulginskas, J. V., & Pless, I. B. (1983). Effects of a seat belt law on child restraint use. *American Journal of Diseases of Children, 137,* 582–585.

Tertinger, D. A., Greene, B. F., & Lutzker, J. R. (1984). Home safety: Development and validation of one component of an ecobehavioral treatment program for abused and neglected children. *Journal of Applied Behavior Analysis, 17,* 159–174.

Thomas, K. A., Hassanein, R. S., & Christophersen, E. R. (1984). Evaluation of group well-child care for improving burn prevention practices in the home. *Pediatrics, 74,* 879–882.

Treiber, F. A. (in press). A comparison of the positive and negative consequences approaches upon car restraint usage. *Journal of Pediatric Psychology.*

United States Consumer Product Safety Commission (1980). *NEISS Data Highlights.* Bethesda, MD: National Injury Information Clearinghouse.

Walker, J. L. (1977). Setting the agenda in the U.S. Senate: A theory of problem selection. *Journal of Political Science, 7,* 423–445.

Westfelt, J. A. R. N. (1982). Environmental factors in childhood accidents. *Acta Paediatrica Scandinavica* (Supp. 291), 1–75.

Williams, A. F. (1976). Factors in the initiation of bicycle-motor vehicle collisions. *American Journal of Diseases of Children, 130,* 370–377.

Williams, A. F., & Wells, J. K. (1981). Evaluation of the Rhode Island child restraint law. *American Journal of Public Health, 71,* 742–743.

Wise, P. H., Mills, M., & Wilson, M. (1983). The influence of race and socioeconomic status on childhood mortality in Boston [Abstract]. *American Journal of Diseases of Children, 137,* 538.

Wolf, M. M. (1978). Social validity: The case for subjective measurement or how applied behavior analysis is finding its heart. *Journal of Applied Behavior Analysis, 11,* 203–214.

12

Biobehavioral Prevention in Primary Care

PATRICK C. FRIMAN AND EDWARD R. CHRISTOPHERSEN

INTRODUCTION

Every major subdivision or section within the formal medical care enterprise in the United States has, as a part of its governing structure, a system of task forces, committees and retreats, the purpose of which is to identify the needs of the population that the subdivision serves and to evaluate the extent to which those needs are currently being met. In order to expedite the service of those needs, the task forces often make recommendations regarding how the relevant medical field can be altered to improve satisfaction of the identified needs.

In 1977, the American Academy of Pediatrics published a revised edition of their Standards of Health Care. The revised standards strongly emphasized prevention as a fundamental goal in primary pediatrics (Committee

Preparation of this manuscript was partially supported by grants from NICHD (HD 03144 and HD 02528) to the Bureau of Child Research, University of Kansas on Standards of Child Health Care, 1977). In order to comply both with the letter and the spirit of the revised standards, pediatric administrators, journals, and practitioners will have to encourage, reward, and conduct effective preventive interventions. Pediatric research is already reflecting changes that have apparently occurred as a function of the renewed emphasis on prevention. (The term "pediatrician," as used in this manuscript, refers to all pediatric primary health care providers. The authors recognize that in many instances preventive strategies such as those discussed in this paper could be implemented by other members of the health care team.)

The field of health education has also influenced preventive pediatrics (Finney & Christophersen, 1984). Health education has been defined as ". . . any combination of learning experiences designed to facilitate voluntary adaptions of behavior conducive to health" (Green, Kreuter, Deeds, & Partridge, 1980, p. 7). Traditionally health education focused on disseminating information that led to informed decisions about health behavior. This distribution of information took place in school, community, and hospital programs designed to teach individuals how to maintain their health (Lazes, 1979). Such health education programs have been effective at increasing knowledge of health issues, but not at changing health behavior (Bergman, 1982; Finney & Christophersen, 1984). The definition of health education provided by Green et al., (1980), however, indicates that health education must not only increase knowledge levels, but must also change behaviors.

Despite the suggestions that many pediatric medical disorders can be prevented, little controlled research demonstrates this. The relative absence of research does not appear to be the result of failed studies but, rather, the result of lack of study. Biobehavioral technology, however, has been applied to prevention of other childhood problems. For example, an established body of research devoted to the prevention of childhood behavior problems exists (Brazelton, 1975; Chamberlin, 1982; Christophersen, 1977; Christophersen & Rapoff, 1980; Cullen, 1976; Yule, 1977). A new but growing body of literature devoted to preventing death and disability in children by increasing car safety also exists (Christophersen, 1983; Christophersen & Gyulay, 1981; Christophersen & Sullivan, 1982). And a body of research devoted to prevention of children's household accidents is emerging (Dershewitz & Christophersen, 1984; Thomas, Hassanein, & Christophersen, 1985). A major task remaining for preventive pediatrics is the development of a biobehavioral technology for prevention of pediatric medical disorders.

The remainder of this chapter will provide a discussion of four pediatric disorders that can occur during the course of child development: obesity, enuresis, encopresis, and testicular cancer. The discussion will provide an overview of the disorders that includes information on definition, incidence, causes and correlates, and treatment. The overviews will be followed by recommendations for pediatricians concerned with prevention of complications due to the disorder (for example, death, disability, or sterility due to testicular cancer) or prevention of the disorder itself.

Of critical interest to prevention of each disorder is the pediatric interview. Once rapport is established in the interview through sensitive interaction with the patient, a wealth of valuable information can be obtained through a simple question and answer format (Boyle, 1978). Such information can be used to plan prevention of future complaints. The dynamics of the pediatric interview will not be a focus of our chapter but we do emphasize the importance of doctor-patient communication, for which there is good information available (Korsch & Negrette, 1972; Pendleton & Hasler, 1983). Furthermore a functional analysis of communication variables within the interview would be a useful behavioral pediatric contribution to child health care.

The recommendations made in this chapter are not based on existing experimental evaluations of preventive interventions for each disorder because, as indicated above, such experiments are rare. The recommendations are based on extrapolations from literature reviewed in each overview. Thus each proposed intervention will ultimately require evaluation. The proposed interventions represent a necessary first step in the development of a validated technology for prevention of childhood medical disorders and the advancement of behavioral pediatrics.

MEDICAL DISORDERS THE PEDIATRICIAN MAY BE ABLE TO PREVENT

Obesity

Definition.   Obese individuals have been described as "unattractive, ungainly, inactive, unpopular and often unhappy" (Brook, 1983, p. 213). Obesity is frequently described as a prevalent disorder that is associated with serious health problems (Woodall & Epstein, 1983). Although some problems with defining obesity exist, the medical diagnosis of obesity is rarely, if ever, a problem (Wright, Schaefer, & Solomons, 1979). Specific definitions of obesity vary from simple one-factor definitions specifying that children who are above a certain percentile in average weight for individuals their same age, height, and sex are obese (Taitz, 1971) to complex multicomponent definitions with criteria for weight, height, and skinfold thickness (Epstein, Wing, Kuller, & Becker, 1983). Despite the variations in definition, that physicians "know a fat person when they see one" is apparent. Therein resides the ease of diagnosis (Wright et al., 1979).

Incidence.   Obesity has been declared a chronic national health problem. Estimates suggest that at least 20 percent of the United States population (more than 40 million people) are overweight. The extent of the problem is revealed by the sheer numbers of individuals that seek treatment for obesity in this country. Stunkard (1979) estimated that over 400,000 people receive some sort of treatment for their weight each week. One of the major reasons so many individuals seek treatment for obesity is obviously because excess weight can be detrimental to physical appearance. But more important than excess weight's effect on appearance is obesity's detrimental effect on health.

The literature showing that obesity is a major health threat is long standing. Mayer (1953) reported that obese individuals have a 50 percent higher incidence of cardiovascular and renal disease and a 100 percent greater incidence of cirrhosis of the liver. More recent studies support the possibility that excess body weight contributes to renal and cardiovascular disease. The recent literature also shows associations between obesity and hyperlipidemia, diabetes mellitus, carbohydrate intolerance, surgical risk, delayed recovery from anesthesia, pulmonary problems, and complications during pregnancy (Bray, 1976; Brownell, 1982; Dawber, 1980; Kannel & Gordon, 1979; Keys, 1979; Van Itallie, 1979). Furthermore while most of the problems associated with obesity occur in adulthood, obesity is the primary cause of pediatric hypertension (Rames, Clarke, Conner, Reiter, & Lauer, 1978). The evidence linking obesity to various health problems indicates that excess weight is so much a risk factor for serious disease processes that it may be considered a disease process itself. Obesity's status as a disease and as a risk factor for disease, coupled with the social and psychological problems that unsightly excess weight can cause, indicate the importance of prevention of obesity.

Causes and Correlates. Several characteristics appear to distinguish those individuals at risk for obesity from those who are not. Primary among these characteristics is excess weight in childhood. Other important characteristics include excess weight gain in mothers during pregnancy (Neuman, 1983), excess weight in one parent (Charney, Goodman, McBride, Lyon & Pratt, 1976), both parents (Garn & Clark, 1976), marital status of parents—children of divorced or separated parents are at greater risk for obesity—(Dietz, 1983) gender—females are more prone to obesity than males—(Abraham & Nordsiek, 1960), and underactivity (Thompson, Jarvie, Lahey, & Cureton, 1982).

The evidence related to risk factors for obesity indicates that pediatricians interested in preventing it should begin their interventions in early childhood. Generally, the research shows that the older children are when they become obese the greater the likelihood obesity will continue into adulthood (Dietz, 1983). More specifically the research focused on the development of adipose (fatty) tissue supports early intervention. Adipose tissue develops as a function of increases in either the size or the number of a person's fat cells (Woodall & Epstein, 1983). But unfortunately for those individuals who begin dieting in late adolescence or adulthood, the number of cells a person has are possibly not reducible, even through weight loss (Knittle, 1978). According to this theory, the number of fat cells that a person develops during the critical period of fat development remain constant for life. Although estimates of when the critical periods of fat development occur vary, investigators who believe that fat cell numbers remain constant agree that the period occurs in childhood.

Other research indicating that prevention should begin in early childhood focuses on infant feeding. For example, bottle feeding has been implicated in excess weight gain in infancy (Trowell, 1975). The amount of formula that is fed to an infant from a bottle can vary widely according to bottle size and the mother's impressions of how much the infant should eat. Mothers without good information about infant needs may feed their infant too much from the bottle. Furthermore, the response requirement is greater for the infant who is breast feeding than for the infant who is fed from a bottle. The bottle fed infant is likely to eat more because feeding from a bottle requires less effort. Thus infants who are breast fed tend to grow more slowly than those who are bottle fed (Hooper, 1965; Taitz, 1971). In addition to bottle feeding, the early introduction of solids is also a contributor to excess weight gain in infants. Generally, solid foods are higher in calories than either breast milk or formula and therefore the infant on solids can receive excess calories and gain excess weight (Neuman, 1983).

Also of interest for pediatricians concerned with prevention of obesity is an apparent relationship between selected mealtime behaviors and child weight. Drabman, Hammer, and Jarvie (1977) showed that overweight children take more bites per unit of time and use fewer chews per bite than children of normal weight. These differences in eating style occur in children as young as 18 months. Other research shows that both child and parent mealtime behaviors influence child weight. Waxman and Stunkard (1980) studied four overweight boys and their normal brothers, and noted that the overweight boys ate faster than their normal weight brothers. Results also showed that the mothers served the overweight boys portions that were larger and that were delivered more frequently than those served to their brothers. Another study showed that the verbal behavior of parents may be related to excess weight in their children (Klesges et al., 1983). Results of this study indicated that parental prompts, particularly encouragements to eat, correlated significantly with the probability that children would eat and with the children's weight.

None of the studies of feeding practices and mealtime behaviors definitively show that such behaviors or practices causes obesity. The studies do show, however, that the behaviors and practices, and the obesity are related. Because of that relationship mealtime behaviors and feeding practices are ideal targets for a prospective intervention for obesity. The studies also provide additional evidence supporting the position that early childhood is the best time to implement prevention for adult obesity.

Treatment. A wide variety of treatment programs are available for obese individuals, including surgery, pharmaceutical regimens, psychotherapy, and behavior therapy. Of the various treatments, behavior therapy has the most experimental documentation (Brownell, 1982). Over 100 controlled studies have been reported and several comprehensive reviews are available (Brownell, 1982; Stunkard, 1979; Stunkard, 1980; Wing & Jeffery, 1979). Behavioral interventions generally involve a group of "sensible" procedures to teach patients changes in eating habits commensurate with weight loss. Despite numerous advances in biobehavioral technology for treatment of obesity, the problems of relatively small weight losses, relapses, and attrition from treatment programs have not yet been resolved (Brownell, 1982).

One aspect of obesity that contributes to its refractory nature is the close relationship between eating habits and lifestyle. Some positive treatment results have stemmed from combining standard behavioral treatment for obesity with social support components. Social support treatment programs typically focus on a salient aspect of a patient's life style. Such programs include self-help groups, spouse involvement, and work site programs (Brownell, 1982). The literature on social support and its influence on obesity treatment shows that eating habits and life style frequently become enmeshed as an individual's life progresses (Brownell, 1982).

An exemplary study showing that behavioral programming with social support components can produce and maintain weight loss in obese children was conducted by Brownell, Kelman, and Stunkard (1983). The study included 42 obese adolescents aged 12 to 16 years. Each child was assigned to one of three treatment groups: mother and child together, mother and child separate, and child alone. Treatment variables included a treatment manual (with information on self-monitoring, exercise, nutrition, stimulus control, cognitive restructuring, behavior chains, etc.) and social support. Dependent variables included direct measures of weight loss and blood pressure. The results showed that children in the mother and child separate group lost more weight (8.4 kg) than did the other two groups (5.3 kg and 3.3 kg). One-year follow-up showed that the weight loss of the mother-and-child-separate group maintained, while the other groups gained weight above baseline levels. Measures of blood pressure in the mother-and-child-separate group also decreased and maintained.

The findings of this study indicate that parent involvement in treatment of obese children is important and that the nature of the involvement is especially important. The limitations on the involvement in the mother-and-child-separate group allowed the parent and child to contend with the sensitive aspects of their relationship in a support group prior to working out problems with each other. The findings of this study shows the effectiveness of using social support to treat childhood obesity, but they also reveal the complexity of the issues involved in the treatment of obese children.

The complicated nature of treatment is an indication of the possible benefits of prevention.

Collectively, the published studies focusing on management of obesity, especially studies involving behavioral and social support components, are increasing the possibility of safe, effective treatment. Currently, however, safe, effective treatment for obesity appears to be more of a goal than a reality. Because obesity is a serious threat to health, is a problem that increases in complexity as life progresses, is a cause of some other serious pediatric disorders, for example, hypertension (Rames et al., 1978), and because effective treatments for obesity remain an elusive goal, prevention may prove at least as productive as treatment.

Prevention.   Controlled studies showing that obesity can be prevented have not been conducted; therefore only tentative recommendations can be made for the pediatrician. Despite the tentative nature of these recommendations, the literature summarized above suggests that pediatricians trying to prevent obesity can have an impact.

The crucial first step in a preventive effort is identification of children who are at risk for obesity. Such children can be identified through a complete medical history which should be part of intake procedures that occur with all newborn infants and with all other new pediatric patients. The features of particular interest include excess weight gain by mothers during pregnancy, excess weight in either parent, and excess weight in the patient at the time of the examination. Following the identification of a child at risk for obesity, the pediatrician should implement health education designed to change as many of the factors that are associated with excess weight gain in childhood as possible. Previous research has shown that in order to be effective such health education strategies should be clearly stated (Korsch & Negrete, 1972), printed in a handout form (Finney, Friman, Rapoff, & Christophersen, 1985), target a health belief that may support obesity (Becker, Maiman, Kirscht, & Haefner, 1978), contain some level of threat for noncompliance (Kirscht, Becker, Haefner, & Maiman, 1978), and not involve an unreasonably large amount of change at one time (Dershewitz & Christophersen, 1984).

Although pediatricians are not trained as psychotherapists or family therapists they can provide health education that changes individual and family behavior. In the case of obesity a primary health education message can be stated clearly to parents: "Fat children will probably get and stay fatter unless something is done." One of the primary health beliefs that needs to be targeted is that large (or fat) children and adults need to eat more than others. In most cases this simply is not true; often they should eat less. Thus the cornerstone of effective treatment for obesity, reduced caloric intake, should be stressed in prevention (Dietz, 1983). Emphasizing the positive aspects of reduced weight may also prove beneficial. Emphasis on the positive aspects of improved child behavior has proven beneficial in other types of interventions (Christophersen, 1977). Some positive points to focus on for parents of children targeted for weight loss include improved appearance, increased access to social reinforcement, and increased capacity for physical activities such as sports (Brownell, 1982; Stunkard, 1979, 1980). The threat component in health education can emphasize the dire health risks the fat child is exposed to because of the excess weight. The handout should also indicate what should be done to aid parents in establishing and maintaining their child's ideal body weight.

The importance of parent health education for control of potential obesity in children is highlighted by the almost total control a parent has over their child's food intake (Neuman, 1983). Thus if pediatricians can motivate parents through health education interventions they can indirectly control the child's weight. The literature suggests that pediatricians should encourage breast feeding, if the mother is capable of it, and restricted bottle feedings, if she is not. If the mother is providing too many breast or bottle feedings the pediatrician should investigate the reasons. When mothers use food to reduce problem behaviors, such as night time crying, the pediatrician should recommend a behavioral intervention that could be substituted for food-based interventions. Protocols for behavioral interventions a pediatrician can recommend in an office visit are available (Christophersen, 1982).

If the infant is already fat and still on the bottle, the introduction of solid foods should be delayed. If solid foods are delayed in infants over six months of age, however, the infant may need an iron supplement (Rohr & Lothian, 1984). When solid foods are introduced the sugar content should be limited. The bulk of solid food can be increased by dietary fiber, which will not produce weight gain and which may ultimately contribute to prevention of other disease processes (Burkitt, Walker, & Painter, 1974) and to bowel control (Levine, 1982). For toddlers and older children, prevention should stress reduced meal sizes, reduced meal durations, smaller and fewer bites, and reduced encouragements to eat in order to control the excess eating that leads to excess weight. For toddlers and older children, intervention may also stress potential increase in children's activity levels. Finally, the health education strategy should emphasize that children who are fat or are at risk for being fat are children who have an increased susceptibility to disease and thus should see their physician more frequently than must children of normal weight. Increased visits to the pediatrician will increase opportunities for the pediatrician to motivate parents to influence their child's eating patterns. This last recommendation is especially important because most of the children will not actually be dieting, but, rather, will be having their growth and physical development monitored carefully by an expert (Neumann, 1983).

As noted previously, that obesity can be prevented has not been proven by controlled research, but the relationship between several modifiable behaviors and obesity has been shown. And a physician's ability to change patient behaviors so as to prevent health problems has also been established (Pomerleau, Bass, & Crown, 1975; Stedman, 1970). By modifying behaviors related to obesity, pediatricians might possibly prevent it. Therefore, a productive research pursuit for behavioral pediatrics would be the formal evaluation of health education interventions designed to reduce caloric intake in children at risk for obesity.

Nocturnal Enuresis

Definition. Nocturnal enuresis (hereafter enuresis) is a disorder in which children over a set age involuntarily, and perhaps unconsciously, pass urine while in bed more than a set number of times per week or month (Wright et al., 1979). Historically the age set for diagnosis of and treatment for enuresis has differed for various investigators studying the problem. Although most investigators seemed to agree that children over the age of six who are not bladder trained are enuretic, some investigators labeled untrained three-year-olds enuretic as well (Crosby, 1950). Cohen (1975) did not set a specific age for treatment of enuresis and recommended only that children who wet the bed be treated when bedwetting begins to interfere with social, emotional, or cognitive development. Although Cohen provided one of the most practical discussions of enuresis, the reluctance to define it by specific age level may impair its value for epidemiologists concerned with incidence. Investigations of incidence are impaired by more than just varying age criteria, however. The number of accidents per time-period necessary for a diagnosis of enuresis also fluctuates from investigator to investigator (de Jonge, 1973). For example Oppel, Harper, and Rider's (1968) criterion for enuresis was one accident per month, where Martin's (1966) was two per week. The resolution of the problems with diagnosis may reside in the more recent criteria for enuresis established by the American Psychiatric Association (1980). They specify that children between five and six years old are enuretic if they wet the bed two or more times a month and that children six and older are enuretic if they wet the bed one or more times a month. Again Cohen's (1975) suggestion does seem more practical from a treatment standpoint, despite the hardship it imposes on the epidemiologist.

One finding consistent across investigations is that the average number of accidents children have, either each week or each month, decreases as they get older (de Jonge, 1982). Another consistent finding is that the physical, social, and emotional hardships imposed by bedwetting increase substantially with age (Wright et al., 1979). Apparently as enuretic children grow older their bedwetting appears more deviant. Therefore the sooner the children stop, the less likely they are to suffer emotional side-effects.

Incidence. Because of the variations in definition and criteria for enuresis, establishing the incidence of the problem is difficult. Estimates range from three million (Wright et al., 1979) to five million (Nunn, 1978). Percentage estimates suggest that 25 percent of all elementary school children exhibit the problem at least once and that 16 percent of all children in the United States between 3 and 15 years of age exhibit enuresis at any one time (Wright et al., 1979). Despite the variability in definitions of enuresis, an examination of even the most conservative set of criteria shows that enuresis is a prevalent clinical problem.

Causes and Correlates.   The literature indicates that several variables correlate with the development of enuresis. Some of the more prominent variables are enuresis in parents, small functional bladder capacity, and socioeconomic status (SES).

In a study of genetics and enuresis, Bakwin (1973) examined the histories of 1815 children and their parents. The results showed that when both parents were enuretic, 77 percent of the children became enuretic. They also showed that 43 percent of the children with one enuretic parent, mother or father, became enuretic. Only 15 percent of children with no enuretic parent became enuretic. Enuresis may be predictable, especially if enuresis in the parents is identified in the medical history of the child.

The literature on functional bladder size and bedwetting provides fairly consistent evidence indicating that reduced functional bladder capacity is often responsible for wet beds (Zaleski, Gerrard, & Shoker, 1973). Urination during sleep has been hypothesized as being caused by deficient production of, or response to, sensory stimuli from the bladder (Yeates, 1973). For urination to occur during sleep, the bladder must fill to its maximum functional capacity and the different stimuli that occur must fail to produce arousal. It has been stated that reduced functional bladder capacity can be attributed only to a deficiency in the central inhibitory response to sensory input from the bladder (Yeates, 1973). This deficiency results in an increased frequency of urinations with reduced volume per urination. Thus children who urinate frequently, but who do not have abnormally large fluid intakes or have polyuria due to some other disorder such as diabetes, are likely to have small functional bladder capacity and are therefore at risk for enuresis. There is no commonly available norm against which parents can compare their child's frequency of urinations or volume per urination. Such normative data would be a valuable contribution to behavioral pediatrics. A parent in collaboration with a pediatrician could conduct input-output assessments and determine whether the child had a small functional bladder capacity. Such collaboration could aid in the detection of children at risk for bedwetting.

Some recent epidemiological research shows that an increased proportion of enuresis occurs in families of lower SES (Gross & Dornbusch, 1983). Obviously a variable as gross or as molar as SES does not yield to functional analysis readily. Numerous problems can be present in a family where social and economic resources are below average. Identifying which of those problems are functionally related to enuresis is a future research agenda for behavioral pediatrics. One variable suggested by Gross and Dornbusch (1983) is a decrease in social resources, or more specifically, the decreased time parents in families with economic problems have to spend with their children. For children not at risk for enuresis, reduced social resources may not be functionally related to continence. But children who are at risk, due to family history or reduced bladder capacity, will probably require increased time and attention in order to promote continence. Thus the aspects of SES that may be relevant to prevention is time and attention. Still these variables are gross and will require further functional analysis. Despite their gross status, time and attention as related to specific training for continence are important variables to study for prevention of enuresis, especially in families with low SES.

Treatment.   The literature on treatment of enuresis is large and still growing. This literature clearly indicates that enuresis can be successfully treated. Treatments for enuresis that have been effective include standard urine alarm treatment (Mower & Mower, 1938), dry bed training (Azrin, Sneed, & Foxx, 1974), self-hypnosis (Olness, 1975), drug therapy (Schmitt, 1982) and urine retention training (Starfield & Mellits, 1968). Of all the available treatments the one of choice appears to be the dry bed training of Azrin et al. (Christophersen & Rapoff, 1979).

Dry bed training is a treatment package that includes a urine alarm, urine retention training, a waking schedule, self-correction of accidents, rewards for correct toileting, and positive practice. In their initial evaluation of dry bed training with developmentally normal children, Azrin et al. (1974) used one night of intensive training in the home and phone follow-up thereafter. Their results showed an average of one accident during the first week, one accident during the second week, and no accidents during the third. At six-month follow-up, none of the children in the study had relapsed to pretraining levels.

Studies by Bollard and his colleagues have systematically replicated these findings, using parents as therapists (Bollard & Woodroffe, 1977). The parents in Bollard and Woodroffe's study were trained in an office setting. Bollard's group went on to show that parents could learn to use dry bed training in a group setting (Bollard, Nettlebeck, & Roxbee, 1982). Bollard also showed that a substantial number of children treated with dry bed training were still dry after two years (Bollard, 1982). Finally, Bollard and Nettlebeck (1982) conducted a component analysis of dry bed training and found that each component of the training decreased accidents, that the effectiveness of the package increased as the number of components increased, and that the entire package was more effective than any other combination. Bollard and Nettlebeck's primary finding, however, was that the urine alarm combined only with the waking schedule was almost as effective as the entire dry bed training package. Collectively the group's findings indicate that dry bed training is effective, and that it can be simplified and used readily by parents trained in individual or group settings. The simplified version of dry bed training validated by Bollard et al. has positive implications for pediatricians concerned with prevention of enuresis.

Prevention. It is logical that at some point in a child's life, intervention to reduce bedwetting would be preventive rather than curative. For example, if a two-year-old is taught not to wet the bed, has the child been cured or has enuresis been prevented? Perhaps the question itself is misdirected. Enuresis is not necessarily a problem in and of itself, but rather can cause developmental and emotional problems (Cohen, 1975). The developmental and emotional problems that are associated with enuresis are more likely to be a function of social response to wetting than a direct result of wetting (Brazleton, 1962, 1973). Thus prevention in relation to enuresis would be prevention of the developmental and emotional problems associated with enuresis (Cohen, 1975).

The best prevention then, would be to begin to toilet train children as soon as they meet the developmental criteria for toileting. Specifically, these criteria include some bladder control (dry for several hours at a time, urination of large amounts at a time), physical readiness (pincer grasp, ambulation), and instructional readiness (several one-step commands) (Azrin & Foxx, 1976; Brazleton, 1962). For children who meet the criteria, but for whom traditional training methods are not effective, special preventive methods adapted from treatment protocols may be effective. It should be noted, however, that training and prevention should not be implemented when a child is going through an intensely negative period due to family, emotional, or health problems. The literature suggests that the children who are most likely to require special procedures are those who have a family history of enuresis or who have small functional bladder capacities. Low SES may also be a factor to consider but further research is necessary to determine how SES interacts with other risk factors. As discussed above, the key variable may be parental time but data are necessary to support this contention. The pediatrician who, after conducting a complete history, identifies a patient with any or all the above mentioned risk factors should prescribe a preventive intervention involving training methods adapted from treatment methods.

The literature focusing on treating enuresis shows that it can be successfully treated even with a modified version of dry bed training. The literature also shows that parents can learn to use dry bed training in either an office or a group setting. Although teaching the entire package would require adujunctive personnel, the pediatrician could probably teach the modified version (alarm and wake schedule) in a busy office setting and follow the treatment by phone.

The modified version of dry bed training is really little more than toilet training (Azrin & Foxx, 1976). The literature also suggests that pediatricians can readily manage modified dry bed training if the cases are not complicated by extreme psychosocial deviancy (Christophersen, 1982). That the training can have positive results is supported not only by the treatment literature, but also by epidemiological literature which shows an inverse relationship between early toilet training and incidence of enuresis (Blomfield & Douglas, 1956). Pediatricians could prescribe such training prior to the fifth birthday, and possibly prior to the third birthday, of children at risk for difficult toilet training and thus for problems associated with enuresis. By so doing they may be able to prevent some cases of enuresis, at least as it is defined by the American Psychiatric Association. Of even greater benefit to children and families is the prevention of the developmental problems that Cohen (1975) indicated may occur secondary to enuresis. As yet such prevention has not been reported; the documentation of benefits that may accrue from prevention is a future direction for behavioral pediatrics.

Psychogenic Encopresis

Definition. Psychogenic encopresis (encopresis) is a disorder without organic pathogenesis in which individuals either voluntarily or involuntarily pass feces into or onto an inappropriate location, usually their clothing (Wright, 1973). The literature specifying the various criteria on which the diagnosis of encopresis is made is much more consistent than the literature on enuresis. Children are encopretic if they are four years or older and regularly pass feces inappropriately (Christophersen & Rainey, 1976; Levine, 1975; Wright, 1975). Also in contrast to the enuresis literature the predominant diagnostic criteria in the encopresis literature are consonant with the criteria set by the American Psychiatric Association (1980). The American Psychiatric Association's criteria specifies that persons over the age of four who pass feces inappropriately more than once a month are functionally encopretic.

Incidence. Estimates of the incidence of encopresis vary from 1.5 percent to 5 percent of the pediatric population, depending on the source of the estimate. Encopresis comprised 1.5 percent of all pediatric referrals from an Israeli kibbutz (Lifshitz & Chovers, 1972) and 5 percent of all child psychiatric referrals from a Scandinavian province (Olatawuria, 1973). In a study of American pediatric patients, Levine (1975) found a 3 percent incidence of encopresis. Despite the higher incidence of encopresis found in psychiatric clinics, pediatricians probably encounter more encopretic children because of larger pediatric case loads (Wright et al., 1979). Another factor that artificially lowers incidence statistics for the psychiatric and pediatric encopretic populations is parental reluctance to report, or parental ignorance of, the condition. Wright (1973) reported that most cases of encopresis are discovered during the assessment of other presenting problems.

Therefore encopresis may be a larger problem for pediatrics than the literature suggests.

Causes and Correlates. A common complaint by the parents of encopretic children is that the children deliberately soil their clothing (Wright et al., 1979). This accusation is usually false (Levine, 1982). The primary cause of excess soiling is fecal retention, which may indeed be deliberate, at least initially (Davidson, 1958). The cause of retention in most cases is not the result of some personality characteristic (for example, stubborness) as is often suggested; retention is the result of a constellation of factors, many of which are beyond a child's immediate control (Levine, 1982, 1983). These factors include a constitutional predisposition, diet, insufficient leverage for passage of hard stools, and occasional or frequent painful passage of hard stools (Christophersen & Rapoff, 1983). The combined effect of these factors is a lowered probability of voluntary stool passage and a heightened probability of fecal retention.

Chronic fecal retention results in fecal impaction, which results in enlargement of the colon. Colon enlargement results in decreased motility of the bowel system; the combined effects result in occasional involuntary passage of large stools and frequent soilings due to seepage of soft fecal matter. This seepage is often referred to as "paradoxical diarrhea" because the children retain large masses of stool and thus are functionally constipated, but their colon allows passage of soft stool around the mass which results in diarrhea (Christophersen & Rapoff, 1983; Levine, 1982).

That fecal impaction is related to encopresis has been established by several investigators, primarily Wright (1975) and Levine (1975). Each independently reported that 80 percent of their patients had fecal impaction accompanying fecal incontinence at the first clinic visit. Subsequent to his 1975 report, Levine and his colleagues developed a simple clinical procedure to identify fecal impactions from a KUB (x-ray of the lower abdomen including the kidneys, ureter, and bladder) (Barr, Levine, Wilkinson, & Mulvihill, 1979). As a result of the improved diagnostic method, Levine revised his initial 80 percent estimate of fecal impaction's coexistence with fecal incontinence to 90 percent (Christophersen & Rapoff, 1979).

Treatment. The most recent literature indicates that effective treatment of encopresis involves several steps. First, parents and pediatricians should "demystify" the entire elimination process (Christophersen & Rapoff, 1983; Levine, 1982). The belief that bowel retention and bowel accidents are generally associated with personality development, and specifically with such characteristics as stubborness, immaturity, or laziness, can result in parents shaming and blaming their children into the bathroom. But a disordered process of elimination such as encopresis should no more be a target for censure and blame than should a disordered process of respiration, digestion, or motor movement. The data-based literature does not support the association between personality characteristics and bowel habits. On the contrary, this literature recommends that parents avoid blaming the child and suggests that they restructure toileting conditions in order to increase the likelihood of proper elimination (Levine, 1982). Second, if there is an anal impaction it should be removed with enemas and/or laxatives (Christophersen & Rapoff, 1983; Levine, 1982). Third, the child should sit on the toilet for about five minutes one or two times a day (Wright, 1975). Fourth, the parents should promote proper toileting with encouragement and not with coercion. They should also not reserve all their praise and affection for proper elimination; a child should be praised just for sitting on the toilet (Christophersen & Rapoff, 1983; Levine, 1982; Wright, 1975). Fifth, a stool softener such as mineral oil (Davidson, 1958) or glycerin suppositories (Wright & Walker, 1977) should be used in order to ease the passage of hard stools. Sixth, dietary fiber should be increased in the child's diet. Seventh, in order to increase and maintain motility in the child's colon, the child's activity levels and fluid intake should be increased (Levine, 1982). Eighth, during toileting episodes the child's feet should be on a flat surface. Foot placement is crucial to the "Valsalva maneuver" (grunting push necessary to produce a bowel movement) (Levine, 1982, 1983). And ninth, the child should be rewarded for all bowel movements in the toilet (Christophersen & Rainey, 1976; Levine, 1982; Wright & Walker, 1977).

One problem with the available evidence supporting the use of such treatment procedures is the lack of controlled study. The research is comprised almost entirely of case reports (Christophersen & Rapoff, 1983). The lack of controls notwithstanding, the body of research devoted to treatment of encopresis is credible because of the large number of subjects discussed and the high percentage of successful treatments reported (Christophersen & Rainey, 1976; Levine, 1975, 1982; Wright, 1975; Wright & Walker, 1977). Thus despite the lack of controls in the treatment literature, the protocols described apparently are useful in the remediation of encopresis. The same literature may also be useful in prevention of encopresis.

Prevention.   As with other medical disorders discussed previously in this chapter, a primary task in preventing encopresis is identifying those children who are most susceptible to it. But encopresis may be distinct from the other disorders in that most, if not all, children may be at risk if the causal conditions are present. Thus prevention should focus on the stages of development of encopresis and how those stages are relevant to pediatric patients. In his discussion of the causes of encopresis, Levine (1982) described three stages of its development. Awareness of these stages could aid in the identification of children most likely to benefit from prevention.

In stage 1 (infants and toddlers), the primary causal variables are simple constipation and parental overreaction. In this stage the pediatrician should use "demystification" to initiate prevention. Demystification instructions for parents should emphasize consistent, nonaggressive, well-informed management of any or all bowel problems, especially constipation. Parents should also be encouraged to follow the toileting readiness criteria established by Azrin and Foxx (1974) before setting up a bowel training program. In general, no reaction at all to a bowel problem is better than an overreaction (Levine, 1982, 1983).

During stage 2 (three to five years) the various stresses associated with toilet training are of paramount concern. Prevention should include continued demystification, which at this stage involves gentle assistance with all toileting tasks, and encouragement to work on, and to talk about, toileting tasks. During stage 2 such aids as toilet seats and small stools for foot leverage may be helpful. Also increased dietary fiber will loosen and moisten stools and help to prevent painful passage of hard stools. Most important, though, is the avoidance of coercion, negative feedback, and inducements to hurry. The child should be encouraged to sit on the toilet at least once a day but for not longer than five minutes. The time for this toileting episode should be consistent across days. And the child should be praised for adherence to the schedule (Christophersen & Rapoff, 1983; Levine, 1983; Wright & Walker, 1977).

During stage 3 (early school years) scheduling toileting episodes becomes the primary concern. Toileting schedules at this stage are especially critical for children whose risk of encopresis has increased because of problems during stages 1 and 2. The psychosocial reactions to bowel movements at school, especially schools without doors on toilet stalls, can be a problem for the child at risk (Levine, 1982, 1983). For such children prevention should involve the regulation of bowel movements so that they occur in the children's home either before or after school. Perhaps the best method of promoting a home schedule for a constipated child is the use of stool softeners such as glycerin suppositories or mineral oil (Christophersen & Rapoff, 1983; Levin, 1983). There is some controversy regarding the use of suppositories, however, and in cases in which this is a concern mineral oil, although less predictable, may be more acceptable. When the regulation of bowel movements becomes consistent as a result of using suppositories, the suppositories should be phased out of the toileting routine. A procedure for this has been established (Christophersen & Rainey, 1976). In addition to regulation of bowel movements, prevention for the school-aged child at risk should include increased dietary fiber, elevated activity levels, increased fluid intake, continued demystification, and praise for the absence of accidents (Levine, 1982, 1983).

As indicated above, the treatment of childhood encopresis has been studied extensively, but not in a controlled experiment. As with enuresis, however, prevention of encopresis has not been studied at all. Yet it seems probable, given the high success rates reported in the treatment literature, that the rates of successful prevention could be just as high.

The prevention recommended here is, at its most burdensome point, a mild treatment procedure, and at its least burdensome point, a mild toilet training procedure. Thus, implementation of the intervention may not require a great deal of extra effort from the parents or the pediatrician. In fact with the exception of those cases where suppositories are needed, prevention is equivalent to ordinary toilet training conducted at an appropriate age level. Therefore the best prevention would be to provide the intervention recommended for children at risk for all children. Bowel training is after all a human experience that is often fraught with complications (Levine, 1982). And it is difficult to ascertain how the interventions used to ease those complications in children at risk for encopresis would cause problems when used with children whose risk is lower. Conversely the procedure might just simplify the entire bowel training process for everyone concerned.

Even in the absence of supportive data, the position of the authors of this chapter is that pediatricians can prevent at least some (perhaps a lot of) encopresis. They could accomplish this by providing health education focused on toilet training for all their patients who are not toilet trained or for whom toileting problems have occurred. The content of this education should contain the information obtained from studies of the biobehavioral treatment of encopresis. A major task remaining for behavioral pediatrics is the documentation of benefits that result from treatment and prevention of encopresis. There are limited data available supporting treatment and none supporting prevention. Much research remains to be done. In addition, some aspects of treatment will require further analysis. For example the use of suppositories versus the use of mineral oil requires further study. If there are side effects that result from the anal manipulation that is required for insertion of suppositories, these effects need to be documented. Overall, the breadth of behavioral pediatrics could be increased by further study of functional encopresis.

Death, Disability, and Sterility Due to Testicular Cancer

Definition and Incidence.   Testicular cancer is a disease involving metastic tumors that first develop on a male's testicles. Testicular tumors are a concern with infants as well as adolescents and young adults but this chapter will not focus on infants. A critical concern for treatment of testicular tumors is early detection. But early detection of testicular tumors has not received the emphasis in health education for men (Cummings, Lampone, Mettlin, & Pontes, 1983) that early detection of breast tumors has in health education for young women (Goldenring & Purtell, 1984).

Testicular cancer is the most frequently occurring cancer in males between the ages of 15 and 35. Testicular cancer is also the leading cause of death by cancer and the second leading cause of all deaths in men between

15 and 35. The incidence has been reported to be as high as 1 in 10,000 in the U.S. Navy but the overall incidence is probably closer to 1 in 50,000 (Droller, 1980; Gault, 1981; Hongladrom & Hongladrom, 1982; Silverberg, 1982).

Causes and Correlates.   The causes of testicular cancer currently appear to be more a product of speculation than of replicable scientific analysis. Epidemiological surveys show that this type of cancer occurs infrequently in blacks—12 to 15 percent of the incidence seen in caucasians (Dixon & Moore, 1953). Correlational studies show that young caucasians with a history of undescended testes are at significant risk for the disease (Droller, 1980). Relationships between testicular cancer and environmental influences have also been suggested (Damjanov & Solter, 1974). But a functional relationship between a specific variable or set of variables and testicular cancer has yet to be established.

Treatment.   Despite testicular cancer's contribution to death in young men, effective treatment is available. The primary factor related to cure, however, is not the method of treatment but when it is treated.

The clinical staging of testicular cancer proceeds through three levels: (1) in which the disease is limited to the testicles, epididiymis, and spermatic cord (sperm collecting vessels); (2) in which the disease spreads to the retroperitoneal nodes (masses of differentiated tissue on the lining of the abdominal cavity); and (3) in which the disease metastisizes (spreads) above the diaphragm into the lungs or beyond the retroperitoneum into other vital organs (Bosl et al., 1981). In stages 1 and 2 the disease is curable through some combination of radiation therapy, chemotherapy, and surgery. Because of advances in all three treatment techniques most patients have an excellent prognosis (Bosl et al., 1981). But for those patients in whom the disease has advanced beyond the retroperitoneum or into the lungs, the prognosis is much more guarded (Goldby, Reynolds, & Vurgin 1979). Thus early detection is critical to effective medical intervention and survival.

Prevention.   Whether testicular cancer can be prevented is doubtful. But prevention of death or major disability due to the disease is an accomplishable goal, the key to which is early detection. The major obstacle to early detection of testicular cancer is ignorance. Knowledge surveys show that most young men, even well educated young men, are either uninformed or misinformed about the symptoms of testicular cancer and what their chances of contracting the disease are (Cummings et al., 1983). Thus an initial task in a preventive effort by pediatricians is early health education focused on the delivery of accurate information about testicular cancer.

The signs and symptoms of testicular cancer are, in most cases, readily detectable. The symptoms include (1) a small, usually painless lump on the front or side of one or both testicles; (2) a heavy feeling in the testes; (3) a dragging sensation in the groin; (4) accumulation of fluid or blood in the scrotal sac; and (5) pain in the more advanced cases (Hongladrom & Hongladrom, 1982).

Although health education materials describing the symptoms of testicular cancer have been available for years (American Cancer Society, 1978) the failure of these materials to affect the knowledge base or behavior of most young men is apparent (Conklin, Klint, Morway, Sawyer, & Shepard, 1978; Cummings et al., 1983). The pediatricians' intervention, then, should involve more than just the provision of written health education materials; it should involve direct physical examination and behavioral training.

According to the literature, testicular self-examination is an easily learned procedure that should emphasize the following: (1) familiarity with the surface, texture, and consistency of one's own testicles in their normal state; (2) that the ideal time for self-examination is during or after a warm bath or shower; (3) that the self-examination should involve both testicles being rotated between the thumb and forefinger until it is determined that the entire surface of each is free of lumps (tumors); (4) that the tube-like structure at the back (epididymis) is not a tumor; and (5) that any detection of a lump should be reported to a physician immediately (Hongladrom & Hongladrom, 1982).

Whether testicular self-examination is, as the literature suggests, an easily learned procedure is an empirical question not yet answered by experimental study. Experimental study has shown, however, that patients can be taught specialized cancer detection procedures (Hall et al., 1980). Hall et al. taught women to detect the presence or absence of breast lesions and to discriminate between normal nodularity and breast lesions by training the women on silicone models. Modeling and guided practice also has had a positive impact on breast self-examination (Marty, McDermott, & Gold, 1983). In all probability young men trained by a pediatrician, via modelling and guided practice, could learn to identify the definitive contrast between a testicle with a normal surface and one with a tumor.

Early detection will not prevent testicular cancer, but it will help to prevent its advanced staging and thus lessen its impact by reducing the severity of the necessary treatment and thereby heighten the chances of survival. Because of the threat delayed detection of testicular cancer presents to the health of young men, special procedures designed to teach such detection should be incorporated fully into pediatric and adolescent care. This incorporation would then require evaluation in order to determine its impact on prevention of problems due to testicular tumors. A major task for behavioral pediatrics is designing effective health education protocols for teaching self-examination skills.

DISCUSSION

A review of the literature devoted to four potentially serious pediatric medical disorders suggests that prevention may substantially reduce the morbidity and/or mortality attributed to each. Prevention of these disorders is important because some of them are life threatening (e.g. obesity, testicular cancer) and all of them have the potential to impair physical and emotional development. Prevention for these disorders should begin at various stages of child development, ranging from early infancy (for obesity) to early childhood (for encopresis and enuresis) to adolescence (for testicular cancer). Because pediatrics is a branch of medicine that covers medical care for children across these age ranges, the pediatrician has been the focus of the information provided here.

A problem with the current literature as it pertains to pediatric medical disorders is its emphasis on cure and its minimal discussion of prevention. Of the disorders discussed, testicular cancer has probably been discussed most frequently in terms of prevention (Bosl et al., 1981; Silverberg, 1982). But the available discussions are more of an exhortation to increase prevention through early detection (Gault, 1981) than a technically specific discussion of how such detection can be implemented. And of the reports devoted to testicular cancer, only one prescribed a complete methodology for detection (Hongladarom & Hongladarom, 1982). Yet the prescribed method has never been evaluated experimentally. Thus although the logic of prevention is apparent, and the utility of the available technology seemingly just as apparent, the paucity of experimental study devoted to prevention of testicular cancer leaves many questions unanswered.

There is even less literature related to prevention of obesity. And the information that is available is, for the most part, a discussion of the benefits of preventing obesity rather than a discussion of how to accomplish this prevention (Abraham & Nordsieck, 1960). Finally, for enuresis and encopresis, very little discussion of prevention has been published and no data are available. Virtually all of the available literature is devoted to either epidemiology, etiology, or treatment.

The lack of literature discussing how to prevent various medical disorders is, in part, an explanation for the minimal practice of prevention in medicine. One of the most unfortunate results of the gap in the literature is an apparent lack of preventive technology. As a result pediatricians have few resources to aid them in conducting effective prevention, whereas they are often provided for when pursuing a cure.

The purpose of this chapter has been to provide a set of suggestions that could be useful in preventing some pediatric medical disorders. But as previously discussed, the methods have not been evaluated experimentally. The proposed methods are either an extrapolation of variables related to the causes and correlates of a disorder or are derivations of direct treatment methods. The literature devoted to etiology and to curative treatment has been, for the most part, experimentally derived. It is plausible that manipulation of events that have been linked to the etiology of a disorder by rigorous experimentation could have an impact on the development of that disorder. It is also plausible that if changing a set of behaviors produces a cure for an afflicted individual, a similar change in behaviors could produce a prevention in an individual at risk. Obviously new experiments are necessary to confirm or disconfirm this hypothesis.

The types of interventions proposed above are only a sample of the many that could be proposed. Combining information obtained from studies of the etiology of a disorder with information obtained from studies of the cure of a disorder could produce a pool of information from which many preventive interventions could be extrapolated.

The biobehavioral literature devoted to the epidemiology and treatment of many disease processes from which such extrapolations could be made is growing (Russo & Varni, 1982; Sexton, 1979; Varni, 1983). Some other disease processes of interest from which such extrapolations could be made include hypertension (Coates et al., 1981), asthma (Masek et al., 1981), peridontal disease (Scheffler and Rovin, 1982), pica (de la Burde & Reames, 1973), cancer (Williams, 1980, and congenital malformations (Warkany, 1983).

An advantageous development that could occur as a result of the development of an effective preventive treatment of a targeted disorder is prevention of other untargeted health problems. For example, the prevention of obesity has the potential to prevent cardiovascular disease, diabetes, hypertension, and blindness as well as many socioemotional problems that can occur secondary to fatness (Addanki, 1981; Coates et al., 1981). The prevention of enuresis and encopresis can prevent urinary tract infection (Stansfield, 1973). The prevention of encopresis can prevent organic disorders of the gastrointestinal tract (Levine, 1975). And prevention of testicular cancer can prevent gastrointestinal pathology, sterility, and death. Thus prevention represents a much more efficient form of medicine than curative interventions.

Just the illumination of the advantages inherent in preventive pediatrics will not resolve all the problems that inhibit its development. The purpose of this chapter has been to suggest some technology for furthering the development of preventive pediatrics. Another purpose has been to emphasize a need for increased research and development. But beyond the provision of technology, other problems remain. Patient compliance is always a concern in medicine. Compliance was not discussed in this chapter however, because it has been thoroughly discussed elsewhere (Haynes & Sackett, 1979; Rapoff & Christophersen, 1982). Another problem in the development of preventive pediatrics is an apparent communication gap between the behavioral sciences and the field of pediatrics; yet increasingly, this gap is narrowing (Christophersen, 1982). A final problem involves the reluctance of third party payers (insurers) to reimburse for preventive services (Terris, 1981). But there is a growing literature showing the cost benefits of effective preventive medical interventions (Kristein, 1982; Terris, 1981). And the possibility exists that effective prevention can be accomplished through biobehavioral strategies. As third party payers are exposed to the data supporting the benefit of preventive strategies, they may be inclined to increase their reimbursement for such strategies (Kristein, 1982). The increased use of Health Maintenance Organizations (HMOs) is also likely to increase the need for preventive services.

Overall, the apparent bias against preventive medicine in favor of curative medicine is still a problem. Generations of physicians have been trained in the biomedical tradition and it is unreasonable to suggest or assume that they should be retrained. But that training programs for new physicians should incorporate the literature outlining the philosophy and the technology of prevention is a reasonable suggestion.

Pediatricians can contribute to the development of preventive medicine and to the training of new preventive practitioners by experimental validation of their preventive efforts. This kind of experimentation could supply some of the literature necessary for the training of new preventive practitioners. The body of this chapter has proposed some preventive technology that would be available for evaluation by pediatricians. By conducting such evaluations, pediatricians would be contributing specifically to the development of preventive pediatrics and generally to the development of behavioral pediatrics.

REFERENCES

Abraham, S., & Nordsiek, M. (1960). Relationship of excess weight in children and adults. *Public Health Reports, 75,* 263–273.

Addanki, S. (1981). Roles of nutrition, obesity, and estrogens in diabetes mellitus: Human leads to an experimental approach to prevention. *Preventive Medicine, 10,* 577–589.

American Cancer Society. (1978). *Facts on testicular cancer.* (Available from the American Cancer Society, Kansas Division, 3003 Van Buren, Topeka, KS 66611).

American Psychiatric Association. (1980). *Diagnostic and statistical manual of mental disorders* (3rd ed.). Washington, DC: Author.

Azrin, N.H.,& Foxx, R.M. (1976). *Toilet training in less than a day.* New York: Simon & Schuster.

Azrin, N.H., Sneed, T.J., & Foxx, R.M. (1974). Dry-bed training: Rapid elimination of childhood enuresis. *Behavior Research and Therapy, 12,* 147–156.

Bakwin, H. (1973). The genetics of enuresis. In I. Kolvin, R.C. MacKeith, & S.R. Meadow (Eds.), *Bladder control and enuresis* (pp. 73–78). Philadelphia: Lippincott.

Barr, R.G., Levine, M.D., Wilkinson, R.H., & Mulvihill, D. (1979). Chronic and occult stool retention: A clinical tool for its evaluation in school aged children. *Clinical Pediatrics, 18,* 674–686.

Becker, M., Maiman, L., Kirscht, J., Haefner, D., & Drachman, R. (1977). The health belief model and dietary compliance: A field experiment. *Journal of Health and Social Behavior, 18,* 348–366.

Blomfield, J.W., & Douglas, J.W. (1956). Bedwetting prevalence among children aged 4 to 7 years. *Lancet, i,* 850–854.

Bollard, J. (1982). A 2-year follow-up of bedwetters treated by dry-bed training and standard conditioning. *Behavior Research and Therapy, 20,* 571–580.

Bollard, J., & Nettlebeck, T. (1982). A component analysis of dry-bed training for treatment of bedwetting. *Behavior Research and Therapy, 20,* 383–390.

Bollard, J., Nettlebeck, T., & Roxbee, L. (1982). Dry-bed training for childhood bedwetting: A comparison of group with individually adminstered parent instruction. *Behavior Research and Therapy, 20,* 209–217.

Bollard, R.J., & Woodroffe, P. (1977). The effect of parent adminstered dry-bed training on nocturnal enuresis in children. *Behavior Research and Therapy, 15,* 159–165.

Bosl, G.J., Vogelzang, N.J., Goldman, A., Fraley, E.E., Lange, P.H., Levitt, S.H., & Kennedy, S.H. (1981). Impact of delay in diagnosis on clinical stage of testicular cancer. *Lancet, 2,* 970–973.

Boyle, W.E. (1978). The pediatric history. In R.A. Hoekelman et al. (Eds.), *Principles of pediatrics: Health-care of the young.* New York: McGraw-Hill.

Bray, G.A. (1976). *The obese patient.* Philadelphia: Saunders.

Brazelton, T.B. (1962). A child oriented approach to toilet training. *Pediatrics, 29,* 121–128.

Brazelton, T.B. (1973). Is enuresis preventable? In I. Kolvin, R.C. MacKeith, & S.R. Meadow (Eds.), *Bladder control and enuresis* (pp. 281–284). Philadelphia: Lippincott.

Brazelton, T.B. (1975). Anticipatory guidance. *Pediatric Clinics of North America, 22,* 533–543.

Brook, C.G.D. (1983). Obesity in childhood. *The Practitioner, 227,* 213–219.

Brownell, K.D. (1982). Obesity: Understanding and treating a serious, prevalent, and refractory disorder. *Journal of Consulting and Clinical Psychology, 50,* 820–840.

Brownell, K.D., Kelman, J.H., & Stunkard, A.J. (1983). Treatment of obese children with and without their mothers: Changes in weight and blood pressure. *Pediatrics, 71,* 515–523.

de la Burde, B., & Reames, B. (1973). Prevention of pica, the major cause of lead poisoning in children. *American Journal of Public Health, 63,* 737–743.

Burkitt, D.P., Walker, A.R.P., & Painter, N.S. (1974). Dietary fiber and disease. *Journal of the American Medical Association, 229,* 1068–1074.

Chamberlin, R.W. (1982). Prevention of behavior problems in young children. *Pediatric Clinics of North America, 29,* 239–247.

Charney, M., Goodman, H.C., McBride, M., Lyon, B., & Pratt, R. (1976). Childhood antecedents of adult obesity: Do chubby infants become obese adults? *New England Journal of Medicine, 245,* 6–9.

Christophersen, E.R. (1977). Children's behavior during automobile rides: Do car seats make a difference? *Pediatrics, 60,* 69–74.

Christophersen, E.R. (Ed.). (1982). Behavioral pediatrics. *Pediatric Clinics of North America, 29.* Philadelphia: Saunders.

Christophersen, E.R. (1983). Automobile accidents: Potential years of life lost. *Pediatrics, 71,* 855–856.

Christophersen, E.R., & Gyulay, J.E. (1981). Parental compliance with car seat usage: A positive approach with long-term follow-up. *Journal of Pediatric Psychology, 6,* 301–312.

Christophersen, E.R., & Rainey, S. (1976). Management of encopresis through a pediatric outpatient clinic. *Journal of Pediatric Psychology, 1,* 38–41.

Christophersen, E.R., & Rapoff, M.A. (1979). Behavioral pediatrics. In O.F. Pomerleau & J.P. Brady (Eds.), *Behavioral medicine: Theory and practice* (pp. 99–123). Baltimore: Williams & Wilkins.

Christophersen, E.R., & Rapoff, M.A. (1980). Biosocial pediatrics. In J.M. Ferguson & C.B. Taylor (Eds.), *The comprehensive handbook of behavioral pediatrics* (pp. 3–21). New York: SP Medical & Scientific.

Christophersen, E.R., & Rapoff, M.A. (1983). Toileting problems of children. In C.E. Walker & M.C. Roberts (Eds.), *Handbook of clinical child psychology* (pp. 583–605). New York: Wiley.

Christophersen, E.R., & Sosland-Edelman, D. (in press). Incorporating child passenger safety into pediatric care. In M.N. Currie (Ed.), *The proceedings: Patient education conference VI.* Kansas City, MO: St. Mary's Hospital.

Christophersen, E.R., & Sullivan, M. (1982). Increasing the protection of newborn infants in cars. *Pediatrics, 70,* 21–25.

Coates, T.J., Perry, C., Killen, J., & Slinkard, L.A. (1981). Primary prevention of cardiovascular disease in children and adolescents. In C.K. Prokop, & L.A. Bradley (Eds.), *Medical psychology: Contributing to behavioral medicine* (pp. 157–196). New York: Academic.

Cohen, M.W. (1975). Enuresis. *Pediatric Clinics of North America, 22,* 545–560.

Committee on Standards of Child Health Care. (1977). *Standards of child health care* (3rd ed.). Evanston, IL: American Academy of Pediatrics.

Conklin, M., Klint, K., Morway, A., Sawyer, J.R., & Shepard, R. (1978). Should health teaching include self-examination of the testes? *American Journal of Nursing, 78,* 2073–2074.

Crosby, N.D. (1950). Essential enuresis—Successful treatment based on physiological concepts. *Medical Journal of Australia, 2,* 533–543.

Cullen, K.J. (1976). A six year controlled trial of prevention of children's behavior disorders. *Journal of Pediatrics, 88,* 662–667.

Cummings, M.K., Lampone, D., Mettlin, C., & Pontes, J.E. (1983). What young men know about testicular cancer. *Preventive Medicine, 12,* 326–330.

Damjanov, I., & Solter, D. (1974). Experimental teratomata. *Current Topics in Pathology, 69,* 69–78.

Davidson, M. (1958). Constipation and fecal incontinence. *Pediatric Clinics of North America, 5,* 749–757.

Dawber, T.R. (1979). *The Framingham study: The epidemiology of athersclerotic disease.* Cambridge, MA: Harvard University Press.

Dershewitz, R.A., & Christophersen, E.R. (1984). Childhood household safety: An overview. *American Journal of Diseases in Children, 138,* 85–88.

Dietz, W.H. (1983). Childhood obesity: Susceptibility, cause, and management. *Journal of Pediatrics, 103,* 676–686.

Dixon, F.J., & Moore, R.A. (1953). Testicular tumors: A clinicopathological study. *Cancer, 6,* 427–431.

Drabman, R.S., Hammer, D., & Jarvie, G.J. (1977). Eating styles of obese and nonobese black and white children in a naturalistic setting. *Addictive Behaviors, 2,* 83–86.

Droller, M.J. (1980). Cancer of the testis: An overview. *Urologic Clinics of North America, 7,* 731–733.

Epstein, L.H. Wing, R.R., Kuller, C., &, Becker, D. (1983). Parent-child obesity and cardiovascular risk factors. *Preventive Medicine, 12,* 437–446.

Finney, J.W., & Christophersen, E.R. (1984). Behavioral pediatrics: Health education in pediatric primary care. In M. Hersen, R.M. Eisler, & P.M. Miller (Eds.), *Progress in behavior modification* (Vol. 16; pp. 185–229). New York: Academic.

Finney, J.W., Friman, P.C., Rapoff, M.A., & Christophersen, E.R. 1985. Improving compliance with antibiotic regimens for otitis media: Randomized clinical trial in a pediatric clinic. *American Journal of Diseases in Children, 139,* 89–95.

Garn, S.M., & Clark, D.C. (1976). Trends in fatness and the origins of obesity. *Pediatrics, 57,* 443–456.

Gault, P.L. (1981). Taking your part in the fight against testicular cancer. *Nursing 81,* May, 47–50.

Goldby, R.B., Reynolds, T.F., & Vurgin, D. (1979). Chemotherapy of metasitic germ cell tumors. *Seminars in Oncology, 6,* 82–86.

Goldenring, J.M., & Purtell, E. (1984). Knowledge of testicular cancer and need for self-examination in college students: A call for equal time for men in teaching of early cancer detection techniques. *Pediatrics, 74,* 1093–1096.

Green, L.W., Kreuter, M.W., Deeds, S.G., & Partridge, K.B. (1980). *Health education planning: A diagnostic approach.* Palo Alto: Mayfield.

Gross, R.T., & Dornbusch, S.M. (1983). Enuresis. In M.D. Levine, W.B. Carey, A.C. Crocker, & R.T. Gross (Eds.), *Developmental-behavioral pediatrics* (pp. 573–586). Philadelphia: Saunders.

Hall, D.C., Adams, C.K., Stein, G.H., Stephenson, H.S., Goldstein, M.K., & Pennypacker, H.S. (1980). Improved detection of human breast lesions following experimental training. *Cancer, 46,* 408–414.

Haynes, R.B., Taylor, D.W., & Sackett, D.L. (Eds.). (1979). *Compliance in health care.* Baltimore: Johns Hopkins University Press.

Hongladrom, T., & Hongladrom, G.C. (1982). The problem of testicular cancer: How health professionals in the armed services can help. *Military Medicine, 147,* 211–213.

Hooper, P.D. (1965). Infant feeding and its relationship to weight gain and illness. *Practitioner, 194,* 391–402.

de Jonge, G.A. (1973). The urge syndrome. In I. Kolvin, R.C. MacKeith, & S.R. Meadows (Eds.), *Bladder control and enuresis* (pp. 66–73). Philadelphia: Lippincott.

Kannel, W.B., & Gordon, T. (1979). Physiological and medical concomitants of obesity: The Framingham study. In G.A. Bray (Ed.), *Obesity in America* (NIH Publication No. 79-359). Washington, DC: U.S. Government Printing Office.

Keys, A. (1979). Is overweight a risk factor for coronary heart disease? *Cardiovascular Medicine, 4,* 1233–1242.

Kirscht, J.P., Becker, M.H., Haefner, D.P., & Maiman, L.A. (1978). Effects of threatening communication and mother's health beliefs on weight change in obese children. *Journal of Behavioral Medicine, 1,* 147–157.

Klesges, R.C., Coates, T.J., Brown, G., Sturgeon-Tisllisch, J., Moldenhauer-Klesges, L. Holzer, B., Woolfrey, J., & Vollmer, J. (1983). Parental influences on children's eating behavior and relative weight. *Journal of Applied Behavior Analysis, 16,* 371–378.

Knittle, J.L. (1978). Adipose tissue development in man. In F. Falkner & J.M. Tanner (Eds.), *Human growth: Postnatal growth* (pp. 295–315). New York: Plenum.

Korsch, B.M., & Negrette, V.F. (1972). Doctor-patient communication. *Scientific American, 227,* 66–74.

Kristein, M.M. (1982). Health care costs and preventive medicine. *Preventive Medicine, 11,* 729–732.

Lazes, P.M. (1979). *The handbook of health education.* Germantown, MD: Aspen Systems.

Levine, M.D. (1975). Children with encopresis: A descriptive analysis. *Pediatrics, 56,* 412–416.

Levine, M.D. (1982). Encopresis: Its potentiation, evaluation, and alleviation. *Pediatric Clinics of North America, 29,* 315–331.

Levine, M.D. (1983). Encopresis. In M.D. Levine, W.B. Carey, A.C. Crocker, & R.T. Gross (Eds.), *Developmental-behavioral pediatrics* (pp. 586–595). Philadelphia: Saunders.

Lifshitz, M., & Chovers, A. (1972). Encopresis among Israeli kibbutz children. *Israel Annals of Psychiatry and Related Disciplines, 4,* 326–340.

Martin, C.R.A. (1966). *A new approach to enuresis*. London: H.K. Lewis.

Marty, P.J., McDermott, R.J., & Gold, R.S. (1983). An assessment of three alternative formats for promoting breast self-examination. *Cancer Nursing, 6*, 207–211.

Masek, B.J., Epstein, L.H., & Russo, D.C. (1981). Behavioral perspectives preventive medicine. In S.M. Turner, K.S. Calhoun, & H.E. Adams (Eds.), *Handbook of clinical behavior therapy* (pp. 475–499). New York: Wiley.

Mayer, J. (1953). Genetic, traumatic, and environmental factors in the etiology of obesity. *Physiological Review, 33*, 472–508.

Mower, O.H., & Mower, W. (1938). Enuresis: A method for its study and treatment. *American Journal of Orthopsychiatry, 8*,436–459.

Neuman, C.G. (1983). Obesity in childhood. In M.D. Levine, W.B. Carey, A.C. Crocker, & R.T. Gross (Eds.), *Developmental-behavioral pediatrics* (536–551). Philadelphia: Saunders.

Nunn, R.G. (1978). Maladaptive habits and tics. *Psychiatric Clinics of North America, 1*, 348–361.

Olatawuria, M.O. (1973). Encopresis: A review of 32 cases. *Acta Pediatrica, 62*, 358–364.

Olness, K. (1975). The use of self-hypnosis in the treatment of childhood nocturnal enuresis. *Clinical Pediatrics, 14*, 273–279.

Oppel, W.C., Harper, P.A., & Rider, R.V. (1968). The age of attaining bladder control. *Pediatrics, 42*, 614–618.

Pendleton, D., & Hasler, J. (Eds.) (1980). *Doctor-patient communication*. New York: Academic.

Pomerleau, O.F., Bass, R., & Crown, V. (1975). The role of behavior modification in preventive medicine. *New England Journal of Medicine, 292*, 1277–1282.

Rames, L.K., Clarke, W.R., Connor, W.E., Reiter, M.A., & Lauer, R.M. (1978). Normal blood pressures and the evaluation of sustained blood pressure evaluation in childhood: The Muscatine study. *Pediatrics, 61*, 245–252.

Rapoff, M.A., & Christophersen, E.R. (1982). Improving compliance in pediatric practice. *Pediatric Clinics of North America, 29*, 377–391.

Rohr, F.J., & Lothian, J.A. (1984). Feeding throughout the first year of life. In R.B. Howard & H.S. Winter (Eds.), *Nutrition and feeding of infants and toddlers* (pp. 65–131). Boston: Little, Brown.

Russo, D.C., & Varni, J.W. (Eds.). (1982). *Behavioral pediatrics: Research and practice*. New York: Plenum.

Scheffler, R.M., & Rovin, S. (1982). Preventing and treating peridontal disease with the Keyes technique: A preliminary assessment. *Preventive Medicine, 11*, 677–695.

Schmitt, B.O. (1982). Nocturnal enuresis: An update on treatment. *Pediatric Clinics of North America, 29*, 21–36.

Sexton, M.M. (1979). Behavioral epidemiology. In O.F. Pomerleau & J.P. Brady (Eds.), *Behavioral medicine: Theory and practice* (3–21). Baltimore: Williams & Wilkins.

Silverberg, I. (1982). Cancer in young adults (ages 15–34). *CA: A Cancer Journal for Clinicians, 32*, 32–42.

Stansfield, J.M. (1973). Enuresis and urinary tract infection. In I. Kolvin, R.C. MacKeith, & S.R. Meadow (Eds.), *Bladder control and enuresis* (pp. 102–103). Philadelphia: Lippincott.

Starfield, B., & Mellits, E.D. (1968). Increase in functional bladder capacity. *Journal of Pediatrics, 72*, 483–487.

Stedman, D.J. (1970). The application of learning principles in pediatric practice. *Pediatric Clinics of North America, 17*, 427–436.

Stunkard, A.J. (1979). Behavioral medicine and beyond: The example of obesity. In O.F. Pomerleau & J.P. Brady (Eds.), *Behavioral medicine: Theory and practice* (pp. 279–298). Baltimore: Williams & Wilkins.

Stunkard, A.J. (1980). *Obesity*. Philadelphia: Saunders.

Taitz, L.S. (1971). Infantile overnutrition among artificially fed infants in the Sheffield region. *British Medical Journal, 1*, 315–316.

Terris, M. (1981). The primacy of prevention. *Preventive Medicine, 10*, 689–699.

Thomas, K.A., Hassanein, R.S., & Christophersen, E.R. (in press). An evaluation of group well-child care for improving parent's home burn prevention practices. *Pediatrics*.

Thompson, J.K., Jarvie, G.J., Lahey, B.B., & Cureton, K.J. (1982). Exercise and obesity: Etiology, physiology, and intervention. *Psychological Bulletin, 91*, 55–79.

Trowell, H. (1975). Pathological growth and maturation in infants associated with modern methods of feeding. *Journal of Tropical Medicine and Environmental Child Health, 21*, 192–198.

Van Itallie, T.B. (1979). Obesity: Adverse effects on health and longevity. *American Journal of Clinical Nutrition, 32*, 2723–2733.

Varni, J.W. (1983). *Clinical behavioral pediatrics*. New York: Pergamon.

Warkany, J.C. (1983). Prevention of congenital malformations. *Current Problems in Pediatrics, 13*, 2–26.

Waxman, M., & Stunkard, A.J. (1980). Caloric intake and expenditure of obese boys. *Journal of Pediatrics, 96*, 187–193.

Williams, C.L. (1980). Primary prevention of cancer beginning in childhood. *Preventive Medicine, 9*, 275–280.

Wing, R.R., & Jeffery, R.W. (1979). Outpatient treatments of obesity: A comparison of methodology and clinical results. *International Journal of Obesity, 3*, 261–279.

Woodall, K.W., & Epstein, L.H. (1983). The prevention of obesity. *Behavioral Medicine Update, 5*, 15–22.

Wright, L. (1973). Handling the encopretic child. *Professional Psychology, 3*, 137–144.

Wright, L. (1975). Outcome of a standardized program for treating psychogenic encopresis. *Professional Psychology, 6*, 453–456.

Wright, L., Schaefer, A.B., & Solomons, G. (1979). *Encyclopedia of Pediatric Psychology*. Baltimore: University Park Press.

Wright, L., & Walker, E. (1977). Treatment of the child with psychogenic encopresis. *Clinical Pediatrics, 16*, 1042–1045.

Yeates, W.K. (1973). Bladder function: Increased frequency and nocturnal incontinence. In I. Kolvin, R.C. MacKeith, & S.R. Meadow (Eds.), *Bladder control and enuresis* (pp. 151–155). Philadelphia: Lippincott.

Yule, W. (1977). The potential of behavioral treatment in preventing later childhood difficulties. *Behavior Analysis and Modification, 2*, 19–32.

Zaleski, A., Gerrard, J.W., & Shoker, M.H.K. (1973). Nocturnal enuresis: The importance of a small bladder capacity. In I. Kolvin, R.C. MacKeith, & S.R. Meadow (Eds.), *Bladder control and enuresis* (pp. 95–102). Philadelphia: Lippincott.

13

Smoking Prevention Programs for Adolescents: Rationale and Review

HERBERT H. SEVERSON AND EDWARD LICHTENSTEIN

Cigarette smoking is the single most preventable cause of death due to cardiovascular disease and cancer (U.S. Department of Health and Human Services [USDHHS], 1982). Yet approximately 1.4 million adolescents begin to smoke cigarettes each year (U.S. Public Health Service [USPHS], 1979). It is estimated that 87 percent of adult smokers begin regular use of cigarettes before leaving high school. Surveys indicate that 26 percent of high school seniors reported daily cigarette use (Johnston, Bachman, & O'Malley, 1980). These rates appear to have remained constant since 1981, although heavy smoking (half pack a day) has decreased from

Preparation of this manuscript was supported in part by grants number HD13409 and HD15825, National Institute of Child Health and Human Development, and by grant number DA03635, National Institute of Drug Abuse.

The authors thank Anthony Biglan and Russell Glasgow for their careful editorial feedback, and Vanita Miller and Lisa James for their typing of the manuscript.

29 percent to 20 percent. Cigarettes are still the most prevalent drug, other than alcohol, used during adolescence.

Surveys of teen smoking behavior reveal that cigarette smoking among girls doubled between 1968 and 1974 (U.S. Department of Health, Education, and Welfare [USDHEW], 1977). Teenage girls' smoking rate is now equal to that for boys, whether one considers daily smoking (26 percent) or heavy smoking (girls, 13.6 percent; boys, 13.1 percent) (Johnston, Bachman, & O'Malley, 1981). Experimentation has continued to move downward to younger grade levels (Chilton Research Services, 1979). Most initial smoking experiences occur before the 10th grade. For example, daily cigarette smoking is reported by 15 percent of teenagers below the tenth grade, and only an additional nine percent of teens report taking up smoking in grades 10 to 12. Our own assessment of middle school children in the state of Oregon determined that smoking rates for seventh grade students vary from a low of 3 percent to a high of 16 percent. On average, approximately 10 percent of seventh graders report having smoked a cigarette in the past week (Severson, Faller, Nautel, Biglan, Ary & Bavry, 1981). In many schools girls report higher levels of smoking than boys at both seventh and ninth grades.

These statistics on the incidence and prevalence of adolescent smoking, coupled with cigarette smoking's demonstrated status as a risk factor, justify the development of primary and secondary smoking prevention programs. In response to this need, several institutes in the National Institutes of Health, including the National Institute of Child Health and Human Development, have supported considerable research on cigarette smoking prevention with young adolescents as the major target group. A lesser but significant amount of research has been conducted on the acquisition of smoking. This chapter describes the major findings in these two areas. The acquisition of smoking is first considered, followed by a description of models of smoking intervention and a review of the extant prevention literature. Since comprehensive reviews of much of the prevention literature have recently been published (Flay, in press; McCaul & Glasgow, in press) we selectively highlight key studies and issues and attempt to offer some directions for future research.

ACQUISITION OF SMOKING

In order to understand adolescent smoking and develop effective prevention programs, it is critical to study the acquisition of smoking behavior. Careful analysis of smoking acquisition and the transition from experimentation to regular smoking should facilitate the implementation of cost-effective interventions that target specific groups of adolescents. There are a wide range of cultural, familial, interpersonal, and organismic factors that could be targeted for such an analysis. Cross-sectional and longitudinal studies have identified peer, parental, and sibling behaviors as important for this smoking acquisition analysis. It is essential, therefore, to elucidate the classes of peer, parental, and sibling behavior that may affect the initiation and maintenance of smoking (Evans, Henderson, Hill, & Raines, 1979). This section examines parent, family, and peer influences on adolescent smoking, and other correlates of smoking behavior.

Parental and Family Influence on Smoking

Parent influence on adolescent smoking was identified as a contributing factor as early as 1960 (Matarazzo & Saslow, 1960). Much of the early work on family influence focused on the relationship between parental smoking status and subsequent teenage smoking. There is a great deal of correlational evidence that smoking practices of parents are related to teenage smoking (Biglan, Severson, Bavry, & McConnell, 1983; Borland & Rudolph, 1975; Levitt & Edwards, 1970). Several studies have shown that the probability of a child smoking is proportional to the number of smoking parents (Banks, Bewley, Bland, Dean, & Pollard, 1978). The 1979 Surgeon General's Report (DHEW, 1979) presents data indicating that in families in which both parents smoke, 22.2 percent of the boys and 20.7 percent of the girls are also smokers, compared with 11.3 percent and 7.6 percent where neither parent smokes. However, this relationship has not always been found (Allegrante, O'Rourke, & Tuncalp, 1977; Ary, Biglan, & Severson, 1983); it has sometimes been found only for one sex (Williams, 1973), and appears to account for less variance in smoking than does peer smoking (Levitt & Edwards, 1970; Mittelmark et al., 1983). On balance, there seems to be an association between parent smoking and the likelihood that a child will smoke. The mechanisms involved in this relationship remain to be investigated.

In addition to parental smoking, it appears that the smoking status of older siblings is also an important factor (Evans & Raines, 1982). The proportion of children who smoke in families which contain a smoking parent *and* an older smoking sibling is more than twice that of families that contain only smoking parents and nonsmoking siblings. Evans and Raines (1982) report that 17 percent of the boys and 20 percent of the girls smoke in families where there is a smoking parent and an older sibling smoking, versus only 7.5 percent of boys and 9.7 percent of girls in families in which there is a smoking parent, but no smoking siblings. Even when parents do not smoke, the presence of an older sibling who smokes also increases smoking rate—19.5 percent and 15.3 percent for boys and girls, respectively. The combined influences of these family members can best been seen in two studies conducted almost a decade apart which found that the lowest rates of smoking children occur in families in which neither parent smokes *and* where there are older nonsmoking siblings (National Institute of Education, 1979; Williams, 1971).

In addition to the smoking status of parents and siblings, recent studies have examined additional family variables that may be relevant to subsequent smoking and drug use in adolescents. These studies suggest that parental rule-setting, attitudes and values toward smoking, the quality of parent-child relations, the discrepancy in parent-child values and perceptions, and closeness to or independence from parents may all be important (Baranowski, 1978, Kandel, Kessler, & Margulies, 1978; McAlister, Gordon, Krosnick, & Milburn, 1982; Pederson, Baskerville, & Lefcoe, 1981; Streit & Oliver, 1972; Tudor, Peterson, & Elifson, 1980). Some data on Norwegian school children supports the potential effectiveness of parental standard-setting regarding smoking (Aaro, Hauknes, & Berglund, 1981). In families where both parents smoked and the children were allowed to smoke by their parents, 72 percent of the children were smokers in the ninth grade (15 years of age). When children in the home of smoking parents were not allowed to smoke, only 21 percent were daily smokers at the same age. When none of the parents smoke and the children were not allowed to smoke, only 10 percent were daily smokers by the ninth grade.

In summary, the smoking of parents and older siblings is statistically associated with smoking of younger children in the family. There is suggestive evidence that parental rule-setting, family closeness, congruent perceptions and values, and parent expectations are important in smoking acquisition. The specific mechanisms by which families have an impact upon smoking decisions remain unclear. Methodological problems with much of the prior research cloud interpretations of the results. The three major deficiencies that pervade the research literature are: (1) the total reliance on adolescents as the source of information (Bentler & Eichberg, 1975); (2) the dependence upon questionnaires or interviews as assessment procedures; and (3) the use of retrospective reports rather than designing prospective studies which longitudinally track the adolescent and family. Direct observation of family interaction would enhance understanding of parental and family influences on adolescent smoking (Biglan & Lichtenstein, 1984). Lichtenstein and his colleagues are currently investigating the mechanisms of family influence on adolescent smoking, using questionnaire, interview, and observational data from both parents and children in a longitudinal study.

Peer Influences on Smoking

Peer influence is the preeminent proximal factor in the initiation of smoking behavior (Severson, 1984). Most adolescents report getting their first cigarette from a peer and being with same-age friends when initially experimenting with cigarettes (Biglan, Severson, Bavry, & McConnell, 1983; Friedman, Lichtenstein, & Biglan, 1985). The influence of peers on adolescent smoking is a direct one. Adolescents smoke when they are with other adolescents who are smoking; adults are seldom present during initial smoking episodes. Friends (57 percent), acquaintances (20 percent), and siblings (11 percent) accounted for 88 percent of those present during initial experimentation, and in about half of the initial smoking incidents, another young person was also trying a cigarette for the first time (Friedman et al., 1985). Authors of a number of cross-sectional studies have concluded that friends' smoking is a primary factor in an adolescent's smoking behavior (Allegrante, O'Rourke, & Tuncalp, 1977; Bewley & Bland, 1977). Krosnick & Judd (1982) conclude that while both parental smoking and peer smoking are important factors in influencing an adolescent to smoke, peer influence appears to increase in importance during adolescence while parental influence decreases. Cross-sectional studies which collect data at a single time point can show the relationship between concurrent behaviors, but cannot show causal relationships.

Longitudinal prediction studies of the factors that predict the onset of smoking also point to the critical role of peer smoking. A hierarchical multiple regression analysis of 506 pretest nonsmoking middle school students demonstrated that, at one-year follow-up, the factors that predict smoking were the number of cigarette offers, daily marijuana use, number of smoking friends, and level of experience with smoking. The amount of variance accounted for (R^2) was 11 percent (Ary & Biglan, 1985).

A one-year follow-up discriminant function analysis of high school pretest nonsmokers yielded a significant R^2 of .192 ($F_{18,235} = 2.85$, $p < .01$). The major predictors were the number of smoking friends and the level of smoking experience (Ary & Biglan, 1985). A recent prospective study by Mittelmark et al. (1983) also concluded that friends' smoking was the most important factor in predicting onset of smoking. Thus to deter experimentation, it makes a good deal of sense to focus upon the peer influence processes.

Peer influence processes continue to be important for the maintenance of smoking (Biglan & Lichtenstein, 1984). Young people are more likely to continue smoking and to become dependent if their friends smoke. In our own work, we have found that the number of friends smoking contributes significant incremental variance to the prediction of smoking rate among adolescents who were already smoking at the initial assessment. Longitudinal studies also confirm the role of peer influence (Ary, Biglan, & Severson, 1983). Here, too, the influence is a direct one, as they frequently smoke as a result of direct modeling from other smoking adolescents. Kniskern, Biglan, Lichtenstein, Ary, & Bavry (1983) experimentally evaluated the impact of smoking models on teenage smokers. The presence of a smoking model produced two significant effects: subjects smoked more cigarettes, but took fewer puffs per cigarette. This implies that teaching students to deal with peer influence processes may be also be valuable for helping young people who have initiated smoking to resist becoming dependent smokers.

There is still much to be learned about the peer social influence processes. Much of the data summarized above comes from self-report questionnaires and are cross-sectional and correlational in nature (Biglan & Lichtenstein, 1984). The transition *process*—from initial experimentation to regular smoking—is not well understood. It is estimated that fully two-thirds of all adolescents try at least one cigarette, but only about 26 percent are regular smokers at the end of high school (Johnston, O'Malley, & Bachman, 1983). Retrospective interview data reported by Hirschman, Leventhal, and Glynn (1984) suggest that there are several different paths to smoking. They found that quick progression was associated with life stress variables, while slower progression was associated with smoking peers. Longitudinal data are needed to test such hypotheses.

Models of the Acquisition Process

The indirect and direct evidence for the role of peer influence on adolescent smoking acquisition is compelling. It is also clear that the effects of peer influence are more substantiated than family influences. The integration of family and peer influences into a comprehensive model remains a task for the future. The useful effort in this direction is exemplified by Flay and his colleagues (Flay, d'Avernas, Best, Kersell, & Ryan, 1983). Their preliminary model considers family, peer, and organismic (personality) variables in relation to the several stages—initiation, experimentation, regular smoking—of adolescent smoking acquisition. An empirically supported model of this sort would provide direction to smoking prevention interventions.

While there is, as yet, no validated theory or model that satisfactorily integrates the data and provides guidelines for interventions, three alternative frameworks have been proposed. These frameworks reflect differing theoretical views of behavior and development.

The behavior analytic framework (Biglan & Lichtenstein, 1984) suggests five classes of variables that are important in understanding the onset of smoking behavior: (1) the modeling effects of the smoking behavior of others; (2) the reinforcing practices of others; (3) the immediate physical and pharmacologic consequences of smoking cigarettes; (4) the teenager's repertoire of behaviors for refusing cigarettes; and (5) countervailing contingencies that reinforce not smoking. The emphasis is on specific, proximal variables: events that occur relatively immediately prior to or after smoking or temptation episodes.

The cognitive-social perspective (Chassin, Presson, & Sherman, 1984; Sherman, Presson, Chassin, & Olshavsky, 1983), like the behavioral framework, emphasizes proximal variables, but they are cognitive in nature. These include specific self-relevant attitudes and beliefs about smoking, normative beliefs, and behavioral intentions. This perspective is based to a large extent on Ajzen and Fishbein's (1970) model of the relationship between attitudes, intentions, and behaviors. Adolescent cognitions and attributions concerning early smoking experiences are also of interest (Hirschman et al., 1984).

The empirical association of attitudes, beliefs, and intentions with smoking is less at issue than the interpretation of directional causality. Persons holding the behavior-analytic view treat attitudes beliefs and intentions as products of adolescents' reinforcement history with peers, siblings, parents, and cigarettes. Intentions, for example, are seen as likely to be a function of prior exposure to discussions of others' smoking or one's own smoking. The expression of an intention may itself increase the probability of the behavior, but this does not seem to be the sense in which intentions are typically said to cause other behavior (Biglan & Lichtenstein, 1984).

The problem behavior theory of Jessor and Jessor (1977) emphasizes more distal variables, including general personality traits and perceived environmental factors not specific to smoking. These variables are seen to define a proneness to deviant behavior and to predict early or premature transition to a variety of adult activities in violation of age norms. The evidence brought to bear support for this theory is the substantial covariation among risk behaviors for the same individuals. Adolescent smoking behavior is a part of a more general class of drug use behaviors and other high risk behaviors such as precocious sexual activity, aggression, and delinquency (Jessor, 1984). In contrast, the behavior-analytic approach emphasizes the role of proximal variables and distrusts the validity and usefulness of dispositional traits.

It is likely that variables from all three theoretical perspectives will have heuristic value in prevention programs. Thus far, only one study has directly compared the three approaches (Chassin et al., 1984). Variables from all three approaches were significant predictors of smoking transition over a one-year period. Further, the three approaches made independent contributions to the prediction of transition. More studies of this sort which compare the relative contributions of differing approaches would be quite informative.

SMOKING PREVENTION

Since smoking cessation efforts with adults have proven disappointing (Glasgow & Bernstein, 1981; Leventhal & Cleary, 1980; Lichtenstein & Brown, 1981), health professionals have turned their attention to the prevention of smoking. Because smoking onset primarily occurs prior to the completion of high school, these efforts have focused largely on adolescent populations. Recent reviews of smoking prevention programs by Flay et al. (in press), Glasgow and McCaul (1984), and Snow, Gilchrist, and Schinke (in press) provide in-depth critical reviews of these prevention programs. We describe the general approach and rationale for current prevention programs, highlight important exemplar programs, and suggest specific factors that appear responsible for programs' effects.

Historical Trends

Emphasis on smoking prevention is not new (Thompson, 1978; Williams, 1971). Early smoking prevention programs typically emphasized information on the risks of smoking, that is, the long-term health consequences. Programs of this type were successful in changing knowledge, and sometimes in changing attitudes, but ineffective in preventing actual smoking behavior (Evans, Henderson, Hill, & Raines, 1979; Williams, 1971).

Recent programs have introduced multicomponent interventions that address a range of psychosocial factors hypothesized to be associated with the development of smoking. Prime consideration is given to the social influence processes that appear to be responsible for the initiation of smoking. Programs have also moved away from an emphasis on long-term health risks (such as lung cancer) as a result of reviews that show that students' knowledge of these negative effects had little effect on their smoking (Goodstadt, 1978). Current programs emphasize short-term, immediate health consequences.

Most programs are aimed toward primary prevention. Their focus is upon trying to prevent young people from trying or ever smoking or, if they have already experimented, from shifting to regular use (Pollich, Ellickson, Reuter, & Kahan, 1984). An additional characteristic of primary prevention programs is their focus upon the general population of adolescents without targeting an "at risk" or problematic subgroup.

There has been more empirical research in smoking prevention than in the prevention of other drug use (Severson, 1984). There are several reasons for this state of affairs. Because cigarette smoking represents the most preventable cause of death due to cardiovascular disease and cancer (USDHHS, 1982), there have been initiatives by the National Institute of Child Health and Human Development, Office of the Surgeon General, and National Cancer Institute to develop and evaluate effective school based smoking prevention programs for adolescents. Some authors have identified the prevention of smoking as a potential model for the prevention of other drug use (McAlister, 1983). An additional reason for studying smoking is the availability of reliable noninvasive biochemical indices of use to corroborate self-reports. In the following sections, we describe the structural characteristics of prevention programs and then describe exemplar programs and summarize the major empirical findings.

An Overview of Prevention Programs

Target Population.   Most recent programs have been aimed at sixth or seventh grade students in classroom settings. Epidemiological data suggest that smoking onset becomes significant at grade seven (U.S. Public Health Service, 1976). An important developmental transition occurs when students move from the elementary school to either a middle school (sixth grade) or junior high school (seventh grade). The new school environment exposes children to different and older classmates and peers. Relatedly, there is increased freedom from parental monitoring and control. In sum, there is the increased potential for experimentation with new behaviors, including drug use.

Assessment. The program or curriculum is typically preceded by a baseline assessment. Subjects are administered questionnaires regarding their smoking behavior and related variables, and also provide expired air and/or saliva samples which they are told can show whether they have smoked. This procedure has come to be known as a "bogus pipeline" procedure (Evans, Hansen, & Mittelmark, 1977). Studies have shown that when students complete questionnaires under these conditions they report higher and more accurate rates of smoking (Bauman & Dent, 1982). The external validation of self-report is an important step in getting accurate information on use and determining the effects of prevention programs. The most common and least expensive biochemical measure is carbon monoxide (CO) from expired air samples. Since the half-life of CO is approximately 2 to 4 hours (Prue, Martin, & Hume, 1980), this measure is only accurate for separating regular smokers from nonsmokers or to determine if a person has smoked cigarettes in the past 24 hours. A second widely used measure is saliva thiocyanate (SCN), which is a by-product of the combustion of tobacco and has a half-life of approximately 14 days (Benowitz, 1983). SCN provides a more accurate assessment of use in the past week, but is considerably more expensive to analyze. There are other reliable physiological indices of smoking, such as plasma nicotine, and urinary or saliva cotinine. However, they are more costly and/or more invasive. None of the biochemical measures are sensitive to very low rate or episodic smoking as is done by many adolescents. Biochemical validation of smoking is itself complex, sensitive to technological advances, and beyond the scope of this chapter. Recent reviews (Benowitz, 1983; Pechacek, Fox, Murray & Luepker, 1984) evaluate the measurement issues.

Structural Characteristics. Most prevention programs have been classroom-based interventions. The access to organized groups of students is one of the advantages of school-based prevention programs. The interventions are usually conducted in health classes, but may involve other teachers as well if health is not a required class at the target grade level. Science, physical education, social studies, and home room teachers have all been enlisted to teach the program in several studies. Most programs involve five to seven class sessions with a range from four sessions (Evans, 1976) to twenty (Botvin et al., 1984). The programs are usually highly scripted and involve teacher training or having trained intervention specialists come into the classroom. Many of the current programs follow initial sessions with "booster" sessions to maintain treatment effects. These are usually scheduled at 3 to 6 month intervals and may occur during subsequent school years. The purpose is to briefly remind students of the key components of the program and prompt them to use the skills they were taught.

Since Evans et al. (1977) pioneered the use of filmed smoking peer messages, many programs use film or videotape to illustrate social pressure situations or teach specific refusal skills or show immediate health consequences of smoking. The Oregon Research Institute program, for example, uses videotaped vignettes enacted by local teens to depict situations in which teens are offered a cigarette or pressured to smoke. The video freezes at the point of the offer and the teacher or peer leader prompts the students to respond as they would in that situation. The advantage of videotaped situations is the standardization of material presented and the realistic nature of the pressure situation (Severson et al., 1981).

Program Components.   There has been a wide range of specific components included in smoking prevention programs. This is a tribute to the creativity of the investigators and the diverse theoretical frameworks on which these programs are built. There is also much commonality across programs. Components that appear to have been universally adopted include (1) awareness of social pressures to smoke, (2) teaching refusal skills, and (3) awareness of immediate physiological consequences. Increasing students' awareness of pressures to smoke includes sensitizing students to peer influence situations, and critiquing media advertisements that promote the sale of cigarettes. The rationale is that before learning to refuse an offer, the students have to comprehend the wide range of factors that may influence them to smoke.

The second basic component is training students how to gracefully refuse a cigarette. The skills are usually modeled by peer leaders or filmed models and the students are given or create role-play situations in which to rehearse their skills. Students are taught several different ways of saying no and are encouraged to try them out in peer role play situations.

The third of the frequently adopted components is instruction in immediate physiological effects of smoking. It is assumed that information on the immediate effects of smoking has stronger pervasive effects on adolescents because the information is "new" (McCaul & Glasgow, in press) and adolescents are more "present oriented" than adults (Mittelmark, 1978). This information may have more salience for adolescents who smoke, but fail to label themselves as smokers and thus may not see long-term health consequences of smoking as personally relevant (McCaul & Glasgow, in press). The primary effects highlighted are the increase in heart rate, blood pressure, blood carbon monoxide levels, and vasoconstriction in hands and feet.

There are several additional components that are sometimes included in prevention programs. Among the most popular of these options are the use of peer leaders, obtaining a public commitment not to smoke, and life skills training, such as stress reduction and decision-making skills. The use of peer leaders was pioneered at Stanford by Perry, McAlister and their colleagues (Perry, Killen, Slinkard, & McAlister, 1980; Perry, Killen, Telch, Slinkard, & Danaher, 1980). The rationale is that teens are more likely to listen to a peer than a teacher, especially with regard to how to handle peer pressure. Such programs use same-age peers who are nominated by classmates and then intensively trained to run small groups or assist the teacher in implementing the program.

The public commitment procedure has been implemented in several ways, ranging from a simple raising of hands in response to a teacher prompt, to a videotaped verbal commitment never to smoke. Hurd et al. (1980) exemplified this procedure when they videotaped students as they completed the sentence, "I'm not going to smoke because. . ." It is hypothesized that once a child makes a public commitment in front of his/her peers, it is more likely that he/she will behave consistently with the commitment.

Another popular option is training in stress management and decision making, as well as general social skills. The premise is that smoking is one of a class of functionally equivalent behaviors through which teens both express themselves and deal with anxiety (Botvin, Baker, Renick, Filazzola, & Botvin, 1984). The purpose of teaching adolescents life skills or coping skills is to provide alternative behavioral repertoires with which to deal with anxiety-provoking stressors common to adolescents. These skills are designed to enhance general personal and social competence (Botvin et al., in press). The stress management procedures usually follow a cognitive rehearsal format, combined with practice in relaxation techniques. Decision-making training includes learning a step-wise decision-making procedure, brainstorming techniques for developing options, and self-instructional techniques (Botvin & Wills, in press). Additional components of assertion training, communication skills, and goal setting are also included in some life skills oriented prevention programs.

REVIEW OF MAJOR STUDIES

A recent review by Flay (1985) identified 26 school-based studies of psychosocial approaches to smoking prevention. Flay identified two major approaches to smoking prevention. The first is the "social influences" model, which focuses on: (1) teaching students about the social influences to smoke, (2) providing them with the behavioral skills with which to resist those influences, and (3) correcting their perceptions of social norms. The second major approach is the "life/social skills" approach, characterized by its emphasis on methods for enhancing general social competence (Glasgow & McCaul, 1984). We have chosen five major research programs for review, four of which illustrate the social influence model, while the fifth illustrates the life skills approach.

The Houston Project

The seminal study of the social influence model was conducted by Richard Evans and his colleagues (Evans et al., 1978). The intervention was based upon McGuire's (1974) social inoculation theory, which postulated that social inoculation is analogous to biological innoculation. Hence an exposure to social influence agents plus counter arguments for these influences will prepare the adolescent to resist later the persuasion or social pressure to smoke (Evans, 1976). Students were shown four 10-minute films in which peers provided information on social influences and modeled resistance techniques. Each film was followed by tests of the students' knowledge of immediate health effects and small-group discussion of resistance to persuasion. Additionally, the classrooms had posters in the room to remind students of resistance strategies.

Two major studies have been reported by Evans and his colleagues (Evans et al., 1978, 1981). In the first, 750 seventh grade students were assigned to one of four groups: treatment (films plus discussion), testing with feedback, testing only, and control. The results showed a 50 percent decrease in smoking onset at the 10-week follow-up when combined treatment and testing groups were compared to control group subjects. The testing with feedback and testing only conditions were as effective as the treatment program. The very short follow-up assessment limits the generalizability of this well-designed study.

Evans et al. (1981) second study was a much larger study involving seventh, eighth, and ninth grade students over a 3-year period. Students in 13 junior high schools were assigned to three experimental and four control groups.

This study also depended upon using four films to trigger discussion on resisting social pressures to smoke. The results again indicated a reduction in smoking onset over the three years. However, the study is difficult to interpret, as individual students were not tracked longitudinally and the results depend upon cross-sectional analyses where the composition of the sample varied. Of interest was the significant relationship found between intention to smoke and subsequent smoking.

Researchers at Stanford, and in New York, Minnesota, Oregon, and Canada quickly followed Evans' pioneering work and produced additional studies testing the psychosocial approach to smoking prevention. These studies used many of the basic components advocated by Evans, such as instruction in resisting peer pressures to smoke, immediate physiological effects of smoking, and eliciting a public commitment to not smoke.

The Stanford Project

Project CLASP, conducted at Stanford, exemplifies prevention programs that followed Evans' work. In a modest study, with only one school per condition (Perry et al., 1980b), the Stanford group found large preventive effects. At a one year follow-up the smoking onset in the treatment group was only a third as much as in the control group. Because of methodological problems, such as only one school per condition, nonequivalence of schools, and large subject attrition, the study cannot be interpreted with great confidence. Of particular interest was the use of older high school peer leaders who were trained to come into the 7th grade classrooms and assist in implementing the 3-consecutive-day program. The program also used peer leaders to assist the four booster sessions that were spread throughout the school year. This influenced subsequent studies, many of which used both older and same-age peer leaders.

Stanford researchers also participated in a collaborative study with Harvard University to test a 12-session, 2-year version of the CLASP curriculum with seventh and eighth grade students (McAlister et al., 1982). This program was taught by high school peer leaders under the supervision of research staff. While the program involved five pairs of matched schools in Massachusetts and California, the study suffered from serious attrition of subjects due to school transfer (30 percent), parent-consent refusal (15 percent), and inconsistent I.D. codes (20 percent). The overall results suggest marginal reduction in smoking rates for weekly and monthly smoking.

Minnesota Studies

The Minnesota group (Luepker, Johnson, Murray, & Pechacek, 1983) was the first to experimentally study the value of same-age peer leaders and a public commitment procedure. The Robbinsdale Anti-Smoking Project (RASP) was initiated in the fall of 1977, and data have been reported for one and two-year follow-ups (Luepker et al., 1983). The design involved five experimental conditions: (1) controls with questionnaire and saliva sample monitoring; (2) minimally measured controls (later dropped from the study); (3) social influences curriculum; (4) social influences curriculum with peer leaders (personalization); and (5) social influences curriculum with peer leaders and a commitment procedure. The social influences curriculum was presented to seventh graders via a combination of video materials and discussion groups over four sessions. A procedure to get personal commitment not to smoke added a fifth session to one group. In the peer-led conditions, same-age peers appeared in some of the video materials and also led classroom discussions. Peer leaders were chosen by their classmates, using sociometric nomination procedures. For the public commitment procedure, students were video recorded making a statement why they were not going to smoke and this was played back to the class.

By the one-year follow-up, the only significant effect was a greater number of never-smokers in the peer-led condition schools. Results of the two- and three-year follow-ups were consistent with the one-year data, showing superior results for the peer leader condition.

The results are difficult to interpret because of nonequivalence of schools, having only one school per condition and dropping one school because of data collection differences. Socioeconomic status (SES) and other risk factors for smoking (for example, parental and friends' smoking) were confounding factors. The control school had the lowest SES, and the school receiving the social influence curriculum had the highest SES. However, this study influenced subsequent smoking prevention efforts, as same-age peer leaders and public commitment procedures have continued to be used in a number of studies. The weight of the evidence does suggest that peer leaders have a beneficial effect on prevention programs, although there are conflicting results (Botvin & Wills, in press; Fisher, Armstrong, & de Klerk, 1983). There was no evidence that the public commitment procedure had an incremental effect.

The present Minnesota program is integral to a large scale community-based heart disease prevention project (Blackburn, Carlton, & Farquhar, 1983). A six-session version of the "Keep it Clean" program has been tested in three schools at the seventh grade level. At one-year post-test, more eighth grade control students than treatment students reported smoking in the past week (8 percent versus 5 percent). When all seventh and eighth grade students in the program and control schools were assessed, it was reported that 8.1 percent of the students in program schools reported smoking compared to 11.8 percent of control students. It is difficult to ascertain whether the treatment effects observed were attributable to the school-based program, or the community-based project (Perry, Murray, Pechacek, & Pirie, 1983).

The Waterloo Project

The Waterloo Smoking Prevention Program (Best et al, 1984; Flay, d'Avernas, Best, Kersell, & Ryan, 1983) followed the basic principles of the social influence approach, but added components on decision-making. Sixth grade students were exposed to six 1-hour, weekly sessions presented by health educators. There were two subsequent maintenance sessions delivered near the end of the school year. Additional booster sessions were provided in grades seven and eight. This program used films showing student actors one or two years older than the subjects.

Twenty-two schools in two school districts in southern Ontario were assigned to experimental and control conditions. The program results were analyzed according to the pretest status of subjects. For students who had never tried smoking prior to the pretest, the smoking prevention program was marginally effective; by the end of grade eight, 53 percent of the control subjects who were never smokers at pretest had tried smoking, while only 40 percent of the program subjects had done so. The program also reported significant reduction of students' transition from nonsmoking to experimental smoking at follow-up. Flay et al. (1983) report the program having greater effects on "high social risk" students. High risk students were defined as those with two or more smoking parents, siblings, and friends. Flay et al. (1983) report a significant reduction of never-smoked students' transition to experimental (0 percent versus 12 percent) smoking. Sixty-one percent of the high risk students in the treatment group who were experimenters in grade six had decided to quit by grade seven, versus only 36 percent in the control group.

The Waterloo study represents one of the more rigorous tests to date of the social influences approach to smoking prevention. The study randomly assigned schools to conditions, and both school and individual served as the unit of analysis. The study trained college students to conduct the intervention, thereby controlling for teacher variability. The 30-month follow-up did a good job of tracking students and included a physiological corroboration of questionnaire data. This program demonstrated strong program effects on those students most at risk to become smokers and this evidence provides support for this approach.

Life Skills Training Project

A second major approach to smoking prevention (Flay, 1985) emphasizes general social skills training. The major assumption behind the Life-Skills Training (LST) approach is that adolescent smoking is one behavior in a constellation of other deviant behaviors, such as truancy and early sexual behavior (Botvin & Wills, 1985; Jessor, 1982). It is postulated that this cluster of behaviors is relatively stable and that underlying cognitive and personality variables such as low self-esteem, high anxiety levels, and poor decision-making skills predispose adolescents toward substance use or other problem behaviors (Botvin, Renick, & Baker, 1983). Therefore, the primary features of the life skills smoking prevention program are (1) utilization of therapeutic strategies to modify an underlying core of intrapersonal cognitive and personality factors, and (2) a focus on general life skills deficits which are thought to determine the use of various substances such as alcohol and marijuana (Glasgow & McCaul, 1984).

Botvin and his colleagues at Cornell University have conducted a number of studies to test the effects of the multicomponent Life Skills Training (LST) program. The second of five studies reported by Botvin & Wills (1985) nicely illustrates this approach. This study involved 902 seventh grade students from seven public junior high schools in suburban New York City. The schools were randomly assigned to three conditions: The

LST curriculum presented once per week for 15 weeks, the LST program presented three times per week for 5 weeks, and a control condition. Two schools were assigned to each intervention, and three schools served as controls. Comparison of the combined-treatment schools with the control schools revealed significant differences in the proportion of new smokers (6 percent versus 13 percent) at the end of one year follow up. No differences were evident between the two presentation formats. The study also reports that experimental effects were greater for students receiving "booster" sessions in next year. As further evidence for the efficacy of this approach, Botvin reports that the prevention program had a significant effect on alcohol and marijuana use as well (Botvin et al., 1983).

The broad spectrum nature of the LST approach is the source of at least three advantages. One advantage is that by including more components one increases the chances of modifying the factors that influence smoking for any given individual. Second, the LST approach may be particularly effective with adolescents who are most predisposed toward substance abuse. Other interventions may be ineffective in providing adolescents with sufficient skills for resisting social pressure to smoke if they are not at least moderately socially competent to begin with (Glasgow & McCaul, 1984). An additional advantage is that the same factors which underlie the use of various substances may be altered. The development of a single-substance abuse prevention program may then have a broad affect on substance abuse.

The complexity of the life skills program presents at least two disadvantages. First, the programs require a very significant commitment from school personnel to cover the requisite number of sessions. Many schools are reluctant to agree to give up 5 to 20 class periods from their tightly scheduled curricula to include this program. A second problem is the lack of evidence as to which components are critical to the program's effectiveness. These programs may have a sound rationale for their components, but the effects are similar to programs lasting only five sessions, and there is no evidence for the incremental affect of the additional segments.

While Botvin & Wills (1985) report 50 percent or greater reduction in smoking initiation rates, alternative statistical analysis methods have examined the differences in terms of percentage of adolescents who smoke in the experimental versus control conditions. This analysis for the same studies show a reduction of adolescent smoking from 3 to 14 percent of the adolescents (Glasgow & McCaul, 1984), which is comparable to other programs. While the LST approach claims generalization effects by reducing reported marijuana and alcohol use (Botvin & Wills, 1985; Pentz, 1983) these results should be interpreted with caution. Glasgow and McCaul (1984) point out that subjects received specific information and social skills pertaining to these substances. Additionally, there was no physiological corroboration of self-report for these substances; hence it is difficult to assess the accuracy of these reports.

Other Studies

There are a number of programs completed and in progress that we have not reviewed in any detail but deserve mention. Research programs are under way in Washington (Schinke & Gilchrist, 1983), Minnesota (Perry et al., 1983), Los Angeles (Flay, 1985), and Oregon (Biglan et al., 1985). The published results to date are similar to those of programs we have reviewed. There are some unique components being used in studies both at USC (Flay, Johnson, & Hansen, 1982) and Oregon (Biglan et al., 1985) that encourage parent involvement. At the University of Southern California, Flay, Johnson, and colleagues tested a social influences model of intervention which included a coordinated series of television segments timed to coincide with school curriculum programs on smoking prevention. Additionally, parents were involved via student homework assignments. A televised cessation program was provided for smoking parents in the week following the intervention. Students who received the classroom program were much more likely to view the television segments than were control students (Flay et al., 1982) While the program produced immediate effects on student knowledge, attitudes, and beliefs, these results dissipated at one-year follow-up. The most significant effect of this study was the change in reported smoking behavior for smoking parents who viewed the cessation programming. Flay (1983) reports that 30 percent of this group of parents attempted to quit or reduce smoking, and 15 percent were not smoking at one-month and one-year follow-up, although there was no corroboration of parental quitting. Nevertheless, it is a creative way to combine televised programming and an in-school prevention program.

Another approach to including parents in prevention programs involves the use of mailed parent messages (Biglan et al., 1985). Four messages were prepared and mailed over a four-week period to randomly selected parents of both treatment and control students. The messages provided information on health risks, and prompted parents to talk to their son or daughter about standards or values they hold on the child's use of cigarettes. The letters also help parents reinforce their child's commitment not to smoke and their use of refusal skills. The letters encourage both smoking and non-smoking parents to set nonsmoking standards at home for their children. While the effect on reduced smoking onset were modest ($p < .10$), these mailed messages may prove to be a cost effective adjunct to a prevention program.

SUMMARY AND CONCLUSIONS

In sum, there have been extensive efforts to develop effective smoking prevention programs. The programs all have multiple components and differ primarily in the emphasis and diversity of components in the program.

Prevention programs based upon the social influences model focus upon sensitizing students to peer and social pressures to smoke and guided practice in how to refuse direct or indirect offers of cigarettes. These programs focus the instruction on behavioral repertoires that are relevant to refusing cigarettes in specific situations. These programs also include components on immediate physiological effects of smoking, and making a commitment not to smoke. The life skills approach exemplified by Botvin treats smoking as a behavior that has functional meaning to the students in terms of their self-esteem and personality. These programs, therefore, are broader in their focus, as they treat smoking behavior as one of a constellation of deviant behaviors.

Irrespective of the theoretical framework, the published results of almost all interventions show significant reduction of reported smoking at the end of at least a 1-year follow-up. These results are encouraging, and indicate progress toward finding effective prevention programs. However, reviewers of this literature have noted important methodological shortcomings that qualify conclusions about cause and effect relationships (Biglan & Ary, 1985; Flay, 1985; McCaul & Glasgow, 1984).

In the next section of this chapter, we review the major limitations of previous smoking prevention programs and provide direction for future research.

LIMITATIONS OF SMOKING PREVENTION RESEARCH

The studies reviewed above provide much basis for optimism. Preventive effects, especially deterring the onset of smoking, have been demonstrated in several studies from several different research programs in different parts of the country. The consistency of the findings strengthens confidence in the effectiveness of the programs. However, smoking prevention studies share some problems of internal validity, as well as external validity or generalizability. In this section, we summarize the major problems and suggest some ways in which further research may deal with them.

Internal validity refers to whether the design and measures employed permit one to draw unambiguous conclusions about cause and effect. The major threat to internal validity in smoking prevention studies is the use of quasi-experimental rather than true experimental designs. In nearly all of the reported research, a small number of schools (though sometimes classrooms) are randomly assigned to either an experimental or control condition, and then subjects or students are used as the unit of analysis. Financial and practical constraints have dictated such practice, but it is well recognized by researchers in this area that such procedure is not optimal (Biglan & Ary, 1985; Flay, 1985). The possibility remains that some unknown idiosyncratic school effect or school process (for example, a charismatic school principal who is opposed to smoking) could have produced the observed differences between treatment and control schools. A true experimental design would require that schools be randomly assigned to condition and be the unit of analysis. Obviously, one would need to study an inordinately large number of schools in order to be able to draw any reasonable statistical conclusions.

Two other threats to internal validity in smoking prevention research are subject attrition and reliance on self-reported smoking rates. Attrition is a threat if it differentially occurs in treated and control schools. This sometimes would appear to have been the case (Biglan et al., in press). If, for example, smokers in a given classroom receiving an intervention transfer schools, leave school, or skip class, they may not be assessed at follow-up. This would lead to an underestimate of the smoking rates in the treatment school. With respect to self-reported smoking, smokers in the treatment schools may feel more social pressure to under-report smoking, because one feature of the intervention program is to make cigarette smoking seem less socially desirable. This possibility is only partially countered by the use of biochemical markers of smoking and bogus pipeline procedures whereby students are led to believe that their self-reports can be corroborated. In fact, the biochemical markers are not very sensitive to the low-rate episodic nature of much adolescent smoking, and provide only a weak check on self-report.

External Validity or Generalizability

Assuming that a study is well-designed, with appropriate measurements, and attains internal validity, there is always the question of whether the effects would generalize to other settings and other occasions. Attrition is perhaps an even more serious problem for external validity. Several studies (Biglan et al., in press; Hansen, Collins, Malotte, & Johnson, 1983) have demonstrated that subjects lost to follow-up are significantly more likely to be smokers or at risk to smoke than those who are retained. It is possible, therefore, that smoking prevention programs do not impact on the high-risk youth that we would most like to influence. Nearly all smoking prevention research thus far has been conducted with largely white, middle-class populations (Flay, 1985). We do not yet know whether these programs would be effective with minority populations, and especially with less socially advantaged youth who are more at risk for smoking and other substance abuse. Finally, it is always uncertain what will happen when programs administered under carefully standardized conditions and research contexts are disseminated and utilized outside of these research settings (Rappaport, Seidman, & Davidson, 1979).

Construct Validity Problems

Construct validity refers to the extent to which we are confident that particular components of a treatment program are responsible for its effects. In other words, do we know how and why a treatment works (McCaul & Glasgow, in press). It is more difficult to establish construct validity, especially in field settings, but some knowledge of this sort is very important for dissemination and for modifying programs to meet changing circumstances. As we have discussed, most smoking prevention programs are based on a social influence model, and would like to assume that the social influence components of the program are responsible for the effects observed. There is virtually no direct evidence in support of this assumption. Most programs have simply compared a multicomponent intervention program with a control or no-treatment condition. The major exceptions to this generalization are some findings that peer leaders significantly improve the effectiveness of the social influence-based intervention (Murray, Johnson, & Luepker, 1983).

Besides not knowing which program components are more or less facilitative, we know little about the characteristics of schools and school environments that promote or inhibit program effectiveness. These problems are well-known to workers in the smoking prevention area (Flay, 1985; McCaul & Glasgow, 1985). On the positive side, one can point to some shared features contained in most of the successful programs (Flay, 1985). This is suggestive evidence that they are at least partly responsible for program effects, but again it is only suggestive, not definitive.

Has Endpoint Smoking been Prevented?

A final issue or shortcoming concerns the clinical meaningfulness of the preventive effects thus far demonstrated. From a public health perspective, it is necessary to prevent endpoint smoking in order for there to be meaningful risk reduction. Endpoint smoking may be defined as high-rate smoking at the end of high school (Biglan & Ary, 1985). Thus far, smoking prevention programs have, at best, reported only two-year follow-up results of programs that were implemented in the seventh grade. We may be able to conclude that the onset of smoking has been deterred until at least the ninth grade, but we do not know whether onset has been deterred, or merely delayed (Biglan & Ary, 1985).

There is further concern here in that the effects most frequently observed in prevention programs have to do with onset in seventh graders. That is, prevention programs show that fewer students who had never smoked at baseline assessment engaged in any smoking when followed up in eighth or ninth grades. It is possible that these preventive effects have occurred in youth who might normally have experimented with cigarettes, but might not have continued on to endpoint smoking without any intervention whatsoever. Students who are already experimenting with cigarettes in the seventh grade are probably more likely to become endpoint adult regular smokers. With few exceptions (Best et al., 1984; Biglan et al., in press), preventive effects have not been demonstrated with youth already experimenting with cigarettes. In sum, we have very little evidence to show that endpoint (that is, regular adult) smoking has been significantly affected by our prevention programs.

FUTURE DIRECTIONS IN SMOKING PREVENTION AND ACQUISITION

The criticisms and limitations noted have direct implications for future research. Needed are large studies where a sufficient number of schools are recruited to permit both random assignment by school and schools as the unit of data analysis, with long-term follow-up that minimizes attrition so that a reasonably intact cohort is followed until the end of high school. If there are too few schools to serve as the unit of analysis, then classrooms may be a reasonable compromise (Biglan & Ary, 1985). Such research must also include a fairly comprehensive process analysis that would demonstrate adequate program implementation and provide suggestive, if not definitive, clues as to what were and were not important program components. Further, it is important that such studies encompass a wide variety of students and schools, both rural and urban, white and minority.

We suggest that school-based programs need to focus more attention on persuading and helping adolescents to *quit* smoking (Biglan & Ary, 1985). There is a moderate amount of spontaneous quitting among adolescents (Chassin et al., 1984). Systematic efforts toward secondary prevention, perhaps aimed at high school students where prevalence rates exceed 20 percent, would pay big dividends.

The problems noted in this chapter are not all due to weak designs or investigator oversight. There are difficulties inherent in longitudinal research in field settings. It is necessary to obtain and maintain the cooperation of relevant school administrators, as well as adolescents and their parents, over long periods of time. This can be difficult. Tracking students across schools (for example, from middle school to high school or even across districts) can be extremely difficult and time-consuming, and contributes to attrition.

The larger the time frame of the intervention and follow-up, the greater the opportunity for extraneous variables—for example, history and maturation—to confound the design and compromise internal validity. In smoking preventions, such confounds might come from local school or school district policy and curriculum changes. For example, a school district might choose to adopt a new drug-abuse curriculum which includes consideration of tobacco. Control schools then receive some intervention, thereby lessening the probability of showing differences between treatment and control schools.

Competent investigators can, to some extent, anticipate and accommodate such extraneous events. But they remain problematic. Prevention research of the sort proposed here is necessarily costly and somewhat risky. While some would question their cost effectiveness, more systematic, large-scale prevention trials are now getting under way. The next few years should provide answers to many of the questions raised here.

The Acquisition of Smoking

Improved intervention research is not necessarily going to provide all the answers. It can reasonably be argued (Chassin et al., 1984; Leventhal & Cleary, 1980; Lichtenstein, 1982) that more effective prevention programs must await the development of a more complete, empirically validated account of acquisition. That is, we need to know more about the developmental processes involved in experimentation and, ultimately, passage to regular use of cigarettes and other tobacco products. While it is clear that peer social influence processes are important, specific ways in which they operate, how they operate at different age levels, and how they interact with other variables is not yet well understood. There is always a tendency to want to intervene with socially significant problems as soon as possible. Such intervention efforts need to be coupled or balanced with corresponding efforts to enhance our understanding of the problem we seek to address.

Below we describe three differing approaches to developing a more comprehensive and useful account of the acquisition of smoking. The approaches reflect the three different theoretical approaches described above: the behavior analytic emphasis on peer social influence processes; the cognitive-social perspective; and the concern with distal personality variables.

The Need to More Fully Specify Social Influence Processes.   As we noted, social influence is the major theme in current prevention programs. This approach assumes that proximal peer and other social influence processes are primary causal factors in smoking acquisition. These social influence processes require further, more specific elucidation (Biglan et al., 1983; Biglan & Lichtenstein, 1984). The recommended research direction, from this perspective, is to study peer influence processes in a more detailed way, and especially to reduce reliance on self-report questionnaire data. The use of structured interviews to yield a description of initial smoking experiences (Friedman et al., 1985), experimental manipulation of smoking models (Kniskern et al., 1983) and the use of a taped situation test to assess refusal skills (Hops et al., in press) illustrate research strategies that follow from this approach. The assumption is that more effective training in resisting social influence processes will emerge from such research.

The Need to Consider Cognitive Factors in Smoking Acquisition. The other two approaches we discuss take a different tack. In these approaches, proximal social influence processes are seen as important causes of smoking that have been overemphasized in current prevention programs. Attitudes toward smoking, perceptions of smoking and nonsmokers, (Sherman et al., 1983) and the cognitive representations of the physical and social reaction to initial smoking episodes (Hirschman et al., 1984) are seen as equally important. Additional research on these variables is urged in order to provide a more comprehensive account of smoking acquisition (Chassin et al., 1984). The use of smoking and other drugs as ways of coping with stress are also deemed important and in need of further investigation (Shiffman & Wills, in press).

Personality Factors and Smoking Acquisition: The Covariation of Smoking and Other Substance Use. The peer social influence and cognitive approaches both emphasize proximal variables: events occurring in temporal proximity to smoking (or nonsmoking) behavior. In contrast, Richard Jessor's data and theory, as described above, suggest the importance of central and distal personality processes. Jessor argues that the covariation among smoking, drinking, marijuana, and other substance use reflect an underlying personality factor that he has labeled "deviant behavior proneness" (Jessor, 1984). He suggests that interventions should, indeed must, focus on this factor if they are to achieve substantial effects. In a sense, Jessor questions the utility of discrete preventive interventions aimed largely at a single substance, be it tobacco, alcohol, or marijuana. Unfortunately, ways to modify "deviant proneness" by means of classroom programs have not been developed. But his data do suggest that the observed covariation among substance use needs to be better understood, and the implications of this covariation for smoking prevention programs cannot be ignored.

SUMMARY AND CONCLUSIONS

This chapter has reviewed research both on smoking acquisition and the prevention programs that have grown out of this knowledge base. We have learned a great deal about factors that are associated with smoking acquisition, but the specific causal mechanisms are not well understood. It is clear that peer-influence processes play a central role in adolescents' initiation into smoking, as well as maintenance during the transition to regular smoking. We do not know how peer influence interacts with adolescent personality and attitudinal variables, developmental levels, or family influence factors. If, as Chassin et al. (1984) suggest, variables from differing theoretical perspectives explain unique variance in the prediction of adolescent smoking, then attempts to integrate both the several classes of variables and the differing theories are overdue.

While there is reason for optimism because of the consistently positive effects provided in more than twenty-five published prevention studies, one should be cautious in the interpretation of those results. Most of the studies share methodological limitations that dampen our enthusiasm. These problems include the use of quasi-experimental designs and considerable attrition which poses a threat to both internal and external validity. There has not yet been sufficiently long follow-up to determine if endpoint (regular) smoking has truly been deterred. Additionally, we do not know which components of these multicomponent interventions are responsible for the observed treatment effects (construct validity). As Flay (1985) points out, current large scale studies under way should provide answers to many of the questions posed with regard to internal, external, and construct validity.

We hope that this review of smoking acquisition and prevention programs provides the reader with a sense of the promise and the problems of this important area of prevention. Since smoking is widely accepted as the number-one preventable cause of death from cardiovascular disease and lung cancer, efforts toward effective prevention remain a high priority. Although the goal of preventing young people from taking up smoking would seem to require a Herculean effort, the health benefit both to individuals and to society make it a goal well worth whatever effort is needed.

REFERENCES

Aaro, L. E., Haunes, A., & Berglund, E. L. (1984). Smoking among Norwegian schoolchildren 1975–1980. II. The influence of the social environment. *Scandinavian Journal of Psychology, 22,* 297–309.

Ajzen, I., & Fishbein, M. (1970). The prediction of behavior from attitudinal and normative variables. *Journal of Experimental Social Psychology, 6,* 466–487.

Allegrante, J. P., O'Rourke, T. W., & Tuncalp, S. (1977). A multivariate analysis of selected psychological variables on the development of subsequent youth smoking behavior. *Journal of Drug Education, 7*(3), 237–248.

Ary, D., & Biglan, A. (1985). *Onset and cessation in adolescent smoking: A prospective analysis.* [Manuscript submitted for publication.]

Ary, D., Biglan, A., & Severson, H. H. (1983, August). *Concurrent correlates and longitudinal predictors of adolescent cigarette smoking.* Paper presented to the 91st Annual Convention of the American Psychological Association, Anaheim, California.

Banks, M. H., Bewley, B. R., Bland, J. M., Dean, J. R., & Pollard, V. (1978). Long-term study of smoking by secondary school children. *Archives of Disease in Childhood, 53,* 12–19.

Baranowski, M. D. (1978). Adolescents' attempted influence on parental behaviors. *Adolescence, 13*(52), 585–604.

Bauman, K. E., & Dent, C. W. (1983). Influence of an objective measure on self-reports of behavior. *Journal of Applied Psychology, 67*(5), 623–628.

Benowitz, N. L. (1983). The use of biologic fluid samples in assessing tobacco smoke consumption. In J. Grabowski & C. Bell (Eds.), *Measurement in the analysis and treatment of smoking behavior*. NIDA Research Monograph 48. Washington, DC: U.S. Government Printing Office.

Bentler, P. M., & Eichberg, R. H. (1975). A social psychological approach to substance abuse construct validity: Prediction of adolescent drug use from independent data sources. In D. J. Lettieri (Ed.), *Preventing adolescent drug abuse*. Rockville, MD: National Institute on Drug Abuse.

Best, J. A., Perry, C. L., Flay, B. R., Brown, K. S., Towson, S. M. J., Kersell, M. W., Ryan, K. B., & d'Avernas, J. R. (1984). Smoking prevention and the concept of risk. *Journal of Applied Social Psychology*, 14(3), 257–273.

Bewley, B. R., & Bland, J. M. (1977). Academic performance and social factors related to cigarette smoking by schoolchildren. *British Journal of Preventive and Social Medicine*, 31, 18–24.

Biglan, A., & Ary, D. (1985). Methodological issues in research on smoking prevention. In C. Bell & R. Battjes (Eds.), *Prevention research: Deterring drug abuse among children and adolescents*. NIDA Research Monograph. Washington, DC: Government Printing Office.

Biglan, A., & Lichtenstein, E. (1984). A behavior-analytic approach to smoking acquisition: Some recent findings. *Journal of Applied Social Psychology*, 14(3), 207–223.

Biglan, A., Severson, H. H., Ary, D. V., Faller, C., Gallison, C., Thompson, R., Glasgow, R. E., & Lichtenstein, E. (in press). Do smoking prevention programs really work? The effects of attrition on the internal and external validity of an evaluation of a refusal skills training program. *Journal of Behavioral Medicine*.

Biglan, A., Severson, H. H., Bavry, J., & McConnell, S. (1983). Social influence and adolescent smoking: A first look behind the barn. *Health Education*, September/October, 14–18.

Blackburn, H., Carleton, R., & Farquhar, J. (1983). The Minnesota Heart Health Program: A research and demonstration program in cardiovascular heart disease prevention. In J.D. Matarazzo, S.M. Weiss, J.A. Herd, N.E. Miller, & S.M. Weiss, (Eds.) *Behavioral health: A handbook of health enhancement and disease prevention*. New York: Wiley.

Borland, B. L., & Rudolph, J. P. (1975). Relative effects of low socioeconomic status, parental smoking, and poor scholastic performance on smoking among high school students. *Social Science and Medicine*, 9, 27–30.

Botvin, G. J., Baker, E., Renick, N., Filazzola, A. D., & Botvin, E. M. (1984). A cognitive-behavioral approach to substance abuse prevention. *Addictive Behaviors*, 9, 137–147.

Botvin, G. J., Renick, N., & Baker, E. (1983). The effect of scheduling format and booster sessions on a broad-spectrum psychosocial approach to smoking prevention. *Journal of Behavioral Medicine*, 6(4), 359–379.

Botvin, G. J., & Wills, T. A. (1985). Personal and social skills training: Cognitive-behavioral approaches to substance abuse prevention. In C. Bell & R. Battjes (Eds.), *Prevention research: Deterring drug abuse among children and adolescents*. NIDA Research Monograph. Washington, DC: U. S. Government Printing Office.

Chassin, L., Presson, C. C., & Sherman, S. J. (1984). Cognitive and social influence factors in adolescent smoking cessation. *Addictive Behaviors*, 9, 383–390.

Chilton Research Services (1979). *Teenage smoking: Immediate and long-term patterns*. The National Institute of Education, U.S. Department of Health, Education and Welfare.

Evans, R. I. (1976). Smoking in children: Developing a social psychological strategy of deterrence. *Journal of Preventive Medicine*, 5, 122–127.

Evans, R. I., Hansen, W. B., & Mittelmark, M. B. (1977). Increasing the validity of self-reports of smoking behavior in children. *Journal of Applied Psychology*, 62(4), 521–523.

Evans, R. I., Henderson, A. H., Hill, P. C., & Raines, B. E. (1979). Smoking in children and adolescents. In *Smoking and health: A report of the surgeon general*. U.S. DHEW. Washington, DC: U.S. Government Printing Office.

Evans, R. I., Henderson, A. H., Hill, P. C., & Raines, B. E. (1979). Current psychological, social, and educational programs in control and prevention of smoking: A critical methodological review. *Atherosclerosis Reviews, 6,* 203–245.

Evans, R. I., & Raines, B. E. (1982). Control and prevention of smoking in adolescents: A psychosocial perspective. In T. J. Coates, A. C. Peterson, & C. Perry (Eds.), *Promoting adolescent health: A dialogue on research and practice.* New York: Academic.

Evans, R. I., Rozelle, R. M., Maxwell, S. E., Raines, B. E., Dill, C. A., Guthrie, T. J., Henderson, A. H., & Hill, P. C. (1981). Social modeling films to deter smoking in adolescents: Results of a three-year field investigation. *Journal of Applied Psychology, 66*(4), 399–414.

Evans, R. I., Rozelle, R. M., Mittelmark, M. B., Hansen, W. B., Bane, A. L., & Havis, J. (1978).
Deterring the onset of smoking in children: Knowledge of immediate physiological effects
and coping with peer pressure, media pressure, and parent modeling. *Journal of Applied
Social Psychology, 8*(2), 126–135.

Fisher, D. A., Armstrong, B. K., & de Klerk, N. H. (1983, July). *A randomized-controlled trial of
education for prevention of smoking in 12-year-old children.* Presented at the Fifth World Conference on Smoking and Health, Winnipeg, Canada.

Flay, B. R. (1985). What do we know about the social influences approach to smoking prevention? Review and recommendations. In C. Bell & R. Battjes (Eds.), *Prevention research: Deterring drug abuse among children and adolescents.* NIDA Research Monograph. Washington,
DC: U.S. Government Printing Office.

Flay, B. R., d'Avernas, J. R., Best, J. A., Kersell, M., & Ryan, K. (1983). Cigarette smoking:
Why young people do it and ways of preventing it. In P. McGrath & P. Firestone (Eds.),
Pediatric and adolescent behavioral medicine. New York: Springer-Verlag.

Flay, B. R., Johnson, C. A., & Hansen, W. B. (1982). *The USC/KABC-TV smoking prevention/ces-
sation program: Preliminary short-term results.* Unpublished manuscript, available at University of Southern California, Los Angeles, California.

Friedman, L. S., Lichtenstein, E., & Biglan, A. (1985). Smoking onset among teens: An empirical analysis of intitial situations. *Addictive Behaviors.*

Glasgow, R. E., & Bernstein, D. A. (1981). Behavioral treatment of smoking behavior. In L. A.
Bradley & C. K. Prokop (Eds.), *Medical psychology: A new perspective* (pp. 355–371). New
York: Academic.

Glasgow, R. E., & McCaul, K. D. (1984). Life skills training programs for smoking prevention:
Critique and directions for future research. In C. Bell & R. Battjes (Eds.), *Prevention re-
search: Deterring drug abuse among children and adolescents.* NIDA Research Monograph.
Washington, D. C.: U. S. Government Printing Office.

Goodstadt, M. S. (1978). Alcohol and drug education: Models and outcomes. *Health Education
Monographs, 6,* 263–279.

Graham, J. W., Johnson, C. A., Flay, B. R., Hansen, W. B., & Sobel, J. (1983). *The synchronous
correlates of drug use: A preliminary correlational analysis of data from Project SMART.* Unpublished manuscript. [Available from Health Behavior Research Institute, University of
Southern California].

Hansen, W. B., Collins, L. M., Malotte, C. K., & Johnson, C. A. (1983). *Attrition in prevention
research.* Paper presented at the 91st Annual Convention of the American Psychological
Association, Anaheim, California.

Hirschman, R. S., Leventhal, H., & Glynn, K. (1984). The development of smoking behavior:
Conceptualization and supportive cross-sectional survey data. Manuscript submitted for
publication.

Hops, H., Weissman, W., Biglan, A., Thompson, R., Faller, C., & Severson, H. H. (in press).
A taped situations test of cigarette refusal skills among adolescents. *Behavioral Assessment.*

Hurd, P. D., Johnson, C. A., Pechacek, T. F., Bast, L. P., Jacobs, D. R., & Luepker, R. V.
(1980). Prevention of cigarette smoking in seventh grade students. *Journal of Behavioral
Medicine, 3*(1), 15–28.

Jessor, R. (1982). Problem behavior and developmental transition in adolescence. *Journal of School Health*, 295–299.

Jessor, R. (1984). Adolescent development and behavioral health. In J.D. Matarazzo, S.M. Weiss, J.A. Herd, N.E. Miller, and S.M. Weiss (Eds.), *Behavioral health: A handbook of health enhancement and disease prevention*. New York: Wiley.

Jessor, R., & Jessor, S. L. (1977). *Problem behavior and psychosocial development: A longitudinal study of youth*. New York: Academic.

Johnston, L. D., Bachman, J. G., & O'Malley, P. M. (1980). *Student drug use in America*. National Institute on Drug Abuse, U.S. Department of Health and Human Services.

Johnston, L. D., Bachman, J. G., & O'Malley, P. M. (1981). *Student drug use in America*. National Institute on Drug Abuse, U. S. Department of Health and Human Services.

Johnston, L. D., O'Malley, P. M., & Bachman, J. G. (1983). *Drugs and American high school students, 1975–1983*. National Institute on Drug Abuse, U. S. Department of Health and Human Services.

Kandel, D. B., Kessler, R. C., & Margulies, R. Z. (1978). Antecedents of adolescent initiation into stages of drug use: A developmental analysis. *Journal of Youth and Adolescence*, 7(1), 13–40.

Kniskern, J., Biglan, A., Lichtenstein, E., Ary, D. V., & Bavry, J. (1983). Peer modeling effects in the smoking behavior of teenage smokers. *Addictive Behaviors*, 8, 129–132.

Krosnick, J. A., & Judd, C. M. (1982). Transitions in social influence at adolescence: Who induces cigarette smoking? *Developmental Psychology*, 18(3), 359–368.

Leventhal, H., & Cleary, P. D. (1980). The smoking problem: A review of the research and theory in behavioral risk modification. *Psychological Bulletin*, 88(2), 370–405.

Levitt, E. E., & Edwards, J. A. (1970). A multivariate study of correlative factors in youthful cigarette smoking. *Developmental Psychology*, 39(1), 5–11.

Lichtenstein, E. (1982). The smoking problem: A behavioral perspective. *Journal of Consulting and Clinical Psychology*, 50(6), 804–819

Lichtenstein, E., & Brown, R. (1981). Current trends in the modification of cigarette dependence. In A. Bellack and M. Hersen (Eds.), *The international handbook of behavioral modification and therapy* (Vol. 2). New York: Plenum.

Luepker, R. V., Johnson, C. A., Murray, D. M., & Pechacek, T. F. (1983). Prevention of cigarette smoking: Three-year follow-up of an education program for youth. *Journal of Behavioral Medicine*, 6(1), 52–62.

Matarazzo, J. D., & Saslow, G. (1960). Psychological and related characteristics of smokers and nonsmokers. *Psychological Bulletin*, 57(6), 493–513.

McAlister, A. L. (1983). Social psychological approaches. In T. Glynn, C. Leukefeld, & J. Ludford (Eds.), *Preventing adolescent drug abuse: Intervention strategies*, NIDA Research Monograph 47 (D.H.H.S. Publication No. ADM83-1280). Washington, DC: U.S. Government Printing Office.

McAlister, A. L., Gordon, N. P., Krosnick, J. A., & Milburn, M. A. (1982). *Experimental and correlational tests of a theoretical model for smoking prevention*. Paper presented at the Society of Behavioral Medicine.

McAlister, A. L., Perry, C., & Maccoby, N. (1979). Adolescent smoking: Onset and prevention. *Pediatrics*, 63(4), 650–658.

McCaul, K. D., & Glasgow, R. E. (in press). Preventing adolescent smoking: What have we learned? *Health Psychology*.

McCaul, K. D., Glasgow, R. E., O'Neill, H. K., Freeborn, V. B., & Rump, B. S. (1982). Predicting adolescent smoking. *Journal of School Health*, 52, 342–346.

McGuire, W. J. (1974). Communication-persuasion models for drug education: Experimental findings. In M. Goodstadt (Ed.), *Research on methods and programs in drug education*. Toronto: Addiction Research Foundation.

Mittelmark, M. B. (1978). *Information on imminent versus long term health consequences: Impact on children's smoking behavior, intentions, and knowledge.* Unpublished doctoral dissertation, University of Houston.

Mittelmark, M. B., Murray, D. M., Luepker, R. V., Pechacek, T. F., Pirie, P. L., & Pallenon, U. (1983). *Adolescent smoking transition states over two years.* Presented as part of the symposium "Becoming a cigarette smoker: The acquisition process in youth," at the annual meeting of the American Psychological Association, Anaheim, California.

Murray, D. M., Johnson, C. A., & Luepker, R. V. (1983). *The prevention of cigarette smoking in children: A comparison of four strategies.* Unpublished manuscript (available at University of Minnesota, Laboratory of Physiological Hygiene, Minneapolis, Minnesota).

National Institute of Education (1979, November). *Teenage smoking: Immediate and long-term patterns.* U. S. Department of Health, Education, and Welfare. Washington, DC: U.S. Government Printing Office.

Pechacek, T. F., Fox, B. H., Murray, D. M., & Luepker, R. D. (1984). Review of techniques for the measurement of smoking behavior. In J. D. Matarrazzo, S. M. Weiss, J. A. Herd, N. E. Miller, & S. M. Weiss (Eds.), *Behavioral health: A handbook of health enhancement and disease prevention* (pp. 729–754). New York: Wiley.

Pederson, L. L., Baskerville, J. C., & Lefcoe, N. M. (1981). Multivariate prediction of cigarette smoking among children in grades six, seven, and eight. *Journal of Drug Education, 11*(3), 191–203.

Pentz, M. A. (1983). Prevention of adolescent substance abuse through social skill development. In T. Glynn, C. Leukefeld, & J. Ludford (Eds.), *Preventing adolescent drug abuse: Intervention strategies,* NIDA Research Monograph No. 47 (D.H.H.S. Publication No. ADM83-1280). Washington, DC: U.S. Government Printing Office.

Perry, C. L., Killen, J., Slinkard, L. A., & McAlister, A. L. (1980a). Peer teaching and prevention among junior high students. *Adolescence, 15,* 277–281.

Perry, C., Killen, J., Telch, M., Slinkard, L., & Danaher, B. (1980b). Modifying smoking behavior of teenagers: A school-based intervention. *American Journal of Public Health, 70,* 722–725.

Perry, C., Murray, D., Pechacek, T., & Pirie, P. (1983). *Community-based smoking prevention: The Minnesota Heart Health Program.* Unpublished manuscript.

Pollich, J. M., Ellickson, P. L., Reuter, P., & Kahan, J. P. (1984). *Strategies for controlling adolescent drug use.* Santa Monica, CA: Rand Corporation.

Prue, D., Martin, J., & Hume, A. (1980). A critical evaluation of thiocyanate as a biochemical index of smoking exposure. *Behavior Therapy, 11,* 368–379.

Rappaport, J., Seidman, E., & Davidson, W. S. (1979). Demonstration research and manifest versus true adoption: A natural history of a research project to divert adolescents from the legal system. In R. F. Muñoz, L. R. Snowden, & J. G. Kelly (Eds.), *Social and psychological research in community settings* (pp. 101–132). San Francisco: Jossey-Bass.

Schinke, S., & Gilchrist, L. (1983). Primary prevention of tobacco smoking. *Journal of School Health, 53*(7), 416–419.

Severson, H. H. (1984). Adolescent social drug use: School prevention programs. *School Psychology Review, 13*(2), 150–160.

Severson, H. H., Faller, C., Nautel, C. L., Biglan, A., Ary, D. V., & Bavry, J. (1981). Oregon Research Institute's smoking prevention program: Helping students resist peer pressure [Monograph]. *Oregon School Study Council Bulletin, 25*(4).

Sherman, S. J., Presson, C. C., Chassin, L., & Olshavsky, R. (1983, August). *Becoming a cigarette smoker: A social psychological perspective.* Paper presented at the annual meeting of the American Psychological Association, Anaheim, California.

Shiffman, S. & Wills, T. (in press). *Coping and substance use.* New York: Academic Press.

Snow, W. H., Gilchrist, L. D., & Schinke, S. P. (in press). A critique of progress in adolescent smoking prevention. *Children and Youth Services Review*.

Streit, F., & Oliver, H. G. (1972). The child's perception of his family and its relationship to drug use. *Drug Forum*, *1*(3), 283–289.

Thompson, E. L. (1978). Smoking education programs 1960–1976. *American Journal of Public Health*, *68*(3), 250–257.

Tudor, C. G., Petersen, D. M., & Elifson, K. W. (1980). An examination of the relationship between peer and parental influences and adolescent drug use. *Adolescence*, *15*(60), 783–798.

U.S. Public Health Service. (1976). *Teenage smoking: National patterns of cigarette smoking, ages 12 through 18, in 1972 and 1974*. Department of Health Education and Welfare, Public Health Service.

U. S. Department of Health, Education, and Welfare (1977). *Research on smoking behavior*,NIDA Research Monograph No. 17 (DHEW Publication No. ADM78-581). Washington, DC: U.S. Government Printing Office.

U. S. Department of Health and Human Services (1982). *The health consequences of smoking: Cancer. A report of The Surgeon General*. Washington, DC: U.S. Government Printing Office.

U. S. Department of Public Health Services (1979). *Smoking and health*. (DHEW Publication No. PHS82-50179). Washington, DC: U.S. Government Printing Office.

Williams, A. J. (1973). Personality and other characteristics associated with cigarette smoking among young teenagers. *Journal of Health and Social Behavior*, *14*, 374–380.

Williams, T. M. (1971, September). *Summary and implications of review of literature related to adolescent smoking*. U. S. Department of Health, Education, and Welfare, Health Services and Mental Health Administration, Center for Disease Control, National Clearinghouse for Smoking and Health.

14

Social and Behavioral Aspects of Obesity in Children

KELLY D. BROWNELL

OBESITY AS A MODEL FOR BEHAVIORAL PEDIATRICS

The management of obesity presents a difficult challenge for behavioral pediatrics. A hallmark of behavioral pediatrics is its multidisciplinary focus on health problems. Obesity is an area where such an approach is vital, not only in research but in practice. Obesity has multiple origins and multiple effects on an individual, and is determined by a complex interaction of genetics, physiology, psychology, and culture.

As an example of this complexity, compare the cases of two patients. Sally and Mary are both 30 years old and weigh 180 pounds—60 percent above ideal weight. Both begin a standard 1200 calorie/day diet. Sally loses two pounds each week and Mary loses one-quarter pound. Sally has been

This work was supported in part by Research Scientist Development Award MH-00319 from the National Institute of Mental Health.

obese for one year, has enlarged fat cells, but has a normal fat cell number. In contrast, Mary has been overweight from birth and has twice the normal number of fat cells. Sally loses weight with no adverse reaction, whereas Mary, even though her weight loss is slight, is preoccupied with food, has dreams about food, and appears extremely sensitive to the sight and smell of food. Sally's resting metabolic rate does not change as she reduces; Mary's decreases by 15 percent, making it even more difficult for her to lose.

This example illustrates some of the physiological complexities of obesity. The psychological aspects of obesity are every bit as complex as the physiological factors, and their interaction complicates the picture even further. Can we conclude that the woman who does not lose weight is weak willed, has inappropriate eating behaviors, or has a psychological need to be fat?

Major advances are being made in the understanding and treatment of obesity in children, partly because of the increasing awareness of its complexity. This has led to its study by experts from many disciplines and has brought together multidisciplinary teams in the best treatment centers. In some cases, these approaches are true to the conceptual foundation of behavioral pediatrics. This chapter will focus on the degree to which this occurs, both in theory and practice.

OBESITY AS A PUBLIC HEALTH PROBLEM

Obesity is a very serious public health problem in adults. There is some dispute about its contribution to health problems in children, (Dietz, 1983), but because most obese children become obese adults, childhood obesity predisposes a person to some of the most serious health problems in adulthood. Therefore, it is a problem which should be taken seriously and treated aggressively (Brownell & Stunkard, 1978,1980a; Coates & Thoresen, 1978; Collipp, 1980; Dietz, 1983).

Prevalence and Seriousness

Prevalence.   Estimates of the prevalence of obesity vary, depending on methodological issues, demographic factors, and the definition of obesity. The Bogalusa Heart Study estimated that the prevalence of obesity, using variations of the body mass index, is less than two percent in school children (Berenson, 1980). Estimates are higher in other studies. The Ten State Nutrition Survey (Garn & Clark, 1976) estimated that 10 to 30 percent of girls were obese, and a study from England gave the figure at 32 percent (Colley, 1974). Huenemann, Hampton, Behnke, Shapiro, and Mitchell (1974) studied school children in Berkeley, California, and found that 8 to

10 percent were at least 20 percent overweight. Forbes (1975) concluded that 25 percent of children are obese.

The exact prevalence of obesity is difficult to determine, but the figure appears to be between 10 percent and 25 percent. The number is higher for girls than for boys, and prevalence increases with age. In addition, prevalence in general has been increasing during the past two decades (Forbes, 1975).

Medical Complications.   The most frequently cited medical complications of obesity in children are carbohydrate intolerance, hypercholesterolemia, elevated blood pressure, increased insulin secretion, and decreased growth-hormone release (Brownell & Stunkard, 1980a; Coates & Thoresen, 1978; Collipp, 1980). However, the effects of obesity are not consistent across individuals or across risk factors. Data from the Bogalusa study in Louisiana showed that height, weight, and age could explain 39 percent of the variance in blood pressure in school age children, but that the same variables could explain only 4 percent of the variance in serum cholesterol (Berenson, 1980; Voors, Foster, Frerichs, Webber & Berenson, 1976).

The most serious risk may result from the tendency of obese children to remain obese throughout life (Abraham, Collins, & Nordsieck, 1971). Obesity in adults is associated with hypertension, hyperlipidemia, diabetes, and, via these factors, with coronary disease (Bray, 1976; Kannel & Gordon, 1979; Van Itallie, 1979). Several of these problems may have definable antecedents in childhood (Dietz, 1983). Kannel and Dawber (1972) note that many atherogenic serum lipid disorders have their origin in childhood, and another study found that adult blood pressure could be predicted by childhood blood pressure patterns (Zinner, Levy, & Kass, 1971).

Psychological and Social Complications.   Being overweight puts a child at a serious social disadvantage (Allon, 1979; Brownell & Stunkard, 1978, 1980a; Millman, 1980). Overweight children are picked last for teams, are teased, and are excluded from many social events. Canning and Mayer (1966) found that overweight high school students were less likely to be admitted to high ranking colleges than were their thin peers, even after controlling for grades and extracurricular activities. As obese children enter adolescence, they are less likely to date and are more likely to be withdrawn.

There are pervasive negative feelings about obesity in our culture (Allon, 1979; Millman, 1980). It is so ingrained that it can be detected among children as young as age five. In one study, children rated pictures of a normal child, an overweight child, and children with a variety of physical handicaps (Staffieri, 1967). The children rated the obese child as least likeable. Even overweight children shared this bias. Feldman (1982) examined the attitudes of 5 to 11 year old children; the children felt that fat children were heavy because of excessive eating and that the fat children could lose weight if they wanted to.

Many overweight children internalize society's view and come to hate themselves and their bodies (Stunkard, 1976). The most common effects of this are constant attention to body weight and body-image disparagement (Stunkard, 1976). The obese suffer from a double disability; their condition has untoward effects physically and socially, but it is the attribution of blame that is most disabling. The notion that obese individuals are responsible for their condition generates the self-doubt that characterizes many heavy adults and children.

Spontaneous Remission and Resistance to Treatment.   If one thing is certain in the obesity field, it is that the problem is resistant to treatment. In a 1959 study, Stunkard and McLaren-Hume found that most obese people would not enter treatment for obesity, that most of those who did enter would not lose weight, and that most of those who did lose weight would regain the weight later. A paper published 23 years later stated that the cure rate for obesity is less than that for many forms of cancer (Brownell, 1982). These statements are based on data from adults. Less is known about children.

It appears that obesity in children does not remit spontaneously and does not yield easily to treatment. Abraham et al. (1971) reported that 80 percent of overweight children become overweight adults, and Stunkard and Burt (1967) estimated that if an overweight child has not slimmed down by the end of adolescence, the odds against he or she doing so as an adult are 28 to 1.

The strength of the relationship between childhood and adult obesity depends on how early obesity is detected in a child (Epstein, in press). Several longitudinal studies have found stronger relationships with older children, and there is some doubt whether obesity in infants carries any special risk for adult obesity (Charney, Goodman, McBride, Lyon & Pratt, 1976; Shapiro, et al. 1984; Stark, Atkins, Wolff, & Douglas, 1981). Epstein (in press) has assembled the figures from the various studies and reached the following conclusions:

> The percentage of obese children who become obese adults is 14% in infancy, 41% at age 7, and about 70% at 10-13 years of age. The percentage of non-obese children who become obese with advancing age increases only slightly. The relative risk at these three ages increases from 2.33 to 3.73 to 6.55. (Epstein, in press).

Most treatments for obese children have not been successful. Coates and Thoresen (1978) reviewed the literature on appetite suppressants, inpatient starvation programs, exercise regimens and other treatments and concluded that the results were discouraging. Brownell and Stunkard (1978,

1980a) found that most treatments were plagued by high attrition, small weight losses, poor maintenance, and untoward emotional effects in the children.

The following actions discuss several new promising treatments for obesity which may improve this picture. It is important to interpret results from any program in light of the difficult nature of the problem, so a "success rate" which may seem lackluster in another area may be a good one for obesity.

PHYSIOLOGICAL FACTORS

There is a vast literature on physiological factors related to the regulation of body weight, the relationship between energy intake and output, mechanisms which influence hunger and satiety, and so forth. To cover these areas is far beyond the scope of this chapter. (See, in particular, Bray, 1976, and the chapters on physiology in Stunkard, 1982). In this chapter, we will consider the importance of physiology in the genesis and maintenance of obesity. In so doing, we will discuss two popular theories—the fat cell theory and the set point theory. Both are useful points of reference to being considering obesity as a disorder with biological determinants and/or biological concomitants.

The Fat Cell Theory

In 1970, Hirsch and Knittle published a paper which stimulated a decade of debate about the role of fat cell size and number in the control of body weight. They hypothesized that adults who were obese as children were hindered by an excessive number of fat cells, and that weight loss was always the consequence of fat cell shrinkage, not disappearance. The theory has led many researchers to study this issue both in clinical and laboratory settings.

The amount of fat in the body is a function of the number of fat cells and the size of those cells (Sjostrom, 1980). A person whose fat cells are larger than normal is considered "hypertrophically" obese, while a person with too many cells is "hyperplastically" obese. In most cases, hyperplastically obese persons have been overweight in childhood: most of one's fat cells are developed before the end of adolescence. Thereafter, weight change occurs as the cells increase or decrease in size, not number. There are exceptions. It is now known that fat cell proliferation can occur in adulthood, but the implications of the theory remain important.

The fat cell theory maintains that each cell has an ideal amount of fat (lipid). If the cells fall below this level, the body responds with a variety of physiological signals to increase energy intake in an effort to replenish the energy supply. A person who is hyperplastically obese may lose a great deal of weight but still be obese by society's standards because of the excessive number of cells. The only way for this person to lose more weight is to deplete the cells to a point below their normal level; but this activates the protective signals and makes it very difficult for weight loss to occur.

The theory has intuitive appeal and helps explain some of the interindividual variance seen in clinical settings. However, fat cell metabolism has been found to be more complicated than believed originally, and it now appears that fat cell multiplication can occur in adult life if positive energy balance is severe and prolonged (Sjostrom, 1980). The theory does suggest that fat cell size and number might present a biological limit beyond which weight loss is very difficult to achieve.

The Set Point Theory

The set point theory has been debated in the physiology literature for many years but has only recently come to the attention of other professionals and the lay public. One reason was the publication in 1982 of a thoughtful book by Bennett and Gurin entitled *The Dieter's Dilemma*. This book took a strong stand in favor of the set point theory, and since the book received considerable media attention, the theory gained wide-spread recognition. Furthermore, some scholars in the field have used the set point theory as a means for explaining the regulation of body weight (Stunkard, 1982).

The set point theory maintains that an organism has an ideal biological weight which the body is "set" to defend. Changes in weight above or below this point trigger internal processes that defend the ideal by stimulating weight gain or weight loss. If a person has an ideal biological weight above society's ideal, movement toward the societal goal would be met by physiological pressure to gain weight. As *The Dieter's Dilemma* puts it: "It is not a fair contest. The set point is a tireless opponent. The dieter's only allies are willpower and whatever incentives there are that make chronic discomfort worthwhile."

Combining Theories

The set point and fat cell theories can merge into a conceptual picture of body-weight regulation. The degree of physiological facilitation or hindrance of weight loss would depend only on where a person stands in relation to the set point. Two women who weigh 200 pounds would be quite different if one was 20 pounds above a set point of 180 and the other was already below a set point of 220 pounds. A person who is above the set point and can afford to reduce may be able to do so until the fat cells reach their lower limit in size. The actual body weight at which this occurs may depend on the number of fat cells. Such a notion is very speculative. The set point and fat cell theories have not received sufficient experimental support to be widely accepted among scientists. However, the theories are interesting and have important implications for obesity in childhood.

One very important implication is that fat cell hyperplasia dooms a person to a lifetime of obesity, or at least to a very hard struggle against a biology that presses for a higher weight. There is speculation that the hyperplasia occurs at specific periods in childhood (Sjostrom, 1980). It may be possible to regulate energy balance (within the confines of adequate nutrition) during these key periods to prevent the fat cell hyperplasia that predisposes an individual to obesity. This is an argument for dealing with childhood obesity in an aggressive fashion.

CLINICAL TREATMENTS

Behavioral approaches to the treatment of overweight children have shown great promise (Epstein, in press), consistently outperforming other treatments, if not in controlled trials, in apparent clinical effectiveness. Reviews of other approaches are available elsewhere (Coates & Thoresen, 1978; Collipp, 1980), but in this chapter, the focus will be on the programs with most applied value and theoretical significance.

Early Behavioral Programs

Dozens of studies of behavior therapy for obese adults were published before a single study with children appeared. The study of children still lags far behind the work with adults, but the picture is changing as more researchers support the case for early intervention.

Research with children can be viewed as occurring in two stages (Brownell, 1982). The first generation of studies involved the transfer to children of techniques developed for adults. This work began with a pilot study in a medical setting conducted in 1970 by Rivinus, Drummond, and Combrinck-Graham. Even though the results were not published until 1976, the procedures received attention earlier. The program involved meetings for mothers and children in which eating behaviors were practiced and instruction was given in self-monitoring and stimulus control. The mean weight loss was 2.8 kg., in contrast to the weight gain occurring before the program.

There were six additional studies in the 1970s testing different aspects of the behavioral approach. Kingsley and Shapiro (1977) investigated the role of mothers in treatment; Aragona, Cassady, and Drabman (1975) studied response cost and reinforcement; and Wheeler and Hess (1976), Gross, Wheeler, and Hess (1976), and Weiss (1977) did controlled studies of multicomponent programs. Epstein and colleagues did a study showing that specific eating behaviors could be observed reliably and could be altered with reinforcement techniques (Epstein, Parker, & McCoy, 1976).

The results from these early studies were promising compared to the poor results reported for other approaches. Weight losses ranged from 4 to 13 pounds and there were no reports of untoward emotional reactions. However, systematic follow-up evaluations were not done and the need to boost weight loss still existed. The second generation of studies followed logically from these early reports.

Comprehensive Behavioral Programs

The studies on behavioral programs published in the 1980s have reported very encouraging results. Weight losses have increased and there are promising reports of maintenance of weight loss.

Epstein and colleagues at the University of Pittsburgh have conducted a systematic research program which has greatly advanced knowledge of the treatment of overweight children. The first two of their studies examined variations of reinforcement procedures with overweight children and their parents (Epstein, Wing, Koeske, Andrasik, & Ossip, 1981; Epstein, Wing, Steranchak, Dickson, & Michelson, 1980). Their most recent study examined the role of exercise (Epstein, Wing, Koeske, Ossip, & Beck, 1982).

Epstein et al. (1980) compared a behavioral program with a nutrition education program for young children and their mothers. The behavioral program included a contingency contract in which the return of a deposit was contingent on weight loss for both the child and mother. Weight losses were significantly greater in the behavior modification group. Epstein et al. (1981) followed with a large study in which the target for reinforcment was the parent and child, just the child, or a nonspecific target. Weight losses for the three groups were equivalent. These two studies, along with the third by this group (Epstein et al. 1982) which is discussed below, reported substantial reductions in the degree of obesity in the children.

Two studies by Coates and his colleagues have helped define the utility of behavioral procedures with obese adolescents. Coates and Thoresen (1981) did an extensive evaluation of three adolescent girls using single-subject methodology. A 10-week behavioral program was used for two subjects whose treatment was staggered, while the third subject served as a control. The program included self-monitoring, stimulus control, modification of eating behavior, exercise management, and reinforcement. The experimenters worked with the families and did a careful analysis of eating and food-storage patterns in the home. The experimental subjects lost 21 and 11.5 pounds, while the control subject gained 5 pounds. There appeared to be an association between specific behavior changes and weight change.

The second study by this group evaluated weekly versus daily sessions and rewards for weight loss versus habit change (Coates, Jeffery, Slinkard, Killen, & Danaher, 1982). The greatest weight losses occured in the group which met daily and was reinforced for weight change. These results suggest that treatment intensity is an important variable and that weight change may be best for the children to use as an index of progress.

Brownell, Kelman, and Stunkard (1983) used a comprehensive behavioral program with obese adolescents. The purpose of the study was to test the role of parental involvement (an issue discussed below). The weight losses, however, were encouraging and support the studies mentioned above in showing that the behavioral program is improving. In the Brownell et al. study, the mean weight loss for all subjects was 12.5 pounds. In the most successful group, the mean loss was 18.5 pounds after 16 weeks of treatment and 17 pounds one year later.

There are several reasons why the behavioral program is producing such favorable results. The first is that the program has expanded and now includes far more than the original stimulus control and reinforcement techniques. Most programs include exercise, parental involvement, cognitive restructuring, and some type of social skills or assertiveness training. Second, the programs are no longer being adapted from programs used with adults. Procedures are being designed specifically for the children, with some appreciation for developmental factors. Third, the programs are emphasizing several key factors, which include exercise, reinforcement, and parental environment.

The Importance of Physical Activity

Energy intake assumes a much more important role than energy expenditure in most treatment programs. The picture is changing, however, with increased appreciation of the metabolic and psychological benefits of exercise (Brownell & Stunkard, 1980b; Donahoe, Lin, Kirschenbaum, & Keesey, 1984; Thompson, Jarvie, Lahey, & Cureton, 1982).

Brownell and Stunkard, 1980b, list five main benefits of increased physical activity in obese persons:

1. Increased energy expenditure
2. Possible appetite suppression
3. Decreased loss of lean body mass during dieting
4. Improvements in psychological functioning (self-concept) and in the physiological correlates of obesity (for example, hypertension.
5. Possible offsetting of the decline in basal metabolic rate which accompanies dieting.

There has been only one systematic study of physical activity in obese children (Epstein et al., 1982). This group compared "lifestyle" and "programmed" activity. Programmed activites are regular bouts of exercises such as jogging, swimming, or attendance at an aerobics class. Lifestyle activities are more routine forms of exercise, which might include riding a bike, playing jumprope, walking to school, or walking the dog. Epstein and colleagues randomly assigned children to receive either lifestyle or programmed activity prescriptions. All subjects received the same treatment otherwise. The results showed that lifestyle activity produced greatest weight losses and better adherence over the long-term and produced better maintenance of exercise tolerance.

The preliminary evidence in this area suggests that treatment programs would benefit from the inclusion of exercise (Brownell & Stunkard, 1980b; Epstein, in press; Epstein et al., 1982; Thompson et al., 1982). The primary clinical issue is how to develop attractive exercise prescriptions and how to motivate children to comply with the prescriptions over the long term.

Reinforcement Programs

Reinforcement procedures have grown increasingly sophisticated in the past several years. Coates et al. (1982) examined the utility of reinforcing weight loss versus habit change, and Epstein et al. (1980, 1981) tested several approaches to contracting. There is not sufficient evidence to be certain that the reinforcement techniques are crucial to behavioral programs, but the clinical experience points in that direction, particularly for younger children.

One danger with reinforcement techniques is the illusion that the procedures are simple in design and are easy to administer. Much research has been devoted to reinforcement procedures, and there are specific principles to follow when using them. The use of reinforcement becomes a complex clinical issue when parents are responsible for administering the procedures outside of the clinical setting. A good starting point for learning about these procedures is the work of Epstein et al. (1980, 1981).

The Role of Parents

Parents play a crucial role in a child's energy intake and expenditure. The parents model eating and physical activity patterns, control much of the food that enters the house, and establish an emotional environment in which thinness may or may not be encouraged. It is logical to assume that parents should be involved in the treatment of their overweight children.

The most successful treatment programs have involved parents in an extensive manner (Brownell et al., 1983; Coates & Thoresen, 1981; Epstein et al., 1980,1981,1982). The programs of Epstein and colleagues use contracting procedures to encourage weight and behavior changes both in parents and in children. Parents receive an intensive training program to help them work with their children.

Several studies have examined parental involvement in a systematic fashion. The first, by Kingsley and Shapiro (1977), found that weight losses in 10 and 11 year old children were similar in groups in which only the child, mother or both mother and child attended. Epstein et al. (1980) found a strong relationship between weight loss in mothers and children when both wanted to lose weight and both earned back deposited money for losing weight. Epstein et al., (1981) found no difference in weight loss between groups in which the parent and child were reinforced for weight loss, only the child was reinforced, or money was refunded for attendance.

A study by Brownell et al. (1983) tested several methods of parental involvement in obese adolescents (ages 12 to 16). Children were assigned to groups in which mothers were not involved, mothers attended the same sessions with their children (Mother-Child Together), or mothers and children attended separate sessions (Mother-Child Separately). Both the short-term losses (18.5 pounds) and the long-term losses after a one-year follow-up (17 pounds) were best for the Mother-Child Separately groups. It was surprising that this seemingly minor manipulation, whether mothers met in the same room with their children or met in the next room, had such a powerful influence on weight change.

These studies show that the parents can be a major source of influence in treatment. More research is needed to define clearly the nature of the parent's role and the specific skills which the parents need to aid their overweight children.

TREATMENT IN THE SCHOOLS

There are several potential advantages to dealing with childhood obesity in the schools. Some researchers feel that an educational context is a more appropriate setting than a medical context in which to deal with obesity (Brownell & Kaye, 1982; Seltzer & Mayer, 1970). This casts the problem in a different light and suggests different approaches to treatment. The second advantage is that large numbers of children can be screened, monitored, and followed longitudinally. Third, treatment can be offered at little or no cost to the parents. Fourth, children who are only mildly obese, or not obese at all, can be identified and instructed in appropriate eating and exercise habits before problems become serious enough to merit professional attention.

Given the promise in this area, and given the recognition by many school officials that obesity is a significant problem, it is surprising that so few programs have been reported. In 1970, Seltzer and Mayer found small but significant decreases in the degree of obesity for school children who participated in a 5-month program of nutrition, exercise, and psychological support. Few studies were done in the entire decade which followed this early report.

The first controlled trial was carried out in New York City by Botvin, Cantlon, Carter, and Williams (1979). Children in an experimental school received a 10-week program of behavior modification, nutrition counseling, and exercise. These children lost more weight than a matched sample of children from a control school. Other positive results have been reported from studies by Collipp (1975), Lansky and Brownell (1982), and Lansky and Vance (1983).

Brownell and Kaye (1982) reported the largest and most consistent losses in a 10-week project carried out in a public school in Florida. Children ages 5 to 12 received a program which emphasized behavior modification, nutrition education, exercise, and social support. The social-support factor seems to have had considerable impact. The program coordinator (a nurse's aide) presented the program in such a positive light that thin children asked to join. The program children had their names posted on a special board and an awards ceremony was held before the entire school in which all participants were given certificates. The anticipated stigma against the overweight children did not occur.

Fully 95 percent of the children in this program lost weight, despite the weight gain that was expected due to growth. The mean weight loss was 9.8 pounds, a significant loss considering the age and size of the children. These results were very encouraging, but as with previous studies, no long-term follow-up was done.

A study done recently in parochial schools in Philadelphia attempted to replicate earlier results and to evaluate the long-term effects of school programs (Foster, Wadden, & Brownell, in press). Children in an experimental school received an expanded version of the program used by Brownell and Kaye (1982). The major change was that older peers were trained and used as counselors for the younger children. These children were compared with a sample of overweight children from a control school having no program.

There were several notable findings from this study. The first was that the experimental children showed significantly greater reductions in percentage overweight after the program and at an 18-week follow-up. However, the weight changes for the program children (0.67 lb) were much smaller than those reported in the earlier study, thus raising the issue of clinical significance. Second, the advantage for the program children was only partially maintained at follow-up, suggesting that specific maintenance approaches may be necessary to sustain the results produced in an initial program. Third, self-concept in the program children improved significantly. This is a positive finding in that factors other than weight change enter into evaluation of a weight-loss program.

It is apparent that school programs are still in their early stages of development. There appears to be the potential for a powerful intervention in an important setting, but many issues must be addressed before the public health implications of these programs are clear. Among these issues are the degree to which parents can and should be involved, the nature of maintenance strategies which might be implemented, the degree to which older children can act as "peer counselors," and the extent to which psychological and social factors change as a result of participation in such a program.

SUMMARY

Obesity in children is a public health problem because of its seriousness, prevalence, and resistence to treatment. It is also a personal problem for those so afflicted. There are physiologiocal and psychological reasons why obesity in children needs to be taken seriously and treated aggressively. Behavior modification programs have shown the most impressive weight-loss records, and, with the recent focus on parental participation, exercise, and reinforcement, the programs may become even stronger. Work in the schools is still in its early stages, but it appears that this could be an effective avenue for reaching large numbers of children once a consistently effective program is devised.

REFERENCES

Abraham, S., Collins, G., & Nordsieck, M. (1971). Relationship of childhood weight status to morbidity in adults. *Public Health Reports, 86*, 273–284.

Allon, N. (1979). Self-perceptions of the stigma of overweight in relationship to weight-losing patterns. *American Journal of Clinical Nutrition, 32*, 470–480.

Aragona, J., Cassady, J., & Drabman, R.S. (1975). Treating overweight children through parental training and contingency contracting. *Journal of Applied Behavior Analysis, 8*, 269–278.

Bennett, W., & Gurin, J. (1982). *The dieter's dilemma: Eating less and weighing more.* New York: Basic Books.

Berenson, G. S. (1980). *Cardiovascular risk factors in children.* New York: Oxford University Press.

Botvin, G. J., Cantlon, A., Carter, B. J., & Williams, C. L. (1979). Reducing adolescent obesity through a school health program. *Journal of Pediatrics, 95*, 1060–1062.

Bray, G. A. (1976). *The obese patient.* Philadelphia: Saunders

Brownell, K. D. (1982). Obesity: Understanding and treating a serious, prevalent, and refractory disorder. *Journal of Consulting and Clinical Psychology, 50*, 820–840.

Brownell, K. D., & Kaye, F. S. (1982). A school-based behavior modification, nutrition education, and physical activity program for obese children. *American Journal of Clinical Nutrition, 35*, 277–283.

Brownell, K. D., Kelman, J. H., & Stunkard, A. J. (1983). Treatment of obese children with and without their mothers. Changes in weight and blood pressure. *Pediatrics, 71*, 515–523.

Brownell, K. D., & Stunkard, A. J. (1978). Behavioral treatment of obesity in children. *American Journal of Diseases of Children, 132*, 403–412.

Brownell, K. D., & Stunkard, A. J. (1980a). Behavioral treatment for obese children and adolescents. In A. J. Stunkard (Ed.), *Obesity.* Philadelphia: Saunders.

Brownell, K. D., & Stunkard, A. J. (1980b) Exercises in the development and control of obesity. In A. J. Stunkard (Ed.), *Obesity.* Philadelphia: Saunders.

Canning, H., & Mayer, J. (1966). Obesity-Its possible effect on college acceptance. *New England Journal of Medicine, 275,* 1172–1174.

Charney, M, Goodman, H. C., McBride, M., Lyon, B., & Pratt, R. (1976). Childhood antecedents of adult obesity: Do chubby infants become obese adults? *New England Journal of Medicine, 295,* 6–9.

Coates, T. J., Jeffery, R. W., Slinkard, L. A., Killen, J. D., & Danaher, B. G. (1982). Frequency of contact and contingent reinforcement in weight loss, lipid change, and blood pressure reduction with adolescents. *Behavior Therapy, 13,* 175–185.

Coates, T. J., & Thoresen, C. E. (1978). Treating obesity in children and adolescents: A review. *American Journal of Public Health, 68,* 143–151.

Coates, T. J., & Thoresen, C. E. (1981). Behavior and weight changes in three obese adolescents. *Behavior Therapy, 12,* 382–399.

Colley, J. R. T. (1974). Obesity in school children. *British Journal of Social and Preventive Medicine, 28,* 221–225.

Collipp, P. J. (1975). An obesity program in public schools. *Pediatric Annals, 4,* 276–282.

Collipp, P. J. (Ed.). (1980). *Childhood obesity* (2nd ed.). Littleton, MA: PSG Publishing.

Dietz, W. H. (1983). Childhood obesity: Susceptibility, cause, and management. *Journal of Pediatrics, 103,* 676–686.

Donahoe, C.P., Lin, D.H., Kirschenbaum, D.S., & Keesey, R.E. (1984). Metabolic consequences of dieting and exercise in the treatment of obesity. *Journal of Consulting and Clinical Psychology, 52,* 827–836.

Epstein, L.H. (in press). Treatment of childhood obesity. In K.D. Brownell & J.P. Foreyt (Eds.), *The physiology, psychology, and treatment of eating disorders.* New York: Basic Books.

Epstein, L. H., Parker, L., & McCoy, J. F. (1976). Descriptive analysis of eating regulation in obese and nonobese children. *Journal of Applied Behavior Analysis, 7,* 402–416.

Epstein, L. H., Wing, R. R., Koeske, R., Andrasik, F., & Ossip, D. J. (1981). Child and parent weight loss in family-based behavior modification programs. *Journal of Consulting and Clinical Psychology, 49,* 674–685.

Epstein, L. H., Wing, R. R., Koeske, R., Ossip, D., & Beck, S. (1982). A comparison of lifestyle change and programmed aerobic exercise on weight and fitness changes in obese children. *Behavior Therapy, 13,* 638–650.

Epstein, L. H., Wing, R. R., Steranchak, L., Dickson, B., & Michelson, J. (1980). Comparison of family-based behavior modification and nutrition education for childhood obesity. *Journal of Pediatric Psychology, 5,* 25–26.

Feldman, B. (1982). Developmental differences in the conceptualization of obesity. *Journal of the American Dietetic Association, 80,* 122–126.

Forbes, G. B. (1975). Prevalence of obesity in childhood. In G.A. Bray (Ed), *Obesity in perspective* (Vol. 2). DHEW Publication No. (NIH) 75-708, Washington, DC: U.S. Government Printing Office.

Foster, G.D., Wadden, T.A., & Brownell, K.D. (in press). A peer-led program for the treatment and prevention of obesity in the schools. *Journal of Consulting and Clinical Psychology.*

Garn, S. M., & Clark, D. C. (1976). Trends in fatness and the origins of obesity. *Pediatrics, 57,* 433–456.

Gross, I., Wheeler, M., & Hess, R. (1976). The treatment of obesity in adolescents using behavioral self-control. *Clinical Pediatrics, 15,* 920–924.

Hirsch, J., & Knittle, J. L. (1970). Cellularity of obese and nonobese human adipose tissue. *Federation Proceedings, 29,* 1516–1521.

Huenemann, R. L., Hampton, M. C., Behnke, A. R., Shapiro, L. R., & Mitchell, B. W. (1974). *Teenage nutrition and physique.* Springfield, IL: Charles C. Thomas.

Kannel, W. B., & Dawber, T. R. (1972). Atherosclerosis as a pediatric problem. *Journal of Pediatrics, 80,* 544–554.

Kannel, W. B., & Gordon, T. (1979). Physiological and medical concomitants of obesity: The Framingham Study. In G. A. Gray (Ed.), *Obesity in America.* Washington, DC: U.S. Department of Health, Education and Welfare, NIH Publication No. 79-359, 1979.

Keesey, R. E. (1980). A set-point analysis of the regulation of body weight. In A. J. Stunkard (Ed.) *Obesity.* Philadelphia: Saunders.

Kingsley, R. G., & Shapiro, J. (1977). A comparison of three behavioral programs for control of obesity in children. *Behavior Therapy, 8,* 30–36.

Lansky, D., & Brownell, K. D. (1982, August). Comparison of school-based treatments for adolescent obesity. *Journal of School Health,* 384–387.

Lansky, D., & Vance, M. A. (1983). School-based intervention for adolescent obesity: Analysis of treatment, randomly selected control, and self-selected control subjects. *Journal of Consulting and Clinical Psychology, 51,* 147–148.

Millman, M. (1980). *Such a pretty face: Being fat in America.* New York: Norton.

Rivinus, T. M., Drummond, T., & Combrinck-Graham, L. (1976). A group-behavior treatment program for overweight children: Results of a pilot study. *Pediatric and Adolescent Endocrinology, 1,* 212–218.

Seltzer, C. C., & Mayer, J. (1970). An effective weight control program in a public school system. *American Journal of Public Health, 60,* 679–689.

Shapiro, L.R., Crawford, P.B., Clark, M.J., Pearson, D.L., & Huenemann, R.L. (1984). Obesity prognosis: A longitudinal study of children from the age 6 months to 9 years. *American Journal of Public Health, 74,* 968–973.

Sjostrum, L. (1980). Fat cells and body weight. In A. J. Stunkard (Ed.), *Obesity.* Philadelphia: Saunders.

Staffieri, J. R. (1967). A study of social stereotype of body image in children. *Journal of Personality and Social Psychology, 7,* 101–104.

Stark, D., Atkins, E. Wolff, D.H., & Douglas, J.W.B. (1981). Longitudinal study of obesity in the National Survey of Health and Development. *British Medical Journal, 283,* 12–17.

Stunkard, A. J. (1976). *The pain of obesity.* Palo Alto, CA: Bull.

Stunkard, A. J. (1980). (Ed.) *Obesity.* Philadelphia: Saunders.

Stunkard, A. J. (1982). Anorectic agents lower a body weight set point. *Life Sciences, 30,* 2043–2055.

Stunkard, A. J., & Burt, V. (1967). Obesity and the body image. II. Age at onset of disturbances in the body image. *American Journal of Psychiatry, 123,* 1443–1447.

Stunkard, A. J., & McLaren-Hume, M. (1959). The results of treatment for obesity. *Archives of Internal Medicine, 103,* 79–85.

Thompson, J. K., Jarvie, G. J., Lahey, B. B., & Cureton, K. J. (1982). Exercise and obesity: Etiology, physiology, and intervention, *Psychological Bulletin, 91,* 55–79.

Van Itallie, T. B. (1979). Obesity: Adverse effects on health and longevity. *American Journal of Clinical Nutrition, 32,* 2723–2733.

Voors, A. W., Foster, T. A., Frerichs, R. R., Webber, L. S., & Berenson, G. S. (1976). Studies of blood pressure in children, ages 5–14 years, in a total biracial community: The Bogalusa Heart Study. *Circulation, 54,* 319–327.

Weiss, A. R. (1977). A behavioral approach to the treatment of adolescent obesity. *Behavior Therapy, 8,* 720–726.

Wheeler, M. E., & Hess, K. W. (1976). Treatment of juvenile obesity by successive approximation control of eating. *Journal of Behavior Therapy and Experimental Psychiatry, 7,* 235–241.

Zinner, S. H., Levy, P. S., & Kass, E. H. (1971). Familial aggregation of blood pressure in children. *New England Journal of Medicine, 284,* 401–408.

15

Primary Prevention of Hypertension in Adolescents

THOMAS J. COATES AND CRAIG K. EWART

INTRODUCTION

Most discussions of blood pressure in adolescents begin with the proviso that hypertension is not a prevalent problem in adolescence and therefore does not require significant attention. We will argue the opposite: because blood pressure tracks and is associated with specific status (e.g., race, sex, socioeconomic class) and modifiable variables (e.g., diet, weight), primary prevention programs should be developed for adolescents. We will present a brief review of the data supporting the tracking hypothesis. Following this will be a discussion of (1) those immutable characteristics which place a person at relatively high risk for hypertension; and (2) potentially modifiable behaviors, the changing of which might be useful

Preparation of this manuscript was supported in part by Grant 5-R01-HL29431 from the National Heart, Lung, and Blood Institute. Presented at NATO Advanced Symposium on "Behavioral Epidemiology and Disease Prevention," Bellagio, Como, Italy. April, 1983.

in the primary prevention of hypertension. Finally, we will present evidence demonstrating the utility of specific programs for lowering blood pressure in adolescents.

BASAL BLOOD PRESSURE AND REACTIVITY

Arterial blood pressure is among the most important factors in increased risk for morbidity and mortality due to cardiovascular disease (Stamler, Stamler, Riadlinger, Algera, & Roberts, 1976). Hypertension left untreated inflicts damage on arterial walls, promotes kidney damage, and places strain on the heart, which is forced to work harder in order to move the blood against higher-than-optimal pressures.

Blood pressure *reactivity* in young persons also may be a significant risk factor for the development of hypertension. It is postulated that hypertension develops in susceptible young persons who respond to environmental or emotional stress by high cardiac output, increased peripheral resistance, or both. When faced with a challenging stimulus, the organism responds with increased output of epinephrine and norepinephrine. The catecholamines cause a rise in peripheral resistance and cardiac output, and acute blood pressure increases result. Fixed hypertension may occur over time as acute increases in blood pressure cause progressive changes in anatomical structures and changes in blood pressure regulation mechanisms.

BLOOD PRESSURE TRACKING

Tracking refers to the phenomenon that a person's relative status on a physiological index is relatively invariant; once elevated, blood pressure will tend to remain elevated relative to others in the population.

Level of elevated blood pressure during adolescence and young adulthood is predictive of later hypertension (Miall & Lovell, 1967; Paffenbarger, Thorne, & Wing, 1968). Remarkable tracking of blood pressure has been observed in the Bogalusa Study. Data from 3524 children, aged 5, 8, 11, and 14 at initial examination, were recollected one year later. The correlation between examination and reexamination was 0.70/0.50 (systolic/diastolic). Observations from a group of 35 fifth-graders examined monthly were pooled to examine intrachild blood pressure and to estimate regression toward the mean. In a multiple-regression analysis, the previous year's blood pressure and an index of present body size accounted for 39 to 55 percent of systolic blood pressure variability, whereas the previous year's systolic blood pressure contributed a partial correlation coefficient of 0.60 to 0.70 for each age cohort.

CORRELATES OF BASAL BLOOD PRESSURE LEVELS

Family History

Family history of hypertension is one the major predictors of hypertension. Paffenbarger et al. (1968), in their longitudinal study of hypertension in college students, reported that history of parental blood pressure contributed to the equation for predicting hypertension in later life. Zinner, Levy, and Kass (1971) extened these observations to a population ranging in age from 2 to 14 years, with a mean of 8.3 years. The sample included 721 children from 190 natural families. Maternal-child correlation coefficients were .16 for systolic and .17 for diastolic pressures; sib-sib- systolic/diastolic correlations were .34 and .32, respectively. Within-family variance of children's blood pressure was significantly lower than between-family variance for both systolic (F = 3.08) and diastolic (F = 2.68) pressures.

Larger epidemiological studies generally have confirmed within-family concordance. Holland and Beresford (1975), for example, studied 501 families selected at random but stratified by family size and social class. The major determinants of blood pressures in children five to eight years of age were parental weight and blood pressure. Children's blood pressures also were correlated highly with those of their siblings. Kass et al. (1975) extended the findings downward to a sample ranging from 3 to 14 years of age. They also studied the sample four years later and found familial aggregations that again were significant. Klein, Hennikens, Jesse, Gourley, and Blumenthal (1975) reported parallel results with black and white families. Langford and Watson (1973) reported similar correlations for diastolic blood pressure among full siblings aged 14 to 20 (.379) and among half-siblings (.354).

Feinleib, Garrison, Borhani, Roseman, and Christian (1975) estimated that as much as 60 percent of the variance in blood pressure may be due to genetic factors. These estimates were drawn by studying 248 monozygous twins and 264 dizygous twins from five study centers across the country. Correlations among monozygous twins' blood pressures (.55/.58) were higher than the correlations found among dizygous twins (.25/.77). Using data from other studies to show the generally lower correlation among siblings, these investigators estimated relative genetic and environmental contributions to blood pressure using a simple additive model.

Genetic differences, alone accounting for blood pressure variance may be questioned on two grounds. First, as Feinleib et al. (1975) pointed out, their results are derived from studying persons in a relatively homogeneous environment. Genetic variance might be inflated because environmental variance has been suppressed. Second, there is a striking similarity in sib-sib and parent-sib relationships found in many different ethnic groups and with different levels of blood pressure and potentially different physical and social environments.

In summary, there is little question that genetic factors are operative in elevated blood pressure and that controversies about the exact contribution of genetic factors will continue. The question does need to be reframed, however, so that the more important factor is not obscured:

What interactions of environmental and genetic factors produce high blood pressure?

Sex

Differences between the sexes in average blood pressure presumably emerge in late adolescence. Average blood pressures among adult males are typically higher than among adult females; this relationship generally holds true across racial groups as well (Stamler et al., 1976). The trends are less clear cut among young persons. The Task Force on Blood Pressure Control (1977) reported no blood pressure differences between males and females from 2 to 14 years of age. After the age of 14, however, average blood pressures and the prevalence of hypertension among males increased above the levels reported for females. Voors, Foster, Frerichs, Webber, and Berenson (1976) also found quite similar pressures among males and females aged 1 to 15 years. Other studies with older adolescents have reported characteristic sex differences both among blacks (Dube, Kapoor, Ratner, & Tunick, 1975) and whites (Miller & Shekelle, 1976).

Race

Blacks in the United States have an unusually high prevalence of essential hypertension and related disorders (Finnerty, Shaw & Himmelsback, 1973; Chenoweth, 1973). Average blood pressure readings for black males and black females exceed those found in white males and females; the prevalence of hypertension in black males is two times greater than that in white males and is associated with higher morbidity and mortality (Stamler et al., 1976).

Voors et al. (1976), in the Bogalusa Study, using six blood-pressure observations, found that black children had significantly higher blood pressure than white children. This difference became obvious beginning at age 10. Comstock (1957) found significant elevations among blacks aged 15 to 24. Krotchen, Krotchen, Schwertman, and Kuller (1974) found significant racial differences among 18 to 19 year olds. With sensitive measurements in large samples, characteristic racial differences might be detected among preadolescent children as well. The National Center for Health Statistics (1973, 1977) also reported small but consistent differences in mean diastolic pressures among black and white children aged 5 to 11 years.

Other studies using casual measures found no differences. The Task

Force on Blood Pressure Control (1977) reported no racial differences among 2 to 5 year olds. Differences may not emerge until middle to late adolescence.

The distribution of pressures among blacks is displaced to the upper end of values in comparison to whites; more blacks than whites may show sustained elevations in blood pressure when rescreened a second time (Miller & Shekelle, 1976). Voors et al. (1976) reported that a significantly greater percentage of black children than would be expected by chance have blood pressures above the 95th percentile.

Socioeconomic Class

Lower socioeconomic class is associated with elevated blood pressure. Langford, Watson, and Douglas (1968), in a study of 5000 black students and 5500 white students reported higher blood pressures in rural than in city students and an inverse relationship between socioeconomic status and blood pressure among urban students. The usual black-white blood pressure differences were abolished when urban black upper-income girls were compared with rural whites, and this relationship also was reversed significantly in males when the same comparison was made. Krotchen et al. (1974) replicated these results among black students only. Inner-city blacks had higher blood pressures than blacks attending a racially integrated school in a middle-class residential area. Among blacks, higher blood pressures were found in children whose parents were laborers or were unemployed than in children of parents in professional occupations. Holland and Beresford (1975) reported inverse relationships among blood pressure and socioeconomic class in studying 501 London families.

Hemodynamics of Hypertension

In some young subjects there appears to be an increased cardiac output and tachycardia indicating a hyperkinetic circulation. Such hyperkinetic or "high output types" also my be hypervolemic. Recent echocardiographic studies in children by Davignon, Rey, Payot, Biron, and Mongeau (1977) have confirmed prior invasive hemodynamic studies of others showing that hypertensive children can be either "hyperkinetic" or "hyperresistant."

Left ventricular hypertrophy characteristically is present at autopsy in patients with established hypertension. Recently myocardial hypertrophy has been described in the spontaneously hypertensive rate before the appearance of elevated pressures and when hypertension is prevented by early immuno-sympathectomy (Cutilletta, Benjamin, Culpepper, & Oparil, 1978). These studies have suggested that myocardial hypertrophy may have a role in the pathogenesis of hypertension.

The echocardiogram has added a new dimension to the study of cardio-vascular performance in hypertension (Sannerstedt, Bjure, & Vannaukas, 1970; Davignon et al., 1977). Measurements of stroke volume, systolic time intervals, and left ventricular wall thickness have shown subtle signs of di-minished left ventricular function in some established hypertensives; but normal or increased cardiac performance in some young or borderline hypertensive subjects has shown them to be assoicated with faster heart rates and shorter preejection fractions and lower ratios of reejection period (REP) and left ventricular ejection time. (LVET).

Zahka, Neill, Kidd, Cutilletta, and Cutilletta (1981) examined 38 normo-tensive subjects of normotensive parents and 44 hypertensive subjects who were referred to a pediatric hypertension center. The average blood pres-sure of the hypertensive patients was 144 + 1.5/95 + 1.3 mmHg, com-pared with 114 + 1.6/61.7 + 1.4 mmHg (p = .001) in the normotensive group. While the difference is certainly significant, the elevated pressures would be considered to be only mildly elevated. Various indices of left ven-tricular mass, however, were significantly greater in the hypertensive pa-tients compared with those of the normotensive controls. Eight percent of the hypertensive patients met criteria of left ventricular hypertrophy. Fur-thermore, the degree of cardiac hypertrophy correlated poorly with either the systolic, diastolic or mean blood pressures. A smiliar lack of correlation between hypertrophy and blood pressure has been reported in adult hy-pertensive patients. Left ventricular hypertophy seems to persist despite good therapeutic control and is present even in borderline hypertension. It could be argued that a degree of hypertrophy could be expected in patients with pressure overload; however, it appears that the degree of hypertophy found by Zahka et al. (1981) is out of proportion to the level of hyperten-sion. Based upon the hypothesis, myocardial hypertrophy may be, at least in part, independent of the degree of hypertension and could have a role in the pathogenesis of the syndrome. The presence of hypertrophy, there-fore, could prove useful in identifying patients who may go on to develop hypertension.

Ponderosity: Weight and Overweight

Weight and weight status are correlated consistently with blood pres-sure across the complete distribution of blood pressures. Londe, Bour-goigne, Robson, and Goldring (1971) reported that the prevalence of obe-sity was higher in hypertensive persons (53 percent) than in normotens-ive controls (14 percent).

Blood pressures are higher among samples of obese perssons than among samples of normal-weight persons. De Castro et al., (1976) studied 320 male high school students. Using 20 pounds above mean weight for height as a criterion for obesity, the obese had average blood pressures of 124/80 mmHg, versus 116/73 mmHg for the nonobese. Court, Hill Dunlop, and Boulton (1974) studied 109 obese persons 1.1 to 17.8 years of age who ranged from 3 to 113 percent overweight. The correlation between measures of subscapular skinfold and pressures were robust (systolic: males = .88, females = .78; diastolic/ m⌐⌐s = .80, females = .70). Coates, Jeffery, Slinkard, Killen, and Danaher (1982a) reported significant relationships in 36 overweight adolescents (13 to 17 years of age; 15 to 100 percent overweight for sex, age, and height) among the factors of weight, percent overweight, and systolic blood pressure. The same relationships were found before and after the students participated in a program designed to reduce their obesity. Epidemiological studies have reported consistently that increases in blood pressure are correlated with increases in weight. These relationships hold true in black and white children and across the entire range of blood pressures and age groups (Dube et al., 1975; Holland & Beresford, 1975; Miller & Shekelle, 1976; Stine, Hepner, & Greenstreet, 1975; Voors et al., 1976). Voors et al. (1976) found that the ponderosity index consistently entered first in stepwise multiple-regression equations in predicting systolic and diastolic blood pressures among all age groups. Bivariate Pearson correlation coefficients between body weight and systolic/diastolic blood pressures were .54/.48.

Diet: Salt Intake

Epidemiological studies have been used to assert that the prevalence of hypertension in populations is related to salt intake (Dahl & Love, 1957). While the populations studied (for example, Polynesia, Micronesia, Africa) differ in many ways, salt intake has been consistenly low in these societies. Animal and physiological studies have been used to support the hypothesis that sodium intake contributes to the determination of arterial pressure over a long period of time within the constraints imposed by an individual genetic endowment (Dahl, 1972).

In general, few topics have stimulated more controversial and inconsistent data than the hypothesis that salt intake elevates blood pressure (Willett, 1981). Many have asserted that because salt intake in the United States is high (2.8 to 6.0 grams of sodium per day), greatly in excess of the 0.4 to 0.8 grams of sodium per day needed, a high prevalence of hypertension has resulted.

Studies elucidating the salt-hypertension hypothesis among children and adolescents have been sparse. Langford et al. (1968) found higher blood pressures among rural than among city students, and inverse relationships between blood pressure and socioeconomic class. Langford and Watson (1973) selected 100 black female sibling pairs for study. Diastolic blood pressures were taken three times per day over eight days in the subjects' homes. Each of the girls also collected a urine specimen every 24 hours for six consecutive days. The sodium to calcium ratio was lower ($\bar{x}$ = 20.4) among those with lower pressures (less than 105 mmHg systolic) than among those with higher pressures ($\bar{x}$ = 34.3; greater than 125 mmHg systolic). The ratio also was higher among rural females than among urban females ($\bar{x}$ = 33.6 versus 24.7, respectively). An inverse relationship also was found between socioeconomic status and sodium/calcium excretion. However, blood pressures and sodium excretion of sodium to calcium ratio were not correlated. An earlier study also failed to confirm correlations between sodium excretion or salt taste threshold and blood pressure, but not according to a direct linear function. Langford and Watson (1975) studied 108 black girls ages 19 to 21, using blood pressures collected over eight days and urine samples collected over six days. One significant correlation emerged: the correlation between diastolic blood pressure and sodium to potassium ratio was .372. The authors concluded that in the salt-sensitive portion of the population, blood pressure may be a direct function of salt intake and an indirect function of potassium and perhaps calcium intake.

Tuthill and Calabrese (1979) demonstrated a statistically significant upshift of 3 to 5 mmHg in mean blood pressure between high-school sophomores in two communities with water containing vastly different amounts of sodium. In a second study (Tuthill & Calabrese, 1981), found identical results among third graders in the same two communities. A confounding factor in the second study was higher sodium intake in the community with higher sodium water. Moreover, the data were supportive of the hypothesis of the sodium blood pressure relationships in the aggregate community level but not in the individual level. For these reasons, Willett (1981) suggested caution in accepting these promising results as definitive.

Data from the Bogalusa Heart Study suggest the hypothesis that a proportion of the population may be sensitive to salt (Berenson, 1980). Blacks with the highest blood pressures had lower levels than whites for similar 24-hour sodium levels. The black males of the high stratum showed a cluster of correlations pointing toward sensitivity of the sodium to potassium intake ratio. Blacks also have positive correlation between blood pressure and sodium intake (Frank, Farris, Major, Webber, & Berenson, 1982).

While the role of salt in the genesis and maintenance of elevated blood pressure among children and adolescents remains controversial, clinical studies among adults support the utility of reducing and controlling mild hypertension by restricting sodium intake (Corcoran, Taylor, & Page, 1951; Dole, Dahl, Cotzias, Eder, & Krebs, 1950). The relative potency of many antihypertensive medications parallels the potency of these drugs in promoting sustained sodium depletion. Finally, several recent clinical studies have supported the utility of reducing mild hypertension by restricting sodium intake. The Stanford 3-Community Study (Farquhar et al., 1977) also reported a significant longitudinal correlation between change in urinary sodium to potassium ratio and a change in blood pressure.

The Task Force on Blood Pressure Control (1977) concluded that the exact significance of salt intake in the genesis of hypertension has not been determined; however, there is general agreement that salt intake should be reduced by individuals with hypertension and by those at risk of developing it. The hypothesis that reduction of salt intake in children and adolescents will result in lower blood pressure remains to be determined.

Behavioral Factors and Blood Pressure Reactivity

It has been noted for some time that individuals differ in their pattern and degree of autonomic response to environmental stimulation.

There are some data to support the hypothesized risk-factor status of cardiovascular activity. Hines (1937) measured blood pressures of 400 normotensive children while they were subjected to a cold pressor test. The children were subdivided into "normal reactors" and "hyperreactors" (those whose pressures rose above 25/20 mmHg; 18 percent of the sample) on the basis of blood pressure increases during the test. Barnett, Hines, Schirger, and Gage (1963) followed 207 of the sample 27 years later. A significant proportion of the hyperreactors became hypertensive, while none of the normal reactors became hypertensive.

Two recent studies have assessed the relation of family variables to exaggerated blood pressure reactivity in adolescents. Falkner, Onesti, Angelakos, Fernandes, and Langman (1979) studied blood pressure response during mental arithmetic in adolescents with varying risk for developing essential hypertension. Three groups were studied: genetic hypertensives ($N = 33$) were those with normal basal blood pressure but at least one parent with essential hypertension; labile genetic hypertensives ($N = 17$) were those who already showed elevated basal blood pressure and also had at least one parent with essential hypertension; controls ($N = 25$) were those who had normal basal blood pressure and no family history of hypertension. (Based on recent studies and reconceptualizations, we would prefer the term "borderline" to the term "labile" used by those investigators; see Insel and Chadwick (1982) and Horan, Kennedy, and Padgett (1981).) Subjects were male and female, black and white, ages 14 to 15 years. Labile genetic hypertensives and normotensive genetic subjects showed greater sustained increases than controls in systolic and diastolic blood pressure during mental arithmetic. Poststress plasma catecholamines were higher in labile and genetic hypertensives than in the control subjects. The investigators concluded that these findings demonstrated increased central nervous system adrenergic activity and cardiovascular responses in labile hypertensives and in normotensive subjects with a genetic risk for developing hypertension.

Baer, Vincent, Williams, Bourianoff, and Bartlett (1980) studied family interactions and posed some interesting questions regarding transmission of hypertension in families. Three-member families (father, mother, and boy or girl aged 8 to 13 years) of hypertensive ($n = 16$) or normotensive ($N = 15$) fathers were videotaped as they interacted under standardized conditions calling for disagreement. Families with hypertensive fathers showed more negative interactions than families with normotensive fathers. Following these interactions, blood pressures of children in hypertensive families rose, whereas blood pressures in normotensive families fell. However, there was a difference between hypertensive and normal families on *one* negative code: "Not Tracking" (i.e., looking away to avoid eye contact). Observers were not blind to subjects' diagnostic status. Patients may have been trying to avoid conflict out of awareness that it affects blood pressure.

Type A (coronary prone) Behavior. The Type A behavior pattern has been associated repeatedly with increased acute blood pressure response to stress. This responsivity is one hypothesized pathway by which Type A might express itself in disease. According to Brand, Rosenman, Sholtz, and Friedman (1976), "Type A behavior is characterized by enhanced aggressiveness and competitive drive, preoccupation with deadlines, and chronic inpatience and sense of time urgency, in contrast to the more relaxed and less hurried Type B behavior pattern." The Western Collaborative Group study (Brand et al., 1976) and the Framingham study (Haynes, Feinleib, & Kannel, 1980) have both provided prospective verification that Type A is a risk factor for cardiovascular disease and that this effect is independent of such traditional risk factors as smoking, blood pressure, and cholesterol. Haynes, Feinleib, Levine, Scotch, and Kannel (1978) developed a 300-item questionnaire for use in the Framingham prospective study. The questionnaire contains 14 subscales (reliability from .64 to .86) in three general areas: (1) behavior types: Type A men, Type A women, emotional lability, ambitiousness, noneasygoing; (2) situational stress: nonsupport from boss, marital disagreement, marital dissatisfaction, aging worries, personal worries; (3) somatic strain: tension state, daily stress, anxiety symptoms, and anger symptoms. There was moderate to good (67 to 80 percent) concordance with the structured interview in discriminating Type A from Type B subjects.

In a cross-sectional study of 1822 persons 45 to 47 years of age, Haynes et al. (1978) found that women 45 to 64 years of age with coronary heart disease (CHD)—mostly angina—scored significantly higher on Type A, emotional lability, aging worries, tension, and anger symptoms scales than did women free of CHD. Among men under 65, Type A, aging worries, daily stress, and tension were associated with prevalence of myocardial infarction.

Haynes et al. (1980) followed 1674 subjects in the Framingham study for eight years. Women who developed CHD scored significantly higher in Framingham Type A, suppressed hostility, tension, and anger than did women remaining free of CHD. The perspective study demonstrates the utility of the Framingham Type A scale in predicting disease.

Type A behavior also has been related to the incidence and prevalence of clinical CHD in men and women (Haynes et al., 1980), angiographically determined severity of atherosclerosis (Blumenthal, Williams, Koenig, et al., 1978; Friedman, Rosenman, Straus, et al., 1968), and the progression of atherosclerosis in men (Krantz, Schaeffer, Daria, Demborski, & MacDougell, 1981).

Type A Behavior and Reactivity in Children. The relationship between Type A behavior and blood pressure reactivity in children and adolescents has been documented in recent research. Siegel and Leitch (1981) found a positive correlation between elevated systolic blood pressure and Type A behavior in adolescents. Children and adolescents in the Bogalusa Heart Study who reported that they felt an exaggerated sense of time urgency had higher mean arterial blood pressure than students who responded negatively to this item (Voors, Sklov, Wolff, Hunter, & Berenson, 1982). Spiga and Peterson (1980) studied fourth- and fifth-grade children in a Catholic school. The Matthews Youth Test for Health (MYTH) was used; the 18 highest- and 18 lowest-scoring males were selected to participate. These students were matched in dyads by Type A and B behaviors so that there were six AA, six AB, and six BB dyads. The dyads played a mixed-motive game in which each player could choose to compete or cooperate on each trial; rewards for individual players were contingent upon both players' choices. Type A's in AA dyads showed more competitiveness than Type A's in AB dyads and Type B's in BB dyads. Type A's in AA dyads also exhibited greater fluctuations in blood pressure during the task than other subjects. Other investigators who have found a relationship between Type A and cardiovascular overresponding in children and adolescent are Lawler, Allen, Critcher, and Standard (1981) and Bergman and Magnusson (1979).

A Multivariate Look

In our laboratory research, we have made an effort to examine in combination the relative contribution of family history, ponderosity, age, and the Type A behavior pattern to basal blood pressure and to blood pressure response in adolescents (Coates, Parker, & Kolodner, 1982). Subjects (21 black and 21 white males ranging in age from 14 to 17 years) were recruited from the Pediatric Blood Pressure Center at The Johns Hopkins Hospital and from local high schools. The characteristics of the subjects are presented in Table 15.1.

Subjects were enrolled in the study after at least three successive blood pressure determinations using suitable cuff sizes had established their basal blood pressure. Approximately one week after the third clinic-based assessment, subjects returned to the Small Group Programmed Environment Laboratory at the Phipps Psychiatric Clinic at The Johns Hopkins Hospital.

TABLE 15.1. PARTICIPANTS IN THE STUDY OF BLOOD PRESSURE
REACTIVITY (N = 42)

	Mean	S.D.
Age	15.60	1.40
Weight (pounds)	153.00	28.50
Average percentage above ideal weight	1.10	0.22
Systolic blood pressure (resting)	122.80	11.60
Diastolic blood pressure (resting)	64.20	13.40
Heart rate (resting)	70.00	9.80
Type A (Jenkins)[a]	−2.19	8.33
Job involvement (Jenkins)[a]	−8.83	8.80
Speed and impatience	−3.54	8.89
Hard-driving and competitive (Jenkins)[a]	−8.30	14.24
Bortner Rating Scale	165.34	34.32
Percent with hypertensive parents	54	
Points on Alluisi Task during 15 minutes on CRT	78.46	22.58

Source: Coates et al., 1982b.

[a]These are standard scores, normalized on a version of the Jenkins Activity Survey developed for adolescents (Spiga & Petersen, 1981).

Each subject was escorted to the recreation area, where he was seated at a desk. An interview took place to collect additional data on family history. The subject was weighted and height was measured. The subject then completed two measures of Type A behavior, the Jenkins Activity Survey (JAS) adapted for adolescents, and the Bortner Rating Scale. The adult version of the JAS is a self-administered questionnaire (60 items) with "Type A," "Hard-driving," "Speed and Impatience," and "Job Involvement" subscales (Demobroski, MacDougall, Shields, Petitto, & Lushene, 1978). Spiga and Peterson (1981) adapted a shortened form (47 items) of this instrument for adolescents, and the adapted version was used in our study.

Following completion of the written tests, the subject was escorted into the small workshop area, where he was seated before the cathode-ray terminal (CRT). He was instructed about the sequence of events to follow and was fitted with a remotely monitored and controlled blood pressure cuff (Vita Stat Model 900-5), a digital thermistor for monitoring skin temperature, and an optically transduced plethysmograph for monitoring peripheral blood flow. Each subject was instructed in how to complete the Alluisi Performance Battery and was given 15 minutes of adaptation to the room and to the monitoring devices. Each subject then was exposed to alternating 15-minute periods of (1) baseline, quiet resting; (2) task performance on the Alluisi Performance Battery on the CRT; (3) baseline, quiet rest, and (4) metronome conditioned relaxation.

The Alluisi Performance Battery required subjects to complete five tasks simultaneously: probability monitoring, horizontal addition and subtrac-

TABLE 15.2.   DEPENDENT VARIABLE: BASELINE SYSTOLIC
BLOOD PRESSURE[a]

Independent Variable	Beta	R
Weight/height^2	.410	.47
Age	.228	.55
Parental hypertension	.298	.58
Job involvement (JAS)	.212	.62
Type A (Bortner)	.149	.64

Source: Coates et al., 1982b.
[a]$R^2 = .41; F = 4.62 (p < .01)$.

TABLE 15.3.   DEPENDENT VARIABLE: BASELINE DIASTOLIC
BLOOD PRESSURE[a]

Independent Variable	Beta	R
Weight/height^2	.608	.56
Type A (Bortner)	.286	.64
Hard driving (JAS)	.307	.67
Age	.275	.69
Type A (JAS)	−.295	.71

Source: Coates et al., 1982b.
[a]$R^2 = .50; F = 7.05 (p < .001)$.

tion of three-digit numbers, matching to sample historgrams, detecting when a stationary signal moves, and detecting when a moving signal becomes stationary (Emuiran, Emuiran, & Brady, 1978).

Stepwise multiple-regression equations with free entry of variables were computed to assess independent variables related to basal blood pressure and to blood pressure change from baseline to Alluisi. The number of variables permitted to enter each equation was limited to five so that models would not be overdetermined. Tables 15.2 and 15.3 present multiple-regression results showing predictors of baseline systolic and diastolic blood pressure. Our findings were simliar to those from the Bogalusa Heart Study (Berenson, 1980) in that we were able to account for 40 percent of the variance in systolic blood pressure. Ponderosity, age, and parental hypertension were significant predictor variables. Most important, measures of Type A behavior entered into the multiple-aggression equations and added significantly to the prediction.

We were able to account for 51 percent of the variance in baseline diastolic blood pressure using both ponderosity and Type A behavior as independent variables.This may represent one of the strongest documentations

TABLE 15.4. DEPENDENT VARIABLE: ABSOLUTE CHANGE IN SYSTOLIC BLOOD PRESSURE[a]

Independent Variable	Beta	B
Alluisi points	− .442	.38
Bortner Type A	.239	.48
Mean baseline systolic pressure	.195	.54
Parental hypertension	− .273	.58

[a]$R^2 = .34; F = 4.57 (p < .01)$.

TABLE 15.5. DEPENDENT VARIABLE: RELATIVE CHANGE IN SYSTOLIC BLOOD PRESSURE[a]

Independent Variable	Beta	B
Bortner Type A	.372	.366
Alluisi points	− .404	.531
Weight/height^2	.254	.575
Parental hypertension	− .214	.606
Age	.078	.617

[a]$R^2 = .381; F = 4.06 (p < .01)$.

TABLE 15.6. DEPENDENT VARIABLE: RELATIVE CHANGE IN DIASTOLIC BLOOD PRESSURE[a]

Independent Variable	Beta	R
Weight/height^2	−.294	.32
Age	.161	.38
Race	.093	.39

[a]$R^2 = .16; F = 3.62 (p < .05)$.

in adolescents of the relation between behavioral factors and baseline blood pressures; certainly it deserves replication.

We were primarily interested in accounting for blood pressure response during performance on the Alluisi Task. Tables 15.4, 15.5, and 15.6 present multiple-regression results showing predictors of the absolute and the relative (percent increase above baseline) changes from baseline to Alluisi in systolic and diastolic blood pressure. Behavioral factors entered most strongly in predicting absolute and relative systolic blood pressure change. Performance on the Alluisi task was negatively related to systolic blood pressure increases (i.e., students who performed better showed smaller relative and absolute increases in systolic pressure), and performance was positively related to Type A as measured by the Bortner inventory. Baseline systolic pressure, parental hypertension, and relative obesity were other variables entering into these questions.

MODIFYING BLOOD PRESSURE IN ADOLESCENTS

Weight Loss

Weight loss can promote blood pressure reduction among adults (Chiang, Perlman, & Epstein, 1969, Tyroler, Heyden, et al., 1975). It has been suggested, however, that drops in blood pressure with weight loss are due entirely to the concomitant reduction in salt intake (Dahl, 1972). Reisin et al. (1978), however, reported reductions in blood pressure concomitant with weight loss and independent of restriction in salt intake among adults. Patients, overweight and hypertensive, fell into three groups: those not receiving antihypertensive drug therapy (Group 1) and those on regular drug therapy but with adequate control of hypertension (Groups 2a and 2b). Groups 1 and 2a received dietary counseling for weight loss, while Group 2b did not. All patients in Groups 1 and 2a lost at least 3 kg; mean losses were 13.5 kg (+ 6.3), and standard deviation was 14.9 (+ 5.3 kg) during the same period. Seventy-five percent of Group 1 and 61 percent of Group 2a returned to a normal blood pressure, and correlations between weight loss and reductions in systolic and diastolic blood pressure were significant in both groups (Group 1 = .42/.56; Group 2a = .24/.30). Mean urinary sodium excretion from a 24-hour sample was similar following treatment among all three groups.

Coates et al. (1982a) examined the relationship between weight loss and changes in blood pressures among normotensive but overweight adolescents. Subjects were 36 adolscents participating in a study of the efficacy of various treatment variables to facilitate weight loss. Prior to their participation in weight-loss classes, subjects reported to the laboratory on two separate mornings. After the subjects had been seated in the laboratory for several minutes, blood pressure was measured in the right arm by a standard sphygmomanometer. The subject was then left alone for 5 minutes, at which time the nurse returned to take a second reading. The same procedure was followed 24 weeks later, following the end of the subjects' participation in the weight-loss classes.

Table 15.7 presents pre- and posttreatment values for weight and blood pressure for all subjects. Blood pressures reported represent the average of the second reading taken at each of two assessment sessions. Pre- and posttreatment values were compared using the t-tests for paired samples.

As can be seen in Table 15.7, there were significant reductions in both systolic and diastolic blood pressures. In addition, the correlation between

TABLE 15.7.   CHANGES IN WEIGHT AND BLOOD PRESSURES DURING WEIGHT LOSS

	Pre	Post	Change
Weight	X = 179.06	169.98	−9.08**
	S.D. = 41.06	40.37	
	R = 136–269	122–182	
Percent overweight	X = 40.62	33.78	−6.84**
	S.D. = 23.13	24.74	
	R = 9–100	2.5–110	
Systolic blood pressure	X = 114.54	107.30	−7.25**
	S.D. = 10.34	14.28	
	R = 98–131	80–129	
Diastolic blood pressure	X = 72.84	66.27	−6.57**
	S.D. = 8.21	9.27	
	R = 75–93	51–85	

$^*p < .05$
$^{**}p < .01$
Source: Adapted from T. J. Coates, R.W. Jeffery, L.A. Slinkard, J.D. Killen, and B.G. Danaher (1982). Frequency of contact and monetary reward in weight loss, lipid change, and blood pressure reduction with adolescents. *Behavior Therapy, 13*(2), 175–185.

change in percent overweight and change in systolic blood pressure was significant (r = .29, p <.05). The correlation between change in percent overweight and change in diastolic blood pressure was not significant ($\approx$.07, n.s.).

Modifying Diet: The Great Sensations Study

Effective nutrition education programs are in short supply. Saylor, Coates, Killen, and Slinkard (1982) conducted an exhaustive review of available empirical evidence on the efficacy of nutrition education programs with children and adolescents. They were able to locate only 25 empirical studies published in the last 12 years. Only five of these met minimal criteria for quality investigations, including adequate follow-up, specification of treatment components, and adequate and reliable dependent measures.

We have conducted three studies demonstrating efficacy of programs based on social learning theory in producing positive nutrition behavior changes in school children. Coates, Jeffery, and Slinkard (1981) developed and evaluated the Heart Health Program for elementary school students to (1) increase their consumption of complex carbohydrates, and decrease their consumption of saturated fat, cholesterol, sodium and sugar; (2) increase their level of habitual physical activity; and (3) generalize these changes to family members. The program produced substantial and maintained changes in students' eating behavior at school, knowledge about heart-health food preferences, and family eating patterns.

Coates, Slinkard, Perry, and Hashimoto (1982e) replicated these effects in a second study. A component analysis revealed that students receiving the instructional program alone showed positive changes in knowledge and preferences, but no changes in behavior. Only those students and their families receiving the full program (containing both instructional and motivational components) showed positive and sustained (across summer vacation) change in diet.

The Great Sensations Program was a nutrition education project developed for high school students (Coates, et al., 1985). It was designed to (1) decrease students' consumption of salty snacks, and (2) increase students' consumption of fresh-fruit snacks. The overall programs were designed following principles of social learning: informative instruction, participatory classroom activities, personal goal setting, feedback and reinforcement. The class program was delivered via six lessons during regular health education classes. A parent involvement program consisted of mailings and telephone calls to parents to teach parents to encourage changes in student snacking habits. A school-wide media program was designed to provide out-of-class peer support for student modification in salty snack foods. The program was evaluated in one high school, using a 2 by 2 design. A second high school served as a no-treatment control. Assessments were taken at baseline, postprogram, at the end of the school year and at the beginning of the next school year following summer vacation. The schoolwide program was effective in decreasing consumption of salty snack foods and of increasing consumption of target snack foods. However, only those students receiving class instruction maintained those changes until the end of the school year. No changes were maintained across summer vacation. These outcomes suggest that school programs using principles of social learning can be effective in facilitating important behavior changes at home and at school. It would be useful to follow this research with (1) studies of methods for enhancing the immediate and longterm reduction of sodium intake; and (2) studies of the impact of these reductions on blood pressure.

The Minnesota Blood Pressure Study

Gillum, Elmer, and Prineas (1981) randomized 80 school children with blood pressures above the 95th percentile for age and sex but below 130/90 mmHg to a family intervention program or to a control group. Twenty children aged 6 to 9 years and their families began a program to modify the family diet toward a goal of 70 mEq sodium per person per day. Families in the treatment group attended four biweekly intensive 90-minute lecture-demonstrations followed by 90-minute maintenance sessions occurring at bimonthly intervals over the remainder of the year. Children and parents attended separate 60-minute sessions, followed by a joint 30-minute low sodium refreshment period with discussion. Adherence was assessed by three-day food records and urine collections in children and adults. Effects were assessed one year following randomization. Results are difficult to interpret, as only 17 of the 41 randomized to treatment completed the full intervention. Twenty-four hour urinary sodium excretion data were available only for 11 intervention families. There was a significant decrease in urinary sodium excretion from the beginning to six months of 34 mmol/24 hr. Poor parent compliance hampered collection and analysis of their data. At one year, urinary sodium excretion data were available on 32 control and 32 intervention families. Both groups showed slight increases in overnight urinary sodium excretion ($+3.7$ and $+2.9$ mmol/10 hr, respectively). There were no significant differences in changes in blood pressure between the two groups. Thus this study demonstrates the difficulty of conducting this kind of intervention and research and suggests that effective programs may require better access to subjects.

Diet and Medication Combined: ADAPT

A Dietary/Exercise Alteration Program, in combination with low dose medication, was developed by the Bogalusa Heart Study as a model pediatric hypertension program (Frank, Farris, Ditmarses, Voors, & Berenson, 1982). ADAPT was designed to accomplish a daily 1-2 g sodium intake. Six core components included private consultation, education classes, self-administered training tool development, school lunch modification, food procurement, and physical activity classes. The objective was to empower children to make judicious choices, using class instruction (12 lessons), regular consultations, and tool usage (sodium counters, recipe books). A supportive environment was fostered by grocery store, restaurant and school-lunch programs. Medication consisted of low-dosage diuretic (chlorthiadone) and β-blocker (propranolol) prescribed at 25 percent of usual therapeutic dose for a given weight. Participants in this study were 100 children, 8 to 18 years of age, who tracked at or above the 90th percentile based on 36 blood pressure readings. These students were randomly assigned to treatment and control groups. Fifty children in the midrange (50th to 60th percentile) served as an additional comparison group. In the first six months of intervention, blood pressures of treatment subjects decreased 8 mmHg systolic and diastolic and remained 5/3 mmHg lower than the risk comparison group. They reached the 50th to 60th percentile for the population. Sodium intake was not decreased significantly. Obese treatment subjects gained less weight than their counterparts in the high obese group.

This program is important because it demonstrates the potential for blood pressure lowering in a segment of the population. It must be noted, however, that the intervention required three full-time nutritionists, a part-time physical activity coordinator, and supporting staff from the Bogalusa Heart Study. Given the effort, it is questionable whether any effect beyond that attributable to the medication can be demonstrated. Moreover, many would question the desirability of administering medications to adolescents and children if other approaches have not been evaluated.

A School-Based Relaxation and Biofeedback Program

Ewart, Coates, and Simon (1983) have been conducting studies in Baltimore City Schools with the following specific aims:

1. To conduct blood pressure screenings in selected high schools in Baltimore City to develop distributions of blood pressure for this population and to identify individuals above the 90th percentile systolic and/or diastolic.
2. To investigate the short- and long-term effects of relaxation on blood pressure when it is taught and practiced regularly in the school classroom (Study 1).
3. To study behavioral correlates of response and nonresponse to treatment (Studies 1 and 2).

School based programs offer several advantages, both scientific and clinical, over more traditional clinic or laboratory based investigations in studying the efficacy of relaxation in lowering blood pressure in adolescents.

1. *Compliance can be enhanced because relaxation will be taught and practiced in the classroom during a regular class period.* This has scientific significance (for an adequate test of hypotheses) and clinical significance (to insure the efficacious use of the strategies). We have attempted previously to conduct clinic-based treatments for elevated blood pressure with adolescents. This was less than optimal. While students reported enjoying relaxation and understood its importance for controlling blood pressure, returning to the hospital for repeated treatments was burdensome. Conducting programs in schools during regular class sessions would enhance correct and consistent application of relaxation.

2. *Maintenance will be enhanced because school and family-involvement programs can be developed and implemented in a cost-effective manner.* Maintenance is one of the key issues in health behavior change. Treatments in schools will facilitate maintenance of change; parents and peers can be encouraged to participate in programs designed to promote maintenance. By working

in the schools, we can develop peer support for use of relaxation and reach parents through existing school-based networks.

In the Fall of 1982 we conducted blood pressure screenings for all students in the ninth and tenth grades at a selected high school. Although 1172 students were listed on school enrollment records, only 866 could be reached by mail or phone to obtain parent consents. Parental refusals were few (9 percent) and 86 percent of the available pool of 866 subjects were screened during the five-week program.

Subjects with a systolic or diastolic blood pressure above the 85th percentile of the screening distribution (> 120 mm Hg systolic or > 73 mmHg diastolic) were screened a second time two months later, and those with either blood pressure above the 120/73 criterion were considered eligible for the PMR intervention study. A total of 79 stduents were randomized to the treatment (class) or no-treatment control group.

The class, offered as an elective in the Health Education program and entitled "High Blood Pressure," was taught for full credit by an accredited teacher. Students attended during regular class hours every day and received credit for participation for the semester-long course.

The class itself covered a full range of topics related to high blood pressure, including basic physiology, factors related to and the consequences of hypertension, and diet, exercise and medication. The unique features of this class were systematic teaching in relaxation and temperature biofeedback. Students were introduced first to progressive muscle relaxation in the following steps:

1. The teacher explained the purpose and goals of the program.
2. The teacher then guided the students through the relaxation procedure.
3. Data were collected on student's ability to attend and complete the procedures with 90 percent accuracy.

Following this, students were introduced to differential relaxation. Differential relaxation teaches discrimination of "tense" versus "relaxed" muscles. It also teaches students to relax on command.

The following steps were used:

1. Teacher read background information, reviewed essential terms and demonstrated the exercise.
2. Students were grouped in two's. One student was on the floor and relaxed his or her body with three complete breaths. The student then followed the teachers' instructions. The partner checked to make sure the student could tense specific muscles while the other muscles remain relaxed.

3. Students changed roles.
4. Data were collected on student's ability to tense and relax muscles.

Finally, students learned to use a finger thermometer as a biofeedback system to assist in monitoring his or her blood pressure during tense or calm situations. (Note: Finger temperature feedback has been used widely in blood pressure reduction; its efficacy rests upon the correlation between temperature increases and vasodilation. Decreased peripheral resistance induced by vasodilation lowers blood pressure.) The following steps were used:

1. The teacher explained the purpose of the finger thermometer.
2. The teacher explained and demonstrated how to use the finger thermometer.
3. The teacher then guided the students as they worked with the finger thermometers.
4. Baseline data were taken during the first few days of the program.
5. Data were taken on students' progress.
6. There was a question and answer period.

Of the 40 students randomized to PMR treatment, 30 attended regularly. PMR sessions were conducted on an average of 4 days per week over a 12 week period; in all, PMR was practiced 45 times. Attendance data showed that subjects participated in an average of 38.4 PMR sessions. Systematic observation showed that during these sessions compliance (as judged from absence of visible movement in 9 muscle groups averaged 80 percent (7 out of 9 groups immobile)).

To evaluate generalization of PMR and finger temperature mastering, behavioral observation and finger temperature data were collected from both treatment and control subjects during the pretest and posttest phases of the study. Subjects were asked to "sit and relax" for five minutes in an unfamiliar school office while temperature and behavioral data were recorded by a trained observer who was unaware of the PMR treatment and was blind to subjects' experimental status. Treatment subjects' breathing rates dropped from a pretest baseline of 17.2 to 11.2 cycles per minute ($t = 5.24$, $p < .001$), whereas breathing of controls increased from 16 to 17.2 per minute. PMR students' finger temperature rose from 91.4 to 94.0 ($t = 1.66$, $p < .06$), while controls dropped from 93.3 to 92.3 (n.s.). PMR students' muscle movement remained stable (60.3 percent to 63 percent motionless), while controls became less quiet at posttest (55.5 percent to 49.4 percent motionless $t = 2.56$, $p < .02$) Analyses of covariance (using pretest as the covariate) revealed statistically significant differences between treatment and controls in breathing rate ($t = 5.75$, $p < .001$); muscle movement ($t = 3.62$, $p < .001$), but not finger temperature ($t = 1.28$, n.s.).

Having shown that students mastered PMR, we next investigated possible BP effects. Fourteen treatment subjects and 17 controls had been eligible for the study on the basis of their systolic pressure. Group pre-post comparisons showed that treatment subjects' systolic pressures dropped from a mean of 127.8 ± 7.8 mmHg to 122.8 ± 7.1 mmHg ($t = 2.33$, $p < .03$), and that corresponding pre and post values for the controls were 127 ± 5.8 mmHg and 127.3 ± 9.7 (n.s.). An analysis of covariance with posttest BP as the dependent variable and the pretest BP as the covariate revealed the difference in systolic pressure to be statistically significant ($t = 1.85$, $p < .04$), suggesting that treated subjects had lowered their BP relative to the assessment-only controls.

Among the treatment subjects, 20 had been eligible on the basis of diastolic pressure, as had 23 controls. Treatment subjects' diastolic pressures dropped from a pretest mean of 78.3 ± 3.7 to 68.7 ± 10.7 ($t = 3.56$, $p < .003$) and corresponding values for controls were 79.0 ± 6.1 and 67.8 ± 8.6 ($t = 6.00$, $p < .001$). Differences between groups were not significant.

Data from behavioral observation and finger temperature measurement demonstrate that adolescent subjects will comply with PMR training offered as a routine exercise in health education classes, that they enjoy this activity, that they can master the PMR technique and that they attain a greater degree of relaxation in a generalization setting than do untrained controls as judged from ratings by a naive observer. We have concluded that our PMR training curriculum is effective in a school classroom context and is ready to be replicated in research with other adolescent school populations during the coming year.

CONCLUSION

Primary prevention of elevated blood pressure in adolescents is important because blood pressure tracks so strongly, and because untreated hypertension in adults is an important risk factor for cerebrovascular and cardiovascular disease. Blood pressure levels can also be lowered through selected lifestyle changes: weight loss, restriction of sodium intake, and relaxation/biofeedback may be effective in lowering blood pressure in adolescents. Aerobic physical activity, blood pressure self-monitoring, and restriction of alcohol intake, effective in lowering blood pressure in adults, may also be effective with adolescents.

Despite the fact that research in this area is quite preliminary, there is enough epidemiological evidence to support prudent clinical practice. At the very least, blood pressures of children and adolescents should be monitored routinely. If more than one casual reading is taken (as is often the case if initial pressures are high) then the blood pressure should be evaluated in relation to appropriate norms. The norms published by the American Academy of Pediatrics are based on casual and not successive pressures. Those devised in the Bogalusa Heart Study (Berenson, 1980), for example, are derived from multiple measurements under relaxed conditions.

If blood pressures are in the elevated ranges, clinicians should counsel and motivate regarding modification of lifestyle factors that influence blood pressure—namely weight, sodium, physical activity, alcohol, and relaxation.

Priority should be placed on the following research questions:

1. The signifance of cardiovascular reactivity remains to be established. It has been hypothesized that reactivity may be a risk factor for the development of hypertension or atherosclerosis. Until the link is established, intervening on this variable is of questionable utility.

2. Nonetheless, it remains an interesting question to determine the most efficacious methods for reducing reactivity. Relaxation may be an effective mode, but our research suggests that increasing competence to perform stressful actions may be equally effective in moderating blood pressure reactivity.

3. Research should be done to examine the relative efficacy of relaxation, biofeedback, weight loss, sodium restriction, and physical activity on blood pressure lowering among adolescents. The effects of these treatments should be examined singly and in combination.

4. Along with this, we need studies of variables which moderate the impact of treatments and of variables which predict differential effectiveness of specific techniques for individual patients.

We believe that a convincing case has been made for the need to develop programs for the primary prevention of hypertension among children and adolescents. The best means of accomplishing that objective, and even whether or not it can be accomplished, remain in question. However, the health implications are enormous and the potential for true prevention of cardiovascular disease is staggering. The effort clearly should be made.

REFERENCES

Baer, P.E., Vincent, J.P., William B.J., Bourianoff, G.G., & Bartlett, P.C. (1980). Behavioral response to induced conflict in families with a hypertensive father. *Hypertension, 2,* 1–70–71.

Barnett, P.H., Hines, E.A., Schirger, A., & Gage, R.P. (1963). Blood pressure and vascular reactivity to the cold pressor test. *Journal of the American Medical Association, 183,* 143–146.

Berenson, G.S. (1980). *Cardiovascular risk factors in children: The early natural history of atherosclerosis.* New York: Oxford University Press.

Berenson, G.S., Voors, A.W., Webber, C.S., Frank, G.C., Farris, R.P., Tobian, C., & Aristimuno, G.G. (1983). A model of intervention for prevention of early essential hypertension in the 1980's. *Hypertension, 5,* 41–53.

Bergman, L.R., & Magnusson, D. (1979). Overachievement and cathecholamine excretion in achievement-demanding situations. *Psychosomatic Medicine, 41,* 181–188.

Blumenthal, J.A., Williams, R. B., Koenig, Y. et al. (1978). Type A behavior patterns and coronary atherosclerosis. *Circulation, 58,* 634–639.

Brand, R.J., Rosenman, R.H., Sholtz, R.I., & Friedman, M. (1976). Multivariate prediction of coronary heart disease in the Western Collaboration Group Study compared to the Framingham study. *Circulation, 53,* 348–355.

Chenoweth, A.C. (1973). High blood pressure: A national concern. *Journal of School Health, 43,* 307–308.

Chiang, B.N., Perlman, L.V., & Epstein, F.H. (1969). Overweight and hypertension. *Circulation 39,* 403–421.

Coates, T.J., Barofsky, I., Saylor, K., Simons-Morton, S., Huster, W., Senergy, E., Straugh, S., Jacobs, H., & Kidd, L. (in press). The great sensations study: Modifying snack food preference of high school students. *Preventive Medicine.*

Coates, T.J., Jeffery, R.W., & Slinkard, L.A. (1981). The heart health program: Introducing and maintaining nutrition changes among elementary school children. *American Journal of Public Health, 71,* 15–23.

Coates, T.J., Jeffery, R.W., Slinkard, L.A., Killen, J.D., & Danaher, B.G. (1982a). Frequency of contact and contingent reward in weight loss, lipid change, and blood pressure reduction in adolescents. *Behavior Therapy, 13,* 175–185.

Coates, T.J., Parker, F., & Kolodner, K. (1982b). Stress and cardiovascular disease. Does blood pressure reactivity offer a link? In T.J. Coates, A.C. Petersen, & C. Perry (Eds.), *Promoting adolescent health: A dialogue on research and practice.* New York: Academic.

Coates, T.J., Slinkard, L.A., Perry, C.P., & Hashimoto, G. (1982c): Heart health eating and exercise: A replication and component analysis. (unpublished manuscript). University of California, San Francisco.

Comstock, G.W. (1957). An epidemiologic study of blood pressure levels in a biracial community in the Southern United States. *American Journal of Hygiene, 65,* 271.

Corcoran, A.C., Taylor, R.D., & Page I.H. (1951). Controlled observations on the effect of low sodium diet therapy in essential hypertension. *Circulation, 3,*1.

Court, J.M., Hill, G.H., Dunlop. M., & Boulton, T.J.C. (1974). Hypertension in childhood obesity. *Australian Pediatric Journal, 10,* 296–300.

Cutilletta, A.F., Benjamin, M., Culpepper, W.S., & Oparil, S. (1978). Myocardial hypertrophy and ventricular performance in the absence of hypertension in spontaneously hypertensive rats. *Journal of Molecular Cardiology, 10,* 689–703.

Dahl, L.K. (1972). Salt and hypertension. *American Journal of Clinical Nutrition, 25,* 231.

Dahl, L.K., & Love, R.A., (1957) Etiological role of sodium chloride intake in essential hypertension in humans. *Journal of the American Medical Association, 164,* 397–400.

Davignon, A., Rey, C., Payot, M., Biron, P., & Mongean, J.G. (1977). Hemodynamic studies of labile essential hypertension. In M.I. New & L.S. Levine (Eds.), *Juvenile hypertension.* New York: Raven.

De Castro, R.J., Besbroeck, R., Erickson, C., Farrell, P., Leong, W., Murphy, D., & Green, R. (1976). Hypertension in adolescents. *Clinical Pediatrics, 15,* 24–26.

Demobroski, T.M., MacDougall, J.M., Shields, J.L., Petitto, J., & Lushene, R. (1978). Components of the Type A Coronary-prone behavior pattern and cardiovascular responses to psycho-motor performance challenge. *Journal of Behavioral Medicine, 1,* 159–176.

Dole, V.P., Dahl, L.K., Cotzias, G.C., Eder, H.A., & Krebs, M.E. (1950). Dietary treatment of hypertension: Clinical and metabolic studies of patients on the rice-fruit diet. *Journal of Clinical Investigation, 29*, 1189.

Dube, S.K., Kapoor, S., Ratner, H., & Turnick, F.L. (1975). Blood pressure studies in black children. *American Journal of Diseases of Children, 129*, 1177–1180.

Emurian, H.H., Emurian, C.S., & Brady, J.V. (1978). Effects of a pairing contingency on behavior in a three person programmed environment. *Journal of the Experimental Analysis of Behavior, 29*, 319–329.

Ewart, C.K., Coates, T.J.C., & Simons, B. (1983). School-based relaxation to lower blood pressure. NHLBI Grant # R01-HL29431.

Falkner, B., Onesti, G., Angelakos, E.T., Fernandes, M., & Langman, C. (1979). Cardiovascular response to mental stress in normal adolescents with hypertensive parents. *Hypertension, 1*, 23–30.

Farquhar, J., Maccoby, N., Wood, P., Alexander, J., Brietruse, H., Brown, B., Hashul, W., McAlister, I., Meyer, A., Nash, J., & Stern, A. (1977). Community education for cardiovascular health. *Lancet I*, 1192–1195.

Feinleib, M., Garrison, R., Borhani, N., Roseman, R., & Christian, J. (1975). Studies of hypertension in twins. In O. Paul (Ed.), *Epidemiology and control of hypertension*. New York: Grune & Stratton.

Finnerty, F.A., Shaw, L.W., & Himmelsback, C. (1973). Hypertension in the inner city II. Detection and follow-up. *Circulation, 47*, 76–78.

Frank, G.C., Farris, R.P., Major, L.R., Webber, L.S., & Berenson, G.S. (1982). Infant feedings patterns and their relationship to cardiovascular risk factor variables in the first year of life. (unpublished manuscript) Louisiana State University.

Frank, G.C., Farris, R.P., Ditmarsen, P., Voors, A.W., & Berenson, G.S. (1982). An approach to primary preventive treatment for children with high blood pressure in a total community. *Journal of the American College of Nutrition, 1*, 357–374.

Friedman, M., Rosenman, R.H., Straus, R. et al. (1968). The relationship of behavior pattern A to the state of the coronary vasculature: A study of 51 autopsied subjects. *American Journal of Medicine, 44*, 525.

Gillum, R.F., Elmer, P.J., & Prineas, R.J. (1981). Changing sodium intake in children: The Minneapolis children's blood pressure study. *Hypertension, 3*, 698–703.

Haynes, S.G., Feinleib, M., & Kannel, W.B. (1980). The relationship of psychosocial factors to coronary heart disease in the Framingham study. *American Journal of Epidemiology, 111*, 37–38.

Haynes, S.G., Feinleib, M., Levine, S., Scotch, N., & Kannel, W.B. (1978). The relationship of psychosocial factors to coronary heart disease in the Framingham Study II. Prevalence of coronary heart disease. *American Journal of Epidemiology, 107*, 384–402.

Heyden, S., de Maria, W., Barbee, S., & Morris, M. (1973). Weight reduction in adolescents. *Nutrition and Metablism, 15*, 295–304.

Hines, E.A. (1937). Reaction of blood pressure of 400 children of standard stimulus. *Journal of the American Medical Association, 108*, 1249–1250.

Holland, W.W., & Beresford S.A.A., (1975). Factors influencing blood pressure in children. In O. Paul (Ed.), *Epidemiology and control of hypertension*. New York: Grune & Stratton.

Horan, M.J., Kennedy, H.L., & Padgett, N.E. (1981). Do borderline hypertensive patients have labile blood pressure? *Annals of Internal Medicine, 94*, 466–468.

Insel, P.M., & Chadwick, J.H. (1982). Conceptual barriers to the treatment of chronic disease: Using pediatric hypertension as an example. In T.J. Coates, A.C. Peterson & C. Perry (Eds.), *Promoting adolescent health: A dialog on research and practice*. New York: Academic.

Kass, E.H., Zinner, S.H., Margolius, H.S., Yhu, L., Rosner, B., & Donner, A. (1975). Familial aggregation of blood pressure and urinary Kallikrein in early childhood. In O. Paul (Ed.) *Epidemiology and control of hypertension.* New York: Grune & Stratton.

Kilcoyne, M. (1978). Natural history of hypertension in adolescence. *Pediatric Clinics of North America, 25,* 47–53.

Klein, B.E., Hennikens, C.H., Jesse, M.J., Gourley, J.E., & Blumenthal, S. (1975). Longitudinal studies of blood pressure in offspring of hypertensive mothers. In O. Paul (Ed.), *Epidemiology and control of hypertension* (pp. 387–395). New York: Grune & Stratton.

Krantz, D.S., Schaeffer, M.A., Daria, J.E., Dembroski, T.M. & MacDougell, J.M. (1981). Investigations of the extent of coronary atherosclerosis, Type A behavioral and cardiovascular response to social interaction. *Psychophysiology, 18,* 654–664.

Krotchen, J.M., Krotchen, T.A., Schwertman, N.L., & Kuller, L.H. (1974). Blood pressure distributions of urban adolescents. *American Journal of Epidemiology, 99,* 315–324.

Langford, H.G., & Watson, R.L. (1973). Electrolytes, environment, and blood pressure. *Clinical Science and Molecular Medicine, 45,* 111s–113s.

Langford, H.G., & Watson, R.L. (1975). Electrolytes and hypertension. In O. Paul (Ed.), *Epidemiology and control of hypertension* (pp. 119–130). New York: Grune & Stratton.

Langford, H.G., Watson, R.L., & Douglas, B.H. (1968). Factors affecting blood pressure in population groups. *Transactions of the Association of American Physicians, 81,* 135–146.

Lawler, K.A., Allen, M.T., Critcher, E.C., & Standard, B.A. (1981). The relationship of physiological response to coronary-prone behavior pattern in children. *Journal of Behavioral Medicine, 4,* 203–216.

Londe, S., Bourgoigne, J.J., Robson, A.M., & Goldring, D. (1971). Hypertension in apparently normal children. *Journal of Pediatrics, 78,* 569–577.

Miall, W.E., & Lovell, H.G. (1967). Relation betwen change in blood pressure and age. *British Medical Journal, 2,* 600–664.

Miller, R.A., & Shekelle, R.B. (1976). Blood pressure in tenth grade students. *Circulation, 54,* 993–1000.

National Center for Health Statistics. (1973). Blood pressure of youths 6–11 years. Publication (HRA) 74-1617, Vital and Health Statistics, Series II, No.135. Washington, DC: U.S. Government Printing Office.

National Center for Health Statistics. (1977). Blood pressure of youths 12-17 years. Publication (HRA) 77-1645, Vital and Health Statistics, Series 11, No.163. Washington, DC: U.S. Government Printing Office.

Paffenbarger, R.S., Thorne, M.C., & Wing, A.L. (1968). Chronic diseases in former college students: VIII. Characteristics of youth predisposing to hypertension in later years. *American Journal of Epidemiology, 88,* 25–32.

Reisin, E., Abel, R., Modaun M., Silverberg, D.S., Eliahou, H.E., & Madou, B. (1978). Effect of weight loss without salt restriction on the reduction of blood pressure. *New England Journal of Medicine, 298,* 1–6.

Sannerstedt, R., Bjure, J. & Vannaukas, E. (1970). Correlation between echocardiographic changes and systemic hemodynamics in human arterial hypertension. *American Journal of Cardiology, 26,* 117–120.

Saylor, K., Coates, T.J., Killen, J.D., & Slinkard, L.A. (1982). Nutrition education research: Fast or famine. In T.J. Coates, A.C. Petersen, & C. Perry (Eds.), *Promoting adolescent health: A dialog on research and practice.* New York: Academic Press.

Siegel, J.M., & Leitch, C.J. (1981). Assessment of the Type A behavior pattern in adolescents. *Psychosomatic Medicine, 43,* 45–46.

Spiga, R., & Petersen, A.C. (1980). The coronary-prone behavior pattern in early adolescence. Presented at the meetings of the American Education Research Association, Boston.

Stamler, J., Stamler, R., Riedlinger, W.F., Algera, G., & Roberts R.H. (1976). Hypertension screening of one million Americans. *Journal of the American Medical Association, 235,* 2299–2306.

Stine, O.C., Hepner, R., & Greenstreet, R. (1975). Correlation of blood pressure with skinfold thickness and protein levels. *American Journal of Diseases of Children, 129,* 905– 911.

Task Force on Blood Pressure Control (1977). *Pediatrics, 59,* 797–820.

Tyroler, H.A., Heyden, S. et al. (1975). Weight and hypertension: Evans County studies of blacks and whites. In O. Paul (Ed.), *Epidemiology and control of hypertension* (pp. 177–204). New York: Grune & Stratton.

Tuthill, R.W., & Calabrese, E.J. (1979). Elevated sodium levels in public drinking water as a contributor to elevated blood pressure levels in the community. *Archives of Environmental Health, 34,* 197–203.

Tuthill, R.W., & Calabrese, E.J. (1981). Drinking water sodium and blood pressure in children: A second look. *American Journal of Public Health, 71,* 722–729.

Voors, A.W., Foster, T.A., Frerichs, T., Webber, L.S., & Berenson, G.S. (1976). Studies of blood pressures in children, ages 5-14 years, in total biracial community: The Bogalusa Heart Study. *Circulation, 54,* 319–327.

Voors, A.E., Sklov, M., Wolfe, T., Hunter, S., & Berenson, G.S. (1982). Cardiovascular risk factors in children and coronary-related to behavior. In T.J. Coates, A.C. Petersen, & C. Perry (Eds.), *Adolescent health: Crossing the barriers.* New York: Academic.

Voors, A.W., Webber, L.S., & Berenson, G.S. (1979). Time course studies of blood pressure in children. The Bogalusa Heart Study. *American Journal of Epidemiology, 109,* 320.

Willett, W.C. (1981). Drinking water sodium and blood pressure: A cautious view of the 'second look.' *American Journal of Public Health, 71,* 729–732.

Zahka, K.G., Neill, C.A., Kidd, L., Cutilletta, M.A., & Cutilletta, A.F. (1981). Cardiac involvement in pediatric hypertension. *Hypertension, 3,* 664–668.

Zinner, S.H., Levy, P.S., & Kass, E.H. (1971). Familial aggregation of blood pressure in childhood. *New England Journal of Medicine, 284,* 401.

PART V

TREATMENT

16

Management of Behavior Problems in Primary Care Settings

EDWARD R. CHRISTOPHERSEN

The field of pediatrics includes a variety of areas to which the behavioral sciences can make and have made significant contributions. Some of the literature on these contributions has been published outside of pediatric journals, in psychological and in behavioral journals, but the importance of these contributions to pediatricians should not be minimized. Pediatricians and family practitioners caring for children (as pediatricians) are the primary professionals who provide child health supervision, or what is commonly referred to as well-baby or well-child care. Anticipatory guidance, the anticipation of potential problems and the accompanying steps that can be taken either to prevent or minimize the impact that these problems will have on any particular child, is the hallmark of well-child care

Preparation of this manuscript was supported by Grants HD 03144 and HD 02528 from the National Institute of Child Health and Human Development. The editorial advice and assistance of Jack W. Finney and Barbara Cochrane is gratefully acknowledged.

(Finney & Christophersen, 1984). Obviously, the most significant examples of effective anticipatory guidance come from the areas of infectious disease and nutrition. Over the years, the field of medicine, primarily through the efforts of pediatricians, has greatly reduced morbidity and mortality from infectious disease and nutritional problems. Within the last 10 years, significant advances have been made that are directly related to general pediatrics and the problems that the pediatrician sees every day.

Dr. Stan Friedman, in the Introduction to his 1975 issue of *Pediatric Clinics of North America*, stated that:

> Behavioral pediatrics maintains the pediatric tradition of emphasizing prevention, with curative and rehabilitative orientation always "second best" to preventing the disease or defect in the first place. Those identified with behavioral pediatrics do not claim expertise in the major psychiatric problems of childhood, but emphasize early intervention and treatment of the less severe problems. (pp. 515–516)

This chapter will review some of the significant contributions that have been made within the field of pediatrics or are directly relevant to the field of pediatrics. Since pediatrics maintains a developmental perspective, so will this review, beginning with assessment and intervention programs for the neonate and progressing through the developmental changes of the child.

INCIDENCE OF BEHAVIOR PROBLEMS IN CHILDREN

A recent and comprehensive study on the incidence of mental health problems in pediatrics was published in 1984 by Goldberg, Roghmann, McInerny, and Burke. They sampled 40 percent of the practicing pediatricians in Rochester County in New York. There probably are regional variations as well as variations due to rural versus urban populations, but a study that included more than 18,000 children is likely to have generality for the overall pediatric population (Christophersen, 1983). The authors found that approximately 5 percent of the total pediatric population presented with some kind of mental health problem. Pediatricians provided the treatment for almost 90 percent of the problems that were diagnosed. The most commonly reported problems were "adaptation reactions" and "conduct disorders." Of the children referred for treatment, the most frequent referral was to psychologists. The authors did caution that they were dealing with "reported" problems, with no data to indicate how closely these reports correlated with actual behavior problems.

The results from the Goldberg study are similar to those of Starfield et al. (1980), who reported occurrence rates from 5 percent to 15 percent. Starfield et al. also depended entirely on physician surveys for their incidence figures. In both the Goldberg and the Starfield studies, however, there were no mechanisms for recording minor, but annoying, behavioral disturbances, such as temper tantrums, eating problems, or thumb-sucking. When such minor problems are included, most researchers agree that the incidence figures would be significantly higher.

RECOGNITION OF BEHAVIOR PROBLEMS BY PEDIATRICIANS

When pediatricians examine a child and interview the child's parent(s), they must be able to recognize behavioral disturbances if they are present. Starfield and Borkowf (1969) conducted a study on physician recognition of behavioral problems in 383 children. They obtained questionnaires from the parent prior to their appointment with the pediatrician and later compared the charting, done by the examining physician, with the questionnaire results. A total of 115 mothers reported concern about their child's physical health. The physicians recognized 90 of these concerns, or 78 percent. Of the total of 48 behavioral concerns that the mothers reported, 20 of these, or 41 percent, were recognized by the physician. The authors concluded that physicians tend to recognize mothers' concerns about their child's physical health much more often than they do mothers' concerns about their child's behavior.

In the Starfield and Borkowf (1969) study, parents were preinterviewed to determine what concerns they had prior to being seen by their physician. Another way to address the same issue is to ask whom the parents will ask if they have behavioral concerns about their children. In the report of the Task Force on Pediatric Education (1978), parents were surveyed to find out, among other questions, whom the parent talked to when they wanted more information about their child's behavior and development. Only 40 percent indicated that they would consult their child's physician. The majority indicated that they would not even contact a professional, but would contact a friend or a family member. This finding may have affected the results reported by Starfield and Borkowf (1980). While there is a tendency to assume that the examining physician either missed the problem or neglected to ask about behavioral problems, it is also possible that the parents, having already decided that their pediatrician was not interested in nor trained in dealing with behavioral problems, elected not to bring the issue up with the pediatrician.

ANTICIPATORY GUIDANCE BY PEDIATRICIANS

In a recent study, Reisinger and Bires (1980) reported on the amount of time pediatricians spent on anticipatory guidance and what topics were discussed with parents during that time. They reported that parents whose children were less than one year of age had the longest appointments, but less than 90 seconds was spent on anticipatory guidance. With teenagers, pediatricians spent only seven seconds. Of the time that pediatricians did spend on anticipatory guidance, the majority of the time with younger patients was spent discussing questions about feeding.

Although some pediatricians, such as Brazelton (1975), report spending substantially greater amounts of time on anticipatory guidance, the data reported by Reisinger and Bires (1980) appears to be representative of the privately practicing pediatrician.

Continuing Education for Parents

Christophersen, Barrish, Barrish, and Christophersen (1984) presented a model for continuing education programs for parents that was predicated on the Standards of Health Care (Committee on Standards of Child Health Care, 1977). Approximately every 5.years the Committee revises their Standards to reflect changes in the field of pediatrics. The authors arrived at their course content by surveying area pediatricians and reviewing the existing literature (Task Force Report on the Future of Pediatrics, 1978) on current well-child care, and organized the course to cover material recommended by the Academy that may not currently be covered by the practicing pediatrician. The topics included normal growth and development, parental coping skills, home injury control, child automobile passenger safety, and behavior management with infants and toddlers; the topics were arrived at by cataloging the actual topics suggested by the Academy and eliminating topics typically covered by pediatricians as a part of well-child care (Reisinger & Bires, 1980).

The classes have been offered for four years. Each class is taught over four weeks, one evening per week, two hours each evening. The four faculty members each teach one class, which means that each faculty member teaches only one class a month. The faculty have terminal degrees; three have Ph.D.'s in Developmental and Child Psychology and one is a pediatric nurse practitioner. The 146 couples who filled our formal, written evaluations, anonymously, provided the following feedback:

Percentage who will or have recommended classes to friends: 100%
What did you like most about the classes?

Discussion about discipline/compliance	31%
Professional faculty	19%
Class discussion/sharing	16%
Coping skills/stress management	14%
Safety	12%
Presenters' personal experiences	12%

How did you find out about the classes?

M.D./Hospital	48%
Friends/Neighbors	31%
Newspaper	9%
Church	2%

Average age of child: 22 months

Obviously, the evaluation of such classes represents a significant challenge to the field, since there are no prior evaluations of this type of program. In Chapter 19 of this book, Medical Compliance in Pediatric Practice by Christophersen, Finney, and Friman, the results of one part of the continuing education offering is discussed. Basically, the area of home injury control (which was selected primarily because it is easier to measure the effects of the program compared to the other topics covered) showed a statistically significant improvement in the safety practices of the experimental families versus the control families. Clearly, they do offer an effective and practical method of providing anticipatory guidance to large numbers of families without altering the way pediatricians structure their practices.

EARLY INTERVENTION PROGRAMS

Intervention during the neonatal period, in cases where there is reason to suspect that a child's development may be compromised (for example, high risk pregnancies, teenage mothers), is the essence of early intervention. Two programs in the United States will be reviewed here as exemplary models for early intervention: The Infant Stimulation/Mother Training Project and the Mailman Center Program

The Infant Stimulation/Mother Training Project

Badger (1977) described an evaluation with 48 mother-infant pairs, half of whom were young mothers (16 years of age and under) and the other half older mothers (18 years of age and older). Each mother-infant pair was then randomly assigned into a group that received class training or a group that received training during home visits. The instruction for the class training consisted of weekly evening sessions during which the instructors covered a multitude of material, mainly through practice and demonstration relevant to parenting an infant. The home visit mothers received monthly home visits during which child development was discussed along with problems related to health and nutrition, but no instruction was provided in the implementation of the infant stimulation program. At the end of one year, the Uzgiris-Hunt Ordinal Scales of Psychological Development (Uzgiris & Hunt, 1975) and the Bayley Scales of Infant Development (Bayley, 1969) were administered. On the Uzgiris scale the infants of the young-mothers-in-classes group scored the highest and the infants of the young-mothers-with-home-visits scored the lowest. The older mothers (both classes and home visits) scored about average. On the Bayley Scales (mental) the infants of the young-mothers-in-classes group averaged a score of 99 versus the infants of the young-mothers-in-home-visits group score of 79. Similarly, on the Bayley Scales (motor) the young-mothers-in-classes group's infants' score of 110 was significantly better than the young-mothers-with-home-visits score of 99.

Dr. Badger and her colleagues have now developed a dissemination program for their Infant Stimulation/Mother Training Project that has made it possible for hospitals to implement the project locally, although no evaluations of the attempts at replication are available at this time.

The Mailman Center

Widmayer and Field (1981) presented the results of a brief intervention program designed for high risk teenage mothers and their preterm neonates. The intervention that they were interested in evaluating consisted of two procedures. The first was a demonstration of the sensory and behavioral capabilities of newborns, which was accomplished by conducting several of the parts of the Brazelton Neonatal Behavioral Assessment Scale (Brazelton, 1973) with the newborn at the mother's bedside while still in the hospital maternity unit. The second was sensitizing the mother to her newborn by asking her to fill out a questionnaire (Mother's Assessment of the Behavior of Her Infant Scale, [MABI]) in the maternity unit and at weekly intervals until the baby reached one month of age.

Thirty mother-infant pairs (who were essentially similar based on birth measures and on Brazelton scores performed at three days of age) were randomly assigned to three groups. The first group was a control group who received no special intervention between routine obstetric/pediatric care, but were asked to complete a weekly assessment of developmental milestones and child rearing attitudes to control for a Hawthorne effect. The second group, the Brazelton Demonstration/MABI group, were administered the Brazelton, in the presence of their mothers, during the postpartum hospital stay. In addition, the mothers of these infants were asked to complete the MABI weekly for the first four weeks of life. The third group did not observe the administration of the Brazelton Scale but were asked to complete the MABI Scale at birth and at weekly intervals for four weeks. The growth and development of the participating infants and their interactions with their mothers were then assessed in their homes when the infants were 1, 4, and 12 months of age (corrected for prematurity).

There were significant differences on the 1- 4- and 12-month measures between the control group and both of the experimental groups, but there were no differences between the two experimental groups. This was contrasted with the fact that there were no significant differences between any combination of the three groups in the postpartum period.

One of the interesting findings in this study was that the mothers who were given the Brazelton demonstration "expressed amazement that their newborn infants were capable of following moving faces, orienting to the sounds of voices, and, in general, of being so aware of their environment" (Widmayer & Field, 1984, p. 714). The authors suggested that the weekly administration of the MABI encouraged the mothers to "rediscover" the behaviors of their infants.

Although Widmayer and Field have not published the results of any dissemination attempts, the clinical applications of their intervention procedures are obvious. Nursing staff on postpartum hospital units can select mothers who appear to be at higher risk than average or mothers who are curious about their infants and want more information about newborns. Christophersen (1984) has prepared a manual for distribution to parents expecting their first child that details how to conduct an examination similar to a Brazelton on their child and includes an adaptation of the MABI questionnaire for the parents to fill out periodically. Also included in the manual are many of the points that are made in the Infant Stimulation/Mother Training Project.

PREVENTION OF BEHAVIOR PROBLEMS

There is little reason to believe that it is possible to raise a child without encountering at least occasional behavior problems. Epidemiological studies have provided normative data on the range and types of problems that are "typically" experienced by parents. Richman, Stevenson, and Graham (1975) interviewed 2,000 parents of three-year-old children to determine whether their children presented with problem behaviors. Of the children who did not present with significant problems, the most common behavior problems identified were bedwetting, toilet training, problems associated with bedtime, and problems at mealtime.

Because pediatricians have responsibility for providing immunizations and all of the episodic acute illness care for children, they are in contact with substantial numbers of young children. It is reasonable therefore, to assert that they are in the best position to provide parents with guidance to prevent or minimize the behavior problems experienced by their children.

Cullen (1976), using a posttest only control group design, examined the effects of 12 parent interviews about child rearing (over a period of five years) that lasted 30 minutes each. The results showed that, at six years of age, the group with the parent interviews had significantly fewer behavior problems (in areas such as eating, sleeping, aggression, lying, and fears) and better family relations. The effects were more pronounced for girls than for boys. There were no significant differences on either learning or intelligence measures (neither of which was addressed in the intervention).

Gutelius, Kirsch, McDonald, Brooks, and McErlean (1977) utilized both the time during well-child care and 28 home visits (over the first three years of care) to provide extensive counseling with experimental families, with the control families receiving regular well-child care. The experimental group families had better dietary habits and better developmental progress (in terms of sleep, toilet training, and shyness) and the experimental families used better child-rearing practices. Interventions by pediatricians can produce behavioral gains, but the amount of time required to produce moderate changes may be impractical to provide, one-on-one, to a large number of families.

Chamberlin, Szumowski, and Zastowny, (1979) conducted a longitudinal analysis of the effects of well-child care on behavioral and developmental problems. Mothers who were seen by pediatricians with high teaching scores had better knowledge of child development and felt more supported in their child-rearing practices. In a recent review of the issue of preventing behavioral problems, Chamberlin (1982) stated that:

> For families in the pediatrician's own practice he or she can help parents cope with troublesome behaviors through education and brief intervention techniques such as behavior modification and link them with community services for more complex problems. In addition the physician can help to promote "competence" by teaching parents how to interact with their children in more affectionate and cognitively stimulating ways. (p. 246)

EARLY TREATMENT OF BEHAVIOR PROBLEMS

The Chapel Hill Pediatrics Program

Schroeder, Gordon, Kanoy, and Routh (1983) published a detailed description of a joint effort of a large pediatric group and a team of mental health professionals from a nearby, hospital-based, university-affiliated facility. The services provided by the team included evening education groups on child development and management, a call-in service in which parents could phone in their questions about their children, and a come-in service in which parents could schedule appointments with the staff. All of the services were available in the pediatrician's office, with the only additional charge being for actual office appointments. The top ten problem areas over a nine-year period were: negative behaviors, toileting, emotional problems, school problems, sleep problems, developmental delay, sibling/peer problems, divorce/separation, family problems, and infant management.

Although the Chapel Hill Program was conducted as a demonstration program and not as a research investigation, the program directors conducted follow-up interviews on parents who had utilized the services over the nine-year period. Their general summation was as follows:

In general, parents gave the suggestions offered ratings of 3 or above (a rating of "1" being not helpful and "5" being very helpful), with the effectiveness of a particular suggestion varying with the specific concern. The advice for negative and sibling/peer problems was seen as consistently more helpful (generally ratings of 4 or more) than the advice given in the categories of sleep or toileting, where the ratings were 3 to 4. (p. 65)

The Chapel Hill Program has evolved over the years to where it is now using specific handouts for problems such as negative behaviors. For example, one handout, based on Forehand and McMahon (1981), focuses on increasing positive parent-child interactions, and another outlines how to issue commands and how to follow through with praise for compliance and time-out by isolation for noncompliance.

Depending on the severity of the problem, the parents are either sent the handouts after a careful, verbal explanation of the procedure, or they are encouraged to make an appointment for further evaluation of the parent-child interaction and possible referral to a one-hour-a-week, 6-week program focusing on the parent-child interaction. (p. 67)

The Chapel Hill Program demonstrates that it is possible for a pediatric group to incorporate mental health services as an adjunctive part of their office offerings, with good acceptance on the part of the families who use that pediatric group. As the authors of the Program stated, the task that lies before them now is to conduct a bona fide experimental investigation of the effectiveness of the intervention program.

The Kansas Program

Christophersen (1982a) described an approach to counseling parents that is based on the following points: (1) pediatricians and family practitioners currently provide the majority of well-child care in the U.S.; (2) office visits are typically very brief (Reisinger & Bires, 1980); (3) their medical practices are well suited to early detection of behavior problems, if the method used for early detection can be applied within the existing constraints of the well-child care setting; and (4) the time needed for the intervention does not negatively impact upon the already hectic schedule of the pediatrician, if the pediatrician can implement the procedures within a brief period of time.

Christophersen (1982a) recommended the use of the Eyberg Child Behavior Inventory (Robinson, Eyberg, & Ross, 1980) for screening child behavior problems, similar to the way the Denver Developmental Screening Test (Frankenburg & Dodds, 1967) is used to screen for developmental delays. The Eyberg can be administered while a parent is in the waiting room or in an exam room waiting to see the pediatrician. Eyberg has provided standardization norms; however, practitioners who routinely use the Eyberg will quickly learn how to scan the parents' answers to determine whether the answers are remarkable in much the same way that many practitioners used the Denver without actually looking up the norms to determine if a child has a remarkable score. If the pediatrician determines, either from a clinical interview or from a screening device like the Eyberg, that a young child presents with minor behavior problems or is a discipline problem for parents, the pediatrician must be able to manage the problem within the time constraints imposed by the primary care setting; that is, they must have procedures that can be implemented in a brief period of time. (Almost by definition, any problem that can be managed in a brief period of time must be one that does not have a long history and one that is not complicated by a variety of psychosocial problems.)

Treatment handouts can also aid the pediatrician in the management of patient behavior problems. Christophersen (1982a) recommended the use of brief written handouts that provide parents with a written summary of management recommendations. One set of handouts, originally published by Christophersen (1982b) included recommendations for minor problems with dressing, mealtime, bedtime, behavior in public places, and automobile travel, as well as handouts for discipline with toddlers and preschoolers. Two of these written handouts were actually subjected to scientific analysis. The automobile travel handout was evaluated in a study by Christophersen and Gyulay (1981). Parents were recruited for the study who were not using child passenger safety seats for their toddler. After research observers rode with the mother-child pairs for several baseline automobile rides, the mothers were given a brief written handout that offered suggestions to make it easier for them to use a child passenger safety seat for everyday travel. During baseline, none of the mothers even used a child passenger safety seat. Immediately after one clinic visit, during which the written handout was presented to the mother and discussed briefly, 62 percent of the children were correctly restrained during automobile rides. Three months later, 75 percent of the children were correctly restrained, six months later 62 percent were correctly restrained, and one full year later, 37 percent were correctly restrained. Although there were only eight mother-infant pairs in this study, the results suggested that, in families where there was no identifiable socioemotional pathology, the use of written handouts with suggestions for parents may be an effective adjunct to office discussion. In a similar analysis, Rapoff, Christophersen, and Rapoff (1982) examined the effectiveness of a written parent handout for use by pediatric nurse practitioners in the management of bedtime problems in toddlers. Battery operated tape recorders were used as the primary source for data collection. That is, the researchers tape-recorded all of the sounds made in the child's room from the time that the parent said, "Good night" until 30 minutes past bedtime. The tapes were then scored to assess both the parents' compliance with the recommended procedures and the child's crying and talking after bedtime. The results indicated that half of the parents in the study used the procedures properly. Furthermore, in those families where the procedures were not used properly, there were significant improvements in child behavior at bedtime.

Although these preliminary analyses do not show that written parent handouts are a panacea for child behavior problems, they do provide objective evidence that, when used in conjunction with office discussion, written handouts can be effective. McMahon and Forehand (1980), in a review of the literature on self-help therapies for parents of behavior disordered children, concluded that evaluations of the effectiveness of written instructions in parent training is in its infancy. They concluded that some of the available research suggests the value of using handouts to train parents to be effective behavior modifiers for their children. Logically, it would seem that a pediatrician who has an established rapport with a family is in a position to make recommendations to that family regarding their child-rearing practices. If written handouts are used in conjunction with such a discussion, they can probably increase the impact that the discussion has on the parents. But it is the combination of the handout and the discussion that appears to make the difference. To date, no one has suggested that a family with an emotionally disturbed or behavior disordered child can actually remedy those problems by reading a book or by following a written handout.

PARENT TRAINING PROGRAMS

There are a variety of parent training programs available for implementation through a traditional office-based practice. The advantages and disadvantages of such programs, as well as descriptions and outcome data, are well presented in a recent book edited by Dangel and Polster (1984), *Parent Training: Foundations of Research and Practice.* Although the majority of parent training programs were not intended for implementation through the pediatrician's office and were not originally evaluated with pediatricians serving as the therapists, many of these procedures can be implemented by practitioners who specialize in the treatment of behavior disordered children. One example of such a program is the program developed by Forehand and McMahon (1981) for treating children who present with problems of noncompliance. These authors selected "noncompliance" as their area of investigation based upon the prevalence of this symptom in their prior research.

Helping the Noncompliant Child

Forehand and McMahon (1981) provide an excellent example of a carefully developed and documented program for provision of services to families with noncompliant children. While they follow the traditional behavioral model of emphasizing the use of praise or reinforcement for appropriate behavior and a mild form of punishment (time-out) for inappropriate behavior, they base their recommendations on a sound data-based foundation. Making use of social learning principles, the authors describe and discuss a two-phase program. The first phase teaches the parents how to provide differential attention, through the use of the "Child's Game." The Child's Game is a highly structured set of procedures for delivering nonjudgmental positive attention to young children, which is designed to teach the parent how to be a more effective reinforcing agent. The second phase consists of training the parents how to use appropriate verbal commands and how to use time-out to decrease noncompliant behavior exhibited by their child.

The authors describe the background necessary for the therapists, the type and length of training sessions, the content of training sessions, assessment of outcome, and criteria for treatment termination. The Forehand and McMahon program for helping the noncompliant child provides a good example of the type of program available to the pediatrician on a referral basis. Obviously, whether the pediatrician chooses to make such services available through his or her office or chooses to refer to such services in the community, the important issue is that the services be available.

REFERRAL OF BEHAVIOR PROBLEMS

Although much has been written about pediatricians functioning as mental health therapists, no data have been published that document the ability of a primary health care provider to incorporate psychotherapy into a busy well-child practice. Typically pediatricians who deliver well-child care do not have the time nor the inclination to become psychotherapists. Conversely, pediatricians who routinely engage in the practice of psychotherapy usually discontinue delivering well-child care. The pediatrician who identifies a significant mental health problem in one of his or her patients usually refers that patient to a mental health professional. Phillips, Sarles, and Friedman (1980) provided useful guidelines for referral. The types of behavior that the authors identified as clearly needing referral are: psychosis (for example, infantile autism) and schizophrenia. Generally they suggested that the pediatrician focus not on the occurrence of a specific behavior, but on the quantity (or rate of occurrence), distribution (or different manifestations of the behavior), severity (judged by the amount of interference that the behaviors cause the patient), and duration (or length of time) that the behavior of concern has been occurring.

Typically pediatricians have different expectations when they refer to medical subspecialists rather than mental health practitioners. When a patient is referred to a medical subspecialist, the pediatrician usually can count on receiving a written report from the subspecialist within a short time after the patient is seen, including a summary of what tests were run and the results of those tests, as well as the recommendations for subsequent treatment. In some instances the patient will be in treatment by the subspecialist and in others the patient will be returned to the pediatrician for treatment. Mental health referrals are often handled very differently. Thorpe and Halpern (1965) in a study of the referral patterns of pediatricians found that 30 percent of the 52 participating pediatricians who used to refer to a mental health clinic had discontinued doing so because of dissatisfaction with the clinic. The major reasons for dissatisfaction were: there were often long delays between referral and treatment; physicians often received little feedback from clinical personnel once a referral was made; and about one-third of the physicians were not even aware of the clinic's services. Eisenberg (1967) even suggested that one reason for the physicians' reluctance to refer to mental health clinic personnel was that such referral involved considerable expense for the family over a long period of time.

Feedback from a mental health facility can be greatly facilitated if the referring physician calls the facility with the referral and specifically requests a written report, much like a report that would be received from other medical subspecialists, of the testing, diagnosis, and treatment recommendations. If the treatment is expected to take a period of time to complete, then interim progress reports can also be requested. The response from the mental health practitioner to these requests can be the basis for the physician's subsequent decision about where to refer the patient/family in need of mental health services.

CONCLUDING REMARKS

Behavioral pediatrics, when practiced in a time- and cost-effective way, can aid considerably in meeting the needs of patients who are seen for primary care. The combination of prenatal education provided by a neighboring hospital, anticipatory guidance provided by the physician, preventive services provided either by the physician or the hospital, early detection of problems (while they are still relatively easy to manage), and referral of behavior problems that are beyond the ability and/or time constraints of a primary care provider, could greatly expand the services that new parents find available to them, at costs that are not prohibitive. The child with severe aberrant behaviors rarely misses detection by the existing health care and public education facilities. Although the problem may not be diagnosed as early as it might be, severe behavior problems rarely go undiagnosed, particularly when compared to the minor behavior problems that normal parents experience with almost every child. Since the physician or nurse who delivers well-baby and well-child care is the only professional who routinely comes into contact with large numbers of infants and young children, he or she must have mechanisms in place to detect behavioral and developmental problems without unduly disrupting the delivery of health services to the patients. Having detected such problems, the decision must then be made whether to treat or to refer the patient. The professional who has not been trained in the detection of minor behavioral and developmental problems is unlikely to detect them in a timely fashion. However, if the procedures for ameliorating such problems are developed for use within pediatric primary care, the pediatrician can begin to address the mild behavior problems encountered by all parents as their children develop.

Perhaps the greatest concern with existing parenting programs stems from the dearth of sound scientific investigations of the programs. Although many research studies have been published that document the effectiveness of highly specialized procedures for particular patient problems, systematic program evaluations have not been forthcoming. In the absence of such evaluations, program dissemination must proceed very cautiously.

REFERENCES

Badger, E. (1977). The infant stimulation/mother training project. In B. Caldwell & D. Stedman (Eds.), *Infant education: A guide for helping handicapped children in the first three years* (pp. 45–61). New York: Walker.

Bayley, N. (1969). *Bayley scales of infant development.* New York: The Psychological Corp.

Brazelton, T.B. (1973). *Neonatal behavioral assessment scale.* Philadelphia.. Lippincott.

Brazelton, T.B. (1975). Anticipatory guidance. *Pediatric Clinics of North America, 22,* 533–544.

Chamberlin, R.W. (1982). Prevention of behavioral problems in young children. *Pediatric Clinics of North America, 29,* 239–248.

Chamberlin,R.W.,Szumowski, E., & Zastowny, T. (1979). An evaluation of efforts to educate mothers about child development in pediatric office practices. *American Journal of Public Health,* 875–885.

Christophersen, E.R. (1982a). Incorporating behavioral pediatrics into primary care. *Pediatric Clinics of North America, 29,* 261–296.

Christophersen, E.R. (1982b). *Little people: Common sense guidelines for child rearing* (2nd ed.). Shawnee Mission, KS: Overland Press.

Christophersen,E.R. (1983). Research issues in developmental and behavioral pediatrics. In M.D. Levine, W.B. Carey, A.C. Crocker, & R.T. Gross (Eds.), *Developmental-behavioral pediatrics.* Philadelphia: Saunders.

Christophersen, E.R. (1984). *Baby owner's manual: What to expect and how to survive the first thirty days.* Shawnee Mission, KS: Overland Press.

Christophersen, E.R., Barnard, S.R., Barnard, J.D., Gleeson, S., & Sykes, B.W. (1981). Home-based treatment of behavior disordered and developmentally delayed children. In M.J. Begab, H.D. Haywood, & H.T. Garber (Eds.), *Psychosocial influences in retarded performance. Vol. II. Strategies for improving competence.* Baltimore: University Park Press.

Christophersen, E.R., Barrish, H.H., Barrish, I.J., & Christophersen, M.R. (1984). Continuing education for parents of infants and toddlers. In R.F. Dangel & R.A. Polster (Eds.), *Parent training: Foundations of research and practice* (pp. 127–143). New York: Guilford.

Christophersen, E.R., Finney, J.W., & Friman, P.C. (1985). Medical compliance in pediatric practice. In N.A. Krasnegor, J.D. Arasteh, & M.C. Cataldo (Eds.), *Child health behavior: A behavioral pediatrics approach.* New York: Wiley.

Christophersen, E.R., & Gyulay, J. (1981). Parental compliance with car seat usage: A positive approach with long-term follow-up. *Journal of Pediatric Psychology, 6*(3), 301–312.

Committee on Standards of Child Health Care. (1977). *Standards of child health care* (3rd ed.). Evanston, IL: American Academy of Pediatrics.

Cullen, K.J. (1976). A six-year controlled trial of prevention of children's behavior disorders. *Journal of Pediatrics, 88,* 662–666.

Dangel, R.F., & Polster, R.A. (Eds.). (1984). *Parent training: Foundations of research and practice.* New York: Guilford.

Eisenberg, L. (1967). The relationship between psychiatry and pediatrics: A disputatious view. *Pediatrics, 39,* 645–647.

Finney, J.W., & Christophersen, E.R. (1984). Behavioral pediatrics: Health education in primary care. In M. Hersen, R.M. Eisler, & P.M. Miller (Eds.), *Progress in behavior modification* (Vol. 16, pp. 185–229). New York: Academic.

Forehand, R.L., & McMahon, R.J. (1981). *Helping the noncompliant child: A clinician's guide to parent training.* New York: Guilford.

Frankenburg, W.K., & Dodds, J.B. (1967). The Denver developmental screening test. *Journal of Pediatrics, 71,* 181.

Friedman, S.B. (1975). Foreword. *Pediatric Clinics of North America, 22,* 515–516.

Goldberg, I.D., Roghmann, K.J., McInerny, T.K., & Burke, J.D. (1984). Mental health problems among children seen in pediatric practice: Prevalence and management. *Pediatrics, 73,* 278–293.

Gutelius, M.F., Kirsch, A.D., McDonald, S., Brooks, M.R., & McErlean, T. (1977). Controlled study of child health supervision: Behavioral results. *Pediatrics, 60,* 294–304.

McMahon, R.J., & Forehand, R. (1980). Self-help behavior therapies in parent training. In B.B. Lahey & A.E. Kazdin (Eds.), *Advances in clinical child psychology* (Vol. 3, pp. 149–176). New York: Plenum.

Phillips, S., Sarles, R.M., & Friedman,S.B. (1980). Consultation and referral: When, why, and how. *Pediatric Annals, 9,* 36–45.

Rapoff, M.A., Christophersen, E.R., & Rapoff, K.E. (1982). The management of common childhood bedtime problems by pediatric nurse practitioners. *Journal of Pediatric Psychology, 7*(2I, 179–196.

Reisinger, K.S., & Bires, J.A. (1980). Anticipatory guidance in pediatric practice. *Pediatrics, 66,* 889–892.

Richman, N., Stevenson, J.E., & Graham, P.J. (1975). Prevalence of behaviour problems in 3-year-old children: An epidemiological study in a London borough. *Journal of Child Psychology and Psychiatry, 16,* 277–287.

Robinson, E.A., Eyberg, S.M., & Ross, A.W. (1980). The standardization of an inventory of child conduct problem behaviors. *Journal of Clinical Child Psychology, 9,* 22.

Schroeder, C.S., Gordon, B.N., Kanoy, K., & Routh, D.K. (1983). Managing children's behavior problems in pediatric practice. In M. Wolraich & D.K. Routh (Eds.), *Advances in developmental and behavioral pediatrics* (pp. 25–86). Greenwich, CT: JAI Press.

Starfield, B., & Borkowf, S. (1969). Physicians' recognition of complaints made by parents about their children's health. *Pediatrics, 43,* 168–172.

Starfield, B., Gross, E., Wood, M., Pantell, R., Allen, C.,Gordon, I.B., Moffatt, P., Drachman, R., & Katz, H. (1980). Psychosocial and psychosomatic diagnoses in primary care of children. *Pediatrics, 66,* 159–167.

Task Force on Pediatric Education. (1978). *The future of pediatric education.* Evanston, IL: American Academy of Pediatrics.

Thorpe, H.S., & Halpern, W. (1965). Pediatricians and a community child guidance center. *Pediatrics, 36,* 773–781.

Uzgiris, I., & Hunt, J. (1975). *Assessment in infancy: Ordinal scales of psychological development.* Urbana, IL: University of Illinois Press.

Walker, H.M. (1970). *Walker problem behavior identification checklist, test and manual.* Los Angeles: Western Psychological Services.

Widmayer, S.M., & Field, T.M. (1981). Effects of Brazelton demonstrations for mothers on the development of preterm infants. *Pediatrics, 67,* 711–714.

17

Biobehavioral Assessment and Management of Pediatric Pain

JAMES W. VARNI AND KAREN L. THOMPSON

Pain in children represents a complex developmental process involving cognitive, emotional, motivational, neurochemical, sensory, socio-environmental, and psychophysiological components which interact to produce differential pain perception and manifestation. The term *pain* is an abstract concept which economically describes a multiplicity of sensations of various etiologies influenced by cultural and social factors (Fabrega & Tyma, 1976). For the young child in the preabstract stage of cognitive development, the term *pain* may be meaningless. Consequently the cognitive-developmental stage of the child, and stage-related misconceptualizations must be considered when assessing and treating pediatric pain (Varni, 1983).

ASSESSMENT

The assessment of pediatric pain requires an interdisciplinary, multidimensional, and comprehensive approach, combining self-report, behavioral, cognitive, socioenvironmental, medical and biological parameters (Schechter, 1984; Varni, 1983). Given the important modeling role parents and other significant adults play in the observational learning of pain responses by children (Craig, 1982; Masek, Russo, & Varni, 1984), the potential socioenvironmental influences not only on the verbal reports of pain intensity and location, but also on such nonverbal expressions as facial grimaces, compensatory posturing, restricted movement, limping, and the absence of developmentally appropriate behaviors, must also be considered in the assessment process. Such a comprehensive and multidimensional assessment process is absolutely mandatory prior to the application of any treatment regimen (Katz, Varni, & Jay, 1984).

COGNITIVE-DEVELOPMENTAL CONCEPTUALIZATIONS

Prior to any intervention, whether pharmacological, psychological, or biobehavioral, effective and efficient management of pain in children depends upon accurate comprehensive assessment (Beales, 1982; Schechter, 1984; Varni, 1983). Evaluation of the pain experience in adults is facilitated by an adult's knowledge and understanding of what pain means, what services are available for relief from pain and how to communicate painful sensations to health care professionals. However, pediatric pain assessment can be confounded by inadequate communication between children and health care providers. Words like "pain" may be entirely absent from a child's vocabulary or given an abstract meaning quite different from that of an adult. Language and specific examples that are appropriate to a child's age and developmental stage should be used in explaining symptoms, procedures, and health instructions (Perrin & Perrin, 1983). Awareness of a child's cognitive-developmental level and cognitively related misconceptions about pain and illness is therefore essential when assessing and treating pediatric pain (Thompson & Varni, in press).

A number of studies have documented stages of childrens' health and illness conceptualizations that seem to mirror Piaget's stages of cognitive development (Bibace & Walsh, 1981; Brewster, 1982; Feldman & Varni, 1985; Perrin & Gerrity, 1981; Steward & Regalbuto, 1975; Whitt, Dykstra & Taylor, 1979); similar stages may exist for children's conceptualizations of pain. To date, age differences in pain conceptions have not been validated; however, a brief review of the stages of health and illness will illustrate the importance of cognitive development for adequate pediatric health care communication.

Briefly six categories are hypothesized: phenomenism and contagion (ages 2 to 6), contamination and internalization (ages 7 to 10), and physiological and psychophysiological (ages 11 and older). Phenomenism is the most developmentally immature explanation. The cause of illness is an external event that may co-occur with the illness but is spatially and/or temporally remote. In the stage of contagion the cause of illness is located in objects or people that are proximate to but not touching the child. People get sick by magic or because they are near certain objects. At approximately age seven, children evolve concrete-logical reasoning. Contamination is a form of concrete reasoning. The cause of illness is viewed as a person, object, or action that is external to the child and that has an aspect or quality that is bad or harmful to the body. Physical contact is necessary for illness to occur. Illness becomes located inside the body in the stage of internalization, even though the ultimate cause of illness may still be external. Confusion still exists about internal organs and functions, but the child can offer vague ideas about his or her internal state. The greatest amount of understanding occurs with children who are able to comprehend physiological and psychophysiological explanations of illness. In the physiological stage the source and nature of the illness lie in specific internal physiological structures and functions. Psychophysiological explanations, the most mature understanding of illness, still describe illness in terms of internal physiological processes, but with the addition of possible psychological causes. The child is aware that a person's thoughts or feelings can affect the way the body functions (see Bibace & Walsh, 1981; Varni, 1983, for comprehensive reviews).

Despite the acknowledgement that cognitive-developmental level will have an affect on pediatric pain assessment (Gildea & Quirk, 1977; Schecter, 1984; Thompson & Varni, in press), developmentally appropriate assessment instruments that measure more than just pain intensity are noticeably lacking. As stated by Melzack (1975), "the word 'pain' refers to an endless variety of qualities that are categorized under a single linguistic label, not to a specific single sensation that varies only in intensity. To describe pain solely in terms of intensity is like specifying the visual world only in terms of light flux without regard to pattern, texture, and the many other dimensions of visual experience." If, as hypothesized, childrens' cognitive-developmental level affects their perception of pain, and traditional assessment methods have been evaluating pain intensity only, then children have not been receiving the most effective intervention because of inadequate pain assessment. The ideal assessment of pediatric pain requires an interdisciplinary, multidimensional and comprehensive approach, combining self-report, behavioral, cognitive, socioenvironmental, medical and biological parameters (Varni, 1983). Rarely have pediatric pain assessments addressed all of these areas.

Self-report measures of pain intensity have been the mainstay of traditional pediatric pain assessment. Self-report measures of pain have included verbal self-report, visual analogue scales, and color cross-modality matching. These measures have been used with varying degrees of success with children. Verbal rating scales of pain intensity are sometimes too complicated for children to understand. Wolff (1980) found that adults often had difficulty using a scale with more than five categories; the implications for children are obvious. The visual analogue scale (VAS) is a form of cross-modality matching, in which line length is the response continuum. The ends are marked with the two extremes for pain, such as "no pain" and "very severe pain" or "pain as bad as it could possibly be." The main advantage of the VAS is the avoidance of numbers or word descriptors and categories (Stewart, 1977). The child is free to indicate on a continuum the intensity of the pain without relating to specific words chosen by the clinician. Abu-Saad (1981) has reported that the VAS is sensitive to medication effects and behavioral indicators of pain in children. Another cross-modality technique involves having children match the pain they are experiencing to a color. Scott (1978) and Eland (1981) have both used the selection of colors to indicate pain intensity with children. Younger children seem to have a more intuitive style in expressing their pain experience than older children (Scott, 1978), so color matching may be more appropriate with this age group.

A major drawback to all these self-report measures is that they are addressing pain intensity only. In an attempt to assess pediatric pain reliably and validly, Varni and Thompson (1985) have developed the Pediatric Pain Questionnaire (PPQ). The Varni/Thompson PPQ is a comprehensive, multidimensional assessment instrument specifically designed for the study of acute and chronic pain in children, with parent, adolescent, and child forms. The PPQ-Child Form addresses the intensity of pain, the sensory, emotive and affective qualities of pain, and the location of pain in a form comprehensible to children. The PPQ has been patterned after the most widely used and respected instrument to measure pain in adults, the McGill Pain Questionnaire (Melzack, 1975). The PPQ-Parent Form consists of components similar to the PPQ-Child Form to allow for cross-validation of the child's reporting of pain. A comprehensive family history section addresses the child's pain history and family pain history, with questions pertaining to symptomatology, past and present treatments for pain, and socioenvironmental situations which may influence pain.

Ongoing research with the Varni/Thompson PPQ has shown it to be effective in providing a comprehensive picture of the child's pain experience (Varni, Thompson, & Hanson, 1985). By using a developmentally appropriate instrument, pain intensity, pain location and the qualitative aspects of the pain experience can be obtained from the child. Socioenvironmental factors that may influence the child's pain can be obtained from the parent, as well as providing further validation of the child's report. By combining an understanding of cognitive-developmental level and conceptualizations of health, illness and pain within a multidimension assessment instrument, pediatric health care professionals will be in a better position to effectively assess and manage acute and chronic pain in children.

ACUTE VERSUS CHRONIC PAIN ASSESSMENT

There are a number of dimensions which can facilitate a differential assessment of acute versus chronic pain in the pediatric population, subsequently determining an appropriate treatment approach.

Acute Pain

Acute pain functions as an adaptive biological warning signal, directing attention to an injury or disease, acting as a deterrent against harmful stimuli, and signalling the necessity for immobilization and protection of an injured area. From a disease perspective, acute pain signals the need for an immediate diagnosis of the underlying pathological process causing the pain, such as acute internal hemorrhaging, which may result from a number of diseases and require immediate and appropriate therapy. However, in some cases of acute pain, the severe intensity of the painful stimulus may be disproportionate to its functional intent as a signalling stimulus. Although neurophysiological mechanisms may differentiate acute and chronic pain (Bonica, 1977; Dennis & Melzack, 1977), it is precisely the severe intensity of acute pain and its associated anxiety which may most parsimoniously distinguish acute and chronic pain (Varni, 1983). Thus the experience of pain contains two components, that is, the original sensation and the emotional reaction to this noxious sensation. This reactive component in acute pain represents the fearful or anxious response which can modulate the pain sensation, and in acute pain often serves to intensify the reaction to noxious stimulation.

Chronic Pain

In chronic pain, the fearful or anxious component is absent or greatly diminished, as the child demonstrates an adaptive response to the initial acute experience, with the distinguishing reactive features of chronic pain characterized by chronic pain behaviors (e.g., compensatory posturing, restricted movement, limping, the absence of developmentally appropriate behaviors), depressed mood, or inactivity (Fordyce, 1976; Varni, 1983). These chronic pain reactions may become reinforced independently of the original nociceptive impulses and tissue damage, being maintained by socioenvironmental influences (Varni, Bessman, Russo & Cataldo, 1980). The potential for narcotic analgesic dependence becomes greater because of this chronicity, which only further maintains the pain reaction process (Fordyce, 1976; Varni & Gilbert, 1982). Eventually, chronic pain reactions may be emitted completely independent of the original organic pathology and persist even after the pathogenic factor has resolved (Bonica, 1977). This stands in marked contrast to the acute pain reaction, which appears to be more closely associated with the pathogenic factor or noxious stimulus. The distinctions between acute and chronic pain will become more evident when illustrated by the treatment descriptions in the following sections on acute and chronic pain management.

TREATMENT

Varni (Varni, 1983; Varni, Katz, & Dash, 1982) has delineated four categories of pediatric pain: (1) pain associated with a disease state (for example, hemophilia, arthritis, sickle cell anemia); (2) pain associated with an observable physical injury or trauma (e.g., burns, lacerations, fractures); (3) pain not associated with a well-defined or specific disease state or identifiable physical injury (e.g., recurrent abdominal pain syndrome, migraine and tension headaches); and (4) pain associated with medical or dental procedures (e.g., lumbar punctures, bone marrow aspirations, surgery, injections).

Although pharmacotherapy may have a role in certain acute and chronic pain cases (Lacouture, Gaudreault, & Lovejoy, 1984), for children nonpharmacologic methods are generally preferred for chronic and recurrent pain. Recently cognitive-behavioral interventions have been the subject of increasing investigation in the management of acute and chronic pain in children (Varni, Jay, Masek, & Thompson, in press). The primary cognitive-behavioral treatment techniques utilized in the management of pediatric pain may be categorized as (1) *pain perception regulation* modalities through such self-regulatory processes as guided imagery, meditation, and progressive muscle relaxation, and (2) *pain behavior regulation* which identifies and modifies the socioenvironmental factors which may influence pain expression and rehabilitation (Varni, 1983). The self-regulation techniques share common features with self-hypnosis, autogenic therapy, meditation, progressive muscle relaxation, and biofeedback training. Laboratory research on experimental pain has indicated the role of distraction, dissociation or refocusing of attention from thoughts concerned with pain, anxiety reduction, suggestions of pain relief, and the imagination of past experiences that are incompatible with pain as potent cognitive variables in the reduction of pain perception (Hilgard, 1975). On the other hand, the pain behavior regulation modality follows the socioenvironmental modification approach initially developed for adult chronic pain patients (Fordyce, 1976). Although similar mechanisms may be operating in both pain perception regulation and pain behavior regulation (e.g., distraction from pain perception as the patient concentrates on emitting developmentally appropriate behaviors or increases in mobility and sleep as pain perception decreases), the focus of treatment has typically identified one or the other treatment modality as the primary management strategy. Following the four pain categories identified by Varni (Varni, 1983; Varni, Katz, & Dash,

1982), the next four sections of this chapter will illustrate some of the current biobehavioral treatment approaches for pediatric pain.

PAIN ASSOCIATED WITH A DISEASE STATE

Chronic Arthritic Pain in Hemophilia

Hemophilia represents a congenital hereditary disorder of blood coagulation, characterized by recurrent, unpredictable internal bleeding episodes affecting any body part, especially the joints and extremities. Repeated hemorrhages into the joint areas (hemarthroses) eventually result in a condition similar to osteoarthritis, a chronic disease characterized by destruction of articular cartilage, pathological bone formation, and impaired function (Sokoloff, 1975). Chronic degenerative arthritis represents the most frequent problem confronting the physician who manages the care of adolescent and adult hemophiliacs, with an estimated 75 percent of hemophilic adolescents and adults demonstrating one or more affected joints (Dietrich, 1976). Antiinflammatory drugs may be employed but are of limited usefulness, with analgesic abuse and dependency of constant concern (Varni & Gilbert, 1982).

Whereas acute pain in the hemophiliac is associated with a specific bleeding episode, chronic arthritic pain represents a sustained condition over an extended period of time. Thus pain perception in the hemophiliac truly represents a complex psychophysiological event, complicated by the existence of both acute bleeding pain and chronic arthritic pain, requiring differential treatment strategies (Varni, 1981a,b). More specifically, acute pain of hemorrhage provides a functional signal, indicating the necessity of intravenous infusion of factor replacement, which temporarily replaces the missing clotting factor and converts the clotting status to normal, allowing a functional blood clot to form. Arthritic pain, on the other hand, represents a potentially debilitating chronic condition which may result in impaired life functioning and analgesic dependence (Varni & Gilbert, 1982). Consequently the development of an effective alternative to analgesic abuse and dependency in the reduction of perceived chronic arthritic pain, while *not* interfering with the essential functional signal of acute bleeding pain, has been the goal of the behavioral medicine approach to hemophilia pain management (Varni, 1981a,b; Varni & Gilbert, 1982).

The following treatment techniques were developed after an intensive preintervention survey with a number of hemophilic patients who experienced severe arthritic pain. All reported reduction in perceived arthritic pain associated with increased body warmth, as experienced during warm weather and hot showers. These findings were consistent with data from 30 patients with rheumatoid arthritis or osteoarthritis, with 27 of these patients reporting pain relief and increased range of motion in the involved joint associated with past experiences of warmth or massage (White, 1973). In the same study, application of a counterirritant (10 percent menthol and 15 percent methyl salicylate) produced a sensation of heat and active tissue hyperemia resulting in decreased pain perception and increased range of motion. A logical extrapolation of this information and the medical literature on arthritis management (Swezey, 1978) subsequently resulted in the training of increased body temperature specific to the affected arthritic joints, with a thermal biofeedback instrument providing the physiological assessment of skin temperature over the targeted arthritic joint. It was further reasoned that increased body temperature specific to a joint area was a function of vasodilation which would not obfuscate the adaptive value of acute hemorrhage pain. Finally, the most severe and intense site of arthritic pain was targeted for initial intervention, with the rationale that other, less severe sites would covary accordingly within a functional, generalized, biophysiological response class. Since earlier findings by Wasserman et al. (1968) had demonstrated abnormal electromyographic readings in muscles adjacent to arthritic joints, relaxation techniques were included as an additional component in the treatment protocol. Following a multiple-baseline design across subjects, training in the self-regulation of arthritic pain consisted of three sequential phases: (1) A 25-step progressive muscle relaxation sequence involving the alternative tensing and relaxing of major muscle groups; (2) Meditative breathing exercises, consisting of medium deep breaths inhaled through the nose and slowly exhaled through the mouth—while exhaling, the patient was instructed to say the word "relax" silently to himself, and to initially describe out loud and subsequently visualize the word relax in warm colors, as if written in colored chalk on a blackboard; and, finally, (3) Guided imagery training was begun after the induction procedures in phases one and two were completed. Initially the patient was instructed to imagine himself actually in a scene previously experienced as warm and pain free, not simply to observe himself there. The scene was evoked by a detailed multisensory description by the therapist, and then subsequently described out loud by the patient. Once the scene was clearly visualized by the patient, the therapist's suggestions included imagining the gentle flow of blood from the forehead down all the body parts to the joint, images of warm colors such as red and orange, and the sensations of warm sand and sun on the involved joint. Further suggestions consisted of statements indicating reduction of pain as the joint progressively felt warmer and more comfortable. As during baseline, the thermal biofeedback unit served as the physiological assessment device rather than as a training instrument, with the thermistor placed on the site of greatest arthritic pain and the patient instructed to attempt actively to increase the temperature at the joint site using the guided imagery techniques. The patients were also instructed to practice the techniques at home a minimum of two daily 15-minute sessions and were encouraged to individualize and actively explore new cognitive strategies in addition to imagining a warm, pleasant scene of their choice, as long as it involved thermal imagery. Self-regulation training was clearly effective in significantly reducing the perceived chronic arthritic pain and analgesic need in all patients, maintained over an extended follow-up (Varni, 1981a,b; Varni & Gilbert, 1982)

Pain and Analgesia Management Complicated by Factor VIII Inhibitor in Hemophilia

The treatment of children with hemophilia has evidenced significant advances in recent years as a result of the development of factor replacement products, home infusion programs, and the opportunity for comprehensive care through regional hemophilia centers (Dietrich, 1976). Unfortunately approximately 10 percent of hemophilic children develop an inhibitor to factor VIII, presenting a serious problem in the management of bleeding episodes. Although the bleeding frequency is no different, the neutralization of factor VIII replacement by an inhibitor (antibody) makes the control of bleeding ineffective. A recent advance in the treatment of hemophilic patients with inhibitors has been the use of prothrombin-complex concentrates (PCC), effecting some level of hemostasis through apparent activated by-products present in the reconstituted preparation. However, clinical reports have indicated the lack of complete effectiveness of these products (Parry & Bloom, 1978). The pain associated with uncontrolled hemorrhage can be extremely severe, with narcotic analgesics traditionally prescribed. Thus although the acute pain of hemorrhage provides a functional signal indicating the necessity of factor replacement therapy, in the hemophilic child with factor VIII inhibitor, the intensity of the pain supercedes its functional intent, with analgesic dependence of constant concern. Consequently, an effective alternative to analgesic dependence in the reduction of perceived pain in the patient with an inhibitor has been greatly needed.

Varni, Gilbert, and Dietrich (1981) reported on a study involving a 9-year-old hemophilic child with factor VIII inhibitor. At 4 years of age, when the inhibitor developed and subsequent factor VIII replacement therapy became impossible, the patient began to require narcotics in order to tolerate the pain of each hemorrhage. Progressively, the need for pain medication increased both for bleeding pain and for arthritic pain in his left knee secondary to degenerative arthropathy. Since the arthritic pain eventually occurred almost daily, the requests for analgesics further increased, so that the acute pain of hemorrhage required ever larger doses for pain relief, even though home PCC therapy and joint immobilization continued for the management of bleeding episodes. As a consequence of bleeding and arthritic pain in the lower extremities, the patient was wheelchair-bound nearly 50 percent of the time, had been hospitalized 16 times in the 4½-year period prior to the study, for a total of 80 days after the development of the inhibitor, with analgesic medication also kept at his school for pain control. The final precipitating event in this steadily worsening cycle occurred during an evening visit to the emergency room because of a very painful and severe left knee hemorrhage which had not responded to home PCC therapy, with the administration of an adult dose of meperidine and I.V. diazepam providing no pain relief.

Training in the self-regulation of pain perception consisted of techniques developed earlier by Varni (1981a,b), with modification in the guided imagery technique (pleasant, distracting imagery rather than thermal imagery) required for the bleeding pain intensity. The patient recorded the severity of pain on a 10-point scale for a 2 ½-week baseline prior to self-regulation training. The average score for both arthritic and bleeding pain during this period was 7, indicating rather intense pain. At a 1-year follow-up after the initiation of the self-regulation training, the patient reported that both arthritic and bleeding pain were reduced to 2 on the scale when he engaged in the self-regulation techniques. In addition to this measure of pain perception, the patient's evaluation at the 1-year follow-up session on a comparative assessment inventory (Varni, 1983) indicated substantial positive changes in arthritic and bleeding pain, mobility, sleep, and general overall functioning. Additional 1-year pre- and post-self-regulation training biobehavioral measures indicated further substantial improvements within a multidimensional assessment paradigm. Narcotic analgesic intake was sharply reduced (meperidine: pre $= 74$ tablets, post $= 0$ tablets; acetaminophen/codeine elixir: pre $= 438$ doses, post $= 78$ doses); physical therapy measures were considerably improved (range of motion of arthritic knee: pre $= 15-105$, post $= 0-140$; quadriceps strength: pre $= 3 +$, post $= 4$); ambulation on stairs was unlimited (pre $= 2-3$ steps maximum, post $=$ no limitation); school days missed were normalized (pre $= 33$ days, post $= 6$); and hospitalizations were not required (pre $= 3$ admissions and 11 total days, post $= 0$).

The analysis of the various parameters assessed in this study suggest a significant improvement across a number of areas. As envisioned by the authors, a deteriorating cycle was evident prior to the intervention, schematically represented as: hemorrhage $\rightarrow$ pain $\rightarrow$ analgesics/joint immobilization $\rightarrow$ atrophy of muscles adjacent to the joints/joint deterioration $\rightarrow$ hemorrhage. Thus as has been previously suggested (Dietrich, 1976), pain induced immobilization results in muscle weakness surrounding the joints, setting the occasion for future hemorrhaging. By breaking this deteriorating cycle at the point of pain severity, the patient was offered the opportunity to decrease immobilization and increase therapeutic activities such as swimming, subsequently improving the strength and range of motion in his left knee, and with this improved ambulatory status, school attendance and general activity level were consequently increased. The possibility that this early intervention may have prevented or reduced the likelihood of later drug abuse must also be considered (Varni & Gilbert,

1982). Finally, it is important to reiterate that these procedures were used for a child with an inhibitor. For the hemophiliac without an inhibitor, bleeding pain serves a functional signal and is best managed with factor replacement therapy. However, in the present case, no effective medical procedure was available to control severe bleeding pain other than powerful narcotic analgesics, clearly an undesirable therapy modality for recurrent pain.

PAIN ASSOCIATED WITH PHYSICAL INJURY

Burns: Chronic Pain Phase

Varni et al. (1980) worked with a 3-year-old child who had been hospitalized for 10 months for the treatment of second and third degree burns to her buttocks, legs, and perineum. The patient's development had been normal previous to the injury; afterward, however, skills were lost and further development was slightly delayed. Scar contractures and subsequent decreased range of motion in both knees made it necessary for the patient to wear Jobst stockings and knee extension splints to prevent contractures, while undergoing a series of operations for plastic surgery. At the time of the initiation of the behavioral program, the patient was exhibiting an array of chronic pain behaviors which interfered significantly with rehabilitation and constructive patient-caregiver interactions. Furthermore, these pain responses appeared to increase both in intensity and frequency of attention seeking and demand avoidance situations. Data were obtained in three different settings: (1) Clinic room where the patient wore the knee extension splints in a contrived setting; (2) Bedroom where the patient wore the splints in the natural hospital environment; and (3) Physical therapy situation during which the physical therapist focused on improved range of motion and independent ambulation.

Three categories of chronic pain behaviors were recorded: (1) Crying, which ranged in intensity from sobbing to screaming; (2) Verbal pain behaviors, which consisted of such statements as "My leg/ankle/foot/stomach hurts," "Ouch," or "I can't stand up"; and (3) Nonverbal pain behaviors consisting of any gestural response expressing pain or discomfort, such as facial grimaces, rubbing her legs or buttocks, or not standing. In addition, a rehabilitative activity measure, number of steps descended, was measured in physical therapy, since it was essential for improving the child's range of motion and independent ambulation.

During the baseline assessment, it became evident that the child's pain behaviors were a function of adult attention and demand situations. In the absence of adult presence or demands for ambulation, chronic pain behaviors were noticeably infrequent. Since the baseline assessment demonstrated that the chronic pain behaviors were influenced by socioenvironmental factors, treatment focused on rearranging the existing contingencies. A combination of an intrasubject multiple-baseline design across settings and a reversal design was employed to determine the functional effects of the behavioral program on the patient's pain behaviors. Multiple baselines were begun simultaneously in all three settings, with treatment implemented first in the physical therapy department, while baseline assessment continued in the clinic and bedroom. Shortly afterward, treatment began in the clinic setting and then subsequently in the bedroom. Brief reversals back to baseline conditions were conducted in the clinic and physical therapy setting to further test the significance of the intervention.

The objective data on the chronic pain and rehabilitative behaviors obtained throughout baseline and treatment conditions demonstrated the therapeutic effectiveness of the behavioral program. In addition, other clinically significant changes were observed. At the beginning of the study, the child's behaviors had severely disrupted her physical as well as her emotional rehabilitation. Physical therapy was essentially terminated because of the patient's interfering pain behaviors. Two patterns emerged when the patient was placed in her bedroom in the crib with knee extension splints on. First, the child would struggle until she had removed the splints, resulting in further contractures and the need for additional plastic surgery. Second, if she failed to remove the splints, her crying would intensify to the point of screaming. At times she would fall asleep, exhausted, and continue sobbing well into the naptime hour. Other times, she would continue screaming until, in consideration of the other children, the nursing staff would remove her to a separate room for the remainder of the hour. Thus pain behaviors during the pretreatment period resulted in the child being isolated from the other children, interfering with the normalization and socialization processes important for a child with a history of prolonged hospitalization. Following the behavioral intervention, a number of concomitant responses were noted. Whereas the child initially resisted splinting attempts, she subsequently began requesting to assist, saying, for example, "I'll do it," "I want to help you." She began to make positive statements about her accomplishments instead of statements of pain and resistance to rehabilitation. Rather than seeking attention from her caregivers for pain behaviors, there was a shift to the utilization of "well" behaviors to attract social attention and praise.

Fordyce (1976), in his extensive work with adult chronic pain, has suggested that during periods of initial trauma and its resultant pain, the patient has many opportunities for the pairing of environmental stimuli to feelings of pain. Whether or not the subjective experience of pain abates over the course of time may be independent of the pain behaviors which the patient displays. While it is not possible to determine if the patient actually feels pain or simply displays the associated behaviors, in the present case no further pain displays were observed in the treatment environments after the onset of the behavioral program. As further suggested by Fordyce

(1976), through learning the patient may actually come to experience pain in certain circumstances in excess of the accompanying physical basis for such pain, or even in the absence of a physical basis for perceived pain. In such cases, or in cases like the present one in which the pain behavior served the patient's immediate needs while hindering long-term rehabilitation, the behavioral program provides an essential component in the comprehensive management of pediatric chronic pain.

PAIN NOT ASSOCIATED WITH PHYSICAL INJURY OR A DISEASE STATE

Migraine and Tension Headaches

Pediatric headache represents an exemplary area demonstrating the necessity for an interdisciplinary assessment in determining the etiology and maintaining conditions of pain perception and pain complaints, and in subsequently selecting an appropriate treatment approach (Shinnar & D'Souza, 1981). For example, headache report may increase once the child discovers that this strategy successfully allows him or her to avoid aversive or negative school situations, such as an impending exam. What may develop is a self-perpetuating cycle whereby the child progressively falls further and further behind in school, subsequently setting the occasion for more negative school situations and resultant headache-avoidance behaviors. This does not imply that the child originally did not experience a headache or that the headaches do not continue to reoccur, but rather that the intensity and frequency of headache perception and complaint may be influenced by stress and other socioenvironmental factors. On the other hand, the chronic, recurrent headache complaint may be a symptom of a brain tumor or intracranial hemorrhage (Curless & Corrigan, 1976; Tomasi, 1979). Evidence of antecedent brain damage or brain dysfunction of possible etiological significance in pediatric recurrent headaches has ranged as high as 69 percent in one clinic sample (Millicap, 1978), whereas other investigators studying pediatric migraine and tension headaches point to socioenvironmental stress factors as the most frequent precipitating event (Bille, 1981; Brown, 1977; Moe, 1978; Shinnar & D'Souza, 1981). Given the rather high prevalence rates of pediatric migraine and tension headaches (Deubner, in a 1977 study of a sample of 600 10- to 20-year olds, found that 22.1 percent of the girls and 15.5 percent of the boys reported migraine headaches), a successful biobehavioral treatment approach may have an impact on a significant number of children in pain.

Masek (1982) utilized a biobehavioral treatment package with 20 children, ages 6 to 12 years, diagnosed as demonstrating migraine headaches. A multiple-baseline across subjects design was used to evaluate the effectiveness of the program, with the children randomly assigned to one of four baseline conditions: 3, 6, 9, or 12 weeks of monitoring headache activity prior to starting treatment. Treatment consisted of frontalis EMG bio-feedback training, meditative breathing and behavioral management/parent training. Treatment effectiveness was determined by examining the daily headache diary, which provided data on headache frequency, duration of attacks, total hours of headache, intensity of pain and medication usage. A total of 18 children experienced at least a 50 percent reduction in both total hours of headache per week and intensity of pain. A subsequent report by Fentress and Masek (1982) involved a controlled group design with children aged 8 to 12 years. The three groups were: (1) Treatment group receiving frontalis EMG biofeedback, meditative breathing training, and behavioral management/parent training; (2) Treatment group receiving the same treatment package as above, except without frontalis EMG biofeedback training and with the addition of progressive muscle relaxation training; and (3) Waiting list control group. The results showed a statistically significant treatment effect for both treatment groups as compared to the control group on the measures: headache frequency, duration of attacks, total hours of headache, and intensity of pain. No effect was found for medication use, which was very low prior to biobehavioral treatment.

Recurrent Abdominal Pain

Oster (1972) studied the prevalence rates of recurrent abdominal pain, headache, and limb pains in an 8-year longitudinal study of school-age children and adolescents between 6 and 19 years of age. The prevalence of recurrent headaches was 20.6 percent; of recurrent abdominal pain, 14.4 percent; and of recurrent limb or "growing" pain, 15.5 percent, with a higher prevalence in all three categories of pain for girls than for boys. From a prognostic perspective, Christensen and Mortensen (1975) conducted a 28-year follow-up investigation of 34 patients who were initially diagnosed during childhood as evidencing recurrent abdominal pain (RAP) in comparison to a control group without childhood RAP. The average age of the clinical and control populations at follow-up was 35.9 and 36.4 years, respectively. At follow-up, 53 percent of the clinical group reported gastrointestinal pain consistent with a diagnosis of irritable colon syndrome, peptic ulcer/gastritis, and duodenal ulcer, as well as milder symptoms such as diarrhea, constipation, and meteorism (abdominal or intestinal distension by gas). Eighty-nine percent of the clinical group reported that these symptoms were provoked by stress. In contrast, only 29 percent of the control group reported gastrointestinal pain as adults. Nongastrointestinal pain symptoms were also more frequent among the clinical patients (32 percent) than among the controls (13 percent), with such complaints as migraine and tension headaches, back pain, and gynecological pain. There were no differences between the clinical and control groups in the incidence of abdominal pain in their children (average age, 8.5 and 9.3

years, respectively). However, in combining the two groups, 28 percent of those children whose parents were complaining of abdominal pain at the time of the follow-up evidenced RAP, whereas only 7 percent of those children whose parents had no abdominal pain at follow-up reported RAP.

Although pediatric chronic, recurrent abdominal pain may be a symptom of a spinal cord tumor (Buck & Bodensteiner, 1981; Eeg-Olofsson, Carlsson, & Jeppsson, 1981), chronic intermittent volvulus (Janik & Ein, 1979), lactose or sorbitol malabsorption (Hyams, 1982; Lebenthal, Rossi, Nord, & Branski, 1981; Wald, Chandra, Fisher, Gartner, & Zitelli, 1982), only an estimated 5 percent of childhood RAP has an organic etiology (Maddison, 1977).

Further, when compared to children not evidencing RAP, childhood RAP patients do *not* show a significant differential biobehavioral response to an acute laboratory induced stress (cold pressor stimulus) on autonomic (peripheral vasomotor and heart rate), somatic (forearm EMG), subjective (pain intensity and distress), and behavioral (facial expression) responses when recorded during baseline, stressor and recovery periods (Feuerstein, Barr, Francoeur, Houle, & Rafman, 1982). Rather, a high frequency of such potential socioenvironmental factors as emotional stress, parental abdominal pain complaints, and recurrent school absences have been implicated as causal factors of childhood RAP (Berger, Honig, & Liebman, 1977; Michener, 1981). Significantly, in a long-term follow-up study of 161 children with RAP, approximately 20 percent underwent surgical or medical treatments of doubtful necessity; that is, no organic cause was evident (Stickler & Murphy, 1979). Thus, as in pediatric headache, an extensive interdisciplinary and comprehensive biobehavioral assessment is mandated prior to any intervention program.

The biobehavioral treatment of pediatric recurrent abdominal pain is relatively unexplored thus far. Sank and Biglan (1974) and Miller and Kratochwill (1979) have reported success with two children utilizing a token economy system to rearrange the socioenvironmental conditions apparently maintaining RAP for these two children. Given the prevalence of RAP, it is somewhat surprising that more intervention studies from a biobehavioral perspective have not been conducted thus far.

PAIN AND ANXIETY ASSOCIATED WITH MEDICAL AND DENTAL PROCEDURES

Even routine well-child examinations may be a source of distress for children, influenced by developmental factors, clinician behavior, and mother-child interactions (Heffernan & Azarnoff, 1971; Hyson, Snyder, & Andujar, 1982; Shaw & Routh, 1982). Although a preventive approach based on modeling in the school setting has been encouraging in reducing medical fears in a general pediatric population (Roberts, Wurtele, Boone,

Ginther, & Elkins, 1982), intervention approaches with clinical populations have emphasized procedural and sensory information regarding the medical procedure (Johnson, Kirchhoff, & Endress, 1975) and relaxation/guided imagery training (Kohen, 1980).

Bone Marrow Aspirations and Lumbar Punctures

Conditioned anxiety in response to recurrent, painful medical procedures such as bone marrow aspirations, lumbar punctures and venipunctures occurs frequently in childhood cancer patients (Kellerman & Varni, 1982). Katz, Kellerman, and Siegel (1980) studied 115 children with cancer undergoing bone marrow aspirations in order to develop a reliable and valid measurement scale of behavioral distress. Given the difficulty in distinguishing between anxiety and acute pain, since these terms refer to constructs, behavioral distress has been defined as a general term encompassing behaviors of negative affect, including anxiety, fear, and acute pain (Katz, Kellerman, & Siegel, 1981). Katz et al. (1980) found that behavioral distress (e.g., crying, clinging, screaming, verbal statements of pain or fear) in response to bone marrow aspirations was virtually ubiquitous and did not habituate in the children studied, clearly suggesting the need for clinical intervention.

Recent work by Jay and her associates (Jay, Elliott, Ozolins, & Olson, 1982; Jay, Ozolins, Elliott, & Caldwell, 1983) typifies the current state-of-the-art in the assessment and management of the extreme anxiety and severe acute pain in pediatric cancer patients undergoing bone marrow aspirations and lumbar punctures (see also Kellerman, Zeltzer, Ellenberg, & Dash,1983; LeBaron & Zeltzer, 1984; Zeltzer & LeBaron, 1982). Jay et al. (1983) developed the Observation Scale of Behavioral Distress (OSBD), a revised version of the Procedural Behavior Rating Scale (Katz et al., 1980), to assess behavioral distress in children with cancer undergoing bone marrow aspiration procedures. The OSBD consists of 11 operationally defined behaviors indicative of anxiety and/or pain in children. Given the difficulty in distinguishing between anxiety and acute pain during noxious medical procedures, behavioral distress has been defined as a general term encompassing both constructs (Katz et al., 1981). The OSBD behavioral categories and their intensity weights are: Cry (1.5), Scream (4.0), Physical Restraint (4.0), Verbal Resistance (2.5), Requests Emotional Support (2.0), Muscular Rigidity (2.5), Nervous Behavior (1.0), and Information Seeking (1.5). The behaviors were recorded in continuous 15-second intervals, with interobserver reliability averaging 84 percent. In addition to the behavioral observations, Jay et al. (1983) also had the children rate their pain on a Pain Thermometer (a numeric scale from 0 to 100). An assessment battery was administered both to the parent and to the child. The child was administered the Norwicki-Strickland Locus of Control Scale for Children and the Spielberger State-Trait Anxiety Inventory for Children. The parent was administered the Parent Evaluation Questionnaire, the Spielberger State-Trait Anxiety Inventory, the Beck Depression Inventory, and the Rotter Internal-External Locus of Control Scale. The OSBD total distress scores were significantly correlated with the children's Trait Anxiety scores and their Pain Thermometer ratings, lending support to the validity of the OSBD as a measure of anxiety and pain. Further, a significant relationship was found between parental anxiety and the children's behavioral distress during the bone marrow aspirations.

Having developed a reliable and valid assessment instrument (the OSBD) (see also Jay & Elliott, 1984), Jay et al. (1982) next developed a cognitive-behavioral treatment package to manage the children's distress during bone marrow aspirations and/or lumbar punctures. The treatment package consisted of the following components: breathing exercises, guided imagery, filmed modeling, behavioral rehearsal, and positive reinforcement. The results indicated that the program was highly effective in reducing behavioral distress for nine of the ten children treated (ages 3 ½ to 9 years), with considerable variability found in the maintenance of the initial therapeutic gains. Current work by Jay and her associates (Jay, Elliott, Katz, & Siegel, 1984) has further developed the cognitive-behavioral treatment package, consisting of stress-inoculation training, distraction, relaxation, altering attributions, emotive imagery, and rehearsal/practice. Preliminary results of an ongoing 3-year treatment-outcome study (1982-85) at Childrens Hospital of Los Angeles further support the efficacy of the intervention package in reducing the distress of 30 children (ages 4 to 14) with leukemia undergoing bone marrow aspirations. Reductions in distress (as compared to a control condition) were observed across a variety of response systems, including behavioral distress, self-reported pain, and physiological arousal.

Finally, Katz, Kellerman and Ellenberg (1984) randomly assigned 36 children (ages 6 to 12 years) with acute lymphoblastic leukemia either to hypnosis or play comparison groups. The children were selected based on their behavioral distress during baseline bone marrow aspirations, and received the interventions prior to their next three procedures. Dependent measures included the revised Procedure Behavior Rating Scale (PBRS-r), nurse ratings, and self-report measures of pain and fear. The major results indicated an interaction effect between sex and treatment group, with girls exhibiting less distress in the hypnosis condition while boys tolerated the procedures better in the play condition. Katz et al. (1984) suggest that future studies on procedural distress include gender as a variable which may facilitate the match between children and intervention techniques.

Dental Procedures

The assessment of children's anxiety during dental procedures has included subjective, behavioral, and physiological measures. The primary anxiety reduction techniques utilized for children in dental situations have included components of filmed modeling, relaxation, and coping-skills training. Melamed, Weinstein, Hawes, and Katin-Borland (1975) found the filmed modeling of a child successfully coping with a dental procedure an effective preparation for children having no prior experience with the actual dental setting.

Siegel and Peterson (1980, 1981) found that teaching specific coping skills and/or providing sensory information about the dental experience were both effective in reducing children's anxiety during dental treatment, as manifested by lower levels of disruptive and uncooperative behaviors, lower ratings of anxiety and discomfort, and lower levels of physiological arousal (radial pulse rate). The children were taught to use several coping techniques in a 30-minute session prior to the dental treatment (anesthetic injection and restoration), consisting of relaxation, distracting (pleasant) imagery, and calming self-instructions. The sensory information provided the children included what to expect at the dentist's office, such as the sights, sounds, and sensations of the dental procedure; they also heard tape-recorded sounds of the dental equipment, such as the drill. Nocella and Kaplan (1982) studied 30 children between the ages of 5 and 13 years with prior dental experience. The majority of the children were scheduled for restorations and the rest were scheduled for extractions, or a combination of restorations and extractions. The children were randomly assigned to a cognitive-behavioral (coping skills) group, an attention-control group, or a no-treatment control group. The children receiving the cognitive-behavioral treatment were taught a combination of coping strategies, including the identification of stimuli (events) which might evoke anxiety, deep breathing exercises, muscle relaxation, and positive self-instructions ("If I get scared or worried I tell myself to 'relax' and I let myself relax my whole body; I tell myself, this is a good dentist, I'm doing good, I can handle this, I'm doing terrific."). Additionally, the children were instructed to imagine their pending visit to the dentist, utilizing their positive self-statements, deep breathing exercises, and the word "relax" to facilitate coping with procedural anxiety. The cognitive-behavioral training session required only 15 minutes prior to the dental treatment. During the dental procedure, the children's behavior was recorded on a behavior checklist consisting of: facial grimaces, restlessness, moving arms and/or legs, sitting up, gripping chair, and verbalizations. The results demonstrated that the cognitive-behavioral treatment group evidenced significantly fewer disruptive behaviors during the dental procedures in comparison to both control groups.

CONCLUSION

The initial success of a substantial body of clinical biobehavioral research across a number of pediatric pain syndromes developed with a relatively small population of children now warrants additional clinical biobehavioral research with larger pediatric population samples. The inclusion of objective parameters (e.g., analgesics, activities of daily living, ambulation, hospitalizations, and school attendance), hypothesized to covary with self-reports of pain intensity, need to be systematically included in all future studies. The interrelationship between these objective measures and child self-report will provide a more comprehensive assessment of the efficacy of the biobehavioral management of pediatric pain within the field of behavioral pediatrics (Varni, 1983).

REFERENCES

Abu-Saad, H. (1981). The assessment of pain in children. *Issues in Comprehensive Pediatric Nursing, 5,* 327–335.

Beales, J.G. (1982).The assessment and management of pain in children. In P. Karoly, J.J. Steffen, & D.J. O'Grady (Eds.), *Child health psychology: Concepts and issues* (pp.154–179). New York: Pergamon.

Berger, H.G., Honig, P.J., & Liebman, R. (1977). Recurrent abdominal pain: Gaining control of the symptom. *American Journal of Diseases of Children, 131,* 1340–1344.

Bibace,R., & Walsh, M.E. (1981). Children's conceptions of illness. In R. Bibace & M.E. Walsh (Eds.), *Children's conceptions of health, illness and bodily functions* (pp. 31–48). San Francisco: Jossey-Bass.

Bille, B. (1981). Migraine in childhood and its prognosis. *Cephalalgia, 1,* 71-75.

Bonica, J.J. (1977). Neurophysiologic and pathologic aspects of acute and chronic pain. *Archives of Surgery, 112,* 750–761.

Brewster, A.B. (1982). Chronically ill hospitalized childrens' concepts of their illness. *Pediatrics, 69,* 355–362.

Brown, J.K. (1977). Migraine and migraine equivalents in children. *Developmental Medicine and Child Neurology, 19,* 683–692.

Buck, E.D., & Bodensteiner, J. (1981). Thoracic cord tumor appearing as recurrent abdominal pain. *American Journal of Diseases of Children, 135,* 574–575.

Christensen, M.F., & Mortensen, O. (1975). Long-term prognosis in children with recurrent abdominal pain. *Archives of Disease in Childhood, 50,* 110–114.

Craig, K.D. (1982). Modeling and social learning factors in chronic pain. In J.J. Bonica, U. Lindblom, & A. Iggo (Eds.), *Advances in pain research and therapy* (Vol. 5). New York: Raven.

Curless, R.G., & Corrigan, J.J. (1976). Headache in classical hemophilia: The risk of diagnostic procedures. *Child's Brain, 2,* 187–194.

Dennis, S.G., & Melzack, R. (1977). Pain-signalling systems in the dorsal and ventral spinal cord. *Pain, 4,* 97–132.

Deubner, D.C. (1977). An epidemiologic study of migraine and headache in 10-20 year olds. *Headache, 17,* 173–180.

Dietrich, S.L. (1976). Medical management of hemophilia. In D.C. Boone (Ed.), *Comprehensive management of hemophilia.* Philadelphia: F.A. Davis.

Eeg-Olofsson, O., Carlsson, E., & Jeppsson, S. (1981). Recurrent abdominal pains as the first symptom of a spinal cord tumor. *Acta Paediatrica Scandinavica, 70,* 595–597.

Eland, J.M. (1981). Minimizing pain associated with prekindergarten intramuscular injections. *Issues in Comprehensive Pediatric Nursing, 5,* 361–372.

Fabrega, H., & Tyma, S. (1976). Language and cultural influences in the description of pain. *British Journal of Medical Psychology, 49,* 349–371.

Feldman, W.S., & Varni, J.W. (1985). Conceptualizations of health and illness by children with spina bifida. *Children's Health Care, 13,* 102–108.

Fentress, D., & Masek, B. (1982, November). Behavioral treatment of pediatric migraine. Paper presented at the Annual Meeting of the Association for Advancement of Behavior Therapy, Los Angeles.

Feuerstein, M., Barr, R.G., Francoeur, T.E., Houle, M., & Rafman, S. (1982). Potential biobehavioral mechanisms of recurrent abdominal pain in children. *Pain, 13,* 287–298.

Fordyce, W.E. (1976). *Behavioral methods for chronic pain and illness.* St. Louis: Mosby.

Gildea, J.H. & Quirk, T.R. (1977). Assessing the pain experience in children. *Nursing Clinics of North America, 12,* 631–637.

Heffernan, M., & Azarnoff, P. (1971). Factors in reducing children's anxiety about clinic visits. *HSMHA Health Reports, 86,* 1131–1135.

Hilgard, E.R. (1975). The alleviation of pain by hypnosis. *Pain, 1,* 213–231.

Hyams, J.S. (1982). Chronic abdominal pain caused by sorbitol malabsorption. *Journal of Pediatrics, 100,* 772–773.

Hyson, M.C., Snyder, S.S., & Andujar, E.M. (1982). Helping children cope with checkups: How good is the "good patient?" *Children's Health Care, 10,* 139–144.

Janik, J.S., & Ein, S.H. (1979). Normal intestinal rotation with non-fixation: A cause of chronic abdominal pain. *Journal of Pediatric Surgery, 14,* 670–674.

Jay, S.M., & Elliott, C. (1984). Behavioral observation scales for measuring children's distress: The effects of increased methodological rigor. *Journal of Consulting and Clinical Psychology, 52,* 1106–1107.

Jay, S.M., Elliott, C., Katz, E.R. & Siegel, S.E. (1984, August). Stress reduction in children undergoing painful medical procedures. Paper presented at the Annual Meeting of the American Psychological Association, Toronto, Canada.

Jay, S.M., Elliott, C.H., Ozolins, M., & Olson, R.A. (1982, August). Behavioral management of children's distress during painful medical procedures. Paper presented at the Annual Meeting of the American Psychological Association, Washington, DC.

Jay, S.M., Ozolins, M., Elliott, C.H., & Caldwell, S. (1983). Assessment of children's distress during painful medical procedures. *Health Psychology, 2,* 133–147.

Johnson, J.E., Kirchhoff, K.T., & Endress, M.P. (1975). Altering children's distress behavior during orthopedic cast removal. *Nursing Research, 24,* 404–410.

Katz, E.R., Kellerman, J., & Ellenberg, L. (1984). Hypnosis in the reduction of acute pain and distress in children with cancer undergoing aversive medical procedures: Does sex make the difference? Manuscript submitted for publication.

Katz, E.R., Kellerman, J., & Siegel, S.E. (1981). Anxiety as an affective focus in the clinical study of acute behavioral distress: A reply to Schacham and Daut. *Journal of Consulting and Clinical Psychology, 49,* 470–471

Katz, E.R., Kellerman, J., & Siegel, S.E. (1980). Distress behavior in children with cancer undergoing medical procedures: Developmental considerations. *Journal of Consulting and Clinical Psychology, 48,* 356–365.

Katz, E.R., Varni, J.W., & Jay, S.M. (1984). Behavioral assessment and management of pediatric pain. In M. Hersen, R.M. Eisler, & P.M. Miller (Eds.), *Progress in behavior modification* (Vol. 18). Orlando, FL: Academic.

Kellerman, J., & Varni, J.W. (1982). Pediatric hematology/oncology. In D.C. Russo & J.W. Varni (Eds.), *Behavioral pediatrics: Research and practice.* New York: Plenum.

Kellerman, J., Zeltzer, L., Ellenberg, L., & Dash, J. (1983). Hypnosis for the reduction of the acute pain and anxiety associated with medical procedures. *Journal of Adolescent Health Care, 4,* 85–90.

Kohen, D.P. (1980). Relaxation/mental imagery (self-hypnosis) and pelvic examinations in adolescents. *Journal of Developmental and Behavioral Pediatrics, 1,* 180–186.

Lacouture, P.G., Gaudreault, P., & Lovejoy, F.H. (1984). Chronic pain of childhood: A pharmacologic approach. *Pediatric Clinics of North America, 31,* 1133–1151.

LeBaron, S., & Zeltzer, L. (1984). Assessment of acute pain and anxiety in children and adolescents by self-reports, observer reports, and a behavior checklist. *Journal of Consulting and Clinical Psychology, 52,* 729–738.

Lebenthal, E., Rossi, T.M., Nord, K.S., & Branski, D. (1981). Recurrent abdominal pain and lactose absorption in children. *Pediatrics, 67,* 828–832.

Maddison, T.G. (1977). Recurrent abdominal pain in children. *Medical Journal of Australia, 1,* 708–710.

Masek, B.J. (1982, March). Behavioral medicine treatment of pediatric migraine. Paper presented at the Annual Meeting of the Society of Behavioral Medicine, Chicago.

Masek, B.J., Russo, D.C., & Varni, J.W. (1984). Behavioral approaches to the management of chronic pain in children. *Pediatric Clinics of North America, 31,* 1113–1131.

Melamed, B.G., Weinstein, D., Hawes, R., & Katin-Borland, M. (1975). Reduction of fear-related dental management problems using filmed modeling. *Journal of the American Dental Association, 90,* 822–826.

Melzack, R. (1975). The McGill Pain Questionnaire: Major properties and scoring methods. *Pain, 1,* 277–299.

Michener, W.M. (1981). An approach to recurrent abdominal pain in children. *Primary Care, 8,* 277–283.

Miller, A.J., & Kratochwill, T.R. (1979). Reduction of frequent stomachache complaints by time out. *Behavior Therapy, 10,* 211–218.

Millicap, J.G. (1978). Recurrent headaches in 100 children: Electroencephalographic abnormalities and response to Phenytoin (dilantin). *Child's Brain, 4,* 95–105.

Moe, P.G. (1978). Headaches in children: Meeting the challenge of management. *Postgraduate Medicine, 63,* 169–174.

Nocella, J., & Kaplan, R.M. (1982). Training children to cope with dental treatment. *Journal of Pediatric Psychology, 7,* 175–178.

Oster, J. (1972). Recurrent abdominal pain, headache and limb pains in children and adolescents. *Pediatrics, 50,* 429–436.

Parry, D.H., & Bloom, A.L. (1978). Failure of factor VIII inhibitor bypassing activity (Feiba) to secure hemostasis in hemophilic patients with antibodies. *Clinical Pathology, 31,* 1102–1105.

Perrin, E.C., & Gerrity, P.S. (1981). There's a demon in your belly: Children's understanding of illness. *Pediatrics, 67,* 841–849.

Perrin, E.C., & Perrin, J.M. (1983). Clinician's assessments of childrens' understanding of illness. *American Journal of Diseases of Children, 137,* 874–878.

Roberts, M.D., Wurtele, S.K., Boone, R.R., Ginther, L.J., & Elkins, P.E. (1982). Reduction of medical fears by use of modeling: A preventive application in a general population of children. *Journal of Pediatric Psychology, 6,* 293–300.

Sank, L.I., & Biglan, A. (1974). Operant treatment of a case of recurrent abdominal pain in a 10-year-old boy. *Behavior Therapy, 5,* 677–681.

Schechter, N.L. (1984). Recurrent pains in children: An overview and an approach. *Pediatric Clinics of North America, 31,* 949–968.

Scott, R. (1978). It hurts red. A preliminary study of children's perception of pain. *Perceptual and Motor Skills, 47,* 787–791.

Shaw, E.G., & Routh, D.K. (1982). Effect of mother presence on children's reaction to aversive procedures. *Journal of Pediatric Psychology, 7,* 33–42.

Shinnar, S., & D'Souza, B.U. (1981). The diagnosis and management of headaches in childhood. *Pediatric Clinics of North America, 29*, 79–94.

Siegel, L.J., & Peterson, L. (1980). Maintenance effects of coping skills and sensory information on young children's response to repeated dental procedures. *Behavior Therapy, 12*, 530–535.

Siegel, L.J., & Peterson, L. (1981). Stress reduction in young dental patients through coping skills and sensory information. *Journal of Consulting and Clinical Psychology, 48*, 785–787.

Sokoloff, L. (1975). Biochemical and physiological aspects of degenerative joint diseases with special reference to hemophilic arthropathy. *Annals of New York Academy of Science, 240*, 285–290.

Steward, R., & Regalbuto, G. (1975). Do doctors know what children know? *American Journal of Orthopsychiatry, 45*, 146–149.

Stewart, M.L. (1977). Measurement of clinical pain. In A. Jacox (Ed.), *Pain: A sourcebook for nurses and other health professionals*, (pp. 107–137). Boston: Little, Brown.

Stickler, G.B., & Murphy, D.B. (1979). Recurrent abdominal pain. *American Journal of Diseases of Children, 133*, 486–494.

Swezey, R.L. (1978). *Arthritis: Rational therapy and rehabilitation*. Philadelphia: Saunders.

Thompson, K.L., & Varni, J.W. (in press). A developmental cognitive-biobehavioral model for pediatric pain assessment. *Pain*.

Tomasi, L.G. (1979). Headaches in children. *Comprehensive Therapy, 5*, 13–19.

Varni, J.W. (1981a). Self-regulation techniques in the management of chronic arthritic pain in hemophilia. *Behavior Therapy, 12*, 185–194.

Varni, J.W. (1981b). Behavioral medicine in hemophilia arthritic pain management. *Archives of Physical Medicine and Rehabilitation, 62*, 183–187.

Varni, J.W. (1983). *Clinical behavioral pediatrics: An interdisciplinary biobehavioral approach.* New York: Pergamon.

Varni, J.W., Bessman, C.A., Russo, D.C., & Cataldo, M.F. (1980). Behavioral management of chronic pain in children. *Archives of Physical Medicine and Rehabilitation, 61*, 375–379.

Varni, J.W., & Gilbert, A. (1982). Self-regulation of chronic arthritic pain and long-term analgesic dependence in a hemophiliac. *Rheumatology and Rehabilitation, 22*, 171–174.

Varni, J.W., Gilbert, A., & Dietrich, S.L. (1981). Behavioral medicine in pain and analgesia management for the hemophilic child with factor VIII inhibitor. *Pain, 11*, 121–126.

Varni, J.W., & Jay, S.M. (1984). Biobehavioral factors in juvenile rheumatoid arthritis: Implications for research and practice. *Clinical Psychology Review, 4*, 543–560.

Varni, J.W., Jay, S.M., Masek, B.J., & Thompson, K.L. (in press). Cognitive-behavioral assessment and management of pediatric pain. In A.D. Holzman & D.C. Turk (Eds.), *Pain management: A handbook of psychological treatment approaches.* New York: Pergamon.

Varni, J.W., Katz, E.R., & Dash, J. (1982). Behavioral and neurochemical aspects of pediatric pain. In D.C. Russo & J.W. Varni (Eds.), *Behavioral pediatrics: Research and practice.* New York: Plenum.

Varni, J.W., & Thompson, K.L. (1985). *The Varni/Thompson Pediatric Pain Questionnaire.* Unpublished manuscript.

Varni, J.W., Thompson, K.L., & Hanson, V. (1985). *The Varni/Thompson Pediatric Pain Questionnaire: I. Chronic musculoskeletal pain in juvenile rheumatoid arthritis.* Manuscript in preparation.

Wald, A., Chandra, R., Fisher, S.E., Gartner, J.C., & Zitelli, B. (1982). Lactose malabsorption in recurrent abdominal pain in childhood. *Journal of Pediatrics, 100*, 65–68.

Wasserman, R.R., Oester, Y.T., Oryshkevich, R.S., Montgomery, M.M., Poske, R.M., & Ruksha, A. (1968). Electromyographic, electrodiagnostic, and motor nerve conduction observations in patients with rheumatoid arthritis. *Archives of Physical Medicine and Rehabilitation, 49,* 90–95.

White, J.R. (1973). Effects of a counterirritant on perceived pain and hand movements in patients with arthritis. *Physical Therapy, 53,* 959–960.

Whitt, J.K., Dykstra, W. & Taylor, C.A. (1979). Children's conception of illness and cognitive development: Implications for pediatric practitioners. *Clinical Pediatrics, 18,* 327–335.

Wolff, B.B. (1980). Behavioral measurement of human pain. In R.A. Sternbach (Ed.), *The psychology of pain* (pp. 129-167). New York: Raven.

Zeltzer, L., & LeBaron, S. (1982). Hypnosis and nonhypnotic techniques for reduction of pain and anxiety during painful procedures in children and adolescents with cancer. *Journal of Pediatrics, 101,* 1032–1035.

18

A Biobehavioral Analysis
of Pediatric Headache

FRANK ANDRASIK, DUDLEY D. BLAKE,
AND MEREDITH STEELE McCARRAN

Meghan Kelly is an 11-year-old who experiences recurrent headache. She has suffered headaches for as long as she can remember; in fact, her mother reports that as an infant, Meghan often became very quiet, and would appear irritable and pale. Meghan would sometimes vomit, as she frequently does now as a 6th grader when she has a headache. She becomes nauseous, feels weak, and appears pale. Although the accompanying headache is especially intense, she prefers the vomiting headaches because they often subside soon after she throws up. Meghan gets headaches every month and usually every week. When the headaches come on, her head throbs. At times the pain is located on the right side of her head, particularly behind the eye, but most times she feels pain in both temples and across her forehead. Normally an outgoing, popular girl, when Meg-

Preparation of this chapter was supported by Research Career Development Award 1 K04 NS00818 and Grant 1 R01 NS16891, both from the National Institute of Neurological Communicative Disorders and Stroke and awarded to the senior author.

394

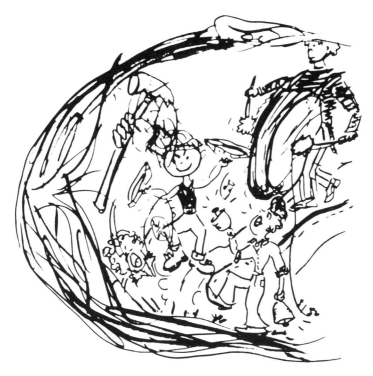

FIGURE 18.1   A child's drawing of how headache pain is experienced.

han feels the headache begin she retreats to her bedroom. There she darkens the room and lies down in order best "to ride out the storm" of her painful headache.

Meghan has seen several physicians and one pediatric neurologist and, while the consensus has been that Meghan suffers "migraine headaches", her mother has chosen not to allow Meghan to take any of the numerous medications recommended. Both parents fear that medications taken at such a young and formative age would create more problems than they might cure.

In describing her headache experience, Meghan was asked to draw a picture which best represented the headache pain she experiences (Figure 18.1). The facial expression drawn on her self-portrait, seen in the lower left-hand corner of the drawing, dramatically illustrates the impact of the headaches on Meghan's life. The surrounding objects in the drawing depict a variety of factors and stressors which Meghan views as critical in the moderation of her headache pain. While not all pediatric headache sufferers experience headaches of the same type or as severe as Meghan's, the life patterns of a significant portion of children appear at least to approximate the description above. It is for these children that this chapter has been written.

This chapter explores four aspects of pediatric headache. The first section describes the epidemiology and natural history of pediatric headache and addresses prevalence, age of onset, sex-age interactions, costs, and prognosis. The second section deals with classification of pediatric headache and describes clinical signs and symptoms, as well as associated conditions. Section three discusses the various etiological influences of pediatric headache, including biological and behavioral aspects. Section four reviews pharmacological and behavioral treatment approaches, and includes a brief focus on issues surrounding measurement of pediatric headache pain.

EPIDEMIOLOGY OF PEDIATRIC HEADACHE

Prevalence

In the past 30 years, a number of epidemiological studies have been conducted to assess the prevalence of pediatric headache. A perusal of Table 18.1 provides an affirmative answer to the question of whether many children experience headache. All epidemiological studies conducted to date have revealed that pediatric headache is not an uncommon phenomenon. In fact, Brown (1977) notes that headache in children is eight times more common than epilepsy; yet the latter—always a serious problem, of course— has received a great deal more attention in published reports and as a clinical phenomenon.

As can be seen from the "Percentage Headache" and "Percentage Migraine" columns of Table 18.1, prevalence estimates vary widely, with a "headache" range of from 6.8 to 78 percent and a "migraine" range of from 2.7 to 18.8 percent. The column labeled "Percentage Migraine" represents a population selected with relative care, in that migrainous features were used as inclusion criteria. (Diagnostic criteria will be described in detail later.) The column for "Percentage Headache," however, represents a uniformly larger subgroup of children who experience recurrent headache of an unspecified type. One may assume that a substantial portion of this pediatric headache population suffer headaches of a tension, or muscle-contraction, type, since that headache class is reported to be two to three times more common than migraine and its variants (Leviton, 1978). In any case, it is important to note that tension and "other" headaches, which are substantially more common than migraine, have received scant attention in pediatric epidemiological studies and clinical research. This situation unfortunately restricts the knowledge base of pediatric headache to results obtained through examinations of migraine headache sufferers. Clearly research is needed to examine more adequately the nonmigrainous head-

TABLE 18.1. DESCRIPTIVE STATISTICS ON EPIDEMIOLOGICAL STUDIES CONDUCTED ON HEADACHE WITH CHILDREN, 1955–1983

Study	Country	Setting	Sample Size	Age of Children	Percentage Headache	Percentage Migraine	Increase with Age?	Sex Diff.
Bille (1962)	Sweden	School	8993	7–15	6.8%	3.9%	Yes	Yes Female
Deubner (1977)	South Wales	Home	600	10–20	78%(a)	18.8%	No	Yes Female
Egermark-Eriksson (1982)	Sweden	School	402	7 11 15	9.6% 16.0% 25.2%	3%	Yes	Yes Older Female
Oster (1972)	Denmark	School phys. exam	18162 2178	6–19	20.6%(b) 20.6%	— 5.5%	No	Yes Female
Sillanpaa (1976)	Finland	School phys. exam	4235	7	37%	3.2%	N/A	No
Sillanpaa (1983a)	Finland	School	3784	13	17.6%	11.3%	—	Yes Female
Sillanpaa (1983b)	Finland	School	2921	7 14	37% 69%	2.7% 10.6%	Yes	Yes Older Female
Sparks (1978)	Great Britain	School	12543 3242	10–18	not assessed	3.4% 2.5%	Yes	Yes —
Vahlquist (1955)	Sweden	School	1236	10–12	13%	4.5%	Yes	No

[a] Presence or absence in past year—no frequency information provided.
[b] 2 sample populations studied.

397

aches, particularly tension headaches, which characterize the pediatric headache population.

Several factors may play a part in the widely varying prevalence rates from the studies surveyed. First, as shown in Table 18.1, the sample sizes of the studies vary considerably. From a methodological standpoint, issues of power and error-variance complicate comparisons across studies in which the sample sizes are more than moderately discrepant. Second, the headache criteria employed varies considerably across the studies. The criteria ranges from asking the child whether he or she experienced any type of headache in the past year (used to determine general headache prevalence in Deubner, 1977) to employing the discrete diagnostic criteria suggested by Vahlquist (1955) (used for determining migraine prevalence in the Bille, 1962, and Sillanpaa, 1976, 1983a, b, studies). Although discrete criteria are useful for reducing the number of "false-positives" and ensuring homogeneous samples, application of overly stringent criteria may increase the number of "false-negatives," which can lead to sample selection biases and limit the generalizability of findings (that is, only the most extreme and/or multisymptomatic cases along the pediatric headache continuum are considered).

Cultural differences pose a third potential confound to the generalizability of the studies reviewed. The countries/cultures assessed, while all Western European nations, are substantially different from one another. In light of the presumed American readership of this volume, it is noteworthy that none of the studies was conducted in the United States, a country even more culturally and economically distinct from those surveyed for the data found in Table 18.1. The validity of generalizing from prevalence rates obtained in other countries/cultures is uncertain; what is clear, however, is that for a more confident extension of the headache epidemiology literature, similar studies are needed in this country.

Finally, the *settings* in which these surveys have taken place may introduce a particular bias into the prevalence rates reported. For example, children may be more willing to "open up" and describe physical problems more carefully when questioned in the home, as opposed to in the school setting, where peer evaluation may inhibit their admission of any personal problem. Similarly, reports obtained in a medical setting or during a physical examination can be expected to differ from descriptions children give in other settings.

The substantial variations in methodologies employed, populations, and settings noted above hamper our ability to make comparisons across studies and to extrapolate findings to new clinical populations. In any event, regardless of the figures used, it is still clear that pediatric headache represents a wide-spread and pervasive phenomenon. For example, by using the lower estimates from the studies summarized above, within an average-sized community in which 25,000 children reside, one can expect that 1700 children will experience recurrent headaches and 675 will suffer

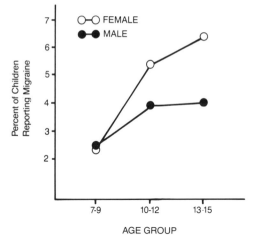

FIGURE 18.2   Age by sex headache incidence rates for a sample of 8,993 Swedish school children. (Values were obtained from Bille, 1962, Table 3, p. 40.)

from migraine headaches. Furthermore, Sillanpaa (1983a) concludes in his explanation of the higher prevalence rates found in his study that headache in children is an increasingly common problem, and that this increase can be attributed to the greater emphasis placed on education in Western society. If this connection is valid, the urgency for ameliorative efforts becomes increasingly critical with the passage of time.

Age of Onset

With few exceptions (Deubner, 1977), the majority of epidemiological studies reported have shown a gradual increase in headache incidence as children get older. This increase is graphically illustrated by the age X incidence schematic by Bille (1981), shown here in Figure 18.2. While most researchers agree that younger children and infants are less likely to experience recurrent headaches, a significant portion of children are thought to experience their first headaches even before they enter school (31 percent in Prensky and Sommer, 1979; 14.7 percent in Hockaday, 1978; and 23.6 percent in Holguin & Fenichel, 1967). However, it is important to note that headache onset data are obtained in an almost exclusively *post hoc* fashion, and descriptions are often obtained many years after initial onset. Relevant to this point is a finding by Bille (1981), in a follow-up study of child migraineurs, in which he reports that the older a headache sufferer becomes, the later the individual dates the onset of headaches. Therefore, headache onset information, gathered in a *post hoc* manner can be expected to show increasing degrees of distortion as the individual becomes older. Alternatively other researchers (Bell, 1968; Brown, 1977; Meloff, 1982) have noted the difficulty inherent in obtaining accurate information from younger subjects whose language and cognitive abilities are not as well developed, that is, infants and very young children who do not have the communicative ability to convey that they are experiencing a headache. Nevertheless, behavioral indicants to ascertain headache occurrence in infants and pre-verbal children have been suggested. These behavioral indicants include: head rolling, head banging, and cyclical vomiting (Meloff, 1982); irritability, fretfulness, and poor food intake (Bell, 1968); and crying, pallor, and vomiting (Bille, 1981). The need for reliability and validity data on these behaviors as headache markers in infants and very young children merits further study. Developing a knowledge base in which headaches can be measured in a preverbal pediatric population may be crucial in furthering a general understanding of the genesis of pediatric headache. As a result of this increased understanding, more efficacious treatments can be developed; preverbal headache sufferers may also reap immense benefit from headache identification based on behavioral markers, in that they may receive treatment early in the natural history of the disorder.

Sex-Age Interactions

Bille's (1962) often-cited monograph, which detailed his findings in an early, yet impressively sophisticated epidemiological study conducted in Uppsala, Sweden, revealed a striking sex-age headache incidence interaction. Up to age 10, boys and girls are equally likely to suffer from migraine headaches; after age 10, girls increasingly predominate as headache sufferers. This finding is graphically illustrated in Figure 18.3 using data extracted from Bille's study involving 8993 children between the ages of 7 and 15.

As was shown in Table 18.1, studies by Deubner (1977), Egermark-Eriksson (1982), and Sillanpaa (1983a, 1983b) substantiate the Bille findings; Sparks (1978) showed an overall higher rate for *males* but did not specifically examine sex as it varies with *age*. However, Sparks reports data showing that 80 percent of the females studied had initial headaches after age 10, while a somewhat smaller percentage of males, 72 percent, experienced their first headaches after that age.

During early adolescence, the most obvious concomitant life event is puberty which, for girls, includes menarche. The few studies which have examined this factor have not found supportive evidence to conclude that this life change contributes to increased headache activity for females. Sparks (1978) reported that only 21 percent of the females he studied felt that their headaches were related in any way to their menstrual cycle. Deubner (1977) found no relationship between menarchal status and the child-patient's recollection of presence or absence of headache or migraine. He did find, however, a statistically significant increase in parent report of headache severity as girls became older, but a *decrease* in severity after

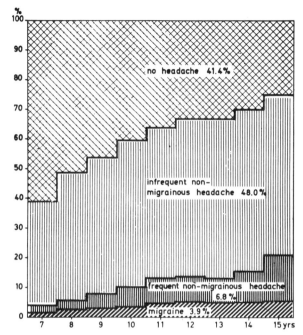

FIGURE 18.3.   Occurrence and type of headache among 8,993 Swedish school children (Reprinted from "Migraine in Childhood and Its Prognosis" by Bo Bille, from *Cephalalgia*, 1981. By permission of Universitetsforlaget, Oslo.)

menarche. To summarize, only a few studies have examined menarche as it may (or may not) relate to age of headache onset with girls, and to date, a direct relationship between these variables is doubtful. Future studies might assess other concomitant life events for girls, for example, intensified sex-role identification and enculturation, cognitive-developmental progression, and so on, in an effort to identify the factors critical to this phenomenon.

In an attempt to explain the higher illness rates found for women in general, Verbrugge (1979) articulated several concerns which may help to explain the sex differential found in pediatric headache. First, as a product of sex-role socialization, women are found to show a greater frequency of "illness behavior." Whereas boys come under increasing pressure to "tough it out" and to minimize expressions of pain, girls are socialized to focus more closely on internal states and symptoms, and to take curative health action. Women also utilize health services to a greater extent than do men and are thus more likely to *find* physical problems. Finally, women are found to be more cooperative during interviews and show more careful attempts to recall past behavior. Thus because women are better interviewees, symptom reporting may be greatly enhanced. While these notions are plausible in accounting for the sex differences evident in pediatric headache reporting, as

Verbrugge (1979) herself notes, attempts at empirical substantiation are needed. In conclusion, however, the consistent age-sex interaction begs for more fine-grained study to explicate the factors responsible for the differential incidence rates.

Cost

In his classic work on pediatric headache, Bille (1962) examined the cost of headache, as measured in time missed from school. Bille found that child headache sufferers missed significantly more school time than other children. Furthermore, Egermark-Eriksson (1982) found that approximately 70 percent of a sample of over 400 children who missed four or more days of school suffered from recurrent headaches. Thus the cost of child headache appears to be substantial, as shown by this single parameter. An examination of other parameters, such as lost parental work-time, child medical costs, time lost from other recreational and psychosocial/educational activities, and so on, should further highlight the urgent need to understand childhood headache and to find safe and effective treatments with which to minimize the impact of this problem.

Prognosis

A critical question with regard to children who suffer from headaches is whether they will outgrow this painful and oftentimes debilitating experience. Several researchers respected in the area of pediatric headache have provided a fairly definitive "no" response to that question. For example, Bille (1981) reported a 23-year follow-up of 73 individuals who reported migraine headaches as children. By age 30, the majority, 60 percent, continued to experience headaches into adulthood. These data are depicted visually in Bille's revealing bar graph shown below in Figure 18.4. In addition, Bille found that the prognosis of remission was better for males (52 percent) than it was for females (30 percent). This finding is consistent with those by other researchers indicating that women outnumber men as adult headache sufferers.

More recently, Sillanpaa (1983b) reported on a 7-year follow-up of 2921 child headache sufferers and obtained results similar to those of Bille. Of the sample of children assessed, 78 percent continued to experience headaches: 41 percent reported that their headaches were either unchanged or worse, while 37 percent believed their headaches were now milder. Only 22 percent of the children were asymptomatic. Similar to the Bille (1981) finding, males were found to have a better headache prognosis than females.

In summary, a substantial percentage of child headache sufferers do not outgrow their headaches, but go on to become adult headache sufferers. This tendency is especially true for females. Furthermore, many of these

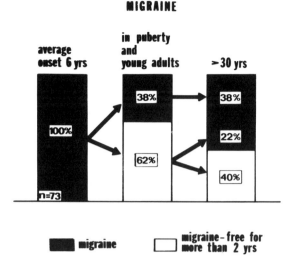

FIGURE 18.4   Twenty-three year follow-up of 73 school children with "more pronounced" migraine symptoms. (Reprinted from "Migraine in Childhood and Its Prognosis" by Bo Bille, from *Cephalalgia*, 1981. By permission of Universitetsforlaget, Oslo.)

children report that the severity of their headaches actually increases over time.

CLASSIFICATION OF PEDIATRIC HEADACHE

The most widely recognized classification system for adult headache is the one developed by the Ad Hoc Committee on the Classification of Headache (1962). Fifteen general headache types are outlined (Table 18.2); those most commonly encountered by the practitioner include vascular migraine headaches, muscle-contraction or tension headaches, and combined headaches (including features of both migraine and tension headaches).

The likelihood of an underlying organic problem for pediatric headache sufferers appears to be slight, and may represent less than 5 percent of the pediatric headache population. Nevertheless, a careful history and physical/neurological examination are essential as a first step in ruling out organic pathology (Bell, 1968; Rothner, 1978). In addition to benefiting the child by identifying early these organic dysfunctions, a thorough assessment will save time and money that might otherwise be wasted by attempting treatment when physical conditions limit the degree of improvement attainable.

Migraine Headaches

Migraine itself has been further subdivided into at least four subtypes: classic migraine, common migraine, cluster headache, and complicated mi-

TABLE 18.2. HEADACHE TYPES FROM THE AD HOC COMMITTEE
ON CLASSIFICATION OF HEADACHE (1962)

1. Vascular headache of migraine type
   a. "Classic" migraine
   b. "Common" migraine
   c. "Cluster" headache
   d. "Hemiplegic" and "opthalmoplegic" migraine
   e. "Lower-Half" headache
2. Muscle-contraction headache
3. Combined headache: Vascular and muscle-contraction
4. Headache of nasal vasomotor reaction
5. Headache of delusional, conversion, or hypochondriacal states
6. Nonmigrainous vascular headaches
7. Traction headache
8. Headache due to overt cranial inflammation
9–13. Headache due to disease of ocular, aural, nasal and sinusal,
   dental, or other cranial or neck structures
14. Cranial neuritides
15. Cranial neuralgias

graine. Classic migraines may be distinguished from common migraines by the inclusion of prodromal symptoms, or "auras," which in most cases appear as visual lines, bars, or shimmerings; occasionally the prodrome is tactile or motor, and may involve parasthesias. Common migraines lack the prodromal symptoms, and the pain more likely occurs bilaterally across the forehead. Cluster headaches, or "Horton's Syndrome," are unilateral, extremely painful headaches of relatively brief duration. Episodes strike in periodic clusters over hours or days, and are described as involving sharp burning or boring sensations. Complicated migraine includes basilar artery, hemiplegic, and opthalmoplegic migraine, as well as the "Alice in Wonderland Syndrome," an acute confusional state (Shinnar & D'Souza, 1981). Rothner (1978) provides a helpful description of the clinical features and assessment procedures both for the subtypes of childhood migraine and for childhood headache of organic etiology.

Migraine headaches, of all types, are presumed to be a vascular disorder. Arteriolar narrowing, or vasoconstriction, both intra- and extracranially, characterizes the prodromal phase. The painful headache phase follows, as vasodilitation occurs in both smaller and large arteries, particularly in the temporal region. The engorgement of these vessels accounts for the pounding or throbbing aspect of migraine pain. Typically, adult migraine involves unilateral throbbing pain located near the temple or eye, with accompanying sensitivity to light or sound, nausea, anorexia, and less frequently, pallor, dizziness, vomiting and parasthesias. Childhood migraine shows similar features, but the pain tends to be located across the forehead rather than near the eye, irritability may be observed, and vomiting and abdominal pain are much more commonly associated with the headache (Bille, 1962). In addition childhood migraines tend to be of shorter duration than adult migraines, and child sufferers seem more prone than adults to related neurologic phenomena, such as hemiparesis, aphasia, vertigo, and confusional states (Barlow, 1978).

In 1979 Prensky and Sommer published criteria for the diagnosis of migraine in children. Although definitive reliability and validity data for the Prensky-Sommer criteria have not been published, the criteria are enumerated here to illustrate a set of inclusion parameters for determining migraine headache in children. These are (1) recurrent headache, separated by symptom-free intervals, and (2) *any three* of the following: (a) abdominal pain, nausea, or vomiting with the headache; (b) hemicrania; (c) a throbbing pulsatile quality of pain; (d) complete relief after a brief period of rest; (e) an aura, either visual, sensory, or motor; and (f) a history of migraine headache in one or more members of the immediate family.

Notice that the only pathognomonic symptom for child migraine is "recurrent headache, separated by symptom-free intervals." The remaining clinical picture allows for $6! \div 3!$ or 120 possible symptom combinations. Thus while child migraine is considered to represent a distinct nosological entity, the Prensky-Sommer criteria, and others as well, encompass a wide range of variations.

Kudrow (1983) links four biochemicals (serotonin, prostaglandins, monoamine oxidase, and estrogen) to the vascular process of migraine. Serotonin levels increase dramatically during the prodromal phase, then fall off during the headache phase of migraines. Serotonin acts to constrict blood vessels; its depletion at the end of the prodromal phase may also serve to lower the pain threshold just prior to the headache. It also stimulates the release of prostaglandins from the lungs; prostaglandins act as potent extracranial dilators leading to painful engorgement of blood vessels. Tyramine also stimulates prostaglandin release, while ergotomine, a commonly used abortive agent, inhibits it. Monoamine oxidase (MAO) has been found to be deficient in some migraineurs; this enzyme is a constituent of blood platelets, whose aggregation lead to the release of serotonin. The fourth biochemical, estrogen, also influences migraine by increasing platelet aggregation and by directly stimulating prostaglandin secretion. The contribution of estrogen to the pathogenesis of migraine may partially explain the higher prevalence of migraine in women, although data earlier reviewed are equivocal.

Tension Headache

Tension, or muscle contraction headache, by its very name implies muscular and/or psychological tension in its etiology. The Ad Hoc Committee

(1962) defined tension headache as an: "ache or sensation of tightness, pressure, or constriction widely varying in intensity, frequency and duration, sometimes long-lasting and commonly suboccipital. It is associated with sustained contraction of the skeletal muscles in the absence of permanent structural change, usually as part of the individual's reaction during life stress." The resulting pain is typically described as bandlike, often bilateral, of insidious onset and a dull, steady ache that is less intense than the pain of migraine. Typically, tension headache sufferers experience headache twice a week or more, unlike migraineurs, whose headache frequency averages less than once per week. Child tension headache sufferers show symptoms similar to those of adults, but can also demonstrate associated symptoms of a migrainous nature, such as throbbing pain, light sensitivity, and nausea (Meloff, 1982). Tension headaches can last for weeks; children may go to sleep with a headache and wake up the next morning with no relief. Pain is believed to result from stimulation of pain receptors in the contracted muscles and ischemia produced by compression of intramuscular arterioles (Haynes, 1980).

In 1981 Jay and Tomasi established criteria for the diagnosis of childhood "chronic scalp muscle contraction headaches." These criteria are: (1) continuous headache of prolonged duration with absence of neurological signs; (2) bilateral distribution of pain; (3) generalized, or "band-like" head pain; (4) absence of nausea or vomiting; and (5) exacerbations temporally related to school performance, social functions, or familial stress. All of the criteria must be met to merit the diagnosis of muscle contraction or tension headache by the Jay-Tomasi classification, despite the frequent overlap of symptoms described above. The validity and utility of these criteria await confirmation.

Numerous studies of the psychophysiological underpinnings of tension headache have failed to uphold the underlying assumptions of the Ad Hoc Committee's description of tension headache. Tension headache sufferers often do not show elevated levels of muscle tension when compared to controls, and muscle tension levels of migraine patients often exceed those of tension patients (Andrasik, Blanchard, Arena, Saunders, & Barron, 1982; Haynes, Cuevas, & Gannon, 1982; Philips, 1977, 1978). Van Boxtel, Goudsward, and Janssen (1983) suggest these negative findings may be attributable in part to the use of unsophisticated measurement approaches. It is also possible that increased muscular involvement may be of etiological significance for only a subset of patients who now end up being diagnosed as muscle tension headache. Adams, Brantley, and Thompson (1982) suggest it may be more accurate to classify individuals revealing normal levels of muscle tension, but otherwise meeting criteria for tension headache, as having "psychogenic" headache. Whether improving psychophysiological assessment techniques and varying current classification practices will lead to more clearcut findings is unknown.

Combined Headache

Combined headache type is essentially a combination of migraine and tension headache, and a sufferer must meet the minimal inclusion criteria for both headache types to be diagnosed as having combined headache. A migraine headache may present first in the child and continue for a long period of time; in response to the sustained head pain, the muscles in the child's neck, shoulders, and forehead become and remain taut, leading to muscle contraction headache symptoms. Conversely, a child originally suffering from a muscle contraction headache may trigger the psychological/physiological prerequisites for migraine. In either case, a combined headache is the result.

An Alternative View of Headache Classification

Ziegler, Hassanein, and Hassanein (1972), upon finding that they could not reliably differentiate between migraine and tension headache by factor analysis, proposed that the two headache types might actually be manifestations of the same underlying cause. This "severity" model of headache, as Bakal (1982) terms it, places migraine and tension headache on the same etiological continuum and attributes differences in symptom presentation merely to severity of underlying vascular involvement. Support for this model as it applies to children emerged in a recent study by Joffe, Bakal, and Kaganov (1983), who showed that child headache sufferers experienced a cross-section of symptoms and that both categories of symptoms increased in frequency as reported intensity and duration of headaches increased. Unfortunately, no effort was made to categorize children by current diagnostic practices to document that these children represented different headache groupings.

Although this continuum model appears to be gaining steadily in appeal, most likely due to its parsimony, it has yet to be subjected to rigorous evaluation. Such an evaluation will require an "unambiguous method of assessing headache severity that is not confounded with the very symptoms that are hypothesized to be consequences of increasing headache severity" (Holroyd, in press). Further, more recent factor analyses of adult headache patients (Arena, Blanchard, Andrasik, & Dudek, 1982; Kroner, 1983) have yielded two stable and valid syndrome factors which resemble the migraine and muscle contraction categories.

Associated Features

Headaches, and migraine headaches in particular, have been linked to motion, or travel sickness. In 1972, Waters surveyed 1718 adult migraineurs in Great Britain about whether they had experienced childhood physical problems, including headache and travel sickness. Waters found a 14 percent concordance rate between children who suffered from the two ailments. In addition, as more migrainous features were reported, so rose the likelihood of a comorbidity with travel sickness; 21 percent of the adults who reported three or more migrainous symptoms as a child also reported experiencing travel sickness. In a study involving 300 child migraineurs, Congdon and Forsythe (1979) found a history of travel sickness in 38 percent (114). Furthermore, 28 children (9 percent of sample) indicated that travel was a precipitant to headache episodes.

Barabas, Matthews, and Ferrari (1983) studied a sample of 222 children from four diagnostic groups: seizure disordered, migraineurs, nonmigraine headache sufferers, and learning disabled children. Travel sickness was reported in 45 percent of the child migraineurs, whereas the incidence was significantly lower for the other groups, ranging from 5.0 to 7.1 percent. Barabas et al. posit that an interplay between peripheral and central nervous system mechanisms accounts for both travel sickness and headaches. Specifically, travel sickness is thought to result from an overstimulation of vestibular mechanisms. Barabas et al. suggest that child migraineurs have hypersensitive peripheral receptors and/or a central dysfunction, involving abnormal neurotransmitter metabolism within emetic regions (vomiting centers of the CNS). The finding that some child headache sufferers have abnormal EEG brain wave activity (Jay, 1982) lends support to the existence of a CNS dysfunction or deviation. Continued study may help towards an increased understanding of this complex disorder.

Assuming that a link exists between travel sickness and (migraine) headaches, Barabas et al. (1983) present a testable hypothesis which may lead to a greater understanding of the pathogenesis of pediatric headache. However, it should be noted that not all studies have provided supportive evidence for a link between travel sickness and headache (Deubner, 1977). In light of some inconsistency found in the literature, the relationship between the two conditions clearly merits further study.

Perhaps closely related to the travel sickness-headache association are reports linking early childhood "cyclical vomiting" to later headache experience. Hammond (1974) studied 23 children (under age 15) who evidenced cyclical vomiting. A second group of 12 individuals between the ages of 17 and 27, who had a similar clinical history as children, served as a follow-up group. Hammond found that six of the younger children (26 percent) reported that they also experienced headaches; in the follow-up group, headache symptoms were reported in eight cases (75 percent). Most importantly, five of the eight individuals in the older group reported that their headaches began during adolescence. The findings reported by Hammond suggest that cyclical vomiting may be a developmental precursor to recurrent headache. Further research, with larger sample sizes, is needed to explicate more fully the relationship between cyclical vomiting and headache. Research should also help determine whether these children constitute a special subtype of pediatric headache. Finally, since both travel sickness and cyclical vomiting have been shown to have a relationship to the headache experience, their utility as reliable behavioral indicants for later headache experience should be explored.

Epilepsy and other seizure disorders have also been linked to headaches, though the relationship does not appear to be as strong as that between headache and travel sickness/cyclical vomiting. Epileptics are known to experience headaches more frequently than nonepileptic children and headache sufferers have a slightly higher frequency of past seizure activity than is seen in the general child population. Since reports examining the relationship between headache and seizure disorders have, for the most part, demonstrated a weak association, only cautious and tentative conclusions can be posited until more empirical verification is obtained.

ETIOLOGICAL FACTORS

Migraine and tension headache might best be conceptualized along three dimensions: precipitants for headache, vulnerability to headache, and maintenance of headache (Holroyd & Andrasik, 1982). It is proposed that an interaction of psychological and biological processes control the experience of pain in recurrent pediatric headache and contribute to each of the three dimensions of precipitants, vulnerability, and maintenance. Bakal (1982) terms this type of conceptualization a "psychobiological model."

Precipitants

The most commonly reported precipitant to headache is stress. For example, Dalsgaard-Nielson (1965) observed that 68 percent of a group of chronic headache patients recognized that psychological stress due to school demands and conflict at home accounted for over half of all childhood migraines. A recent assessment study of headaches in young people (Leviton, Slack, Masek, Bana, & Graham, 1984) noted that the most commonly acknowledged contributor to headache in children up to age 16 was "an especially hard day," with "worrying a lot" and "unexpected excitement or pressure" following closely behind.

Are children and adults with problematic headaches victims of an overstressful lifestyle? Preliminary data collected with child headache sufferers at our clinic indicate, on the contrary, that they are exposed to equivalent levels of stress as are children who are headache-free (Andrasik, Kabela, Quinn, Blanchard, & Rosenblum, 1985). Data from a group of adult headache sufferers and their controls similarly found no significant difference between recently experienced life stresses in the two groups (Andrasik, Blanchard, Arena, et al., 1982). Therefore, it appears that migraine and tension headaches are both precipitated by typical everyday stresses to which the headache-prone person responds in a psychologically and biologically atypical and extreme manner. Unfortunately, all analyses of the link between stress and headache have been retrospective in nature; prospective studies with repeated assessment are needed to explicate more fully the role of stress as a trigger for pediatric headache.

Other precipitants to headaches include physical stressors, such as exertion, eye strain, fatigue, and hunger (Bille, 1962). The consumption of certain foods, such as chocolate, cheese, Chinese food, and citrus fruit, often reportedly trigger migraine headaches. Dalton and Dalton (1979), using retrospective food diaries, found that these foods accounted for 38 percent of the headaches listed by a group of children. Much interest has been generated by Hanington's (1967) oral tyramine hypothesis, which postulates that consumption of tyramine, a vasoactive amine, reliably leads to headache in a select group of migraineurs. Tyramine, it will be recalled, stimulates prostaglandin release, which causes active vasodilation. Congdon and Forsythe (1979) administered capsules containing tyramine or placebo to 80 child migraineurs (in double-blind fashion) and found tyramine was no more likely to cause headache than placebo. However, food records kept by parents for a 3-month interval identified seven children (or 9 percent) whose headaches were reliably associated with ingesting fish, chocolate, gravy, meat, onions or semolina. The link between dietary triggers and migraine remains intriguing, yet controversial (Kohlenberg, 1982, Medina & Diamond, 1978). Our speculation is that food substances serve as headache precipitants for only a minority of children.

Vulnerability

One component of biobehavioral vulnerability to headache includes the genetic, or heritability factor. Migraine has long been considered to be transmitted genetically; several studies have found a high incidence, up to 95 percent, of recurrent headaches in blood relatives (Lance & Anthony, 1966; Ziegler, 1978). The majority of such prevalence studies, however, have used data based upon retrospective information gleaned from the patient, not from the relatives themselves. As seen above, fully 78 percent of the general population may suffer from some sort of headache at some time; careful questioning would be necessary to determine a more exact diagnosis among relatives of probands. Bakal (1982) notes that the reported prevalence rates tend to decrease to levels as low as 5 percent as the criteria used become more rigorous. Waters (1971), for example, directly interviewed migraineurs' relatives for prevalence of migraine, rather than relying upon retrospective information supplied by the headache sufferers themselves; he found a prevalence of only 10 percent in the families of probands.

Heritability of migraine has also been proposed to be sex-linked. Bell

(1968) suggests that migraine headaches may be transmitted through the mother's side of the family. Bille (1981) reports that in a prospective follow-up of former child migraineurs, the females were more likely to have offspring who also suffered from headaches. In addition these headache-prone offspring were likely to be female, suggesting a mother-daughter heritability link. However, this may be a premature conclusion based upon a limited sample. In a sample of 600 randomly selected children, Duebner (1977) found that both sons and daughters of migrainous mothers had an equal chance of having migraine. On the other hand, if the father were a migraineur, the son had a significantly greater likelihood than the daughter of experiencing migraines. Deubner's results suggest that, rather than being inherited, headache behaviors may be learned by children imitating behaviors exhibited by their parents. The role of social learning of the migraine experience by children from their parents clearly merits further research.

Despite the higher frequency of tension headaches in the population at large, genetic factors have not been implicated in their transmission. Conclusions on the heritability of headache based on the data from migraineurs must be qualified, due to a potentially serious confound. One of the criteria for establishing a diagnosis of migraine is the presence of migraine in one or more first-degree relatives; this selection bias probably artificially inflates the family concordance rate (Waters, 1971).

Another component of a biobehavioral vulnerability is the psychological disposition of sufferers to headache. As early as 1937, Wolff described a "headache personality" for migraineurs. He portrayed adult migraineurs as being perfectionistic, ambitious, inflexible, reserved, and orderly. Subsequent studies with child migraineurs tended to support Wolff's observations; Bille (1962) found youthful migraineurs, particularly females, to be significantly more anxious and cautious than nonmigraineurs; Krupp and Friedman (1953) found a tendency in childhood headache sufferers toward sensitivity, need for approval, cleanliness, thoroughness, and a serious approach to responsibilities. In addition, the children were generally of superior intelligence. Prensky and Sommer (1979), in a retrospective chart review of migrainous children, reported heightened levels of depression, overactivity, compulsive features, and anxiety.

The chief methodological problems with such reports include their use of retrospective information and their incomplete descriptions of the procedures used both to select and to test their subjects. These include the use of nonstandardized rating scales and no mention of how matching of subjects occurred. Since the children being described suffered from headaches severe enough for them to have sought medical help, one cannot attribute causality to the personality features found. Indeed one might speculate that the experience of frequent, unexplainable, severe head pain would tend to lead to heightened levels of depression, anxiety, and caution.

Headaches and depressive symptomatology have often been associated in the case of chronic tension headache (Diamond 1983, Martin, 1978). Of a group of 25 children presenting with either tension or migraine headache to a neurology clinic, 10 met the criteria for depression (Ling, Oftedal, & Weinberg, 1970). (Four of these ten, it might be noted, presented with migrainous symptoms). Unfortunately the authors made no attempt to determine whether the depressive symptoms preceded or postdated the onset of problem headaches. Several of the vegetative signs of depression (anorexia, sleep disturbance, lack of energy, and somatic complaints) may be attributable to the headaches themselves; association of the problems cannot be construed as causality.

The depression-headache association has led to trials with antidepressant medications as a prophylaxis for headache; seven of ten child headache sufferers treated by Ling et al. with either amitriptyline or imipramine demonstrated marked clinical improvement. On the other hand, successful treatments for headache symptoms alone have shown concomitant decreases in depression (Cox & Thomas, 1981; Gerber, Miltner, Birbaumer, & Lutzenberger, 1983), adding evidence for the notion that with a decrease in pain, depressive symptoms also decrease.

Results of psychological tests conducted in our clinic on 32 child migraineurs and 32 carefully matched nonheadache controls revealed higher scores on all scales measuring depression and somatic complaints among the migraineurs (Andrasik et al. 1985). Given the high rate of concurrent somatic complaints in children with headache, including nausea, abdominal pain, dizziness, and related neurological involvement as noted above, a finding of increased reported somatic complaints in these children is not surprising. Consistent with the notion that depression may be a consequence of rather than a precursor to migraine, the older children in this sample showed higher levels of depression than did the younger migraineurs. Clearly, research is needed to determine whether depression in these children precedes or follows the development of chronic headache symptoms, and whether children experiencing other forms of unexplained chronic pain exhibit similar depressive reactions.

Melzack's (1973) studies of pain have demonstrated that pain is not a unidimensional sensory phenomenon, but rather a multidimensional experience which includes such factors as sensory intensity, affectivity, and evaluative components which are highly influenced by social experience. The multiplicity of these factors and their differential contribution to the pain experience help explain the frequently contradictory results of psychophysiological studies of headache. It follows that the cognitive-evaluative reactions of the headache sufferer will contribute to the experience of pain. The population of children seen for headache complaints may consist of those individuals who catastrophize their experiences: "Oh, no, I can't bear this pain"; "The pain is out of my control"; "Here comes a headache, I'm sure it's going to hurt terribly." It is possible to speculate that many children experience headache without the accompanying catastrophic thinking; these children just cope with the occasional distress and do not present to clinics for headache.

Maintenance

The factors which precipitate headache need not be the same factors which maintain it. A child's reporting of head pain rarely meets a neutral response from the environment. In some cases, secondary gains, in the form of excused absences from school or stressful events, parental sympathy and attention, and increased opportunities to engage in preferred activities, such as watching television and lying in bed, may serve as powerful reinforcers for the child. A common finding for child migraineurs, for example, is that headache frequency decreases sharply in the school vacation months.

Although childhood headaches initially appear to be clearly associated with life stresses, as headache severity and frequency increase, a growing autonomy of headache symptoms from identifiable stressors also increases (Joffe et al., 1983). Bakal (1979, 1982) and colleagues have attempted to explain this phenomenon by suggesting that one consequence of recurrent attacks is a physiological and psychological shift in which the symptoms and anticipation of the pain act as triggers themselves. Thus, those with the most severe and more frequent attacks often awaken with a headache in the morning before an anticipated stressful event (Joffe et al., 1983).

The importance of psychological factors in the precipitation of, vulnerability to, and maintenance of headache in children has been seen to be a recurring theme. The cognitive coping patterns of the child play a large part in the headache experience; treatment of childhood headache would best take psychological factors into account.

TREATMENT OF PEDIATRIC HEADACHE

Medical reassurance, over-the-counter preparations, and prescribed medications constitute the dominant approach for managing recurrent pediatric headache at present; but behavioral techniques have begun to show much promise as viable treatment alternatives. The pharmacological and behavioral treatments currently under investigation are based on extensive knowledge acquired with adult headache sufferers over the past 15 years and represent downward extensions of existing procedures to children. An important promise of effective treatment is that it will save the child from a life-time of chronic pain and emotional suffering.

Measurement of Pediatric Headache Pain

Valid measures of pain are essential for evaluating efficacy of treatment. Pain is a very private experience and it can be accessed only through verbal reports of the patient or by inferences based on observed behaviors. Headache measurement is woefully underdeveloped in general and virtually unaddressed for children in particular. The headache diary has become the "gold standard" for assessing headache pain of adults. The headache diary, which is completed each day, asks the subject periodically to note the presence or absence of headache, to assign an intensity value if pain is present, and to record any medications taken as a result of pain, and any other desired information. Preliminary research suggests that the headache diary, although in wide use, has one particular shortcoming in that its focus may be restricted largely to a single aspect of the pain experience (Andrasik, Blanchard, Ahles, Pallmeyer, & Barron, 1981). This data collection procedure has been adopted in many studies of pediatric headache sufferers, with little attention being given to its appropriateness. Basic measurement investigations are needed to determine the extent to which the adult headache diary can validly be "down-sized" to children and to assess whether a child's developmental progression alters the experience and report of pain (Jeans, 1983).

Two investigations have been conducted thus far. The first, (Richardson, McGrath, Cunningham, & Humphreys, 1983) compared diary ratings of headache intensity provided by parents and their children. High levels of agreement were noted, helping to begin to establish concurrent validity of the headache diary for children. The second investigation (Andrasik, Burke, Attanasio, & Rosenblum, in press) replicated the findings of Richardson et al., and, additionally, examined the correspondence between diary measures of headache activity and independent estimates of the same measures obtained from children and parents during interviews. Interview based measures for children and parents alike were markedly discrepant from diary-based measures. Caution appears in order when judging outcome from interview data alone.

Pharmacological Treatment

Medication serves two chief functions for headache sufferers, symptomatic and preventive (Diamond & Dalessio, 1982). Abortive and palliative agents commonly recommended for symptomatic treatment of pediatric headache include peripheral vasoconstrictors, anticonvulsants, antiemetics, antispasmodics, sedatives, and analgesics (ranging from aspirin and related compounds to narcotics). Prophylactic agents consist of antihypertensives, anticonvulsants, serotonin antagonists, and antidepressants. Research with adults suggests the benefits of antidepressants may result in large part from the alterations in serotonergic activity and metabolism they induce, rather than from the alleviation of depressive symptomatology that might underlie headache (Couch & Hassanein, 1979).

Nearly all of the medications commonly used with adult headache sufferers have been advocated for use with children. Table 18.3 provides cita-

TABLE 18.3   UNCONTROLLED TRIALS OF MEDICATION FOR PEDIATRIC MIGRAINE HEADACHE

Medication	Authors
Ergotamine	Krupp & Friedman (1953)
	Bille (1962)
	Hinrichs & Keith (1965)
	Holguin & Fenichel (1967)
	Prensky (1976)
	Millichap (1978)
	Congdon & Forsythe (1979)
	Shinnar & D'Souza (1981)
Phenobarbital/Phenytoin	Hinrichs & Keith (1965)
	Ling, Oftedal, & Weinberg (1970)
	Prensky (1976)
	Millichap (1978)
	Buda & Joyce (1979)
	Congdon & Forsythe (1979)
	Shinnar & D'Souza (1981)
Methysergide	Holguin & Fenichel (1967)
	Congdon & Forsythe (1979)
Cyproheptadine	Bille, Ludvigsson, & Sanner (1977)
Clonidine	Congdon & Forsythe (1979)
Amitriptyline/Imipramine	Ling, Oftedal, & Weinberg (1970)

Uncontrolled Trials of Medication
for Pediatric Tension Headache

Diazepam	Millichap (1978)
Phenobarbital/Phenytoin	Ling, Oftedal, & Weinberg (1970)
Amitriptyline/Imipramine	Ling, Oftedal, & Weinberg (1970)
Chlordiazepoxide	Millichap (1978)

tions to anecdotal or otherwise uncontrolled claims for efficacy of various medications for pediatric migraine and tension headache.

Unfortunately, only a few of the published investigations include controlled designs. Results from three double-blind, placebo-controlled investigations are summarized in Table 18.4. All 3 medications were found to be efficacious for the short-term prophylaxis of migraine; the only study including a longer-term follow-up revealed maintenance of effects. In both studies by Sillanpaa, children administered placebos revealed substantial clinical improvement as well, and these improvements stand in marked contrast to the virtual absence of improvement for children receiving placebo in Ludvigsson's study (1974). It is difficult to account for these varied response rates to placebo. The only major discernable methodological difference was that Ludvigsson evaluated outcome from diary records kept by children and parents, while Sillanpaa and colleagues determined outcome from interviews conducted with patients. Perhaps patients receiving placebo overestimated actual improvement (Cahn & Cram, 1980). Alternatively, varied patient characteristics may also account for some of the differences.

It is obvious that pharmacological treatments are underevaluated in the area of pediatric headache. Although practitioners assume children will respond to medication in a manner similar to adults, research is needed to define the parameters of effective treatment and to identify possible side effects and contraindications. Certain medications may have increased negative side effects when administered to children during their critical growth period. The medications studied thus far appear to have been well tolerated. Minor side effects (hypersensitivity, lethargy, sleep disruption, and so on) were reported in only 7 percent of patients receiving propranalol (Ludvigsson, 1974), 10 to 11 percent for anticonvulsants (Buda & Joyce, 1979; Millichap, 1978), and 11 percent for papaverine (Sillanpaa & Koponen, 1978). Sillanpaa (1977) reported a much higher rate of side effects for children receiving Clonodine (in 39 percent of patients); most common side effects were fatigue and nausea, but additional problems included disruption of the sleep/wake and menstrual cycles, vomiting, and a paradoxical intensification of pain for one child. However, one of the uncontrolled pharmacological trials reported a very serious consequence of methysergide for a child who subsequently developed thrombophlebitis. Diamond and Dalessio (1982) recommend that this medication be used only as a last resort for particularly resilient cases because of the possibility of such side effects.

There are several shortcomings to use of medication with children. First, abortive agents must be administered in a timely manner for optimal effects. Children experience warning symptoms less frequently than do adults and auras (when they do occur) often are of briefer duration, making it difficult to administer abortive agents in an optimal manner. Further, effective administration requires that children possess these medications at all times, and many children may find it inconvenient to carry medications with them during play, school, and so on (Shinnar & D'Souza, 1981). Second, as earlier stated, side effects from chronic use of these medications by children during their key growth years are really not known, because of the absence of systematic research. Third, research with adult headache sufferers reveals that chronic overuse of certain recommended medications

TABLE 18.4. CONTROLLED TRIALS OF MEDICATION FOR PEDIATRIC MIGRAINE

Author(s)	Number of Subjects	Type of Headache	Age	Study Design	Pharmacological Agents	Results Short-Term	Results Long-Term
Ludvigsson (1974)	28	Migraine	7–16	Double-blind Placebo-controlled Crossover	Propranolol	70% reduction in frequency of attacks averaged across both 3-month trials	Not evaluated
					Placebo	9% reduction in frequency of attacks averaged across both 3-month trials	
Sillanpaa & Koponen (1978)	37	Migraine	6–15	Double-blind Placebo-controlled	Papaverine	74% of children obtained improvement in excess of 50% after 2 months of treatment	62% of children obtained improvement in excess of 50% at a mean follow-up of 4.5 months
					Placebo	50% of children obtained improvement after 2 months of treatment	53% of children obtained improvement in excess of 50% at a mean follow-up of 4.5 months
Sillanpaa (1977)	57	Migraine	0–15	Double-blind Placebo-controlled	Clonidine	57% of children were "greatly improved" after 2 months of treatment	Not evaluated
					Placebo	42% of children were "greatly improved" after 2 months of treatment	

(analgesics, Kudrow, 1982, and ergotamine, Ala-Hurula, Myllyla, and Hokkanen, 1982) can lead to paradoxical effects and actually serve to intensify pain, a phenomenon referred to as "rebound headache." Uncontrolled use of analgesics can even compromise outcome for an otherwise effective medication. Kudrow speculates that analgesics sustain pain by suppressing central serotonergic pathways concerned with regulation of dull pain. Whether these paradoxical effects will be more or less likely for children is unknown; however, regular reliance on such medication at a young age would seem to place children at increased risk for subsequent abuse during adulthood.

The above caveats suggest it may be particularly fruitful to explore nonpharmacological approaches, either as adjunctive or alternative treatments to medical management. In the adult area, at least one investigation (Mathew, 1981) has shown that an optimal treatment effect occurs with the combination of pharmacological and behavioral treatment procedures. Whether this will hold with children as well awaits further investigation. If findings from the adult area are a useful guide, caution seems indicated when exploring pharamacological-behavioral treatment combinations. Preliminary data collected by Jay, Renelli, and Mead (1984) revealed that regular use of propranolol or amitriptyline impeded the progress of adult patients receiving biofeedback therapy. All patients were able to reach the training criterion established by the researchers, but with significantly greater difficulty and increased frustration.

Behavioral Treatment

Two types of behavioral treatment predominate in the literature investigating efficacy for adult headache patients: biofeedback and relaxation. Both have as their chief aim the reduction of physiological arousal underlying headache. Biofeedback uses what may be called the "rifle" approach (targeting specific response systems), whereas relaxation training uses the "shotgun" approach (seeking to effect an overall state of relaxation). The more precise focus of biofeedback has led investigators to advocate specific approaches for specific headache types. However, recent data are beginning to question the validity of this practice (Daly, Donn, Galliher, & Zimmerman, 1983).

Two separate forms of treatment exist for the biofeedback management of migraine headache. The first, and by far the most popular, encompasses thermal biofeedback, wherein migraineurs are taught voluntarily to raise the temperature of their hands. Developers of this biofeedback approach (Sargent, Green, & Walters, 1972, 1973) recommend it be combined with certain aspects of autogenic training (Schultz & Luthe, 1969) and term the resultant combination "autogenic feedback." This treatment owes its development to a serendipitous laboratory finding, which accounts for its lack of face validity. Early explanations of therapeutic effects were based on a hydraulic model of blood flow; researchers speculated that hand warming shunted blood from the cranium to the extremities, thereby counteracting the cephalic vasodilitation phase of headache. There are two problems with this account. First, studies that have compared handwarming to handcooling have found similar treatment outcomes (Kewman & Roberts, 1980; Largen, Mathew, Dobbins, & Claghorn, 1981), which should not be possible. Gauthier, Bois, Allaire, and Drolet (1981) hypothesize, alternatively, that thermal biofeedback may serve to stabilize the vasomotor response system. Second, recent research suggests that digital vasodilitation may result more from increased (beta-adrenergic) rather than decreased (alpha-adrenergic) sympathetic activity (Cohen & Coffman, 1981). Only further research can confirm the viability of these more contemporary views.

The second biofeedback approach for migraine headache follows from a more logical treatment rationale. Cephalic vasomotor biofeedback teaches individuals to decrease blood flow directly in the temporal artery as a means for aborting headache (i.e., the biofeedback equivalent to ergotamine). Acquiring control of the pulse amplitude of the temporal artery is difficult, and the instrumentation for monitoring this response is complex. Although the limited published investigations all convey positive outcomes, this biofeedback treatment remains experimental.

Biofeedback treatment for tension headache involves teaching individuals to control muscle contractures believed to underlie the headache (Budzynski, Stoyva, & Adler, 1970; Budzynski, Stoyva, Adler, & Mullaney, 1973). Stoyva and Budzynski (1974) claim that electromyographic (EMG) biofeedback leads to a generalized state of relaxation, which they term "cultivated low arousal," but evidence does not support this conclusion (Thompson, Haber, & Tearnan, 1981). Further, process analyses of EMG biofeedback have found treatment effects to be independent of direction of change for EMG levels (Andrasik & Holroyd, 1980; Cram, 1980). It is possible that Gauthier et al.'s notion of biofeedback leading to response stability can account for findings in the area of EMG biofeedback as well. Alternatively, it has been argued (Holroyd & Andrasik, 1982) that improvements in headache resulting from biofeedback treatments may be more a consequence of cognitive and behavioral changes stimulated by contingent successes patients experience during biofeedback, than a direct result of their efforts to control the relevant physiological parameter. Recent research provides support for this cognitive-behavioral mediational account (Holroyd et al., 1984).

Relaxation therapies used for headache are varied and range from passive forms (such as meditation and autogenic therapy by itself) to active forms (such as progressive muscle relaxation). Research has not been conducted to examine change processes underlying relaxation treatment for headache.

Two recent meta-analyses of biofeedback and relaxation training for adult headache permit a quick and efficient examination of the extensive research base with adults (Blanchard & Andrasik, 1982; Holroyd & Penzien, 1985). In a meta-analysis, groups of subjects receiving a common treatment become the unit of analysis, rather than data from individual subjects. Average group improvement for biofeedback and relaxation treatments and various control procedures are summarized in Table 18.5. For migraine, autogenic feedback is the only treatment statistically superior to psychological placebo, although all active behavioral treatments exceed results for pharmacological placebo. Although autogenic feedback was not statistically distinguishable from relaxation training alone, the magnitude of the difference was 17 percent, which seems to be of clinical significance. Turning to tension headache, relaxation, EMG biofeedback or combinations of both were found to be statistically superior to both psychological control conditions. Holroyd and Penzien (1985) did not consider results from investigations of pharmacological placebos. We have included average group improvement from eight pharmacological examinations of placebos administered in double-blind fashion for comparison (from Blanchard & Andrasik, 1982). It is obvious from examining the range of improvement across studies and treatment conditions that no one behavioral treatment is uniformly effective across headache types and investigational settings. Whether carefully matching patients to treatments can reduce this excessive variability is not known.

Cognitive stress-coping training is a third psychological treatment for headache. Cognitive-based treatments have much appeal because of their broader and more flexible focus. Treatment directly targets cognitive, affective, and sensory components of headache, as well as any depression, frustration, and despair resulting from unremitting pain. Evaluations of this approach are limited in number, which accounts for it not being included in the meta-analyses. Further, all but a few of the published outcome investigations of cognitive therapy (Gerhards et al., 1983; Holroyd & Andrasik, 1978; Holroyd, Andrasik, & Westbrook, 1977; Knapp & Floin, 1981) have confounded treatment by including biofeedback, relaxation, or both. Additional research is needed to document the independent contributions of this new but promising behavioral treatment alternative.

Our search of the pediatric behavioral literature uncovered the treatment reports summarized in Table 18.6 (convention presentations were excluded unless we were able to obtain a more complete manuscript from authors). Review of these studies leads to the following conclusions. Although treatment research is at an early stage of development, results are uniformly encouraging. In fact, outcomes obtained by children far exceed those obtained by adults receiving essentially identical procedures (see Table 18.5). Improvements for migraineurs receiving behavioral treatment range from 5 percent to complete elimination of headache; success rates for tension headache sufferers all exceed 75 percent. Additionally, the behavioral procedures have been found to be readily adaptable to children, requiring only minor adjustments (Attanasio et al., in press). These highly positive findings led Diamond and Franklin (1975) to conclude: "Autogenic training accompanied with biofeedback is the treatment of choice in children with migraine. We feel that it will prevent these children from developing into drug habituated and depressed adults and is the best prophylactic-type therapy available" (p. 192). Further tests of behavioral treatment procedures, including larger samples and longer follow-up intervals, are necessary to substantiate the strong claims of Diamond and Franklin, however. Evaluations of behavioral treatments for tension headache are particularly needed. Table 18.6 reveals only three investigations of behavioral treatment for pediatric tension headache, involving a total of only 12 children. This stands in marked contrast to the 37 separate studies reviewed by Holroyd and Penzien (1985).

Many of the treatments included multiple components, which we term the "kitchen sink approach." This practice is not unusual when research is at an early stage of development. Further, some investigators included treatment components that would be difficult to deliver in a fairly standard fashion across subjects (e.g., individualized behavior therapy for problems encountered at school or home, as done in Mehegan, et al., 1984). The isolation of components contributing most to outcome may not be a major concern to clinical practitioners, but it merits a high priority for researchers. Children treated by Labbé and Williamson (1984) evidenced no meaningful abilities to regulate their hand temperatures in the absence of feedback (reliable increases occurred only in the presence of the feedback stimulus). Biofeedback remains an effective treatment in search of an explanation.

Although the role of secondary gains has been much researched for other forms of chronic pain, little attention has been accorded their role in pediatric headache, except in the form of three case reports. Ramsden, Friedman, and Williamson (1981) reported on the successful reduction of head pain reports with contingency management procedures. Similarly, Lake (1981) increased the school attendance of an 11-year-old migraineur through attention to and modification of consequent events in the boy's environment. Yen and McIntire (1971) successfully reduced headaches in a 14-year-old female by applying a response cost contingency. Ramsden et al. included punishment in their treatment procedure. The potential for abuse and unpleasant emotional side effects may limit widespread use of this procedure. Further research is warranted on the general role of secondary gains in the maintenance of headache in childhood, but care should be taken that not just the *reports* of pain show behavioral decrease.

Results from the two studies including no-treatment controls (Andrasik et al., 1984; Labbé & Williamson, 1984) are fairly consistent and reveal minimal change as a function of time alone. However, the only investigation to include a placebo control (Richter, McGrath, Humphreys, Goodman, Firestone, & Keene, 1984) found a fairly sizeable change in symptom report.

TABLE 18.5. META-ANALYSIS OF BIOFEEDBACK AND RELAXATION TREATMENT FOR ADULT HEADACHE

A. Migraine Headache

	Treatment Conditions[a]						
	Autogenic Feedback	Relaxation	Vasomotor Biofeedback	Thermal Biofeedback	Psychological Placebo	Headache Monitoring	Pharmacological Placebo
Average Group Improvement (%)	64.9	47.9	42.3	34.6	27.6	17.2	16.5
Number of Groups	11	7	4	7	5	6	6
Range of Improvement (%)	35 to 82	16 to 83	11 to 63	21 to 45	8 to 54	−3 to 47	

B. *Tension Headache*

	Treatment Conditions[a]					
	Relaxation & EMG Biofeedback	EMG Biofeedback	Relaxation	Noncontingent EMG Biofeedback	Headache Monitoring	Pharmacological Placebo[b]
Average Group Improvement (%)	57.1	46.0	44.6	15.3	−3.9	34.8
Number of Groups	9	26	15	6	10	8
Range of Improvement (%)	29 to 88	13 to 87	17 to 94	−14 to 40	−28 to 12	19 to 62

Source: A, Blanchard and Andrasik, 1982; B, Holroyd and Penzien, 1985.

[a]Treatment conditions sharing an underline do not differ at the .05 level of significance.

[b]From Blanchard and Andrasik, 1982.

TABLE 18.6. BEHAVIORAL TREATMENT OF PEDIATRIC HEADACHE

Authors	Number of Subjects	Age	Study Design	Treatment Procedure	Results
			A. Migraine		
Diamond & Franklin (1975)	32	9–18	Collection of case studies	Thermal BF, EMG BF, Autogenic TR, Relaxation TR	81% judged to show "good response" over 30-month period
Feuerstein & Adams (1977)	1	15	Systematic Case Study	EMG BF & Vasomotor BF	Headache activity increased during EMG BF; 86% reduction in HA frequency at 9-week follow-up for vasomotor BF
Sallade (1980)	8	8–11	Single Group Outcome	Dietary management, Relaxation TR, & Client-Centered Therapy (delivered in group format)	50% reduction in headache frequency at end of treatment
Lake (1981)	1	11	Case Study	Contingency management: reinforcement for increasing school attendance	School attendance regular and headache-free intervals lasting up to 3 weeks at 1-year follow-up
	1	15	Systematic Case Study	EMG BF, Autogenic TR, & Anxiety Management TR	Headache free at 3-month follow-up
Olness & MacDonald (1981)	3(15)[a]	9, 11 & 13	Collection of Case Studies	Thermal BF & Self-Hypnosis	Headaches "no longer problematic" at varied follow-ups

N	Study	Age	Design	Treatment	Outcome
2	Andrasik, Blanchard, Edlund, & Rosenblum (1982)	12 & 14	Multiple Baseline Across Subjects	Thermal BF & Autogenic TR	67 and 57% reduction in headache sum through follow-ups of 7 to 10 weeks
1	Houts (1982)	11	Systematic Case Study	Thermal BF & Relaxation TR	75% reduction in headache frequency at 1-year follow-up
3	Labbé & Williamson (1983)	9, 12, 13	Multiple Baseline	Thermal BF & Autogenic TR	Each child headache free at 2-year follow-up
1 (combined with tension HA)	Marrazo, Hickling, & Sison (1983)	15	Case Study	EMG BF, Thermal BF, & Rational Emotive Therapy	Headache free at 18-month follow-up (for preceeding 3 months)
1	Ramsden, Friedman, & Williamson (1983)	6	Multiple Baseline Across Settings: School and Home	Contingency management: reinforcement for well behavior and punishment for pain behavior	Headache free at 10-month follow-up in both settings
14	Andrasik, Attanasio, Blanchard, Burke, Kabela, McCarran, Blake, & Rosenblum (1984)	8–16	Controlled Group Outcome	Thermal BF & Autogenic TR	90% of children thus far seen for 6-month follow-up ($n = 9$) were improved
16				Relaxation TR	70% of children thus far seen for 6-month follow-up ($n = 9$) were improved
18				No treatment; Wait-List Control	25% of children improved at end of wait-list interval

TABLE 18.6. *(Continued)*

Authors	Number of Subjects	Age	Study Design	Treatment Procedure	Results
Labbé & Williamson (1984)	14	7–16	Controlled Group Outcome	Thermal BF & Autogenic TR	63% of children seen for 6-month follow-up (*n* = 8) were improved
	14			No treatment; Wait-List Control	14% of children improved at end of wait-list interval
Mehegan, Masek, Harrison, Russo, & Leviton (1984)	20	6–12	Multiple Baseline Across Groups of Subjects	EMG BF, Meditative Relaxation TR, & "Behavior Therapy" (primarily contingency management and therapy for school and family problems)	91% reduction in headache activity at 1-year follow-up
Werder & Sargent (1984)	19	7–17	Single Group Outcome	Thermal BF, EMG BF, Autogenic TR, Relaxation TR, Self-Awareness, & Guided Imagery	92% of children seen for 2–3 year follow-up (*n* = 13) could "successfully regulate their headaches"
	2 (combined with tension HA)			Same as above	50% of children seen for 2–3 year follow-up (*n* = 2) could "successfully regulate their headaches"

Study	N	Age	Design	Treatment	Outcome
Richter, McGrath, Humphreys, Goodman, Firestone, & Keene (1984)	15 (8 high severity, 7 low severity)	9–18	Controlled Group Outcome	Relaxation TR	66% reduction in headache activity for high severity and 65% for low severity groups at 4-month follow-up
	15 (7 high severity, 8 low severity)			Cognitive TR; Cognitive Restructuring, Stress-Innoculation TR, Rational Emotive Therapy, & Cognitive Control of Pain	67% reduction in headache activity for high severity and 59% for low severity groups at 4-month follow-up
	12 (5 high severity, 7 low severity)			Attention Placebo Control	33% reduction in headache activity for high severity and 70% for low severity groups at 4-month follow-up
B. Tension					
Yen & McIntire (1971)	1	14	Systematic Case Study	Response cost: record certain information after each headache complaint	92% reduction in headache frequency through 5-week follow-up
Andrasik, Blanchard, Edlund, & Attanasio (1983)	1	11	Systematic Case Study	EMG BF	79% reduction in HA Sum at 1-year follow-up; 75% reduction in HA frequency at 1-year follow-up
Werder & Sargent (1984)	10	7–17	Single Group Outcome	Thermal BF, EMG BF, Autogenic TR, Relaxation TR, Self-Awareness, & Guided Imagery	80% of children seen for 2–3 year follow-up ($n = 5$) could "successfully regulate their headaches"

[a]The authors state 15 subjects were treated, but they discuss results for only 3 children.

Richter et al., divided subjects in each experimental condition into groups revealing low severities and high severities of headache during baseline. Children with low severity headaches were highly responsive to placebo treatment (mean improvement = 70%), whereas children with high severity headaches were not (mean improvement = 33%). Further tests of the unique contributions of behavioral procedures appear warranted.

As in the adult area, cognitive treatments are especially underdeveloped. The only large scale investigation of cognitive treatment found it to be equivalent in effectiveness to relaxation training alone; effects were similar for children with low and high severity headaches alike (Richter et al., 1984).

Even with these especially promising results, a proportion of children are not being helped to any meaningful degree. The search for factors predictive of response to a particular treatment is helpful to better match patients to treatments. Diamond and Franklin (1975) found the presence of depression to be predictive of a poor response to behavioral treatment. McGrath (1984) also found a significant relationship between depression and outcome; however, the relationship he noted was much more modest (correlation = .26) and was in a direction opposite that of Diamond and Franklin. Diamond (1979) later reported that age had a bearing on outcome, with children under 12 showing the best response. The subsequent reports by Werder and Sargent (1984) and Andrasik et al. (1984) were unable to substantiate this age effect. Preliminary analyses we conducted to assess effects due to gender, chronicity, and familial headache status likewise proved to be of no predictive value. The search will have to continue for factors effective in predicting treatment response.

CONCLUDING REMARKS

Headache control is a relatively new endeavor for behavioral pediatrics. Given this, we were mindful of several questions as we approached this chapter. First, how typical is headache among children? Meghan, whom we discussed at the outset of this chapter, is a dramatic case, but just how representative is her problem? Second, is headache likely to subside as a child matures? We uncovered literature that reveals headache is widespread among children and is unlikely to yield to the passage of time alone. The remaining question foremost in our minds was what can pediatric behavioral practitioners do about headache? It seems there is much that can be done, although we have just begun to scratch the surface. We attempted to outline what is currently known about treatment, where gaps are located, and how these gaps might be filled. As our understanding of the myriad biological and behavioral aspects of pediatric headache becomes more complete, widespread application of this knowledge will, it is hoped, help Meghan and the thousands of other headache sufferers better realize their life potential.

REFERENCES

Ad Hoc Committee on Classification of Headache. (1962). Classification of headache. *Journal of the American Medical Association, 179*, 717–718.

Adams, H. E., Brantley, P. J., & Thompson, K. (1982). Biofeedback and headache: Methodological issues. In L. White & B. Tursky (Eds.), *Clinical biofeedback: Efficacy and mechanisms* (pp. 358–367). New York: Guilford.

Ala-Hurula, V., Myllyla, V., & Hokkanen, E. (1982). Ergotamine abuse: Results of ergotamine discontinuation, with special reference to the plasma concentration. *Cephalalgia, 2*, 189–195.

Andrasik, F., Attanasio, V., Blanchard, E. B., Burke, E., Kabela, E., McCarran, M., Blake, D. D., & Rosenblum, E. L. (1984). *Behavioral treatment of pediatric migraine headache.* Paper presented at the meeting of the Association for Advancement of Behavior Therapy, Philadelphia, Pennsylvania.

Andrasik, F., Blanchard, E. B., Ahles, T., Pallmeyer, T., & Barron, K. D. (1981). Assessing the reactive as well as the sensory component of headache pain. *Headache, 21*, 218–221.

Andrasik, F., Blanchard, E. B., Arena, J. G., Saunders, N. L., & Barron, K. D. (1982). Psychophysiology of recurrent headache: Methodological issues and new empirical findings. *Behavior Therapy, 13*, 407–429.

Andrasik, F., Blanchard, E. B., Arena, J. G., Teders, S. J., Teevan, R. C., & Rodichok, L. D. (1982). Psychological functioning in headache sufferers. *Psychosomatic Medicine, 44*, 171–182.

Andrasik, F., Blanchard, E. B., Edlund, S. R., & Attanasio, V. (1983). EMG biofeedback treatment of a child with muscle contraction headache. *American Journal of Clinical Biofeedback, 6*, 96–102.

Andrasik, F., Blanchard, E. B., Edlund, S. R., & Rosenblum, E. L. (1982). Autogenic feedback in the treatment of two children with migraine headache. *Child and Family Behavior Therapy, 4*, 13–23.

Andrasik, F., Burke, E. J., Attanasio, V., & Rosenblum, E. L. (in press). Child, parent, and physician reports of a child's headache pain: Relationships prior to and following treatment. *Headache.*

Andrasik, F., & Holroyd, K. A. (1980). A test of the specific and nonspecific effects in the biofeedback treatment of tension headache. *Journal of Consulting and Clinical Psychology, 48*, 575–586.

Andrasik, F., Kabela, E., Quinn, S., Blanchard, E. B., & Rosenblum, E. L. (1985). *Psychological functioning of children who have recurrent migraine.* Manuscript submitted for publication.

Attanasio, V., Andrasik, F., Burke, E. J., Blake, D. D., Kabela, E., & McCarran, M. S. (in press). Clinical issues in utilizing biofeedback with children. *Clinical Biofeedback and Health.*

Arena, J. G., Blanchard, E. B., Andrasik, F., & Dudek, B. C. (1982). The Headache Symptom Questionnaire: Discriminant classificatory ability and headache syndromes suggested by a factor analysis. *Journal of Behavioral Assessment, 4*, 55–69.

Bakal, D. A. (1979). *Psychology and medicine. Psychobiological dimensions of health and illness.* New York: Springer.

Bakal, D. A. (1982). *The psychobiology of chronic headache.* New York: Springer.

Bakal, D. A., & Kaganov, J. A. (1979). Symptom characteristics of chronic and nonchronic headache sufferers. *Headache, 19*, 285–289.

Barabas, G., Matthews, W. S., & Ferrari, M. (1983). Childhood migraine and motion sickness. *Pediatrics, 72*, 188–190.

Barlow, C. F. (1978). Migraine in childhood. *Research and Clinical Studies in Headache, 5*, 34–46.

Bell, W. E. (1968). Headache in childhood. *Headache, 8,* 127–132.

Bille, B. (1962). Migraine in school children, *Acta paediatrica scandinavica, 51,* 1–151.

Bille, B. (1981). Migraine in childhood and its prognosis. *Cephalalgia, 1,* 71–75.

Bille, B., Ludvigsson, J., & Sanner, G. (1977). Prophylaxis of migraine in children. *Headache, 17,* 61–63.

Blanchard, E. B., & Andrasik, F. (1982). Psychological assessment and treatment of headache: Recent developments and emerging issues. *Journal of Consulting and Clinical Psychology, 50,* 859–879.

Brown, J. K. (1977). Migraine and migraine equivalents in children. *Developmental Medicine and Child Neurology, 19,* 683–692.

Buda, F. B., & Joyce, R. P. (1979). Successful treatment of atypical migraine of childhood with anticonvulsants. *Military Medicine, 144,* 521–523.

Budzynski, T., Stoyva, J., & Adler, C. (1970). Feedback-induced relaxation: Application to tension headache. *Journal of Behavior Therapy and Experimental Psychiatry, 1,* 205–211.

Budzynski, T. H., Stoyva, J. M., Adler, C. S., & Mullaney, D. J. (1973). EMG biofeedback and tension headache: A controlled outcome study. *Psychosomatic Medicine, 35,* 484–496.

Cahn, T., & Cram, J. R. (1980). Changing measurement instrument at follow-up: A potential source of error. *Biofeedback and Self-Regulation, 5,* 265–273.

Cohen, R., & Coffman, J. (1981). Beta-adrenergic vasodilator mechanisms in the finger. *Circulation Research, 49,* 123–146.

Congdon, P. J. & Forsythe, W. I. (1979). Migraine in childhood: A study of 300 children. *Developmental Medicine and Child Neurology, 21,* 209–216.

Couch, J. R., & Hassanein, R. S. (1979). Amitriptyline in migraine prophylaxis. *Archives of Neurology, 36,* 695–699.

Cox, D., & Thomas, D. (1981). Relationship between headaches and depression. *Headache, 21,* 261–263.

Cram, J. R. (1980). EMG biofeedback and the treatment of tension headaches: A systematic analysis of treatment components. *Behavior Therapy, 11,* 699–710.

Dalsgaard-Nielson, T. (1965). Migraine and heredity. *Acta neurologica scandinavica, 41,* 287–300.

Dalton, K., & Dalton, M. E. (1979). Food intake before migraine attacks in children. *Journal of the Royal College of General Practitioners, 29,* 662–665.

Daly, E. J., Donn, P. A., Galliher, M. J., & Zimmerman, J. S. (1983). Biofeedback applications to migraine and tension headaches: A double-blinded outcome study. *Biofeedback and Self-Regulation, 8,* 135–152.

Deubner, D. C. (1977). An epidemiologic study of migraine and headache in 10-20 year olds, *Headache, 17,* 173–180.

Diamond, S. (1979). Biofeedback and headache. *Headache, 19,* 180–184.

Diamond, S. (1983). Depression and headache. *Headache, 23,* 123–126.

Diamond, S., & Dalessio, D. J. (1982). *The practicing physician's approach to headache* (3rd ed.). Baltimore: Williams & Wilkins.

Diamond, S., & Franklin, M. (1975). Biofeedback: Choice of treatment in childhood migraine. In W. Luthe & F. Antonelli (Eds.), *Therapy in psychosomatic medicine* (Vol. 4). Rome: Autogenic Therapy.

Egermark-Eriksson, I. (1982). Prevalence of headache in Swedish school-children. *Acta paediatrica scandinavica, 71,* 135–140.

Feuerstein, M., & Adams, H. E. (1977). Cephalic vasomotor feedback in the modification of migraine headache. *Biofeedback and Self-Regulation, 2,* 241–254.

Gauthier, J., Bois, R., Allaire, D., & Drolet, M. (1981). Evaluation of skin temperature biofeedback training at two different sites for migraine. *Journal of Behavioral Medicine, 4*, 407–419.

Gerber, W. D., Miltner, W., Birbaumer, N., & Lutzenberger, W. (1983). Cephalic vasomotor feedback therapy: A controlled study of migraineurs and normals. In K. A. Holroyd, B. Schlote, & H. Zenz (Eds.), *Perspectives in research on headache.* (pp. 163–170). Lewiston, NY: C. J. Hogrefe.

Gerhards, F., Rojahn, J., Boxan, K., Gnade, C., Petrick, M., & Florin, I. (1983). Biofeedback versus cognitive stress-coping therapy in migraine headache patients. In K. A. Holroyd, B. Schlote, & H. Zenz (Eds.), *Perspectives in research on headache* (pp. 171–182). Lewiston, NY: C. J. Hogrefe.

Hammond, J. (1974). The late sequelae of recurrent vomiting of childhood. *Developmental Medicine and Child Neurology, 16*, 15–22.

Hanington, E. (1967). Preliminary report on the tyramine headache. *British Medical Journal, 1*, 550–551.

Haynes, S. N. (1980). Muscle contraction headache: A psychophysiological perspective of etiology and treatment. In S. N. Haynes & L. R. Gannon (Eds.), *Psychosomatic disorders. A psychophysiological approach to etiology and treatment.* New York: Gardner.

Haynes, S. N., Cuevas, J., & Gannon, L. R. (1982). The psychophysiological etiology of muscle-contraction headache. *Headache, 22*, 122–132.

Hinrichs, W. L., & Keith, H. M. (1965). Migraine in childhood: A follow-up report. *Mayo Clinic Proceedings, 40*, 593–596.

Hockaday, J. M. (1978). Late outcome of childhood onset migraine and factors affecting outcome, with particular reference to early and late EEG findings. In R. Greene (Ed.), *Current concepts in migraine research,* New York: Raven.

Holguin, J., & Fenichel, G. (1967). Migraine. *Journal of Pediatrics, 70*, 290–297.

Holroyd, K. A. (in press). Recurrent headache. In K. A. Holroyd & T. Creer (Eds.), *Self-management of physical disease: Developments in health psychology and behavioral medicine.* New York: Academic.

Holroyd, K. A., & Andrasik, F. (1978). Coping and the self-regulation of chronic tension headache. *Journal of Consulting and Clinical Psychology, 46*, 1036–1045.

Holroyd, K. A., & Andrasik, F. (1982). A cognitive-behavioral approach to recurrent tension and migraine headache. In P. C. Kendall (Ed.), *Advances in cognitive-behavioral research and therapy* (pp. 275–320). New York: Academic.

Holroyd, K. A., Andrasik, F., & Westbrook, T. (1977). Cognitive control of tension headache. *Cognitive Therapy and Research, 1*, 121–133.

Holroyd, K. A., & Penzien, D. B. (1985). *Client variables and the behavioral treatment of recurrent tension headache: A meta-analytic review.* Unpublished manuscript.

Holroyd, K. A., Penzien, D. B., Hursey, K. G., Tobin, D. L., Rogers, L., Holm, J. E., Marcille, P. J., Hall, J. R., & Chila, A. G. (1984). Change mechanisms in EMG biofeedback training: Cognitive changes underlying improvements in tension headache. *Journal of Consulting and Clinical Psychology, 52*, 1039–1053.

Houts, A. C. (1982). Relaxation and thermal feedback treatment of child migraine headache: A case study. *American Journal of Clinical Biofeedback, 5*, 154–157.

Jay, G. W. (1982). Epilepsy, migraine, and EEG abnormalities in children: A review and hypothesis. *Headache, 22*, 110–114.

Jay, G. W., Renelli, D., & Mead, T. (1984). The effects of propranolol and amitriptyline on vascular and EMG biofeedback training. *Headache, 24*, 59–69.

Jay, G. W. & Tomasi, L. G. (1981). Pediatric headaches: A one year retrospective analysis. *Headache, 21*, 5–9.

Jeans, M. E. (1983). Pain in children—A neglected area. In P. Firestone, P. J. McGrath, & W. Feldman (Eds.), *Advances in behavioral medicine for children and adolescents*. Hillsdale, NJ.. Erlbaum.

Joffe, R., Bakal, D. A., & Kaganov, J. (1983). A self-observation study of headache symptoms in children. *Headache, 23*, 20–25.

Kewman, D., & Roberts, A. H. (1980). Skin temperature biofeedback and migraine headache: A double-blind study. *Biofeedback and Self-regulation, 5*, 327–345.

Knapp, T. W., & Florin, I. (1981). The treatment of migraine headaches by training in vasoconstriction of the temporal artery and a cognitive stress-coping training. *Behaviour Analysis and Modification, 4*, 267–274.

Kohlenberg, R. J. (1982). Tyramine sensitivity in dietary migraine.. A critical review. *Headache, 22*, 30–34.

Kroner, B. (1983). The empirical validity of clinical headache classification. In K. A. Holroyd, B. Schlote, & H. Zenz (Eds.), *Perspectives in research on headache* (pp. 56–65). Lewiston, NY: C. J. Hogrefe.

Krupp, G. R., & Friedman, A. P. (1953). Recurrent headache in children: A study of 100 clinic cases. *New York State Journal of Medicine, 53*, 43–45.

Kudrow, L. (1982). Paradoxical effects of frequent analgesic use. In M. Critchley, A. P. Friedman, S. Gorini, & F. Sicuteri (Eds.), *Advances in neurology: Headache: Physiopathological and clinical concepts* (Vol. 33). New York.. Raven.

Kudrow, L. (1983). Pathogenesis of vascular headache. In W. H. Rickles, J. H. Sandweiss, D. Jacobs, & R. N. Grove (Eds.), *Biofeedback and family practice medicine* (pp. 41–59). New York: Plenum.

Labbé, E. E., & Williamson, D. A. (1983). Temperature biofeedback in the treatment of children with migraine headaches. *Journal of Pediatric Psychology, 8*, 317–326.

Labbé, E. L., & Williamson, D. A. (1984). Treatment of childhood migraine using autogenic feedback training. *Journal of Consulting and Clinical Psychology, 52*, 968–976.

Lake, A. E. (1981). Behavioral assessment considerations in the management of headache. *Headache, 21*, 170–178.

Lance, J. W., & Anthony, M. (1966). Some clinical aspects of migraine. *Archives of Neurology, 15*, 356.

Largen, J. W., Matthew, R. J., Dobbins, K., & Claghorn, J. L. (1981). Specific and non-specific effects of skin temperature control in migraine management. *Headache, 21*, 36–44.

Leviton, A. (1978). Epidemiology of headache. In V. S. Schoenberg (Ed.), *Advances in neurology* (Vol. 19, pp. 341–352). NY: Raven.

Leviton, A., Slack, W. V., Masek, B., Bana, D., & Graham, J. R. (1984). A computerized behavioral assessment for children with headaches. *Headache, 24*, 182–185.

Ling, W., Oftedal, G., & Weinberg, W. (1970). Depressive illness in childhood presenting as severe headache. *American Journal of Diseases of Children, 120*, 122–124.

Ludvigsson, J. (1974). Propranolol used in prophylaxis of migraine in children. *Acta neurologica scandinavica, 50*, 109–115.

Marrazo, M. J. Hickling, E. J., & Sison, G. F. P. (1983). *The psychological treatment of childhood migraine: A review and case presentation*. Paper presented at the meeting of the Biofeedback Society of America, Denver, Colorado.

Martin, J. J. (1978). Psychogenic factors in headache. *Medical Clinics of North America, 62*, 559–570.

Martin, P. R. (1983). Behavioural research on headaches: Current status and future directions. In K. A. Holroyd, B. Schlote, & H. Zenz (Eds.), *Perspectives in research on headaches* (pp. 204–215). Lewiston, NY: C. J. Hogrefe.

Mathew, N. T. (1981). Prophylaxis of migraine and mixed headache: A randomized controlled study. *Headache, 21,* 105–109.

Medina, J. L., & Diamond, S. (1978). The role of diet in migraine. *Headache, 18,* 31–34.

Mehegan, J. E., Masek, B. J., Harrison, R. H., Russo, D. C., & Leviton, A. (1984). *Behavioral treatment of pediatric headache.* Unpublished manuscript.

Meloff, K. L. (1973). Headache in pediatric practice. *Headache, 13,* 125–139.

Meloff, K. L. (1982). Headaches in children: Cause for parental concern but commonly benign. *Postgraduate Medicine, 72,* 195–202.

Melzack, R. (1973). *The puzzle of pain.* Harmondsworth, England: Penguin.

Millichap, J. G. (1978). Recurrent headache in 100 children: Electro-encephalograhic abnormalities and response to phenytoin (dilantin). *Child's Brain, 4,* 95–105.

Olness, K., & MacDonald, J. (1981). Self-hypnosis and biofeedback in the management of juvenile migraine. *Developmental and Behavioral Pediatrics, 2,* 168–170.

Oster, J. (1972). Recurrent abdominal pain, headache and limb pains in children and adolescents. *Pediatrics, 50,* 429–436.

Philips, C. (1977). A psychological analysis of tension headache. In S. Rachman (Ed.), *Contributions to medical psychology.* Oxford: Pergamon.

Philips, C. (1978). Tension headache: Theoretical problems. *Behaviour Research and Therapy, 16,* 249–261.

Prensky, A. L. (1976). Migraine and migraineous variants in pediatric patients. *Pediatric Clinics of North America, 23,* 461–471.

Prensky, A. L., & Sommer, D. (1979). Diagnosis and treatment of migraine in children. *Neurology, 29,* 506–510.

Ramsden, R., Friedman, B., & Williamson, D. (1983). Treatment of childhood headache reports with contingency management procedures. *Journal of Clinical Child Psychology, 12,* 202–206.

Richardson, G. M., McGrath, P. J., Cunningham, S. J. & Humphreys, P. (1983). Validity of the headache diary for children. *Headache, 23,* 184–187.

Richter, I. L., McGrath, P. J., Humphreys, P. J., Goodman, J. T., Firestone, P., & Keene, D. (1984). *Cognitive and relaxation treatment of pediatric migraine.* (Under Review)

Rothner, A. D. (1978). Headaches in children: A review. *Headache, 18,* 169–175.

Sallade, J. B. (1980). Group counseling with children who have migraine headaches. *Elementary School Guidance and Counseling,* 87–89.

Sargent, J. D., Green, E. E., & Walters, E. D. (1972). The use of autogenic training in a pilot study of migraine and tension headaches. *Headache, 12,* 120–124.

Sargent, J. D., Green, E. E., & Walters, E. D. (1973). Preliminary report on the use of autogenic feedback training in the treatment of migraine and tension headaches. *Psychosomatic Medicine, 35,* 129–135.

Sargent, J. D., Walters, E. D., & Green, E. E. (1973). Psychosomatic self-regulation of migraine headache. *Seminars in Psychiatry, 5,* 415–428.

Schultz, J. H., & Luthe, W. (1969). *Autogenic training* (Vol. 1). New York. Grune & Stratton.

Shinnar, S. & D'Souza, B. J. (1981). The diagnosis and management of headaches in childhood. *Pediatric Clinics of North America, 29,* 79–94.

Sillanpaa, M. (1976). Prevalence of migraine and other headache in Finnish children starting school. *Headache, 16,* 288–290.

Sillanpaa, M. (1977). Clonidine prophylaxis of childhood migraine and other vascular headache: A double blind study of 57 children. *Headache, 17,* 28–31.

Sillanpaa, M. (1983a). Prevalence of headache in prepuberty. *Headache, 23,* 10–14.

Sillanpaa, M. (1983b). Changes in the prevalence of migraine and other headaches during the first seven school years. *Headache, 23,* 15–19.

Sillanpaa, M., & Koponen, M. (1978). Papaverine in the prophylaxis of migraine and other vascular headache in children. *Acta paediatrica scandinavica, 67,* 209–212.

Sparks, J. P. (1978). The incidence of migraine in schoolchildren: A survey of the Medical Officers of Schools Association. *The Practitioner, 221,* 407–411.

Stoyva, J., & Budzynski, T. (1974). Cultivated low arousal—An antistress response? In L. V. DiCara (Ed.), *Limbic and autonomic nervous system research* (pp. 369–394). New York. Plenum.

Thompson, J. K., Haber, J. D., & Tearnen, B. H. (1981). Generalization of frontalis electromyographic feedback to adjacent muscle groups: A critical review. *Psychosomatic Medicine, 43,* 19–24.

Vahlquist, B. (1955). Migraine in children. *International Archives of Allergy and Applied Neurology, 7,* 348.

Vahlquist, B. & Hackzell, G. (1949). Migraine of early onset: A study of thirty-one cases in which the disease first appeared between one and four years of age. *Acta paediatrica scandinavica, 38,* 622–636.

Van Boxtel, A., Goudswaard, P., & Janssen, K. (1983). Absolute and proportional resting EMG levels in muscle contraction and migraine headache patients. *Headache, 23,* 215–222.

Verbrugge, L. M. (1979). Female illness rates and illness behavior: Testing hypotheses about sex differences in health. *Women & Health, 4,* 61–79.

Waters, W. E. (1971). Migraine: Intelligence, social class, and familial prevalence. *British Medical Journal, 2,* 77–81.

Waters, W. E. (1972). Migraine and symptoms in childhood: Bilious attacks, travel sickness and eczema. *Headache, 12,* 55–61.

Werder, D. S., & Sargent, J. D. (1984). A study of childhood headache using biofeedback as a treatment alternative. *Headache, 24,* 122–126.

Wolff, H. G. (1937). Personality features and reactions of subjects with migraine. *Archives of Neurology and Psychiatry, 37,* 895–921.

Yen, S., & McIntire, R. W. (1971). Operant therapy for constant headache complaint: A simple response-cost approach. *Psychological Reports, 28,* 267–270.

Ziegler, D. K. (1978). The epidemiology and genetics of migraine. *Research Clinical Studies in Headache, 5,* 21–33.

Ziegler, D. K., Hassanein, R., & Hassanein, K. (1972). Headache syndromes suggested by a factor analysis of symptom variables in a headache prone population. *Journal of Chronic Diseases, 25,* 353–363.

19

Medical Compliance in Pediatric Practice

EDWARD R. CHRISTOPHERSEN, JACK W. FINNEY, AND PATRICK C. FRIMAN

As pediatric health care expands to include not only the treatment of disease but also the prevention of disease and disability, the effectiveness of health care remains dependent on medical compliance by parents and their children. Numerous studies have documented the problem of noncompliance with regimens for the treatment of acute illnesses (Bergman & Werner, 1963; Charney, Bynum, & Eldredge, 1967), for chronic diseases (Gordis, Markowitz, & Lilienfeld, 1969; Lund, Jorgensen, & Kuhl, 1964), and for preventive strategies to protect and promote child health (Gordis & Markowitz, 1971; Reisinger, Williams, John, Roberts, & Podgainy, 1981). Medical compliance has been extensively reviewed in the literature (Dunbar & Stunkard, 1979; Haynes, Taylor, & Sackett, 1979; Rapoff

The research reported herein and the preparation of this manuscript were supported by grants to ERC (NICHD HD 03144 and NICHD HD 02528; NHTSA 7-A02; and Kansas Department of Transportation Grant 84-02-02). The editorial assistance of Barbara Cochrane and Ruth Cargo is gratefully acknowledged.

435

& Christophersen, 1982) and in this volume. The present chapter will highlight findings from the authors' ongoing research and then illustrate, through discussion of recent research findings, some issues that are relevant for pediatric primary health care providers.

Experimental research on compliance improvement strategies suggests that a variety of educational, organizational, and behavioral variables can be identified and implemented to improve patient compliance with physician recommendations (Dunbar, Marshall, & Hovell, 1979; Rapoff & Christophersen, 1982). Educational strategies that explain the patient's disease or its treatment regimen have been developed for pediatric practice. Organizational strategies, such as decreasing patient's waiting time for seeing the provider or care by a consistent physician, have been used in some health care settings. Behavioral strategies, such as the use of pill dispensers, patient monitoring sheets, regimen tailoring, and token economies have also been used. Although compliance problems in some health care settings have allowed for only one procedure to be implemented by the provider, other settings may allow more flexibility or may allow for more comprehensive programming to enhance compliance.

As is often the practice in new areas of inquiry, the search for variables that correlate with compliance was made by early researchers (Becker, Drachman, & Kirscht, 1972). Numerous variables, such as patient demographics, disease characteristics, and regimen requirements, were identified through correlational research. Unfortunately these variables are usually very difficult to change or manipulate (Cataldo, 1982). Therefore correlational studies have not provided information on which to base compliance improvement strategies.

The choice of a compliance improvement strategy must be based on the presenting problem and on the activities of the providers who are responsible for patient care if the research on medical compliance is to be truly useful to primary providers. The strategies must be compatible with the primary providers' role in improving the ease of interventions based on these findings. Pediatric outpatient appointments are generally brief visits (5 to 15 minutes), during which the patient's history is taken, the physical examination is conducted, and recommendations are made. Thus compliance-improvement strategies for pediatric practitioners must be easy to explain and capable of being implemented quickly. Many previously recommended procedures are effective but are not feasible for pediatricians (Christophersen & Rapoff, 1979). For example, token economy procedures to increase regimen compliance have been effective for children with insulin-dependent diabetes (Lowe & Lutzker, 1979) and juvenile rheumatoid arthritis (Rapoff, Lindsley, & Christophersen, 1984). Such intensive procedures require considerably more time for implementation and follow-up than is usually available in pediatric practice.

Much of the early research on medical compliance has been characterized by a lack of theoretical structure or direction. There has been little recognition that in many areas of interaction between professionals and parents, dependence on traditional health education strategies such as lectures or "pep talks" is not adequate to ensure patient compliance. This is not to say that accident prevention or other areas of health education should or can be treated as behavioral deficiencies (Williams, 1982). However, the effectiveness of health education for improving health status will always depend, at least in part, on behavior change of parents or caregivers that results from health education.

Janis (1983) reviewed the published literature on medical compliance and stated that "the most serious medical problems that today plague the majority of Americans and Europeans are not primarily medical; they are behavioral problems requiring the alteration of personal habits, preferences, and decisions" (p. 146). Janis postulated that, while health care providers want their patients to comply with their recommendations, patients will weigh the benefits of a recommended course of action against the perceived costs of or barriers to taking that action only when their dominant coping pattern is vigilance. This vigilance pattern occurs only when three conditions are met: (1) the person is aware of the serious risks of not complying (conflict), (2) the person is optimistic about finding a satisfactory solution (hope), and (3) the person believes that there is adequate time to search and deliberate before a final decision is made (adequate time). It is only when the person conducts an adequate information search and appraisal of the corresponding consequences, without overlooking or ignoring crucial information about relevant costs and benefits, that we can actually expect compliance.

Janis states that most of the patient activities that are positively related to compliance involve positive incentives for carrying out the recommended action, and most of the patient activities that are negatively related involve negative incentives (the difficulties and deprivations expected if one carries out the course of action recommended by the health professional).

Thus Janis's work suggests that the minimum requirements for compliance would be that the patient understands the seriousness of the problem, knows the benefits and the costs of complying and not complying, and has time in which to ponder the options available to him. Obviously, the "pep talks" and "scare tactics" of many health care professionals are unlikely, given Janis's minimum requirements, to lead to compliance.

For example, in the typical well-child visit, the pediatric health care provider may warn a parent of the dangers associated with automobile travel for infants and young children. However, in the 97 seconds that Reisinger and Bires (1980) found is usually devoted to anticipatory guidance, there is no opportunity for all of the conditions that Janis posits to be met. Janis's work would predict that the patient, if provided with the pros and cons of a particular health education strategy, given a positive rationale for complying with the recommendations and the time to think it through, would comply with the recommendations. In a recent paper on compliance with the use of child restraint seats, Treiber (in press) compared three approaches: positive consequences (wherein the parent was told of the advantages of using child restraint seats); negative consequences (wherein the parent was told of the risks that accompany not using child restraint seats); and a combination approach (wherein the parent was told of both the positive and negative consequences of child restraint seat usage). His results showed that the combination-group results were superior to those of the other two groups. There are numerous other areas within the general area of health education where such a "combination" of strategies is appropriate and applicable. The inclusion of the strategies recommended in Janis's work, similar to those strategies investigated in research by the present authors and others, certainly merits consideration by individuals and institutions responsible for planning health education efforts for expectant parents and parents of young children.

The series of studies described later were conducted in busy clinical pediatric settings, without substantially changing the existing care structure. Furthermore, patients from lower, middle, and upper socioeconomic levels were served in these clinical settings. The findings suggest that socioeconomic and demographic characteristics were not predictive of an individual patient's response to a compliance improvement strategy.

The first study was an evaluation to increase appointment-keeping in a hospital-based ambulatory pediatrics clinic. Broken appointments are a prime source of disruptions to child health supervision and acute illness follow-up care. A second study evaluated a child-passenger safety program to increase the use of child restraint seats and thereby reduce, ultimately, morbidity and mortality from automobile accidents, the greatest single threat to children in the United States. The third study was an evaluation of a group well-child education strategy to improve parental efforts to reduce the likelihood of a home accident that would result in the child being burned. The fourth study, adherence with short-term regimens, was conducted with children undergoing treatment for otitis media, one of the most common illnesses encountered in pediatric practice. Short-term antibiotic regiments are frequently prescribed for acute infections, but many children do not receive the complete treatment.

COMPLIANCE WITH PEDIATRIC HEALTH CARE APPOINTMENTS

A health care appointment that is neither kept nor cancelled is a broken appointment. As many as one-third of all health care appointments are broken (Jonas, 1971). Broken health care appointments can cause a failure of continuity of care, waste valuable professional time, prevent the delivery of prophylactic medical services and thereby increase the risk of communicable disease, and generally reduce the productivity of medical service providers (Alpert, 1964; Frankel & Hovell, 1978; Hertz & Stamps, 1977; Oppenheim, Bergman, & English, 1979). Broken appointments are a problem in most medical settings, but they are particularly chronic in pediatric outpatient clinics. Of the studies devoted to reducing broken appointments, those using appointment reminders have been the most common. But, reminders are not always effective in pediatric settings (Morse, Coulter, Nazarian, & Napodano, 1981).

In their 1985 study, Friman, Finney, Rapoff, and Christophersen employed a within-subjects experimental analysis to determine the effects of experimental procedures on the percentage of appointments kept and the percentage broken in a pediatric outpatient clinic. The procedures consisted of mailed and telephoned reminders plus an added component, reduced response requirements (in the form of parking in the lot adjacent to the clinic).

Experimental procedures were sequentially introduced to the patient population of individual pediatric providers in the general outpatient clinic. Providers included pediatric nurse practitioners and board-certified pediatricians. Data were obtained from the appointment schedule sheets in the clinic and were validated by direct observation and chart review. Broken appointments were defined as those marked DNKA, which stood for Did Not Keep Appointment (appointments cancelled before the appointment time were not included as broken appointments). Kept appointments were defined as those marked kept. The percentage of appointments kept was determined by the ratio of appointments made and appointments kept. A similar method was used for the percentage of broken appointments. The results showed that the experimental procedures increased the percentage of appointments kept and decreased the percentage of broken appointments with each provider. A total of approximately 5600 appointments were included in this study. Data on social validity showed that the providers and patients thought that the procedures were helpful in improving show-rates and thereby in improving the quality of medical care for children. Finally, a financial analysis revealed that the amount of money billed per appointment scheduled increased during the experimental period for all providers. The increase averaged 16 percent with a range from 6 percent to 30 percent. From a discussion with the administrator of the outpatient clinic, it was determined that the 16 percent increase in the amount billed per scheduled appointment would more than offset the costs incurred by implementation of the intervention procedures.

COMPLIANCE IN CHILD PASSENGER SAFETY

Automobile accidents pose the greatest threat to the health and well-being of children in the United States. No other single factor accounts for as many children killed or injured each year (Christophersen, 1983a). No other factor accounts for as many children with permanent spinal cord injuries, facial disfigurements, or permanent brain dysfunction (Christophersen, in press). Although every major organization and society that represents the interests of professionals who care for children has endorsed child passenger safety as a primary concern, the development of a comprehensive program for encouraging parents to acquire and use child passenger safety restraint devices correctly, over an extended period of time, has remained an elusive and frustrating goal (Pless, 1978).

Christophersen, Sosland-Edelman, and LeClaire (1985) have completed the initial evaluation of an effective and inexpensive child passenger safety program, including one-year follow-up data (collection of continued follow-up data is proceeding at this time). A total of 129 mother-infant pairs were entered into the study, with one-third started in April, one-third in August, and one-third in December. This design provided controls for the season of the year and the weather and also provided an original program and two direct replications. There are five basic components to the program. The first component, a child passenger safety law, was passed in the State of Kansas in 1981 and went into effect in 1982. Previous research on the effects of such laws has produced favorable results in other states (Sanders, 1982). The second component, a hospital-based restraint-seat loaner program, had been in effect at the participating hospital for approximately one and one-half years at the time the evaluation was begun. Previous research on loaner programs has produced favorable results, although there have been numerous unsolved problems with these types of programs (Christophersen & Sullivan, 1982; Reisinger & Williams, 1978). The third component, physician involvement, has also previously produced favorable results, especially when the physician provided prompts to and discussion with the parents at intervals beginning with the birth of the baby and continuing until the child was one and one-half years or two years old (Reisinger et al., 1981). The fourth component, nurse involvement, is made necessary by the design of loaner programs, which require that the nurse serve as the primary educator/motivator for new parents (Christophersen & Sullivan, 1982). The fifth component, community involvement, has historically been recognized as a possibly important component, although little, if any, previous research on this component has been conducted.

The five-component child passenger safety program has been a success. The parent compliance of 93 percent at one year follow-up makes this the most successful child passenger safety program that has ever been evaluated in the United States. If these results can be replicated in other settings, under similar conditions, then pediatrics will have an effective, cost-efficient program to aid in the prevention of the deaths and injuries that occur each year as a result of automobile accidents. Of course, the ultimate evaluation must also include a demonstration that the families who participated in programs to increase compliance also have a lower level of injuries sustained from automobile accidents.

COMPLIANCE IN HOME INJURY CONTROL

Burn injuries rank second only to automobile accidents as a major cause of accidental death in children from birth to 15 years of age (Vaughn, McKay, & Behrman, 1979). In children aged one to four, burns are the leading cause of death in the home (Reisinger, 1980). Specifically, flame burns account for 20 to 30 percent of burns in the pediatric population, while scald burns are responsible for 40 to 50 percent of burns in children (Vaughn et al., 1979). Tap water burns account for 7 to 17 percent of all scald burns in children requiring hospitalization (Feldman, Schaller, Feldman, & McMillon, 1978).

Reliable and inexpensive smoke detectors are widely available and are known to reduce injuries and deaths resulting from home fires by alerting occupants while they can still escape (Bright, 1978; Feldman et al., 1978). In addition, Feldman et al. (1978) and Baptiste and Feck (1980) have suggested that reduction of home hot water heater temperatures to below 130 degrees Farenheit would prevent accidental and deliberate (as in child abuse) tap water burns of children.

Generally, pediatricians are left with the major responsibility for educating parents of young children about the dangers of burns from home accidents. Evaluation of the effectiveness of the pediatrician's efforts at education is always difficult and sometimes impossible. For example, when a physician instructs a parent to provide a nutritionally balanced diet or to practice accepted dental hygiene procedures, compliance data are rarely available. The area of home injury control has been selected for the present research focus because it offers the unique opportunity to assess the effectiveness of the provider's recommendations. The ease of assessment exists because the recommendations, if followed, produce a permanent observable change in the living environment.

A group well-child format was selected for this research (Thomas, Hassanein, & Christophersen, 1984), because previous research (Casey, Sharp, & Loda, 1979; Osborn & Woolley, 1981) has shown that a group format is at least as effective as individual well-child care and because the group format is more efficient (i.e., the entire parent education portion can be done by one nurse practitioner). The 58 families who participated in the study were randomly assigned to an experimental and control group. Both groups received the same general information (primarily information on normal child development, nutrition, dental care, and so on.) and the experimental group received an additional protocol on home injury control. The protocol included instructions for obtaining and installing at least one smoke detector and instructions for changing the setting on their hot water heater to 125 degrees or less (in an effort to reduce the probability of a scald-type injury).

To correspond with Janis's (1983) considerations for enhancing compliance, the parents in the experimental group were given written and verbal information on the advantages of complying (e.g., less risk of injury or death to their children, lower utility bills etc.). Disadvantages of complying (e.g., that the hot water would run out much sooner if baths, dishwashers, and washing machines were used in succession) were also discussed, but some disadvantages that had appeared in popular and professional literature (e.g., that clothes and dishes could not be washed as well because of the lowered hot water heater setting) were countered with information provided by soap manufacturers. Parents were given adequate time to make their decisions regarding compliance: home observations were conducted at least several weeks after the well-child class.

All home safety outcome data were obtained during unannounced home visits, during which the observer(s) not only asked the parents if they had made the changes recommended during their well-child classes, but actually checked the operation of the smoke detector, using certified procedures from the local fire department. Hot water temperatures were checked at the kitchen faucet, using an electronic thermometer. Results of the home observations indicated that the experimental portion of the group well-child classes was effective in convincing parents to lower their hot water-heater settings, while the control group well-child classes were not. Although these procedures did not convince the entire experimental group to comply with the recommendation to change their hot water heater settings, the results were significant at the .0001 level.

The other measure made during the unannounced home visit involved observing at least one smoke alarm. The results of this portion of the study showed an increase in smoke detector usage in the experimental group that was not significant ($p > .1232$ level). That the results were better for the water-heater settings than for the smoke alarm installation is consistent with the literature. Dershewitz and Christophersen (1984) stated that the more actual effort a provider's recommendation requires for parents, the less likely they are to comply with it. For some safety measures (e.g., smoke detectors, locking medications), more intensive motivational systems may need to be developed to improve parents' adoption of safety measures that have a greater response requirement.

COMPLIANCE WITH A SHORT-TERM REGIMEN

Prescription of an antibiotic for an acute infection is the most frequent medical treatment provided by pediatricians (Aronson, 1981). Most parents purchase the prescribed medicine, but many of their children do not receive the complete antibiotic course (Bergman & Werner, 1963). Brief, specific health education messages, delivered orally and in written form, appear to be effective in increasing adherence to short-term regimens by pediatric patients. Counseling by the pediatrician and written instructions on the importance of completing the regimen have been shown to improve adherence by patients who received a 10-day penicillin prescription (Colcher & Bass, 1972). Furthermore, several strategies implemented by pharmacists who dispense the prescriptions have improved compliance. These strategies include written reminders, self-monitoring calendars, pill-dispensing devices, and calibrated measuring devices (Linkewich, Catalano, & Flack, 1974; Mattar, Markello, & Yaffee, 1975).

Many pediatric studies of compliance have been correlational and have not specified a standardized strategy that can be used in pediatric practice. Therefore, a study of enhancing parent compliance with short-term regimens was conducted in an ambulatory pediatrics clinic (Finney et al., 1985). Acute otitis media, one of the most common diagnoses made by pediatricians, accounts for a significant portion of antibiotic prescriptions. About 70 percent of children have had at least one episode of acute otitis media by the age of three. Because an antibiotic regimen is a frequent medical recommendation that often results in noncompliance by parents, a practical strategy that increases the percentage of patients who receive the full treatment regimen would be useful for most pediatric practices.

The effectivness of a simple compliance improvement protocol was evaluated by recruiting children with otitis media who received an antibiotic prescription to participate in a prospective randomized clinical trial. Parents and their children were randomly assigned to experimental and control groups. All children received standard medical management of otitis media. The experimental group parents received (1) a written educational handout that described the common symptoms of ear infections and the importance of the child receiving all prescribed medication, (2) a month-long self-monitoring calendar on which to record dosages of medicine given each day, and (3) a midregimen telephone prompt by a secretary. To control for the therapist contact received by the experimental group, the experimenters administered the Eyberg Child Behavior Inventory (Eyberg & Ross, 1978) to the control group patients. Health outcome measures included a two-week follow-up ear examination, with completion of the Otoscopic Examination Form by the pediatric health care staff (Bluestone & Cantekin, 1979). Compliance was measured during an unannounced home visit by determining the amount of medicine remaining in the bottles and obtaining a urine sample for assay.

The results showed that compliance with the antibiotic regimen was significantly higher for parents who received the compliance-improvement strategies. Eighty-two percent of the experimental children received 80 percent or more of the recommended doses at the time of the home visit, whereas only 49 percent of the control children had received most of their doses. This difference between groups was significant at the .01 level.

Antibiotic assays were completed for a sample of control and experimental children. The assay results showed a high correspondence with the medication measure, with 78 percent agreement for control children and 74 percent agreement for experimental children. Thus, the two methods of compliance assessment—the indirect medication measure and the direct urine assay—produced similar indications of patient compliance. The high correspondence of the two measures suggests that a relatively simple assessment, the amount of medication remaining at the end of an antibiotic regimen, could be completed by pediatric providers during follow-up appointments to assess patient compliance. Further experimental validation of this compliance assessment technique would be a useful contribution to compliance research.

Compliance with short-term regimens can be improved by providing parents with an educational handout, a self-monitoring calendar, and a brief telephone reminder. Based on the criteria suggested by Sackett et al. (1975), the results of the present study are clinically significant: the experimental group was significantly more compliant, and the difference between the two groups was greater than 25 percent. These results are similar to those produced by other compliance-improvement strategies that have involved supplementary verbal and written instructions (Colcher & Bass, 1972; Linkewich et al., 1974) and somewhat better than pharmacy-based counseling and reminder interventions (Lima, Nazarian, Charney, & Lahti, 1976; Mattar et al., 1975). These procedures also appear to be simple and easily incorporated into routine pediatric practice and thus appear feasible for pediatricians to include in standard practice (Christophersen & Rapoff, 1979).

The majority of compliance-improvement interventions that have been evaluated in pediatric practice have involved strategies designed to motivate parents to give children their medicine. Another area for future research is the design of procedures to assist parents in motivating their children to comply with regimen requirements. Many children refuse to take oral medicines because of their taste or texture. Simple behavior management guidelines may be useful for distribution with other compliance interventions to facilitate parent management of their children's behavior (Christophersen, 1982). Other more intensive procedures may be required for more complicated regimens, such as exercise for juvenile rheumatoid arthritis (Rapoff et al., 1984), diabetes (Lowe & Lutzker, 1979), and dietary management (Magrab & Papadopoulou, 1977).

COMPLIANCE AND PEDIATRIC PRACTICE

Many methods used to improve compliance in pediatrics can be classified as primarily informational and instructional; the methods designed to teach parents about health behaviors have also been expected to motivate parents to adopt these health behaviors (Finney & Christophersen, 1984). Informational and instructional procedures have been the least effective strategies for increasing adherence to long-term regimens (Haynes, 1979). Therefore, additional procedures must be developed to improve adherence. The work of Janis (1983) suggests that the minimum requirements for compliance would be that the patient understands the seriousness of the problem, knows both the benefits and the costs of complying and not complying, and has time in which to ponder available options. Frequently health care providers will inform a patient that some behavior patterns present a risk to health. They will then make health-related recommendations without addressing the inconveniences that may accompany such compliance. For example, in the research discussed above on child passenger safety, most programs do not mention that a child restraint seat may be inconvenient to use, that the seat may get extremely hot while in an automobile in the sun, or that the child may not want to ride in the restraint seat. Similarly, in the research on hot water-heater temperature settings, most programs do not tell parents that lowered temperature settings will not affect the cleanliness of dishes or clothes washed in an automatic machine.

Two studies have directly addressed the issue of incentive systems for health behaviors. Christophersen (1977) suggested that improvements in toddler behavior when child passenger safety restraints are used may serve as an immediate reinforcer for parents' continued use of child restraints. And a subsequent study showed that continued use of child restraints resulted from an educational intervention that emphasized improved child behavior (Christophersen & Gyulay, 1981). Lund et al. (1964) used a social reinforcement approach to maintain compliance with a long-term regimen and suggested that the use of incentives for compliance by parents and patients could be feasible in pediatric care settings. Treiber's recent paper (in press) on compliance with the use of child restraint seats showed that the results from the combination group (wherein the parent was told both the positive and negative consequences of child restraint seat usage) were superior to those of both the other groups. These results are consistent with Janis's (1983) recommendations and were superior to most of the published outcomes with child passenger safety programs.

Social Reinforcement.   The use of social reinforcement to enhance compliance is one strategy that may be useful in primary care. The pediatrician usually has a personal rapport with families that may facilitate adherence to the pediatrician's recommendations (Sammons, 1982). Monitoring of parent compliance by direct observation (e.g., use of child restraints on trips to doctor), by indirect measure (e.g., receipts or cartons for smoke detectors), and by office-based assessment (e.g., assays, mother-child interactions) would provide the necessary information for the pediatrician to deliver social reinforcement contingent on compliance with earlier advice. This is in sharp contrast to the procedure of simply asking a parent to verbally report on compliance. A system of public posting for the pediatric office may also serve as an effective motivator (Quilitch, 1975). The names of parents and children who have adopted the various health promotion and protection strategies taught by the pediatrician could be posted in the waiting room. Practical assessment strategies that provide objective indicators of adherence are needed to improve the use of incentives in pediatric health care.

Social Support.   Scheduling parents to meet in groups for well-child care has produced increased attendance at appointments (Osborn & Woolley, 1981). The use of groups of parents may be an effective strategy for increasing adherence with other health behaviors. Baer (1982) discussed the use of groups as a generalization strategy based on the Method of Common Stimuli (Stokes & Baer, 1977). Baer's recommendation was to choose the group systematically to include friends and acquaintances who could serve as "adherence stimuli" for each other. The group members' interactions in the community (outside the well-child group) may serve to cue the performance of the health behavior taught in the group.

Cobb (1976) has also identified social support as a promising strategy for increasing adherence. He defines social support as a belief that one is cared for and loved, is esteemed and valued, and belongs to a network of communication and obligation. The technology for measuring socially supportive behavior is developing (Wahler, 1980); future research on social support and its influence on adherence to health advice should be extended into health education research (Colletti & Brownell, 1982).

Mass Media.   Media programs have been designed to inform large numbers of people about health behavior, and the use of mass media to influence health behavior of children and their parents has been proposed (Lehman, 1979). Two levels of effectiveness must be evaluated for media presentations: changes in knowledge and attitudes and changes in behavior (Green, Kreuter, Deeds, & Partridge, 1980).

Media presentations can be effective in producing changes in knowledge. The Stanford Heart Disease Prevention Project produced a well-designed series of television programs and messages that were highly effective in increasing knowledge of cardiovascular risk factors (Farquhar et al., 1977).

Behavior change, however, has not resulted from most health education media programs. The Stanford Project found that the televised programs and messages did not produce changes in "complex" behaviors, such as smoking, although some "simple" behavior changes, such as using margarine and skim milk, occurred (McAlister & Berger, 1979). An expensive television campaign for seat belt usage had no measurable effect on the use of seat belts (Robertson et al., 1974). Recently, a structured health-education counseling program for smoking cessation appeared to be effective in reducing smoking (McAlister, Puska, Koskela, Pallonen, & MacCoby, 1980), but a highly structured community support group who watched the shows together served as a facilitator of behavioral change. Media programs alone do not appear to produce behavior change, but, with the addition of support groups, media programs may contribute to the effectiveness of health education.

Modeling.   Because children and parents watch large amounts of television (Lehman, 1979), modeling of appropriate health behavior on television may be a relatively low-cost, supplementary adherence strategy. Social learning approaches are effective teaching strategies (Bandura, 1969), and their use in health education has been recommended (Christophersen & Sullivan, 1982; Pless, 1978). Modeling of desired health behavior on television programs (e.g., using seat belts, purchasing smoke detectors, serving healthy food), combined with other health education efforts, may increase the knowledge of children and parents about significant issues in child health and may improve adherence with a variety of practices that will improve child health.

Finney and Christophersen (1984) suggested numerous directions for future compliance research, including the development of programs that target health behaviors associated with the most significant morbidity and mortality (Young & Reisinger, 1980), programs directed towards one or two specific behaviors (Dershewitz, 1979; Dershewitz & Christophersen, 1984), that provide explicit and directive advice (Casey et al., 1979), that incorporate written organizational protocols (Christophersen, 1982), and programs that include feasible and cost-effective adherence improvement strategies (Cataldo, 1982).

SUMMARY AND RECOMMENDATIONS

The present series of experiments on compliance were all conducted in a busy pediatric outpatient clinic, without substantially altering the existing clinic practices. Specific interventions were chosen, based on how readily they could be incorporated into the daily clinic routine as well as on their consistency with Janis's (1983) recommendations on compliance-improvement strategies. Thus the experiments were not contrived for the convenience of the research staff but were conducted under "real world" conditions. Conducting the experiments under routine clinic conditions resulted in findings that are more likely to generalize to other outpatient departments (cf. Baer, 1982).

Several aspects of the research discussed in this paper indicate the success of this large-scale venture into medical compliance. The study on appointment-keeping showed that the behavior of an entire pediatric clinic was amenable to assessment and to change. The appointment keeping study was conducted with more than 5,600 scheduled appointments and produced not only substantial increases in the percentage of appointments kept, but also a substantial increase in the amount of money billed by the clinic for the clinical services rendered. This study replicates numerous prior studies on appointment-keeping and extends previous findings by adding reduced response requirement to the intervention and social and financial validation procedures to the anlaysis of the data. The child passenger safety program has been adopted by the original hospital that participated in the evaluation program, and by several other hospitals in the metropolitan area as well. The home injury control program, which employed a group well-child setting to impart information to new parents, represents one of the first anticipatory guidance programs to accomplish measurable goals. Most of the previous research on the topic of parent education has produced less than satisfactory results, leading many researchers to conclude that pediatricians' attempts to educate parents is virtually a waste of time. Perhaps future investigators will be less skeptical and will conclude that parent education can succeed if it is conducted properly. The study on compliance with an antibiotic regimen for otitis media also builds on and extends earlier research on this topic. The procedures studied both in the appointment keeping study and the otitis study can easily be implemented by pediatric health care providers without substantially altering their type or style of practice.

Each of these studies included actual observation of the behavior of the recipient of the procedures, rather than relying on either a verbal or written report, or an analogue to the actual implementation of the procedures. Each study also included frequent interobserver reliability checks to verify that the observation procedures were a valid indication of the behavior of the patients. Because each study was conducted in the setting for which the procedures were ultimately intended, the problem of generalization is greatly reduced (Christophersen, 1983b).

Future research efforts aimed at analyzing compliance in pediatric care could benefit by including social validation and financial analysis measures. That the protocols are still in use, long after the research monies have run out and the research staff has terminated its efforts, is perhaps the best indicator of social validity. Collectively, our findings indicate that the integration of compliance-improvement strategies into pediatric practice will result in the benefits of higher compliance by patients and will provide opportunities for objective evaluation of the standard regimens that are prescribed for pediatric health problems.

REFERENCES

Alpert, J.J. (1964). Broken appointments. *Pediatrics, 34,* 127–132.

Aronson, S.A. (1981). The health needs of infants and children under 12. In Dept. of Health and Human Services, *Better health for our children: A national strategy: Vol. 4, Background papers* (DHHS Publication No. PHS 79-55071, pp. 243–283). Washington, DC: U.S. Government Printing Office.

Baer, D.M. (1982). The role of current pragmatics in the future analysis of generalization technology. In R.B.Stuart (Ed.), *Adherence, compliance, and generalization in behavioral medicine.* New York: Brunner/Mazel.

Bandura, A. (1969). *Principles of behavior modification.* New York: Holt,Rinehart & Winston.

Baptiste, M.S., & Feck, G. (1980). Preventing tap water burns. *American Journal of Public Health, 70,* 727.

Becker, M.H., Drachman, R.H., & Kirscht, J.P. (1972). Predicting mother's compliance with pediatric medical regimens. *Journal of Pediatrics, 81,* 843–854.

Bergman, A.B., & Werner, R.J. (1963). Failure of children to receive penicillin by mouth. *New England Journal of Medicine, 268,* 1334–1338.

Bluestone, C.D., & Cantekin, E.I. (1979). Design factors in the characterization and identification of otitis media and certain related conditions. *Annals of Otorhinolaryngology, 88*(Supp. 60), 13–28.

Bright, R.G. (1978). *Technical development of domestic fire detectors.* Washington, DC: National Bureau of Standards.

Casey, P., Sharp, M., & Loda,F. (1979). Child health supervision for children under two years of age: A review of its content and effectiveness. *Journal of Pediatrics, 95,* 1–9.

Casey, P., & Whitt, K. (1980). Effect of the pediatrician on the mother-infant relationship. *Pediatrics, 65,* 815–820.

Cataldo, M.F. (1982). The scientific basis for a behavioral approach to pediatrics. *Pediatric Clinics of North America, 29,* 415–423.

Charney, E., Bynum, R., & Eldredge, D. (1967). How well do patients take oral penicillin? A collaborative study in private practice. *Pediatrics, 40,* 188–195.

Christophersen, E.R. (1977). Children's behavior during automobile rides: Do car seats make a difference? *Pediatrics, 60,* 69–74.

Christophersen, E.R. (1982). Incorporating behavioral pediatrics into primary care. *Pediatric Clinics of North America, 29*(2), 261–296.

Christophersen, E.R. (1983a). Automobile accidents: Potential years of life lost. *Pediatrics, 71,* 855–856.

Christophersen, E.R. (1983b). Research issues in developmental and behavioral pediatrics. In M.D. Levine, W.B. Carey, A.C. Crocker, & R.T. Gross (Eds.), *Developmental-behavioral pediatrics* (pp. 1197–1209). Philadelphia: Saunders.

Christophersen, E.R. (in press). The prevention of developmental disabilities through child passenger safety. In R.I. Jahiel, J. Byrne, R. Lubin, & J. Gorelick (Eds.), *Handbook of prevention of mental retardation and developmental disabilities.* New York: Van Nostrand Reinhold.

Christophersen, E.R., & Gyulay, J.E. (1981). Parental compliance with car seat usage: A positive approach with long-term follow-up. *Journal of Pediatric Psychology, 6,* 301–312.

Christophersen, E.R., & Rapoff, M.A. (1979). Behavioral pediatrics. In O.F. Pomerleau & J.P. Brady (Eds.), *Behavioral medicine: Theory and practice* (pp. 990–923). Baltimore.. Williams & Wilkins.

Christophersen, E.R., & Sullivan, M.A. (1982). Increasing the protection of newborn infants in cars. *Pediatrics, 70,* 21–25.

Christophersen, E.R., Sosland-Edelman, D., & LeClaire, S. (1985). An evauation of two comprehensive infant car seat loaner programs with one-year follow-up. *Pediatrics, 76*(1), 36–42.

Cobb, S. (1976). Social support as a moderator of life stress. *Psychosomatic Medicine, 38,*300–314.

Colcher, I.S., & Bass, J.W. (1972). Penicillin treatment of streptococcal pharyngitis: A comparison of schedules and the role of specific counseling. *Journal of the American Medical Association, 222,* 657–659.

Colletti, G., & Brownell, K.D. (1982). The physical and emotional benefits of social support: Application to obesity, smoking, and alcoholism. In M. Hersen, R.M. Eisler, & P.M. Miller (Eds.), *Progress in behavior modification* (Vol. 13). New York: Academic.

Dershewitz, R.A. (1979). Will mothers use free household safety devices? *American Journal of Diseases of Children, 133,* 61–64.

Dershewitz, R.A., & Christophersen, E.R. (1984). Childhood household safety: An overview. *American Journal of Diseases of Children, 138,* 85–88.

Dunbar, J.M., Marshall, G.D., & Hovell, M.F. (1979). Behavioral strategies for improving compliance. In R.B. Haynes, D.W. Taylor, & D.L. Sackett (Eds.), *Compliance in health care* (pp. 174–190). Baltimore: Johns Hopkins University Press.

Dunbar, J.M., & Stunkard, A.J. (1979). Adherence to diet and drug regimen. In R. Levy, B. Riftkind, & S. Dennis, (Eds.), *Nutrition, lipids, and coronary heart disease.* New York: Raven.

Eyberg, S.M., & Ross, A.W. (1978). Assessment of child behavior problems. The validation of a new inventory. *Journal of Clinical Child Psychology, 7,* 113–116.

Farquhar, J.W., Maccoby, N., Wood, P., Alexander, J., Breitrose, H., Brown, B., Haskell, W., McAlister, A., Meyer, A., Nash, J., & Stern, M. (1977). Community education for cardiovascular health. *Lancet, 1,* 1192–1195.

Feldman, K.W., Schaller, R.T., Feldman, J.A., & McMillon, M. (1978). Tap water scald burns in children. *Pediatrics, 62,* 1–7.

Finney, J.W., & Christophersen, E.R. (1984). Behavioral pediatrics: Health education in pediatric primary care. In M. Hersen, R.M. Eisler, & P.M. Miller (Eds.), *Progress in behavior modification* (Vol. 16, pp. 185–229). New York: Academic.

Finney, J.W., Friman, P.C., Rapoff, M.A., & Christophersen, E.R. (1985). Improving compliance with antibiotic regimens for otitis media: Randomized clinical trial in a pediatric clinic. *American Journal of Diseases of Children, 139,* 89–95.

Frankell, B.S., & Hovell, M.F. (1978). Health service appointment keeping: A behavioral and critical review. *Behavior Modification, 2,* 435–464.

Friman, P.C., Finney, J.W., Rapoff, M.A., & Christophersen, E.R. (in press). Improving pediatric appointment keeping with reminders and reduced response requirement. *Journal of Applied Behavior Analysis.*

Gordis, L., & Markowitz, M. (1971). Evaluation of the effectiveness of comprehensive and continuous pediatric care. *Pediatrics, 48,* 766–776.

Gordis, L., Markowitz, M., & Lilienfeld, A.M. (1969). The inaccuracy in using interviews to estimate patient reliability in taking medications at home. *Medical Care, 7,* 49–54.

Green, L.W., Kreuter, M.W., Deeds, S.G., & Partridge, K.B. (1980). *Health education planning: A diagnostic approach.* Palo Alto, CA: Mayfield.

Haynes, R.B. (1979). Determinants of compliance: The disease and the mechanics of treatment. In R.B. Haynes, D.W. Taylor, & D.L. Sackett (Eds.), *Compliance in health care* (pp. 49–62). Baltimore: Johns Hopkins University Press.

Haynes, R.B., Taylor, D.W., & Sackett, D.L. (Eds.). (1979) *Compliance in health care.* Baltimore: Johns Hopkins University Press.

Hertz, P., & Stamps, P.C. (1977). Appointment keeping behavior re-evaluated. *American Journal of Public Health, 67,* 1033–1036.

Janis, I.L. (1983). The role of social support in adherence to stressful decisions. *American Psychologist, 38,* 143–160.

Jonas, S. (1971). Appointment breaking in a general medicine clinic. *Medical Care, 9,* 82–88.

Lehman, P. (1979). Health education. In U.S. DHEW, *Healthy people: The Surgeon General's report on health promotion and disease prevention.* Washington, DC. U.S. Government Printing Office.

Lima, J., Nazarian, L., Charney, E., & Lahti,C. (1976). Compliance with short-term antimicrobial therapy: Some techniques that help. *Pediatrics, 57*, 383–386.

Linkewich, J.A., Catalano, R.B., & Flack, H.L. (1974). The effect of packaging and instruction on outpatient compliance with medication regimens. *Drug Intelligence and Clinical Pharmacology, 8*, 10–15.

Lowe, K., & Lutzker, J.R. (1979). Increasing compliance to a medical regimen with a juvenile diabetic. *Behavior Therapy, 10*, 57–64.

Lund, M., Jorgensen, R.S., & Kuhl, V. (1964). Serum diphenylhydantoin (phenytoin) in ambulant patients with epilepsy. *Epilepsia, 5*, 51–58.

Magrab, P.R., & Papadopoulou, Z.L. (1977). The effects of a token economy on dietary compliance for children on hemodialysis. *Journal of Applied Behavior Analysis, 10*, 573–578.

Mattar, M.E., Markello, J., & Yaffee,S.J. (1975). Pharmaceutic factors affecting pediatric compliance. *Pediatrics, 55*, 101–107.

McAlister, A., & Berger, E.D. (1979). Media for community health promotion. In P.M. Lazes (Ed.), *The handbook of health education*. Germantown, MD: Aspen Systems.

McAlister, A., Puska, P., Koskela, K., Pallonen, U., & Maccoby, N. (1980). Mass communication and community organization for public health education. *American Psychologist, 35*, 375–379.

Morse, D.L., Coulter, M.D., Nazarian, L.F., & Napodano, R.J. (1981). Waning effectiveness of mailed reminders on reducing broken appointments. *Pediatrics, 68*, 846–849.

Oppenheim, G.L., Bergman, J.J., & English, E.C. (1979). Failed appointments: A review. *Journal of Family Practice, 8*, 789–796.

Osborn, L.M., & Woolley, F.R. (1981). Use of groups in well child care. *Pediatrics, 67*, 701–706.

Pless, I.B. (1978). Accident prevention and health education: Back to the drawing board? *Pediatrics, 62*, 431–435.

Quilitch, H.R. (1975). A comparison of three staff-management procedures. *Journal of Applied Behavior Analysis, 8*, 59–66.

Rapoff, M.A., & Christophersen, E.R. (1982). Compliance of pediatric patients with medical regimens: A review and evaluation. In R.B. Stuart (Ed.), *Adherence, compliance and generalization in behavioral medicine* (pp. 79–124). New York: Brunner/Mazel.

Rapoff, M.A., Lindsley, C.B., & Christophersen, E.R. (1984). Improving compliance with medical regimens: A case study with juvenile rheumatoid arthritis. *Archives of Physical Medicine and Rehabilitation, 65*, 267–269.

Reisinger, K.S. (1980). Smoke detectors: Reducing deaths and injuries due to fire. *Pediatrics, 65*, 718–724.

Reisinger, K.S., & Bires, J.A. (1980). Anticipatory guidance in pediatric practice. *Pediatrics, 66*, 889–892.

Reisinger, K.S., & Williams, A.F. (1978). Evaluation of programs designed to increase the protection of infants in cars. *Pediatrics, 62*, 280–287.

Reisinger, K.S., Williams, A.F., John C.E., Roberts, T.E., & Podgainy, H.J. (1981). Effects of pediatrician's counseling on infant restraint use. *Pediatrics, 67*, 201–206.

Robertson, L.S., Kelley, A.B., O'Neill, B., Wixom, C.W., Eiswirth, R.S., & Haddon, W., Jr. (1974). A controlled study of the effect of television messages on safety belt use. *American Journal of Public Health, 64*, 1071–1080.

Sackett, D.L., Haynes, R.C., Gibson, E.S., Hackett, B.C., Taylor, D.W., Roberts, R.S., & Johnson, A.L. (1975). Randomised clinical trial of strategies for improving medication compliance in primary hypertension. *Lancet, 1*, 1205–1207.

Sammons, J.H. (1982). Written instructions and patient compliance. *Journal of the American Medical Association, 248*, 2890.

Sanders, R.S. (1982). Legislative approach to auto safety: The Tennessee experience. In A.B. Bergman (Ed.), *Preventing childhood injuries*, Report of the Twelfth Ross Roundtable on Critical Approaches to Common Pediatric Problems (pp. 29–33). Columbus: OH: Ross Laboratories.

Stokes, T.F., & Baer, D.M. (1977). An implicit technology of generalization. *Journal of Applied Behavior Analysis, 10*, 349–367.

Thomas, K.A., Hassanein, R.S., & Christophersen, E.R. (1984). An evaluation of group well-child care for improving parents' home burn prevention practices. *Pediatrics, 74*, 879–882.

Treiber, F.A. (in press). A comparison of the positive and negative consequences approaches upon car restraint usage. *Journal of Pediatric Psychology.*

Vaughn, V.C., McKay, R.J., & Behrman, R.E. (1979). *Nelson textbook of pediatrics.* Philadelphia: Saunders.

Wahler, R.G. (1980). The insular mother: Her problems in parent-child treatment. *Journal of Applied Behavior Analysis, 13*, 207–219.

Williams, A.F. (1982). Passive and active measures for controlling disease and injury: The role of health psychologists. *Health Psychology, 1*, 399–499.

Young, T.L., & Reisinger, K.S. (1980). Wall socket electrical burns: Relevance to health education. *Pediatrics, 65*, 825–827.

20

Parent Compliance with Medical and Behavioral Recommendations

JOHN M. PARRISH

Parent noncompliance with professional recommendations is perhaps the most pervasive problem in the delivery of health care to children. Such noncompliance takes many forms, including delays in seeking care, nonparticipation in community screening or immunization programs, erratic involvement in ongoing services marked by missed appointments, and failure to implement prescribed medical, educational, or behavioral regimens. This noncompliance may jeopardize the success of any professional's therapeutic efforts by minimizing or erasing possible benefits of preventive or curative services. As one consequence, children may undergo additional and otherwise unnecessary diagnostic and treatment procedures, thereby generating added health care costs and possible

The development of this chapter was supported by Grants No. 00917-15-0 and MCJ-243270-01-0 from the Maternal and Child Health Service of the U.S. Department of Health and Human Services.

iatrogenic effects. Furthermore poor adherence may disrupt the professional/patient relationship and adversely influence the parent's satisfaction with services, making subsequent compliance with professional recommendations less likely. Moreover, low levels of compliance obscure or even preclude attempts to evaluate accurately the quality of care rendered (Becker, 1979).

Parent noncompliance also significantly hinders research aimed at assessing treatment efficacy (Dunbar, 1983). If investigators of specific treatment regimens for children do not take into account the extent of parent compliance, it is not possible to determine whether the advice or prescription is an effective intervention. In addition, the safety of treatment and the incidence of side effects cannot be assessed unless noncompliance with the regimen under investigation is taken into account. This applies to the assessment of both medical and behavioral intervention.

Approximately a decade ago, Becker & Maiman (1975) stated that patient noncompliance with professional recommendations is "the best documented but least understood health-related behavior" (p. 11). Despite an exponential increase in the number of adherence studies since then, this statement may still apply to the issue of parent compliance. Most of the compliance literature pertains to adult patients (Cohen, 1979; Haynes, Taylor, & Sackett, 1979; Sackett & Haynes, 1976; Stuart, 1982). Studies with adults suggest that at least one-third of patients fail to follow professional advice completely (Blackwell, 1973; Gillum & Barsky, 1974; Podell, 1975). In cases where the intervention is preventive in nature, and/or the patients are without symptoms, and/or the prescribed regimen is long-term, only about one-half of the patients are usually compliant (Podell, 1975; Sackett, 1976). In clinics primarily serving low-income populations, noncompliance with professional recommendations is frequently reported to be at or above 60 percent (Becker, 1979; Becker & Maiman, 1975).

Less attention has been given to compliance with recommendations for pediatric populations, where the central concern is with parent management of the child's medical prescription and/or behavior therapy program. Litt and Cuskey (1980) estimated the overall parent compliance rate to be 50 percent, with a range from 20 to 80 percent. In a recent review of 23 pediatric studies, Dunbar (1983) reported that compliance with short-term antibiotic therapy was judged to range between 18 and 58 percent. Presenting problems included otitis media and streptococcal pharyngitis and measures consisted of interviews, home pill counts, or urine assays. According to Dunbar, the percentage of compliance in cases of chronic pediatric conditions was similar, ranging from 11 to 89 percent. Among the chronic conditions examined were asthma, cancer, cystic fibrosis, epilepsy, and rheumatic fever. Measures employed included urine, saliva or serum assays, interviews, and clinical judgment. Dunbar concluded that the overall compliance rates reported in the pediatric literature concerning both acute and chronic conditions were no better than those rates found with adult patients.

This chapter reviews the literature pertaining to parent compliance with professional recommendations, addressing medical and behavioral treatments for children either with acute or chronic conditions. References are drawn from the adult as well as the child literature and have been chosen to provide a representative sample of studies regarding the measurement of compliance, the determinants of compliance, strategies for improving compliance, and priorities for future research. References that involve adult patients are included to supplement topics that have hitherto received little attention by researchers investigating parent adherence.

MEASUREMENT OF PARENT COMPLIANCE

Definition of Parent Compliance

Parent compliance can be defined as the extent to which a parent's behavior, in terms of administering prescribed medications or implementing suggested behavioral strategies, coincides with professional advice. The term "adherence" is often used interchangeably with "compliance." As Dunbar (1983) points out, operational definitions of compliance typically fall within three categories. One consists of simply clustering parents into nominal (i.e., qualitative) groups, such as "good," "moderate," or "poor" compliers, or "noncompliers." Another type of definition offers a composite index of compliance that yields an overall score for compliance for each parent based on a set of recommended behaviors. For example, in an often-referenced study of doctor-patient communications, Francis, Korsch, and Morris (1969) combined medication consumption, attendance at follow-up appointments, and adherence with a variety of recommendations into a single composite compliance index. A third definition expresses compliance as a percentage based upon the quantitative amount of the prescribed regimen that has been followed by the parent. For instance, in the case of a drug regimen, compliance could be defined as the number of prescribed doses administered by the parent divided by the number of doses prescribed for the child, with the ratio multiplied by 100.

Of the three definitions, the one most frequently employed in the pediatric literature is the qualitative categorization of individuals into groups labelled, for example, "good" and "poor" adherers (Arnhold et al, 1970; Buchanan & Mashigo, 1977; Colcher & Bass, 1972). Such categorization is problematic in many respects. Frequently there is no scientific basis for defining the "good compliance" category. Many investigators have employed arbitrary cut-offs for various qualitative compliance categories. Often patient populations have been divided into compliers and noncompliers on a strictly statistical basis, without concern for external validity (e.g., a relationship with therapeutic outcome). For instance, a median split may result in a cut-off level that has no biological significance (Gordis, 1979). Such arbitrary cut-offs have resulted in a high degree of variability in classifications employed, thereby severely limiting conclusions drawn from across-studies comparisons.

Ideally when parent compliance with a prescribed medication is being investigated, there would be a validated biological basis for selecting the cut-off point between compliance and noncompliance. Noncompliance would be idiographically defined as the point below which the desired preventive or therapeutic result is unlikely to be achieved with the medication prescribed for the clinical condition exhibited by the child under study (Gordis, 1979). One step toward a solution would require investigators to develop a uniform definition of "satisfactory" compliance for each intervention recommended for various clinical illnesses or disorders.

Another problem associated with categorical definitions is instability in an individual's compliance. There is frequently a question of whether compliance levels remain consistent for a given patient over time, and, therefore, whether it is ever justified to label a parent as a "complier" or "noncomplier." The compliance level of an individual parent is likely to be so variable that the parent cannot be classified once and for all with any reliability. Every parent's level of compliance must be reexamined periodically to determine whether it has changed. In this fashion, the characterization of parents as compliers or noncompliers would be based optimally on periodic assessments.

The second most frequently employed definition of compliance is an index, which is typically a summation compliance score across a set of behaviors or regimens that the parent or patient is asked to complete (Durant, Jay, Linder, Shoffitt, & Litt, 1984; Jay, Durant, Shoffitt, Linder, & Litt, 1984). As with the qualitative classification of parents, there are many problems associated with an index definition of parent compliance. For instance, while such a definition measures compliance with an entire set of professional recommendations, it obscures compliance with individual components of the prescribed regimen. There is evidence to suggest that compliance with one aspect of a regimen is not necessarily predictive of compliance with other aspects (Webb, et al., 1984). Also it is unclear in most cases whether the components comprising the index, such as appointment keeping and medication adherence, are sufficiently related to be considered as a unitary measure of compliance.

Of the three definitions cited by Dunbar (1983) the one which is the most informative, yet the one most seldom utilized, is the percentage definition of compliance (Lima, Nazarian, Charney, & Lahti, 1976). Here, as stated above, the ratio of prescribed pills taken to not taken within a specified interval is calculated. This measure yields data regarding the range or distribution of compliance levels among parents for a given drug or intervention program. Importantly, a percentage measure allows comparisons across studies, prescriptions, and populations, even though the denominator, such as total pills to be taken, changes from one investigation or sample to another.

Nonetheless, the percentage definition of compliance also has its problems. For the majority of medical or behavioral regimens prescribed for children, there is little or no knowledge of what percentage of the prescription needs to be implemented by the parent to achieve the desired therapeutic outcome. In a frequently cited study, Gordis, Markowitz & Lilienfeld (1969a) reported that children taking as little as 30 percent of their prescribed prophylactic penicillin were protected substantially from recurrences of rheumatic fever, suggesting that the determination of what constitutes an acceptable percentage of compliance is not as straightforward as typically assumed.

Methods of Measurement

Investigators have developed numerous methods of measuring parent compliance, including biological indices, informal assessments (e.g., clinical judgments) on the part of the professional service provider, evaluations of therapeutic outcomes, pill counts, semistructured interviews, self-monitoring by parents, and direct observations (Dunbar, 1983, Gordis, 1976). Selected literature regarding each method of measurement will be reviewed, with methods ordered from most to least objective (Rapoff & Christophersen, 1982).

Biological Indices.   When the prescription involves the administration of a medication or diet by the parent to the child, biological measures taken from the child constitute an indirect method of assessing parent compliance with a drug or diet regimen. These measures have been frequently cited in the pediatric literature (Eney & Goldstein, 1976; Gordis et al. 1969a; Smith, Rosen, Trueworthy, & Lowman, 1979) and can be collected in at least three ways. One is to detect the presence of the medication itself in the child's blood, urine, or saliva, through tests such as urine assays for the presence of antibiotics, blood serum levels of phenobarbital, or theophylline levels in the child's saliva. The timing of such assays is critically important. Another is to examine for the presence or absence of a metabolite of the medication or specific dietary substance.

A third biological procedure is to determine the presence or absence of a tracer or marker, that is, a substance that has been added to the medication that can be detected in the child's blood or urine if the medication has been administered by the parent. Most tracers and markers are detected through urine assays. Such indices must be inert, nontoxic, and freely excreted. Examples of agents meeting these criteria include riboflavin, phenosulfonphthalein (phenol red), and phenazopyridine (Epstein & Cluss, 1982).

Tracers and markers can either be used by adding them to all of the medication, with compliance assessed by determining the percentage of tests that contain them or by adding such substances only to a portion of the total doses in a particular known random order, thereby permitting a more precise measure of compliance patterns (Epstein & Masek, 1978).

Although these biological indices may offer an indirect indication of whether or not a child has been given the prescribed medication, there are problems associated with their use and, therefore, caution is recommended when relying upon these measures. An important issue when measuring compliance by biological indices is that of pharmacokinetic variations (Gordis, 1979). There are known individual differences among children in the absorption, distribution, metabolism, and excretion of drugs. Such individual differences may be attributable to the bioavailability of a drug (Chasseaud & Taylor, 1974) or to genetic differences (Vessel, 1974) among children in how they metabolize and excrete a drug.

Bioavailability refers to the amount of a drug absorbed following a specific formulation relative to the amount of the drug absorbed from a standard formulation. For example, the form in which a drug is administered (i.e., capsule, tablet, or parenteral) will have an effect upon its absorption. The rate of release of an orally administered drug will vary, with slowest rates usually associated with tablets, and the most rapid rates with aqueous solutions and syrups. Thus the absence of a therapeutic level of a drug prescribed for the child may result because the parent did not administer the medication *or* because the form or amount of the medication administered was insufficient to reach a therapeutic level (Gordis, 1979).

Also, biological indices may not accurately measure the degree of parent compliance. Such measures may simply indicate whether or not some amount of the medication was administered. One does not know if the entire prescribed amount was administered or only a part of it. Moreover biological indices cannot usually be employed to measure compliance over extended periods of time, but only to indicate whether or not a child was administered the medication within some relatively short time prior to the assessment. In addition some investigators have noted a discrepancy between specimens obtained at home and those obtained during clinic visits (Gordis et al., 1969a).

Assay procedures for all medications are not yet available and those that have been developed are sometimes prohibitively expensive or time consuming. At this time, given their relative intrusiveness, in addition to the limitations just cited, biological measures appear to serve best as random periodic indicators of compliance (Dunbar, 1979). Preferably, these spot checks would be conducted so as to reduce the reactive effects of the biological measurement on the parent's compliance behavior. For example, to minimize such effects in the case of urine assays for marker substances, the marker selected would not affect the child's urine in any way observable by the parent. In addition the schedule for collection of the biological measures would be randomized and the parent would be informed of the rationale for the collection of specimens but not of the specific collection schedule.

Direct Observation. Another method of measurement, that of direct observation, consists of having an individual in the home other than the parent record parent behaviors that are indicative of the extent to which the parent is administering a prescribed treatment. For example, a family member, neighbor, public health nurse, or some other trained professional would periodically observe and record the parent's implementation of treatment. From a methodological viewpoint, direct observation is preferable to many other measures of compliance, including clinical judgment, therapeutic outcome measures, pill counts, and parent self-report via interview or parent self-recordings. Because of the complexity of pharmacokinetic variations (Gordis, 1979) and temporal limitations associated with the use of many blood and urine assays, direct observation is sometimes preferable over indirect biological indices as well. Reliable direct observations eliminate the need to depend upon the more indirect assessment strategies. Although direct observation strategies consisting of event, interval, outcome, and time-sample recordings are employed frequently in the applied behavior analysis literature to assess the effects of systematic training on parent behavior, use of direct observation methods has not been reported extensively in the pediatric literature concerned with parent compliance.

Although presenting clear methodological advantages, direct observation strategies are often ruled out primarily on the basis of inconvenience and expense, and the reactive (including therapeutic) effects of direct observations are sometimes difficult to control. As more applied behavior analysts develop an interest and an expertise in behavioral pediatrics in general and in parent compliance with medical recommendations in particular, the use of direct observation strategies is likely to become more prevalent in the pediatric literature. The refinement and increased availability of audiovisual devices, such as portable videotaping equipment and audio cassette recorders with automatic timers, plus further development of a calibration model of reliability assessment involving paraprofessionals and family members are also likely to promote this trend.

Pill Count. Another frequently employed measure of parent compliance is the pill count. This method provides a comparison between the amount of medication remaining in the child's bottle or other dispenser and the amount that should be remaining based on the amount and dosage of the initial prescription and the length of time since the prescription was filled. The pill count provides a simple, yet inexpensive, quantitative assessment of compliance and permits a crude estimation of the effect of varying compliance levels on therapeutic outcome.

The pill count may yield an inaccurate measure of compliance for several reasons, however. For example, the parent may not leave all unused pills in the bottle or dispenser in an effort to falsely increase the apparent level of compliance and thereby please the clinician. Alternatively the parent may simply forget to return all pills after dividing them into different containers placed at different sites. Furthermore, pill counts may result in inflated estimates of parent compliance when the prescribed medication is ingested by other family members as well as the child. There is some evidence that pill counts are more reliable when they are conducted unobtrusively or without prior announcement (Linkewich, Catalano, & Flack, 1974; Porter, 1969).

Another problem is that the correlation between pill counts and biological indices of compliance is low, with pill counts often providing a higher estimate of compliance (Bergman & Werner, 1963; Roth, Caron, & Hsi, 1971) than biological measures. For instance, Bergman and Werner (1963) presented compliance distribution data based both on urine assays and pill counts in a study of compliance by parents of children prescribed a ten-day pencillin regimen for streptococcal pharyngitis. By the ninth day of the regimen, the urine tests indicated that only 8 percent of the children were being administered the antibiotic, while the estimate based on the pill count was 18 percent.

One possible explanation for this low correlation is that pill counts and biological indices measure distinct aspects of compliance. Pill counts provide an assessment of the extent of compliance over a relatively long period of time, while the biological indices assess only whether or not any medication was consumed in a relatively brief time interval just prior to assessment. On the positive side, pill counts typically yield more conservative estimates of compliance than self-report measures (Dunbar, 1977; Francis et al., 1969; Park & Lipman, 1964).

In summary, pill counts are a relatively convenient, inexpensive method of measuring compliance and are generally preferable to parent self-report measures. However, pill counts do not typically identify variability in parent compliance over time and are likely to provide an overestimate of parent compliance. Therefore, conclusions based on pill counts should be forwarded tentatively, especially when unannounced or inobtrusive checks are not possible.

Therapeutic Outcome. A frequently employed measure of compliance is the outcome of the treatment regimen. Based on the assumption that the recommended regimen would be effective if followed, therapeutic outcome initially appears to be a reasonable measure of compliance. While few would disagree that compliance is a mediator of therapeutic outcome, there are a number of problems associated with using outcome as a measure of compliance. Some components of effective professional assistance are not mediated solely through compliance. For example, in the case of a phobia, the child's anxiety may be alleviated by the support received from the professional care provider in addition to parent compliance with and child participation in *in vivo* relaxation exercises. Consequently, clinical outcome may be a partial product of aspects of professional care not mediated by compliance with instructions.

Another problem is that there is not necessarily a one-to-one correspondence between compliance and therapeutic outcome. Categorizing parents as compliant or noncompliant on the basis of the child's clinical outcome may be misleading. For instance, a parent may be complying with an inappropriate therapy or an inappropriate dose of the correct medication and thus not be achieving the desired outcome. Conversely a child may be indicating an adequate response to treatment, despite poor parent compliance with the prescribed treatment, because of the child's idiosyncratic response to a lowered dose. Even when there is a correspondence between compliance and outcome, the nature of this relationship requires much further study. For instance, it may be that a parent is likely to stop a medication regimen when the clinical outcome is favorable. Relatively little is known about the association between improvements in the child's health and parent compliance.

As indicated above, the compliance-outcome relationship may be a function of the prescribed dosage. For instance, the effect of noncompliance on outcome may depend on how closely the prescribed dosage approximates the minimal dosage required to obtain a therapeutic effect. If the dosage prescribed far exceeds the minimum effective prescribed medication and the parent's compliance with the medication dose is low, this low compliance may not reduce the effectiveness of therapy. Also a child may have been prescribed multiple medications and the parent's compliance with the medication under investigation may differ considerably from compliance with other medications that, although not being studied, are effective. Given these many problems, the use of therapeutic outcome as exhibited by the child as an indirect measure of parent compliance is not typically recommended.

Clinical Judgment.   Several studies, most of which have involved adult patients, have documented the inability of professionals to predict patient compliance (Caron & Roth, 1968; Davis, 1966; Mushlin & Appel, 1977). There are a few investigations of physicians' estimates of parent compliance that corroborate this finding (Charney et al., 1967; Wood, Feinstein, Taranta, Epstein, & Simpson, 1964). In general the literature suggests that clinicians do no better than chance when determining whether or not an adult patient is compliant. For example, Caron and Roth (1968) investigated the ability of physicians to identify a group of adult peptic ulcer patients who were noncompliers with a prescribed antacid regimen. They reported a correlation of .01 between physicians' estimates of patient compliance and a bottle count. Twenty-two of 27 physicians overestimated patient compliance, even when their assessment was restricted to patients about whom they were confident.

In a study appearing ten years later, Roth and Caron (1978) reported a higher correlation (.48); yet physicians still overestimated compliance. In a similar project, Mushlin and Appel (1977) examined the ability of physicians to predict patient compliance in returning for follow-up appointments and in taking a prescribed dosage of digitalis and diuretics. While physicians were judged to be correct in 145 of 187 patients, their predictions were accurate for only 14 of 40 patients who did not return for follow-up appointments, and their ability to predict compliance with the medication regimen was even poorer. More studies specific to parents are needed. However, the present literature with adults suggests that professional estimates of parent compliance are unlikely to be of practical value in day-to-day delivery of health services.

Self-Monitoring.   Another compliance measure is that of self-monitoring, which consists of having the parent maintain a written record of the parent's completion of the professionally recommended regimens using either a repeated event recording or time-sampling observational system. Self-monitoring has several advantages over an interview with the parent, including the collection of data at the time compliance occurs and thereby reducing the problem of poor recall upon retrospective questioning. In addition, self-recording by the parent permits an investigation of individual variation in compliance behavior among parents over time. Parent-collected records, if sufficiently detailed, may serve to identify specific environmental factors that may influence parent compliance. Information regarding the overall percentage of compliance will not provide these data in that varying patterns associated with different obstacles to compliance may lead to the same level of compliance overall. Moreover, self-monitoring often results in significant treatment benefits (Nelson, 1977a).

As with other self-report measures, daily records kept by parents are especially subject to bias. In order to satisfy the clinician, parents may record inaccurately so as to inflate their apparent level of compliance. Alternatively, because of competing activities, parents may simply fail to keep records, thereby producing an incomplete, often uninterpretable measure of parent compliance. Factors documented to be related to improvements in the reliability of self-recordings include: operational definitions of discrete target behaviors, training in self-monitoring skills, immediate recordings of target behaviors, differential reinforcement of accurate self-recording responses, preannounced accuracy checks, and minimal distractions at the time of self-recording (Nelson, 1977b). The assessment of the reliability of self-recordings is problematic because of reactive effects of simultaneous direct observation by another individual.

Most recently, mechanical monitoring devices have been employed to monitor compliance. For example, mechanical counters that record the number and time sequence of pills removed from prescription bottles are available (Moulding, Onsted, & Sbarbaro, 1970). Dunbar (1983) reports that mechanical monitors designed to measure compliance with medications such as bronchodilators are under development. As yet, use of these devices has been limited, to a large extent, to controlled experimental demonstrations and has not become widespread in clinical practice.

In conclusion, self-monitoring as a measure of parent compliance is not frequently reported in the pediatric literature, although there are numerous references in the child behavior therapy literature (Herbert & Baer, 1972). Self-monitoring by parents, particularly when judged to be reliable through the collection of independent, simultaneous recordings by paraprofessionals or other family members, could be employed as a means of collecting more detailed information regarding parent compliance. However, it would be unwise to assess compliance solely on the basis of self-monitoring by the parent.

Parent Self-Report via Interview.   Many practitioners rely on parent self-report to yield an estimate of compliance. The parent is simply asked whether he or she followed professional recommendations. A few investigators have examined the validity of conclusions drawn from parent self-report during interviews. For instance, Feinstein et al. (1959) compared conclusions based on interviews with those based on a pill count when measuring parent compliance with a prescribed penicillin prophylaxis for children. There was a high level of agreement between the two measures in identifying "poor" compliers. However, there was a large discrepancy in the classification of "good" compliers. Based upon interview responses, 73 percent of parents were classified as "good" compliers, while pill counts resulted in the placement of 55 percent of parents in the same category.

In a study conducted in a pediatric outpatient clinic, Francis, Korsch, and Morris (1969) examined mothers' compliance with physicians' advice primarily through the mother's responses to interview questions. In addition, they completed pill counts with 129 of the 330 parents who had received prescriptions for oral medication. There were few discrepancies between the interview and pill-count assessments of compliance. In each discrepant case, however, the interview responses suggested a higher level of compliance than that substantiated by pill count. Gordis, Markowitz, and Lilienfeld (1969b) compared interview data with urine tests to assess parent compliance with an oral prophylaxis for rheumatic fever. The results indicated that the parent's interview responses overstated compliance and understated noncompliance in comparison with the urine assays.

These three studies raise questions concerning the validity of parents' interview responses. It appears that many parents overestimate their level of compliance. Even so, interviews have been shown to be an effective means of identifying some noncompliers, and there is little evidence that compliant patients misrepresent themselves as noncompliers (Gordis et al., 1969b). There are some data suggesting that the patient who admits to being noncompliant is likely to respond favorably to an intervention designed to increase compliance (Sackett, 1979). Interviews, therefore, may result in the identification of some parents who are receptive to compliance-enhancing strategies. Dunbar (1979) suggests that the validity of interview responses can be enhanced through employing skilled interviewers who provide differential reinforcement to respondents for accuracy, rather than just for statements indicating high levels of compliance or clinical progress. Dunbar (1979) also recommends that the interviewer provide cues that it is acceptable for the parent to report deviations from the prescribed regimen.

The advantages of the interview as a measure of parent compliance are that it is relatively inexpensive, it can be conducted easily on a regular basis, and it does serve to identify some noncompliers. In addition, it allows for an in-depth examination of problems encountered by the noncompliers who attempt to follow recommendations. There is evidence, however, that parent's interview responses yield an overestimate of compliance in comparison with pill counts and urine tests, especially when the parent exhibits a high degree of variability in adherence to the prescribed regimen.

Summary and Recommendations Regarding Measurement of Parent Compliance

To date, numerous methods have been employed to assess parent compliance, including biological indices obtained from the children, direct observations of parent behavior, pill counts, assessment of treatment outcome, estimates by professionals of compliance, self-monitoring by parents, and semistructured interviews. Because each method has some disadvantages, it is advisable for research investigators and practitioners to employ a combination of measures, with each measure selected to provide a unique bit of complementary information not available through the other methods (Dunbar, 1979; Dunbar & Agras, 1980).

For example, when there is a question about the adequate therapeutic level or actual consumption of a prescribed drug, biological indices should be taken periodically. When possible, direct observation or self-monitoring should be included in the assessment package to provide information about specific environmental factors that routinely influence parent compliance. In addition, periodic semistructured interviews should be conducted to acquire detailed information regarding adherence solutions as well as obstacles to compliance encountered by parents. Based on the literature, exclusive reliance on clinical judgment or therapeutic outcome is extremely questionable. Where only short-term measures are needed, biological indices and direct observation appear to be the assessment methods of choice. Where long-term measures are required, pill counts, self-monitoring and interviews, calibrated by periodic direct observations and biological indices, would appear sufficient.

DETERMINANTS OF PARENT COMPLIANCE

Much of the literature regarding the determinants of compliance is based upon research with adult patients. Only a few such studies have specifically investigated factors associated with parent compliance. For the purpose of this review, it is assumed that variables found to influence adult compliance in general are likely to be similar to those influencing parent compliance in particular. Table 20.1 provides a list of selected determinants found to correlate with compliance.

Demographic Factors

Much of the early research on compliance examined high and low rates of adherence to medical advice in terms of easily quantifiable dimensions, such as the demographic, personal, and social characteristics of the specific population studied. Taken as a whole, this emphasis has resulted in a morass of disparate findings that are either not predictive of compliance (Charney et al., 1967; Davis, 1968a; Davis, 1968b) or are contradictory (Marston, 1970; Mitchell, 1974). Few studies have found an association between demographic factors and compliance (Haynes, 1976). In general investigators have not shown that compliance is consistently related to sex, income, intelligence, level of education, or marital status (Arnhold et al., 1970; Charney et al., 1967., Davis, 1968b; Elling, Whittemore, & Green, 1960). Demographic factors appear to be associated with the likelihood of initiating or gaining access to health services, but not with compliance to professional recommendations among patients already in the health delivery system (Haynes, 1976). The major finding to date is that noncompliance is observed among adults of all demographic categories (Becker, 1979).

There are at least four problems inherent in a demographic approach to predicting compliance (Becker, 1979). First, even if a consistent relationship between one or more demographic factors and adult compliance were documented, it is unlikely that any of the detected associations would explain the phenomenon. Demographic studies, at best, are likely to yield variables similar to risk factors. The resultant data may assist in identifying groups of parents toward which interventions designed to increase compliance should be directed, but they would not specifically provide information regarding the form or content of the needed intervention(s). Second, most characteristics identified by demographic studies are relatively immutable and, therefore, knowledge about them seldom points toward oppor-

TABLE 20.1. DETERMINANTS OF COMPLIANCE

Determinants	Effects on Compliance		
	Hinder	Promote	No Effect
Demographic factors			
Age			X
Sex			X
Intelligence		X	X
Education		X	X
Socioeconomic status	X		X
Marital status			X
Features of disease			X
Features of therapeutic regimen			
Patient understanding of recommendations		X	X
Duration of treatment	X		
Complexity of regimen	X		
Frequency of dosage	X		
Side effects	X		X
Cost of treatment	X		
Parenteral administration		X	
Lifestyle changes/restrictions required	X		
Degree of supervision		X	
Continuity of care		X	
Consumer satisfaction		X	
Features of referral process			
Time lag between referral and first appointment	X		
Length of clinic waiting time	X		
Other			
Health beliefs of parents			
Perception of child's vulnerability		X	
Perception of child's illness		X	X
Severity of symptoms			
Low	X		
Medium		X	
High	X		
Increased disability		X	
Perceived efficacy of care		X	
Social support		X	
Differential consequences		X	

tunities for interventions to increase compliance. Third, even in the few instances where relationships between demographic factors and compliance have been found, such findings do not explain why a large number of adults who present one or more identified risk factors nonetheless routinely comply with professional advice. Finally, the findings regarding demographic variables are unlikely to result in unified theories or testable hypotheses regarding differential rates of compliance among adults. Consequently, freestanding demographic studies should receive a low research priority.

Features of the Disease

Very few studies in the pediatric literature have examined the relationship of parent compliance with features of the child's disease. Findings taken from the adult literature suggest that disease factors are relatively unimportant determinants of compliance (Haynes, 1979a). In general, an adult's previous experience with a disease, including its duration and previous hospitalization for it, does not appear to influence the adult's compliance. Some studies have been reported indicating that compliance varies directly with symptom severity (Haynes, 1979a). However, contrary to expectations, increasing symptoms are sometimes associated with decreased parent compliance (Charney et al., 1967). There is some evidence that increased disability may be associated with increased compliance (Hayes, 1979a). When taken as a whole, the literature suggests that one cannot identify an adult noncomplier based on diagnostic or disease features. It is unlikely, therefore, that noncompliant parents can be routinely selected on the basis of the child's diagnosis or disease. Since examination of the features of the child's disease are not expected to result frequently in the detection or improvement of parent compliance, future research in this area should also have a relatively low priority.

Features of the Therapeutic Regimen

Several features of the therapeutic regimen have been associated with compliance.

Patient Knowledge and Compliance.   One explanation for poor compliance is that the adult does not have an adequate understanding of the prescribed regimen. For example, in a study involving low-income patients receiving care at a neighborhood health center, Svarstad (1974) found that 50 percent of the patients could not correctly state how long they were to take prescribed medications, 26 percent did not know the prescribed dosage, 17 percent could not identify the prescribed frequency of administration, 16 believed "prn" drugs were to be taken regularly, and 23 percent could not state a rationale for taking each prescribed drug. Seventy-three percent of the patients who correctly recalled their physician's instructions were adhering to the recommended regimen, while only 16 percent of those who erroneously recalled the instructions ultimately complied. The clarity of the physician's instructions was also examined. Among those patients receiving instructions judged to be clear, 62 percent understood the instructions and 54 percent complied. Among patients receiving relatively unclear instructions, 40 percent understood them but only 29 percent complied.

Findings regarding the relationship of patient knowledge and compliance are not consistent, however. For instance, based on a study of compliance with a ten-day course of prescribed penicillin for streptococcal infections among children, Bergman and Werner (1963) reported that 95 percent of the parents correctly identified the proper directions for drug administration, yet only 45, 30 and 18 percent of the children were receiving their medication as prescribed by the third, sixth, and ninth days, respectively. As Becker (1979) points out, it is reasonable to view a parent's knowledge of certain aspects of the regimen to be an essential prerequisite for compliance but also to recognize that such information may not often be sufficient to elicit adequate parent cooperation.

Podell (1975), in a book instructing physicians how to enhance compliance with medical regimens for hypertension, noted that more than twice as many studies suggest that there is no relationship between patient knowledge and compliance as suggest that there is a positive association. In attempting to explain these inconsistent findings, Podell contended that the provision of information is helpful to individuals who are motivated to comply but who are ignorant of the prescribed procedures, whereas for already knowledgeable but insufficiently motivated patients, additional information about the recommended procedures is not likely to improve compliance.

Duration of Regimen and Compliance.   The literature suggests that compliance with medications prescribed for short periods declines rapidly, as illustrated by the Bergman and Werner (1963) study. The duration of prescribed treatment appears to have an effect upon compliance: adherence to treatment typically decreases over time (Charney et al., 1967; Gordis & Markowitz, 1971; Sackett & Haynes,1976). The decline in compliance over time argues for the selection of therapeutic alternatives of short duration, when such alternatives are available and not contraindicated by other considerations.

Complexity of Regimen and Compliance.   Compliance typically declines as the complexity of the prescribed regimen increases (Haynes, 1976). The number of medications or treatments prescribed usually has an important effect upon compliance: the more treatments prescribed, the lower the compliance rate (Francis et al., 1969; Hulka, Kupper, Cassel,

Efird, & Burdette, 1975,. Weintraub, Au, & Lasagna, 1973). There is consistent evidence that prescription of multiple drugs is associated with a reduction in compliance. Compliance declines sharply when the number of daily medications to be administered is three or more (Blackwell, 1979; Greenberg, 1984). It is unclear whether this performance decrement is solely a function of noncompliance or is a result of poor comprehension (medication errors) as well as noncompliance.

Dosage Schedule and Compliance.   The influence on compliance of the number of times per day a medication is to be taken is not clear. For example, with adult patients, Gatley (1968) and Brand, Smith, and Brand (1977) have reported a steep decline in compliance as the frequency of dosing increased from one time to four times per day. However, also with adult patients, Parkin, Henney, Quirk, & Crooks (1976) found little to no correlation between compliance and the number of daily doses. One of the few studies concerned specifically with parent compliance also did not reveal a high correlation (Lima et al., 1976). Therefore, despite the emphasis given by some investigators to "once daily" doses (Clark & Troop, 1972), there is no consistently documented linkage between higher dosage frequency and low compliance.

Side Effects and Compliance.   One of the most frequent contentions made by clinicians and pharmaceutical companies alike is that negative side effects decrease compliance. However, the findings of some studies do not support this notion (Latiolais & Berry, 1969). Furthermore, in studies in which patients have provided reasons for their noncompliance, side effects as a cause of noncompliance have usually been mentioned by only five to ten percent (Daschner & Marget, 1975; Weintraub et al., 1973). Overall, negative side effects do not appear to have a major influence upon compliance among adults as patients. Little is known about whether parents are more or less compliant when the child exhibits such side effects.

Cost of Treatment and Compliance.   There is surprisingly little research on the effect of cost of therapy upon compliance. Costs associated with recommendations have usually been found to be negatively associated with compliance (Alpert, 1964; Antononsky & Kats, 1970). Previous studies do not typically distinguish between the cost of the treatment and the actual cost to the patient in terms of time from work, transportation and child-sitting expenses. Much more research into the impact of costs upon compliance, especially compliance of parents of children with chronic disorders, is needed (Mosher, Rafter, & Gajewski, 1984).

Type of Drug/Route of Administration and Compliance.   Several studies, most with adults as patients, have found differences in compliance rates for alternative drugs or alternative routes of administration for the same drug. Use of procedures requiring only passive cooperation by the patient, such as parenteral administration by professionals in a clinic or hospital, obviously results in higher levels of compliance. Active cooperation, in which the adult is typically requested to comply with instructions in the home, is less easily achieved, and a steep gradient has been demonstrated in which compliance among adults who must acquire new habits—for example, taking a prescribed medication—is much greater than that shown by adults who must alter old behaviors, such as dietary habits (Haynes, 1976). In turn this is less difficult to accomplish than recommendations requiring the withdrawal of reinforcers such as cigarettes. Additional studies of the features of therapeutic regimens as they relate to degree of parent compliance are needed and should receive a relatively high research priority.

Degree of Supervision and Compliance. Several investigators have reported a positive association between the degree of supervision provided by the professional and the extent of compliance on the part of adult patients. As might be expected, in general, hospitalized patients are more compliant than day patients, who are in turn more compliant than outpatients. Parent compliance would be predicted to parallel this according to the level of supervision afforded the child's case. Some studies have shown improvements in compliance when the frequency of outpatient visits is increased, when professionals maintain periodic telephone contact with the patient, when home visits are made, when family members are enlisted to assist in supervision of the prescribed regimen, or when feedback regarding objective evidence of noncompliance is shared with the patient (Haynes, 1976).

Continuity of Care and Compliance. Parent compliance appears to be enhanced when continuity of care is provided (Gordis & Markowitz, 1971). In a private practice setting, Charney et al. (1967) demonstrated that mothers are more likely to comply with recommendations offered by the regular family physician than with those extended by the physician's partner or another doctor. Becker, Drachman, and Kirscht (1972a) documented that clinic mothers are more compliant both in keeping appointments and following the prescribed regimen when seen by a familiar physician.

Consumer Satisfaction and Compliance. The patient's stated level of satisfaction with the service provider and the service delivery system has been found to correlate positively with compliance (Alpert, 1964; Becker et al. 1972a; Becker, Drachman, & Kirscht, 1972b; Haynes, 1976., Korsch & Negrete, 1972; Litt & Cuskey, 1984). Based upon a review of 35 studies, Baekeland and Lundwall (1975) concluded that the clinician's relationship with the patient significantly influences subsequent adherence. The successful clinician has a warm, empathetic manner, engages in social conversation with the patient, and permits patients to participate actively in the design of the prescribed regimen (Korsch & Negrete, 1972).

Francis et al. (1969) reported that a parent's level of compliance with a regimen prescribed for the child is higher when the parent is pleased with the initial contact, perceives the physician to be friendly, and believes the physician understands the presenting complaint. While the patient's attitudes toward health professionals in general and the health care system as a whole do not appear to influence compliance (Haynes, 1976), compliance has been found to be positively related to the patient's conclusions that the therapist has met his or her expectations. For excellent reviews of issues pertaining to parent satisfaction with professional services, the reader is referred to McMahon and Forehand (1983) and Lebow (1982).

Features of Referral Process and Compliance.   There are several studies regarding the features of the referral process as possible determinants of compliance. One aspect of the referral process that has been examined is the time lag between the referral contact and the clinic appointment. Although some investigators have reported that the call-appointment interval is unrelated to appointment keeping (Alpert, 1964; Gates & Colburn, 1976; Schroeder, 1973), other researchers have documented that the longer the time lag between the receipt of the referral and the initial appointment, the lower the probability that the first appointment will be kept (Benjamin-Bauman, Reiss, & Bailey, 1984; Finnerty, Shaw, & Himmelsbach, 1973; Glogow, 1970).

For example, in one experiment, Benjamin-Bauman et al. (1984) assigned patients referred to a family planning unit of a public health department to appointments within either one or three weeks of the referral call. Show rates for patients assigned to the one-week group were significantly higher than those for the three-week group. In a second experiment, patients were given appointments either the next day or two weeks from the date of the referral contact. Show rates for patients in the next-day group were significantly above those for patients in the latter group. Additional research into the impact of the referral process on compliance should be assigned a high research priority, given the evidence suggesting that straightforward changes in referral procedures can dramatically improve compliance.

Clinic Structure and Compliance.   Some attention has been directed toward the effect on compliance of the mechanics of establishing appointments and the structure of the service delivery system. For instance, the length of the parents' waiting time in the clinic area appears to be inversely related to compliance. Decreased clinic waiting time has been found to be associated with an increase in appointments kept (Alpert, 1964; Finnerty, Mattie, & Finnerty, 1973). Also Rockart and Hoffman (1969) observed that when outpatients were scheduled at the same time for an appointment at a hospital and seen on a first-come, first-serve basis, the no-show rate was 27 percent. When all patients were scheduled for the same time but assigned to specific physicians, the no-show rate was 22 percent. When patients were given individual appointment times but were not scheduled to see a specific physician, the percentage of missed appointments was 13. The mean waiting time was 85, 57, and 33 minutes in these three groups, respectively. However, it is impossible to clearly attribute the results solely to the method of appointment scheduling, to the method of physician assignment, or to the length of the waiting time, given that each variable was allowed to vary with the others.

Health Beliefs of Parents.   Much of the medical literature pertaining to parent compliance has investigated various aspects of the health belief model, a theory initially proposed by a group of social psychologists attempting to explain an individual's propensity toward a recommended preventive health action (Rosenstock, 1974). The theory suggests that whether or not an individual will comply with a professional's recommendation is a function of the individual's perception of the level of personal susceptibility to a particular illness or condition, the degree of severity of the clinical course of a disease if contracted, the prescribed regimen's potential effectiveness in preventing or reducing the individual's susceptibility, and the physical, psychological, and financial costs related to undertaking or continuing the recommended behavior. Becker and Maiman (1975) have adapted this model to the issues surrounding parent compliance. They have added factors related to the parent's general motivation to promote the child's health, concern with the child's possible resusceptibility to previously contracted illness or conditions, and general faith in the health delivery system, as well as characteristics of the doctor-patient relationship.

In the pediatric literature, there are a number of studies (Becker et al. 1978) demonstrating positive correlations between a parent's estimate of the child's vulnerability to illness and the parent's subsequent compliance with medical recommendations. In addition, several studies of preventive health behaviors have obtained positive correlations between the parent's perception of the child's illness and compliance with health-related recommendations (Becker, 1976; Becker, Drachman, & Kirscht, 1974; Charney et al., 1967; Francis et al., 1969; Gordis, Markowitz, & Lilienfeld, 1969c).

However, other studies have found no significant relationships between perceptions of the child's illness and actual participation in a variety of preventive screening programs (Haefner & Kirscht, 1970; Kirscht, Haefner, Kegeles, & Rosenstock, 1966). Additional research suggests an inverted U-shaped function among asymptomatic individuals—that is, very low levels of perceived severity do not sufficiently motivate action, while very high levels are inhibitory (Becker, Kaback, Rosenstock, & Ruth, 1975).

The health belief model predicts that compliance is partially a function of perceived benefits and costs. Several studies of preventive health behaviors have reported positive correlations between perceived efficacy of the preventive care and subsequent compliance. For example, Elling et al. (1960) and Heinzelmann (1962) both found that the parent's belief in the ability of penicillin to prevent the recurrence of rheumatic fever was predictive of the parent's adherence to the recommended medical regimen. Becker et al. (1974) presented results suggesting that the parent's belief in the efficacy of the prescribed medication predicted regular administration of penicillin to the child. The degree of required behavioral change is negatively correlated with patient cooperation. Patients are more likely to comply with proscribed behaviors than with prescribed ones (Collette & Ludwig, 1969; Elling et al., 1960; Francis et al., 1969; Gillum & Barsky, 1974).

The proponents of the health beliefs model contend that the bulk of data taken from research examining compliance with medical recommendations indicate relationships between such compliance and the parent's perceptions of susceptibility, severity, benefits, and costs. Less enthusiastic supporters point out that while both prospective and retrospective studies substantiate the predictive value of the model, prospective studies typically reveal a weaker relationship than retrospective ones, suggesting that changes in compliance may precede as well as follow changes in the parent's health beliefs.

Social Support and Compliance. Several studies have shown that compliance is higher among adult patients with supportive, intact families, and lower among those with unstable or no families (Elling et al., 1960; MacDonald, Hagberg, & Grossman, 1963). Other studies cite the positive contributions made by friends or peers (Gray, Kesler, & Moody, 1966; Jay et al., 1984). Wahler (1980) has examined the relationship of a mother's contact with other adults with her compliance to professional recommendations regarding management of her child's oppositional behavior. He has reported that on days of frequent mother contacts with other adults, mother-child problems were lower in frequency than on days characterized by infrequent contacts. His findings suggest that a parent's social contacts may influence the extent of parent compliance with professional instructions in the home. In 1983, Wahler and Graves reviewed several studies indicating that parent compliance may be a function of myriad elements of the parent's social network.

The family can influence adherence in multiple ways. Dunbar and Agras (1980) suggest that the family's expectations of change and the family's attitudes toward the regimen itself may be significant factors. Based upon these expectations and attitudes, family members may be more or less likely to encourage, remind, and provide differential consequences for compliance. In addition, the family may effect changes in the home environment in order to promote compliance. For instance, the family may alter its shopping patterns, resulting in the decreased stockpiling of high-calorie foods in the home as a means of assisting a child to comply with recommendations for weight reduction. Furthermore, various members of the family may share responsibility for implementing the prescribed regimen. There is a need for more investigations of social factors that affect parent-child interactions as well as those social factors specific to the child and the prescribed treatment.

Differential Consequences and Compliance. The provision of differential consequences is one of the most influential determinations of compliance. In the context of medical treatment, patients who become noncompliant without any negative health consequences may be prone to repeat their noncompliance in the future (Dunbar, 1983). Conversely, those patients with a history of compliance with a previous regimen resulting in health improvements may be more likely to be compliant with present and future recommendations (Haynes, 1976). Little research has focused upon the impact of a patient's compliance history on the patient's present performance. In addition, few investigations have examined whether compliance with one aspect of a prescribed regimen is predictive of compliance with other aspects.

With respect to facilitating the acquisition and maintenance of skills required of parents in order for them to be compliant with professional directives, there is voluminous behavioral parent training literature which suggests that the delivery of differential consequences is an essential determinant (Dangel & Polster, 1984). Given this literature, it is surprising that so many professionals assume that parents, especially those with poor compliance histories, will follow recommendations in the absence of differential consequences. The highest research priority should be assigned to the identification of environmental factors related to compliance.

A behavioral analysis of compliance would center on the isolation of stimulus factors that set the occasion for compliance and of consequences that increase or decrease the probability of compliance (Zifferblatt, 1975). As Rapoff and Christophersen (1982) point out, there are situations in which the importance of stimuli and consequences is obvious. They cite the case of compliance with antacid regimens, where there are salient cues (an "upset" stomach) that set the occasion for ingestion of antacid tablets and positive consequences (relief of discomfort) following this ingestion. Unfortunately, such salient cues and immediate consequences are not present in many compliance situations. Research aimed at identifying cues and differential consequences for an extensive array of problems and procedures is urgently needed. Following such identification, programmatic research designed to assess the relative influence of these environmental factors will be critically important.

Summary and Recommendations Regarding Determinants of Parent Compliance

Research attempting to identify factors that correlate with and predict compliance may be useful in several ways. Such research may continue to suggest new directions to scientists and practitioners interested in developing compliance-improving strategies. In addition, investigations of possible determinants may eventually yield risk factor profiles that may serve to define target populations and point toward more timely and economical interventions. Moreover, identification of determining factors may further research into compliance-enhancing strategies by indicating on which key variables subjects should be matched prior to assignment to experimental and control conditions. Given the paucity of research to date pertaining to parent compliance, each of the variables examined with adults as patients warrants further study. Based on the available literature, it appears that highest research priorities should be assigned to features of the referral process, clinic structure, and therapeutic regimen, and to the roles of social support and differential consequences in promoting parent compliance.

STRATEGIES FOR IMPROVING PARENT COMPLIANCE

The literature is replete with strategies that have been shown to be effective in improving adult compliance with medical and/or behavioral recommendations. These strategies differ in the degree to which they focus on didactic instruction, use of behavioral procedures to promote acquisition and maintenance of skills required for compliance, adjustments to the regimen, and the organizational aspects of the health delivery system. Table 20.2 presents a list of commonly employed interventions.

Educational Strategies

In general, educational strategies aim to improve compliance via the transmission of information about a disease or condition and its treatment. Related to the use of prescribed medications and compliance with other facets of a medical regimen, patient education approaches have frequently involved group lectures and demonstrations, and/or individual instructions and counseling. No educational strategy has been routinely successful in increasing compliance. Many approaches typically increase the parent's knowledge about the child's condition, but do not result in improvement in the parent's compliance or in the child's therapeutic outcome. For example, in one study, (Bowen, Rich & Schlotfelt, 1961) a group of diabetic patients attended a series of lectures and demonstrations regarding their recommended daily regimen. Following participation in this

TABLE 20.2. COMMON COMPLIANCE INTERVENTIONS

Educational strategies
    General information about disease and its treatment
    Counseling

Combined educational and behavioral strategies
    Verbal step-wise instructions
    Instructional manuals
    Written protocols
    Modeling
    Behavioral rehearsal
    Media-assisted training
    Performance-based feedback
    Prompting
Self-management
    Goal setting
    Self-monitoring
    Problem solving
Environmental rearrangements
Contingent reinforcement

Adjustment to regimen
    Reduced complexity
    Lowered costs
    Individual tailoring
    Dose packaging
    Prolonged action drugs
    Parenteral formulations
    Pill containers with signal alarms

Organizational strategies
    Employment of referral clerks
    Preintake counseling
    Extended supervision
    Use of health management specialist
    Promotion of appointment-keeping
        Shortened time lags between referral and appointment
        Telephone/Mail reminders
        Monetary/Cash-equivalent incentives
        Waiting list contingencies
        Increased convenience

series, most patients demonstrated improved skills related to the administration of insulin. However, there was no measure of daily compliance and there were no reported differences from control patients in blood sugar levels, weight change, or clinical complications.

Haynes (1979b) reviewed several studies attempting to educate adults about their own or their child's disease and its management. Educational strategies included programmed instruction, lectures and demonstrations, and individual instruction and counseling. These strategies consistently resulted in increases in the adults' knowledge about the conditions, but few concomitant improvements in either compliance or therapeutic outcome. Other studies have reported more positive results. For instance, in two studies of parent compliance with the prescribed use of oral antibiotics for streptococcal pharyngitis, individual counseling was supplemented with written instructions. This combination resulted in improvements in compliance and therapeutic outcome in comparison with a control group in one study (Colcher & Bass, 1972). Although the other study (Leistyna & Macaulay, 1966) did not include a control group, 89 percent of parents receiving this intervention were judged to be compliant with the oral penicillin prescription, a higher percentage than that predicted by control groups given similar recommendations in other studies (Bergman & Werner, 1963; Charney et al., 1967).

A number of studies in the social psychology literature focus on the motivational effects of *how* information is transmitted to adults, in contrast with *what* information is presented. In the studies reviewed by Haynes (1979b), for example, educational materials identical in content were presented in various ways to several groups of adult patients. Across these studies, no one message type, whether it was considered "high or low in fear" or whether it provided "no information" versus "minimal" or "in-depth" information, was consistently successful in effecting changes in the adults' attitudes or behavior.

The literature regarding educational strategies suggests that the clinician would be well advised to emphasize the specific procedures that the parent is to follow, in addition to the provision of general information about the child's illness, condition, or problem. This recommendation is based on the lack of consistent evidence that general information about the child's presenting complaint or the action of a medication is sufficient to promote parent compliance, although understanding of the treatment regimen does appear to influence parent behavior positively.

Green (1979) offers several practical suggestions to improve patient comprehension, recall, and compliance when educational strategies are employed. He advises that the verbal instructions be brief—that is, that the clinician be extremely selective and only present information that the parent needs to know in order to carry out the recommended regimen. In addition he suggests that the more important information be presented first as opposed to later in the discussion with the parent, based on the experimental literature pertaining to retention and recall. He contends that all information, be it conveyed orally or through a written protocol, should be clearly organized, categorized, and labelled.

Moreover, Green recommends that, whenever possible, verbal instructions be supplemented by written suggestions. This is predicated on what he refers to as the "principle of repetition," which holds that repeated information is more likely to be retained than information which is not repeated. Written instructions, especially when specific to the particular child, can be referred to over and over again by the parent. Written protocols that are generally stated, in contrast to those that are child- or problem-specific, may not be as effective.

Combined Educational and Behavioral Strategies

According to Epstein and Ossip (1979), parent compliance with a prescribed therapeutic regimen is dependent upon at least two factors: (1) that requested behaviors be in the repertoire of the parent, and (2) that motivational contingencies be sufficient to produce and maintain the prescribed actions. The first factor, until recently, has been relatively overlooked because noncompliance has typically been attributed to poor motivation or "willpower." However, compliance with professional recommendations becomes an issue only after it has been established that the parent has all the requisite behaviors to carry out the instructions. It may be that many prescriptions are not followed because parents have not acquired the skills necessary to implement them. A growing body of literature suggests that an analysis of behavioral competence, that is, an analysis of behaviors required to implement a treatment, may be central in some cases in which the parent is noncompliant (Bernstein, 1982; Budd & Fabry, 1983; Budd, Riner, & Brockman, 1983; Zifferblatt, 1975).

The use of behavioral principles to teach skills to parents has proliferated over the past two decades. There is a resultant voluminous literature pertaining to behavioral approaches to parent education and training. For extensive reviews of this literature, the reader is referred to Berkowitz & Graziano (1972), Dangel & Polster (1984), Forehand & Atkeson (1977), Graziano (1977), Johnson & Katz (1983), McMahon & Forehand (1980), Moreland, Schwebel, Beck & Wells (1982), and O'Dell (1974).

Several studies have examined the relative efficacy of various techniques employed to train parents, teachers, and paraprofessionals. One of the most consistent findings is that verbal instruction alone does not always result in the acquisition and/or maintenance of skills needed by parents and others to comply with recommendations (Bowen et al., 1961; Gardner, 1975; Sanders & Glynn, 1981; Sepler & Myers, 1978).

Instructional manuals based upon detailed task analyses (Resnick, Wang, & Kaplan, 1973) of requisite skills have been shown to be effective in promoting the satisfactory completion of complex tasks (Fawcett &

Fletcher, 1977; Heifetz, 1977; Matthews & Fawcett, 1979). Such manuals typically include a set of learner instructions, a statement of training objectives, a rationale for the overall task, special skills needed for task completion, when and by whom each activity should be conducted, illustrations of situations calling for performance, concrete descriptions of each step in the task, reading comprehension quizzes, and practice examples.

The use of brief, problem-focused written protocols as a supplement to orally delivered instruction is becoming more prevalent (Christophersen, 1982; Lowe & Lutzker, 1979; McMahon & Forehand, 1978) and is likely to be found more feasible (Rapoff & Christophersen, 1982) than the employment of instructional manuals. The protocols are usually one to two pages in length. They typically specify what treatment is to be delivered, when, and by whom. Furthermore, instructions regarding what not to do are often included. Recommendations are frequently presented in a step-wise fashion, along with a few interspersed examples of how the recommendations are to be applied. Christophersen (1982) presents an extensive array of sample protocols that are relevant to promoting parent compliance with professional directives.

There are several other training techniques and, on occasion, many of them have been shown to be superior to didactic instruction in the form of lectures. Numerous investigators have presented evidence supporting the effectiveness of modeling (Peed, Roberts, & Forehand, 1977) and modeling plus behavioral rehearsal *in vivo* or in role play situations (Flanagan, Adams, & Forehand, 1979; Forehand & McMahon, 1981; Koegel, Glahn, & Nieminen, 1978; Nay, 1975; O'Dell, Flynn, & Benlolo, 1977; O'Dell, Mahoney, Horton, & Turner, 1979).

There is a growing body of literature suggesting that media-assisted parent training consisting of videotape modeling or individual videotape feedback is quite effective (Bernal, Williams, Miller, & Reagor, 1972; Dowrick & Raeburn, 1977; Griffiths, 1974; Nay, 1975; Webster-Stratton, 1981a, 1981b, 1982) and is sometimes superior to training via a written manual or via *in vivo* modeling and behavior rehearsal (Flanagan, Adams, & Forehand, 1979; Nay, 1975; O'Dell et al., 1979). For example, O'Dell et al. (1979) randomly assigned sixty parents to one of six groups: (1) no treatment control, (2) training via a written manual, (3) training via a film, (4) training via a film plus a performance test, (5) training via modeling and rehearsal, and (6) brief training by modeling and rehearsal. Each training intervention was superior to no treatment in promoting the acquisition of performance skills as demonstrated in role play situations. A film combined with a performance test was most effective, followed by a film alone. The results of this study, among others, suggest that training films may enhance parents' acquisition of the skills necessary to comply with professional recommendations.

With respect to establishing motivational contingencies, the pediatric, rehabilitation, and behavior therapy literatures present numerous alternative strategies for facilitating compliance. Such interventions include prompting (Bates, 1977; Meyers, Thackwray, Johnson, & Schleser, 1983; Nazarian, Mechaber, Charney, & Coulter, 1974; Turner & Vernon, 1976), self-management training involving goal setting, self-monitoring, problem-solving, and rearranging the home environment (Burg, Reid, & Lattimore, 1979; Herbert & Baer, 1972; Loeber & Weisman, 1975; Sanders & Glynn, 1981), contingent reinforcement in the form of differential attention, praise, points, tokens, and money (Fleischman, 1979; Gardner, 1975, 1976; Iwata, Bailey, Brown, Foshee, & Alpern, 1976; Lowe & Lutzker, 1979; Rapoff, Lindsley, & Christophersen, 1984) alone and in conjunction with response cost.

Monitoring of parent administration of prescribed medication to children is also a useful strategy for promoting compliance. Dawson and Jamieson (1971) reported that routine monitoring of serum levels of anticonvulsant medication was associated with increases in parent compliance. Eney and Goldstein (1976) evaluated the effects of monitoring salivary levels of theophylline prescribed for children with chronic asthma. They found that clinician-provided feedback to parents on the drug levels obtained resulted in increased parent compliance, particularly when the parents were informed beforehand that salivary levels would be monitored.

A number of investigators have tested the efficacy of various combinations of the training techniques and motivational contingencies cited above with adult clients, service providers, or parents of children receiving services. Combinations employed successfully have included: programmed instruction, lecture, modeling, group discussion, and homework (Burkhart, Behles, & Stumphauzer, 1976); role playing, feedback, and self-management (Komaki, 1977); lecture, rehearsal, feedback, and homework (Stern & Golden, 1977); lecture, modeling, and homework (Schinke, 1979); instructions, role playing, and feedback (Jones, Fremouw, & Carples, 1977); self-monitoring plus feedback (Sanson-Fisher, Seymour, & Baer, 1976); instructional manual, lecture, modeling, role playing, and feedback (Willner et al., 1977); lecture, discussion, modeling, videotapes, behavior rehearsal to criterion, and feedback (Dancer, et al. 1978); programmed text with study guide and worksheets, review of graphs of target behaviors, and feedback (Kelley, Embry, & Baer, 1979); instructional manual, videotapes, feedback, and modeling (Koegel, Russo, & Rincover, 1977); workshops and social reinforcement (Montegar, Reid, Madsen, & Ewell, 1977); and instructional manuals, self-monitoring, feedback, reinforcement via a point economy, and praise for symptom reduction (Epstein et al., 1981).

Unfortunately despite the plethora of literature pertaining to combinations of training techniques and incentives, there are relatively few studies examining the incremental contributions made by the various components of these packages. One well-controlled component analysis was conducted by Epstein and Masek (1978). They examined the relative efficacy of several behavioral interventions in increasing college students' compliance with a Vitamin C regimen. Each subject was assigned randomly to one of four groups: self-monitoring, taste, taste plus self-monitoring, and a no-treatment control group. Subjects who engaged only in self-monitoring recorded the time the Vitamin C tablets were taken. Those assigned to the taste only condition received flavored tablets to increase the saliency of tablet taking, while those participating in the self-monitoring and taste procedure received flavored tablets and recorded the flavor of each tablet ingested. Six weeks later, one-half of the subjects in each group received a portion of a monetary deposit contingent upon meeting a preset compliance criterion, while the other half in each group continued their previous procedures.

Epstein and Masek (1978) found that self-monitoring alone and taste plus self-monitoring were most effective during the first six weeks. The introduction of the monetary incentive resulted in significant increases in compliance, regardless of the subject's previous history of noncompliance. Increasing the saliency of the tablets through flavoring alone did not increase compliance. The results suggested that self-monitoring was more effective than increased salience, with monetary contingencies as effective as self-monitoring and taste combined. The Epstein and Masek study provides a useful methodology for partialing out the relative effects of a multicomponent compliance intervention and illustrates that all components of an intervention package may not be active ingredients.

As a function of the combined educational/behavioral strategies noted above, some parents may acquire the skills necessary to follow professional recommendations. However, such acquisition does not guarantee that parents will employ their newly learned skills in the home and community or maintain the prescribed actions over time. It is critically important to discover training procedures that result in high levels of parent compliance across settings, tasks, persons, and time. Many studies regarding the issues of generalization and maintenance have been reported in the child behavior therapy literature. For excellent reviews of research into these issues, the reader is referred to Forehand and Atkeson, (1977), McMahon, Forehand, and Griest (1982), and Stokes and Baer (1977).

In a seminal discussion article, Stokes and Baer (1977) highlight several approaches to facilitating generalization, including training for each required skill one at a time, training with materials and under the conditions likely to be found in the home, training through the use of multiple examples while varying the instructions and cues, training for self-management skills, and use of intermittent or delayed reinforcement. When taken as a whole, the literature addressing generalization of skills is somewhat encouraging. For example, didactic instruction combined with modeling, role playing, and feedback has been shown to result in generalization of training effects from clinic to home (Forehand et al., 1979).

When didactic instruction is employed as one component of a training package, some research indicates that the incorporation of general principles in addition to specific problem-specific procedures enhances skill generalization as well as training outcome (Glogower & Sloop, 1976; McMahon, Forehand, & Griest, 1981; O'Dell et al., 1977; Schinke, 1979). In order to facilitate generalization, Koegel, Glahn, and Nieminen (1978) recommend teaching general procedures rather than, not in addition to, problem-specific techniques.

Some literature suggests that increasing the degree of parent involvement in the design of the prescribed treatment protocol would increase the probability of compliance (Gardner, 1975). For instance, parents would participate in the determination of goals and in the selection of treatments, schedules, and supplies. Moreover, involving parents in the training of other parents being asked to follow the same directives is likely to promote skill generalization (Jones et al., 1977). Furthermore, the probability of compliance may be increased occasionally through environmental rearrangements in the home. For example, Twardosz, Cataldo, and Risley (1974) found that a rearrangement of the physical environment of a day care center resulted in significant increases in the frequency of desirable staff behaviors.

Another means of enhancing generalization of skills may be through the establishment of formal feedback systems that regularly evaluate whether parents are completing prescribed actions. It is likely that training parents to self-monitor, record, and manage their own efforts (Loeber & Weisman, 1975; McMahon et al., 1981) would result in increased compliance, especially if a review of such records was a routine part of the agenda during clinic or home visits. The impact of periodic telephone contacts between clinic appointments, in order to review previously extended recommendations and to assess parent compliance, in addition to providing reminders has not yet been investigated widely.

The literature pertaining to maintenance permits even more optimism. For example, trainee performance has been maintained via public posting (Hutchinson, Jarman, & Bailey, 1980), personal or written feedback (Ford, 1980; Loeber & Weisman,1975), public posting plus feedback (Greene, Willis, Levy, & Bailey, 1978), contingent reinforcement via praise, tokens, and/or money (Bates, 1977); peer competition plus cash prizes (Patterson, Griffin, & Panyan, 1976); reward opportunities (Iwata et al., 1976); self-recording (Burg et al., 1979); and didactic instruction, modeling, role-playing, and feedback (Baum & Forehand, 1981; Forehand et al., 1979; Peed et al., 1977).

Future research pertaining to combined educational/behavioral approaches is needed to address the following questions (Bernstein, 1982): (1) What problems must parents be able to solve in order to be compliant with professional directives? (2) What skills must parents employ to solve these common problems? (3) What training procedures are most likely to facilitate acquisition of these skills? (4) What procedures are most likely to promote generalization and maintenance of these skills? Of these four questions, the first two have received less attention to date than the latter two. The first question is especially important because the use of common compliance problems as examples during training may be beneficial, and there is no need to train parents to solve problems they are unlikely to encounter. Interviews, questionnaires, diaries, and direct observation can be employed to ascertain descriptions and relative frequencies of problems faced by parents. There are several approaches to determine skills required by parents to solve the problems identified. One is to ask parents what they do and/or what skills they consider useful. An alternative is to utilize interviews, questionnaires, diaries, and direct observation to collect descriptions of effective problem-solving methods employed by parents. A third is to identify two groups of parents—those who comply and those who do not comply—followed by a systematic evaluation of what variables discriminate the two groups (Bernstein, 1982).

With respect to training procedures, it is not yet known what specific combinations of strategies are optimally effective. Furthermore, few studies have investigated whether the efficacy of training techniques varies as the parameters of these techniques vary. For instance, as Ford (1980) indicates, modeling involves a message (is the model competent or incompetent?), a valence (is the model rewarded or punished for the behavior demonstrated?) and a medium (for example, *in vivo*, audiotape, or videotape). Finally, little is known about the relative efficiency or cost-effectiveness of procedures designed to promote generalization and maintenance of skills acquired by parents.

Adjustments to the Regimen

The medical literature points toward several characteristics of prescribed regimens that can be manipulated to improve parent compliance, including reduced complexity and costs of scheduled medications, individual tailoring, dose packaging, prolonged-action drugs, and parenteral formulations. Becker (1979) advises that, whenever feasible, every effort should be made to reduce the regimen's complexity, duration, and cost, as well as the parent's need to alter habits. As discussed above, each of these factors has been found to be a determinant of compliance.

It appears that increased convenience to the parent of any kind increases compliance. For example, individual tailoring, which may involve fitting the recommended regimen to the parent's daily schedule to maximize convenience, has been found to be somewhat facilitative of compliance (Dunbar, Marshall, & Hovell, 1979). Norell (1979) tailored the use of eye drops for glaucoma patients to routine events in the patient's lives and found that tailoring resulted in significant decreases in missed doses. Simplification of the medication schedules, which may consist of packaging medication in single doses rather than in an amount that requires two or three administrations per day (Brand et al., 1977), combining drugs in single tablets to reduce the number of pills to be taken (Clark & Troop, 1972), use of sustained-action preparations to reduce the frequency of doses (Colcher & Bass, 1972; Feinstein et al., 1968), presentation of drugs in calendar packs (Linkewich et al., 1974; Peterson, McLean & Millingen, 1984), employment of pill containers with signal alarm devices (Azrin & Powell, 1969), utilizing pills with unique features to minimize confusion, and providing measuring tools for liquid medications (Mattar, Markello, & Yaffee, 1975) have been sometimes associated with improvements in compliance.

Another strategy shown to be effective in increasing compliance is the use of a suitable parenteral formulation to be administered either by the medical staff or by the parents themselves. This method, when feasible, circumvents several compliance problems. In two studies of prophylaxic interventions for rheumatic fever, children who received penicillin injections once a month had fewer relapses than children receiving oral medications (Feinstein et al., 1968; Feinstein et al., 1959). Finally Sackett (1976), among others, has recommended that medications be added to the prescribed regimen to counteract the side effects of the primary drug in order to reduce the possible deleterious effects of aversive conditioning.

Much more research is needed to examine the relative efficacy of various manipulations on the characteristics of the regimen. Although many of the interventions listed above have much intuitive appeal, surprisingly few studies have yet documented sizeable clinical effects with some of them. For example, the limited research regarding individual tailoring suggests that this strategy does not always have a powerful effect (Sackett, 1976). The systematic manipulation of variables found to have the highest positive as well as negative correlations with compliance, based upon the literature pertaining to determinants, is likely to yield the most effective results.

Strategies Directed at Organizational Aspects of the Service Delivery System

The research literature suggests that parent compliance can be enhanced through certain organizational strategies that are feasible in most pediatric service delivery systems. When the compliance problem involves a referral to another service within the health care system, strategies such as letters from the referral source to the patient as well as to the receiving clinic, and the employment of a referral clerk in the receiving clinic to assist patients with the establishment of an initial appointment and to provide the patient information about the implications of the referral, the nature of the services to be offered, and how the patient can assist in the provision of beneficial services have been shown to be successful (Barry & Daniels, 1984; Glogow, 1970; Haynes, 1979b; Kluger & Karras, 1983; Larsen, Nguyen, Green, & Attkisson, 1983). Furthermore, the use of referral clerks to provide preintake counseling and to assist consumers of service, including parents, to overcome obstacles related to scheduling and transportation difficulties has been shown to be effective (Fletcher, Appel, & Bourgois, 1974; Hoehn-Saric et al., 1964).

In general, the literature suggests that the more supervision provided by the clinician in regard to the implementation of the prescribed regimen, the greater the degree of parent compliance. Extended supervision may involve increasing the frequency of clinic visits, including home visits in the treatment program, and assigning responsibility to a team member to monitor compliance. Home visits have been employed in several studies with, reportedly, a high degree of success. For example, in a pediatric clinic (Anderson, Rowe, Dean, & Arbisser, 1971), families of children who did not keep appointments were visited in their home by paraprofessionals who arranged more convenient appointment times, transportation, and childsitters. In this case, home visits resulted in a marked increase in the percentage of kept appointments.

A few studies have examined the effectiveness of a family health management specialist to promote parent compliance. For instance, one research team (Fink, Malloy, Cohen, Greycloud, & Martin, 1969) randomly assigned parents appearing in a pediatric ambulatory care clinic to a series of meetings with a public health nurse. The nurse assessed the parents' ability to follow medical recommendations, devised a feasible set of recommendations along with the physician, provided information regarding the child's medical condition and its treatment, and assisted the parents to implement the management plan and to attend follow-up appointments. In comparison with the performance of parents assigned to a control group, parents receiving assistance from the nurse exhibited greater knowledge of and compliance with recommended procedures.

One of the most pervasive examples of parent noncompliance with professional health recommendations is the failure to keep scheduled appointments (Adebojono, 1973; Alpert, 1964; Badgley & Furnal, 1961; Mindlin & Densen, 1971; Smiley, Byres, & Roberts, 1972). Such parent noncompliance adversely affects continuity of care, training of professionals, and the fiscal solvency of many ambulatory clinics. Appointments initiated by the parent during periods when the child is exhibiting symptoms, in contrast to well-child appointments, are more likely to be kept (Sackett, 1976; Sackett & Snow, 1979). As mentioned earlier, there is a growing literature indicating that a reduction in the length of the interval between the referral and the date of the initial appointment is directly related to compliance (Benjamin-Bauman et al., 1984; Finnerty, Shaw, & Himmelsbach, 1973; Hoffman & Rockhart, 1969). For example, Finnerty, Shaw, and Himmelsbach (1973) reported a sizeable increase in the percentage of kept initial appointments when these appointments were scheduled only one or two days in advance instead of one or two weeks. Benjamin-Bauman et al. (1984) suggest that appointments should be scheduled within seven days of a referral.

When the time lag between referral and initial appointment cannot be so short, a telephone or mailed reminder within a few days of the appointment has been found to be very effective in increasing appointment-keeping (Brigg & Mudd, 1968; Duer, 1982; Gates & Colburn, 1976; Nazarian et al., 1974; Reiss & Bailey, 1982; Reiss, Piotrowski, & Bailey, 1976; Turner & Vernon, 1976; Yokley & Glenwick, 1984). Such reminders have also been used somewhat successfully to promote attendance at follow-up appointments (Ossip-Klein, Vanlandingham, Prue, & Rychtarik, 1984; Rice & Lutzker, 1984). However, there is some evidence that the effectiveness of reminders decreases over time (Morse, Coulter, Nazarian, & Napadono, 1981). In general, postcard reminders are the easiest and least expensive method (Schroeder, 1973). While telephone contacts may be somewhat more effective (Shepard & Moseley, 1976), they are more time-consuming and expensive than mailed reminders.

Methods involving differential consequences including monetary or cash-equivalent incentives (Parrish, Charlop, & Fenton, in press; Reiss et al., 1976; Rice & Lutzker, in press; Yokley & Glenwick, 1984), and waiting list contingencies (Parrish et al., in press) have also resulted in a higher percentage of appointment-keeping. The evidence supporting the efficacy of these behavioral interventions has been obtained in medical settings such as family planning clinics (Benjamin-Bauman et al., 1984; Duer, 1982) and health departments (Nazarian et al., 1974; Reiss et al., 1982), family practice centers (Rice & Lutzker, 1984), dental screening clinics (Reiss et al., 1976), mental health centers (Brigg & Mudd, 1968), and behavior management clinics in pediatric hospitals (Parrish et al., in press).

Most studies have not found a relationship between time since last appointment and the probability of keeping the next one (Gates & Colborn, 1976; Nazarian et al., 1974; Schroeder, 1973). Neither the time of day nor the day of the week for the scheduled appointment appears to influence keep rates (Gates & Colborn, 1976; Mattar et al., 1975; Nazarian et al., 1974; Schroeder, 1973). Length of waiting time in the clinic for each appointment is associated with subsequent rates of appointment-keeping (Haynes, 1976). Long waiting times before and during appointments are frequent reasons given by patients for not keeping later appointments (Alpert, 1964; Badgley & Furnal, 1961; Davis, 1968b; Finnerty, Mattie, & Finnerty, 1973). As indicated above, the convenience of receiving services, particularly with respect to the method of scheduling appointments, is also an important determinant of appointment-keeping (Rockart & Hoffman, 1969). It appears that individual appointment times, in contrast to block appointments, would result in a higher percentage of kept appointments.

Summary and Recommendations Regarding Compliance Interventions

Numerous strategies for improving compliance with medical and behavioral recommendations have been investigated. General information pertaining to the child's disorder and its management is seldom sufficient. Parent compliance is likely to be facilitated through the use of experimentally validated behavioral training procedures designed to promote the acquisition of skills required for adherence. Such procedures typically involve the provision of brief, well-organized, and task-specific verbal instructions and corresponding written protocols. These verbal and written instructions are supplemented, when appropriate, by therapist modeling of the recommended treatment strategies, followed by an opportunity for the trainee (parent) to imitate the observed behaviors. The therapist then provides performance-based feedback and, if necessary, remedial training consisting of additional instruction, modeling, behavioral rehearsal, and feedback. When feasible, media-assisted training via videotape modeling is sometimes employed.

Once the parent has acquired the requisite skills, environmental interventions designed to further the maintenance and generalization of parent compliance are established. Such interventions may consist of periodic prompting, self-management training, contingent reinforcement, monitoring of compliance by the parent and/or others, and feedback. Generalization is enhanced through training with materials and under the conditions typically found in the home. Whenever possible, parent participation in the design of the prescribed treatment protocol is encouraged.

Parent adherence to medical recommendations may be increased further through the employment of medication calendars, special pill packages, prolonged-action drugs, parenteral administrations, signal alarm devices, and by feedback based upon periodic assessments of drug levels. Reinforcement contingent upon well-documented medication use and/or symptom control may also prove to be effective.

Regardless of whether the recommendations are medical or behavioral in nature, the clinician should attempt to reduce the complexity, duration, and cost of the prescribed regimens. Regimens can be adjusted in multiple ways, for example, through individual tailoring the regimen to the parent's daily routine. Parent compliance is also likely to be augmented through extended supervision, involvement of family members, employment of a compliance specialist, provision of information regarding the severity of the child's condition and the potential benefits of treatment, and repeated monitoring of adherence.

Furthermore, parent compliance can be improved through organizational tactics, such as the use of reminders and differential consequences to increase appointment keeping, reductions in waiting time before appointments, minimization of inconvenience factors, and scheduling of individual appointments. Much more research regarding the relative efficacy of and costs-benefits associated with each of the strategies described above is needed. In addition, more frequent collection of follow-up data in order to assess the durability of changes in parent compliance with long-term regimens is highly important.

PRIORITIES FOR FUTURE RESEARCH

There are several gaps in the literature pertaining to parent compliance. Indeed, the literature on parent compliance *per se* is surprisingly sparse. At present, many conclusions regarding parent compliance with medical and behavioral recommendations are based in part upon inferences drawn from studies of adult patients. Relatively few investigations outside of the behavioral parent training literature have been completed that target specific parameters of or interventions for parent compliance. Conclusions pertaining to parent adherence are also limited by several methodological weaknesses that are evident throughout the literature. The most basic flaws rest with the differing definitions of compliance used inconsistently across studies, the arbitrary cutoffs for establishing "good" versus "poor" adherence, and the variability in reported compliance rates using different measurement procedures with the same population. As Epstein and Cluss (1982) point out, a common method for measuring parent adherence across a variety of target problems is needed. Pill counts, parent self-report, and estimates of compliance by professionals are not sufficiently reliable. Biological assays are more reliable, but individual differences in responsivity to drugs and the fact that many biological measures are too expensive and/or invasive to be taken repeatedly pose significant problems. In the case of measuring pill-taking behavior, for example, Epstein and Cluss recommend the widespread use of biological tracers or flavored pills.

Although particular studies of compliance pose idiosyncratic methodological problems that require solutions, a few issues frequently occur across studies. In addition to precise and uniform definitions of compliance, the literature would be furthered if investigators were to provide more detailed information about (1) the selection and demographics of parent samples, (2) the disease, condition, or behavior problem presented by the child, (3) the prescribed therapeutic regimen, and (4) the measures of compliance employed. Such information would assist current researchers in their efforts to systematically replicate previous studies and would facilitate an assessment of the generality of the findings. There is need to establish the comparability and relative validity, reliability, and cost of various direct and indirect methods of measuring compliance. For now, because of the problems inherent in each of the most frequently employed methods of measurement, it is advisable that investigators utilize multiple measures whenever possible.

More studies involving inception cohorts are required. Many previous investigations have not followed all parents who began implementing a specific therapeutic regimen, possibly resulting in a systematic loss of the more noncompliant parents, who either drop out completely or rarely keep appointments, thereby biasing the study sample and perhaps invalidating any conclusions drawn. Through presenting data for every parent present at the beginning of a particular therapeutic regimen for children, later determinations of group compliance are more likely to be valid.

In parallel with the need to examine complete inception cohorts is the need for more studies reporting compliance distributions within and across various parent samples, therapeutic regimens; and diseases, conditions, and problems at different stages of the therapeutic process. Given that some determinants may have more pronounced effects upon compliance when adherence is relatively high and others only when it is relatively low, compliance studies should include tables of the extent of compliance exhibited by individual parents, so that the correlates of compliance/noncompliance as well as the variability associated with specific interventions can be assessed more easily. Compliance distributions may point to differing compliance levels among those who admit and those who deny a compliance problem. In addition, different compliance-improving strategies may be more effective at different levels of compliance, suggesting that more favorable clinical results may occur when specific strategies are paired with specific distributions (Sackett, 1979). Also needed are a series of community-based as well as hospital-based studies to assess compliance distributions within different health care delivery systems and different public assistance and private insurance programs.

In addition there is a need for further studies of the correlation of compliance with the achievement of therapeutic goals. Although adherence and clinical outcome are not necessarily predictive of one another, it is likely that at least some interventions designed to increase adherence will result in improved levels of symptom control. Whenever possible, investigations of compliance-improving interventions should include clinical outcome measures. The degree of compliance required for attainment of a desired clinical effect is likely to vary from regimen to regimen. For instance, a frequently reported illustration concerns children who were given by their parents as little as one-third of prescribed oral penicillin and were subsequently found to be adequately protected against recurrences of rheumatic fever (Gordis et al., 1969a). If outcome measures are obtained along with compliance measures, it may be possible in some instances to rule out noncompliance as the critical factor responsible for variability in treatment outcome. In these situations, researchers could then shift the focus to biological differences, such as variations across individuals in pharmacokinetics. As is, many examinations of the efficacy of medical and behavioral prescriptions are often equivocal because treatment failures may be the result of parent noncompliance.

Of critical importance are additional studies of the relationship between attendance at scheduled appointments and compliance with prescribed regimens. It should not be assumed that the higher the percentage of kept appointments the greater the extent of parent compliance with recommendations, or the greater the likelihood of a therapeutic outcome (Bigby, Pappius, Cook, & Goldman, 1984; Smith, Seale, & Shaw, 1984). More research is needed regarding the effectiveness of various methods to increase the efficiency of service delivery, for example, reducing the lag between referral and first contact as well as availability of subsidized transportation and child sitters and reductions in waiting time for individual appointments. Also, some additional studies of the effects of improved continuity of care are needed.

Furthermore, additional research is indicated to document the relationship between compliance and various parameters of the prescribed regimen, including alternative forms of treatment, such as oral versus parenteral administrations of medications, size of individual doses, dosage scheduling, medication side-effects, use of safety containers, reductions in the complexity of regimens, and gradual introduction of multicomponent prescriptions. It may be that reducing the number of unnecessary prescriptions may reduce noncompliance. There is also a need for extensive interdisciplinary research regarding the impact of attitudinal characteristics of parents, specifically those factors hypothesized to be important by the adaptation of the health belief model to pediatric issues, and characteristics of parent/therapist interactions upon parent compliance.

One major gap in the literature on parent compliance is the measurement of long-term adherence. Many previous studies have investigated adherence only to short-term regimens, such as administering antibiotics for acute infections. Studies that have employed sound measures of compliance have not continued, typically, for more than a few months, and those studies reporting follow-up data have not often employed repeated measures of compliance. Because many children served in the health care delivery system have chronic disorders, the investigation of parent compliance over extended periods is obviously very important.

Investigations into the acceptability of alternative assessment and treatment procedures as judged by parents themselves may offer useful information to the clinician selecting among these alternatives (Kazdin, 1980; Kazdin, 1981). Moreover, with respect to specific compliance-improving strategies, the social validity of the observed changes requires scrutiny. In the case of parent compliance, social validity refers to an evaluation of whether demonstrated changes in parent adherence are deemed clinically important by the parents involved and by an impartial panel of noninvolved parents and professionals. According to Kazdin (1977) and Wolf (1978), parent satisfaction with a particular intervention is likely to be a factor in the maintenance of the intervention by parents.

A high priority should be given to investigations of the natural history of compliance, that is, the consistency in extent of compliance exhibited by individual parents over a long period of time in response to a variety of regimens for a variety of pediatric disorders. Also much research attention should be given to the application of compliance-improving strategies found to be effective among parents for improving the clinical behavior of practitioners.

Finally, the issue of practicality is of central importance. Although many promising intervention strategies have been identified, it is still unclear whether these strategies can be implemented by clinicians not working in research settings. Service providers are chiefly responsible for delivering patient care and, therefore, may not have enough time to assess compliance and, when indicated, select and implement interventions designed to improve adherence. In addition to facing time constraints, many service providers are unlikely to have sufficient professional training to employ the full array of available assessment and treatment procedures. To date, few investigators have reported information that permits an analysis of the feasibility of the procedures utilized. Consequently, a high priority should be given to research into the feasibility of alternative strategies, with increased attention to details pertaining to the amount of time typically required to complete procedures and the professional training of those who conducted the procedures. Optimally, this feasibility research would be conducted in representative service delivery settings.

REFERENCES

Adebojono, F.O. (1973). A comparative study of child health care in urban and suburban children. *Clinical Pediatrics, 12,* 644–648.

Alpert, J.J. (1964). Broken appointments. *Pediatrics, 34,* 127–132.

Anderson, F.P., Rowe, D.S., Dean, V.C., & Arbisser, A. (1971). An approach to the problem of noncompliance in a pediatric outpatient clinic. *American Journal of Diseases of Children, 122,* 142–143.

Antonovsky, A., & Kats, R. (1970). The model dental patient: An empirical study of preventive health behavior. *Social Science Medicine, 4,* 367–380.

Arnhold, R.G., Adebonojo, F.O., Callas, E.R., Callas, J., Carte, E., & Stein, R.C. (1970). Patients and prescriptions: Comprehension and compliance with medical instructions in a suburban pediatric practice. *Clinical Pediatrics, 9,* 648–651.

Azrin, N.H., & Powell, J. (1969). Behavioral engineering: The use of response priming to improve prescribed self-medication. *Journal of Applied Behavior Analysis, 2,* 39–42.

Badgley, R.F., & Furnal, M.A. (1961). Appointment breaking in a pediatric clinic. *Yale Journal of Biological Medicine, 34,* 117–123.

Baekeland, F., & Lundwall, L. (1975). Dropping out of treatment: A critical review. *Psychological Bulletin, 82,* 738–783.

Barry, S.P., & Daniels, A.A. (1984). Effective change in outpatient failed appointments. *Journal of Family Practice, 18*(5), 739–742.

Bates, P. (1977). The search for reinforcers to train and maintain effective parent behaviors. *Rehabilitation Literature, 9,* 291–295.

Baum, C.G., & Forehand, R. (1981). Long term follow-up assessment of parent training by use of multiple outcome measures. *Behavior Therapy, 12,* 643–652.

Becker, M.H. (1976). Sociobehavioral determinants of compliance. In D.L. Sackett & R.B.

Haynes (Eds.), *Compliance with therapeutic regimens* (pp. 40–50). Baltimore: Johns Hopkins University Press.

Becker, M.H. (1979). Understanding patient compliance: The contributions of attitudes and other psychosocial factors. In S.J. Cohen (Ed.), *New directions in patient compliance* (pp. 1–40). Lexington, MA: Heath.

Becker, M.H., Drachman, R.H., & Kirscht, J.P. (1972a). Predicting mothers' compliance with pediatric medical regimens. *Medical Care, 81*(4), 843–854.

Becker, M.H., Drachman, R.H., & Kirscht, J.P. (1972b). Motivations as predictors of health behavior. *Health Services Reports, 87*, 852–861.

Becker, M.H., Drachman, R.H., & Kirscht, J.P. (1974). A new approach to explaining sick-role behavior in low-income populations. *American Journal of Public Health, 64:* 205–216.

Becker, M.H., Kaback, M.M., Rosenstock, I.M., & Ruth, M.V. (1975). Some influences on public participation in a genetic screening program. *Journal of Community Health, 1*, 3–14.

Becker, M.H., & Maiman, L.A. (1975). Sociobehavioral determinants of compliance with health and medical care recommendations. *Medical Care, 13*, 10–24.

Becker, M.H., Radius, S.M., Rosenstock, I.M., Drachman, R.H., Schuberth, K.C., & Teets, K.C. (1978). Compliance with a medical regimen for asthma: A test of the health belief model. *Public Health Reports, 93*, 268–277.

Benjamin-Bauman, J., Reiss, M.L., & Bailey, J.S. (1984). Increasing appointment keeping by reducing the call-appointment interval. *Journal of Applied Behavior Analysis, 17*, 295–301.

Bergman, A.B., & Werner, R.J. (1963). Failure of children to receive penicillin by mouth. *New England Journal of Medicine, 268*, 1334–1338.

Berkowitz, B.P., & Graziano, A.M. (1972). Training parents as behavior therapists: A review. *Behavior Research and Therapy, 10*, 297–317.

Bernal, M.E., Williams, D.E., Miller, W.H., & Reagor, P.A. (1972). The use of videotape feedback and operant learning principles in training parents in management of deviant children. In R. Rubin, H.F. Fensterheim, J. Anderson, & L. Ullmann (Eds.), *Advances in behavior therapy.* New York: Academic.

Bernstein, G.S. (1982). Training behavior change agents: A conceptual review. *Behavior Therapy, 13*, 1–23.

Bigby, J.A., Pappius, E., Cook, E.F., & Goldman, L. (1984). Medical consequences of missed appointments. *Archives of Internal Medicine, 144*(6), 1163–1166.

Blackwell, B. (1973). Drug therapy: Patient compliance. *New England Journal of Medicine, 289*, 249.

Blackwell, B. (1979). The drug regimen and treatment compliance. In Haynes, R.B., Taylor, D.W., & Sackett, D.L. (Eds.), *Compliance in health care.* (pp. 144-156). Baltimore: Johns Hopkins University Press.

Bowen, R.G., Rich, R., & Schlotfeldt, R.M. (1961). Effects of organized instruction for patients with the diagnosis of diabetes mellitus. *Nursing Research, 10*, 151–159.

Brand, F., Smith, R., & Brand, P. (1977). Effect of economic barriers to medical care on patients' noncompliance. *Public Health Reports, 92*, 72–78.

Brigg, E.H., & Mudd, E.H. (1968). An exploration of methods to reduce broken first appointments. *Family Coordinator, 17*, 41–46.

Budd, K.S., & Fabry, P.L. (1983). Behavioral assessment in applied parent training: Use of a structured observation system. In R.F. Dangel & R.A. Polster (Eds.), *Parent training: Foundations of research and practice.* New York: Guilford.

Budd, K.S., Riner, L.S., & Brockman, M.P. (1983). A structured observation system for clinical evaluation of parent training. *Behavioral Assessment, 5*, 373–393.

Burg, M.M., Reid, D.H., & Lattimore, J. (1979). Use of a self-recording and supervision program to change institutional staff behavior. *Journal of Applied Behavior Analysis, 12,* 363–375.

Burkhart, B.R., Behles, M.W., & Stumphauzer, J.S. (1976). Training juvenile probation officers in behavior modification: Knowledge, attitude change, or behavioral competence? *Behavior Therapy, 7,* 47–53.

Caron, H.S., & Roth, H.P. (1968). Patient's cooperation with a medical regimen. *Journal of the American Medical Association, 203,* 922–926.

Charney, E., Bynum, R.,Eldredge, D., Frank, D., MacWhinney, J.B., McNabb, N., Scheiner, A., Sumpter, E., & Iker, H. (1967). How well do patients take oral penicillin? A collaborative study in private practice. *Pediatrics, 40,* 188–195.

Chasseaud, L.F., & Taylor, T. (1974). Bioavailability of drugs from formulations after oral administration. *Annual Review of Pharmacology, 14,* 35–46.

Christophersen, E.R. (1982). Incorporating behavioral pediatrics into primary care. In E.R. Christophersen (Ed.), *The Pediatric Clinics of North America, 29* (2). Philadelphia: Saunders.

Clark, G.M., & Troop, R. (1972). One tablet combination drug therapy in the treatment of hypertension. *Journal of Chronic Diseases, 25,* 57–64.

Cohen, S.J. (1979). *New directions in patient compliance.* Lexington, MA: Heath.

Colcher, I.S., & Bass, J.W. (1972). Penicillin treatment of streptococcal pharyngitis: A comparison of schedules and the role of specific counseling. *Journal of the American Medical Association, 222,* 657–659.

Collette, J., & Ludwig, E.G. (1969). Patient compliance with medical advice. *Journal of the National Medical Association, 61,* 408–411.

Dancer, D.D., Braukmann, L.J., Schumaker, J.B., Kirigin, K.A., Willner, A.G., & Wolf, M.M. (1978). The training and validation of behavior observation and description skills. *Behavior Modification, 2,* 113–134.

Dangel, R.F., & Polster, R.A. (Eds.) (1984). *Parent training: Foundations of research and practice.* New York. Guilford.

Daschner, F., & Marget, W. (1975). Treatment of recurrent urinary tract infection in children. Compliance of parents and children with antibiotic therapy regimen. *Acta Paediatrica Scandinavia, 64,* 105–108.

Davis, M.S. (1966). Variations of patients' compliance with doctors' orders: Analysis of congruence between survey responses and results of empirical investigations. *Journal of Medical Education, 41,* 1037–1048.

Davis, M.S. (1968a). Variations in patients' compliance with doctors' advice: An empirical analysis of patterns of communication. *American Journal of Public Health, 58,* 274–288.

Davis, M.S. (1968b). Physiologic, psychological and demographic factors in patient compliance with doctors' orders. *Medical Care, 6,* 115–122.

Dawson, K.P., & Jamieson, A. (1971). Value of blood phenytoin estimation in management of childhood epilepsy. *Archives of Diseases in Childhood, 46:247,* 386–388.

Dowrick, P.W., & Raeburn, J.M. (1977). Video-editing and medication to produce a therapeutic self model. *Journal of Consulting and Clinical Psychology, 45,* 1156–1158.

Duer, J.D. (1982). Prompting women to seek cervical cytology. *Behavior Therapy, 13,* 248–253.

Dunbar, J.M. (1977). Adherence to medication: An intervention study with poor adherers to a medication regimen. Unpublished dissertation, Stanford University.

Dunbar, J.M. (1979). Issues in assessment. In S.J. Cohen (Ed.), *New directions in patient compliance* (pp. 41–57). Lexington, MA: Heath.

Dunbar, J.M. (1983). Compliance in pediatric populations: A review. In P.J. McGrath & P.

Firestone (Eds.), *Pediatric and adolescent behavioral medicine* (pp. 210–230). New York: Springer.

Dunbar, J.M., & Agras, W.S. (1980). Compliance with medical instructions. In Ferguson, J.M., & Taylor, C.B. (Eds.), *The comprehensive handbook of behavioral medicine* (Vol. 3; pp. 115–145). New York: Spectrum.

Dunbar, J.M., Marshall, G.D., & Hovell, M.F. (1979). Behavioral strategies for improving compliance. In R.B. Haynes, D.W. Taylor, & D.L. Sackett (Eds.), *Compliance in health care* (pp. 174–190). Baltimore: Johns Hopkins University Press.

Durant, R.H., Jay, M.S., Linder, C.W., Shoffitt, T., & Litt, I. (1984). Influence of psychosocial factors on adolescent compliance with oral contraceptives. *Journal of Adolescent Health Care, 5*(1), 1–6.

Elling, R., Whittemore, R., & Green, M. (1960). Patient participation in a pediatric program. *Journal of Health and Human Behavior, 1,* 83–89.

Eney, R.D., & Goldstein, E.D. (1976). Compliance of chronic asthmatics with oral administration of theophylline as measured by serum and salivary levels. *Pediatrics, 57* (4), 513–517.

Epstein, L.H., Beck, S., Figueroa, J., Farkas, G., Kazdin, A.E., Daneman, D., & Becker, D. (1981). The effects of targeting improvements in urine glucose on metabolic control in children with insulin dependent diabetes. *Journal of Applied Behavior Analysis, 14,* 365–375.

Epstein, L.H., & Cluss, P.A. (1982). A behavioral medicine perspective on adherence to long-term medical regimens. *Journal of Consulting and Clinical Psychology, 50,* 950–971.

Epstein, L.H., & Masek, B.J. (1978). Behavioral control of medicine compliance. *Journal of Applied Behavior Analysis, 11,* 1–10.

Epstein, L.H., & Ossip, D.J. (1979). Health care delivery: A behavioral perspective. In J.R. McNamara (Ed.), *Behavioral approaches to medicine: Application and analysis* (pp. 9–32). New York: Plenum.

Fawcett, S.B., & Fletcher, R.K. (1977). Community applications of instructional technology: Teaching writers of instructional packages. *Journal of Applied Behavior Analysis, 10,* 739–746.

Feinstein, A.R., Spagnuolo, M., Jonas, S., Kloth, H., Tursky, E., & Lemitt, M. (1968). Prophylaxis of recurrent rheumatic fever. *Journal of the American Medical Association, 206,* 565–568.

Feinstein, A.R., Wood, H.F., Epstein, J.A., Taranta, A., Simpson, R., & Tursky, E. (1959). A controlled study of three methods of prophylaxis against streptococcal infection in a population of rheumatic children. II. Results of the first three years of the study, including methods for evaluating the maintenance of oral prophylaxis. *New England Journal of Medicine, 260,* 697–702.

Fink, D., Malloy, M.J., Cohen, M., Greycloud, M.A., & Martin, F. (1969). Effective patient care in the pediatric ambulatory setting: A study of the acute care clinic. *Pediatrics, 43,* 927–935.

Finnerty, F.A., Jr., Mattie, E.C., & Finnerty, F.A. III (1973). Hypertension in the inner city. I. Analysis of clinic dropouts. *Circulation, 47,* 73–75.

Finnerty, F.A., Shaw, L.W., & Himmelsbach, C.K. (1973). Hypertension in the inner city. II. Detection and follow-up. *Circulation, 47,* 76–78.

Flanagan, S., Adams, H.E., & Forehand, R. (1979). A comparison of four instructional techniques for teaching parents to use time-out. *Behavior Therapy, 10,* 94–102.

Fleischman, M.J. (1979). Using parenting salaries to control attrition and cooperation in therapy. *Behavior Therapy, 10,* 111–116.

Fletcher, S.W., Appel, F.A., & Bourgois, M. (1974). Improving emergency-room patient follow-up in a metropolitan teaching hospital. *New England Journal of Medicine, 291,* 385–388.

Ford, J.E. (1980). A classification system for feedback procedures. *Journal of Organizational Behavior Management, 2,* 183–191.

Forehand, R.L., & Atkeson, B. (1977). Generalization of treatment effects with parents as therapists: A review of assessment and implementation procedures. *Behavior Therapy, 8,* 575–593.

Forehand, R.L., & McMahon, R.J. (1981). *Helping the noncompliant child. A clinician's guide to parent training.* New York: Guilford.

Forehand, R.L., Sturgis, E.T., McMahon, R.J., Aguar, D., Green, K., McMahon, R., Wells, K.C., & Breiner, J. (1979). Generality of treatment effects resulting from a parent training program to modify child non-compliance. *Behavior Modification, 3,* 3–25.

Francis, V., Korsch, B.M., & Morris, M.J. (1969). Gaps in doctor-patient communication. *New England Journal of Medicine, 280,* 535–540.

Gardner, J.M. (1975). Training non-professionals in behavior modification. In T. Thompson & W. Dockens (Eds.), *Applications of behavior modification.* New York: Academic.

Gardner, J.M. (1976). Training parents as behavior modifiers. In S. Yen & R.W. McIntire (Eds.), *Teaching behavior modification.* Kalamazoo, MI: Behaviordelia.

Gates, S.J., & Colburn, D.K. (1976). Lowering appointment failures in a neighborhood health center. *Medical Care, 14,* 263–267.

Gatley, M.S. (1968). To be taken as directed. *Journal of the Royal College of General Practice, 16,* 39–44.

Gillum, R.F., & Barsky, A.J. (1974). Diagnosis and management of patient non-compliance. *Journal of the American Medical Association, 228,* 1563–1567.

Glogow, E. (1970). Effects of health education methods on appointment-breaking. *Public Health Reports, 85,* 441–450.

Glogower, F., & Sloop, E.W. (1976). Two strategies of group training of parents as effective behavior modifiers. *Behavior Therapy, 7,* 177–184.

Gordis, L. (1976). Methodologic issues in the measurement of patient compliance. In D.L. Sackett & R.B. Haynes (Eds.), *Compliance with therapeutic regimens* (pp. 51–66). Baltimore: Johns Hopkins University Press.

Gordis, L. (1979). Conceptual and methodological problems in measuring patient compliance. In R.B. Haynes, D.W. Taylor, & D.L. Sackett (Eds.), *Compliance in health care* (pp. 23–45). Baltimore. Johns Hopkins University Press.

Gordis, L., & Markowitz, M. (1971). Evaluation of the effectiveness of comprehensive and continuous pediatric care. *Pediatrics, 48,* 766–776.

Gordis, L., Markowitz, M., & Lilienfeld, A.M. (1969a). Studies in the epidemiology and preventability of rheumatic fever. Part IV. A quantitative determination of compliance in children on oral penicillin prophylaxis. *Pediatrics, 43* (2), 173–182.

Gordis, L., Markowitz, M., & Lilienfeld, A.M. (1969b). The inaccuracy in using interviews to estimate patient reliability in taking medications at home. *Medical Care, 17,* 49–54.

Gordis, L., Markowitz, M., & Lilienfeld, A.M. (1969c). Why patients don't follow medical advice: A study of children on long-term antistreptococcal prophylaxis. *Journal of Pediatrics, 75,* 957–968.

Gray, R.M., Kesler, J.P., & Moody, P.M. (1966). Effects of social class and friends' expectations on oral polio vaccination participation. *American Journal of Public Health, 56,* 2028–2032.

Graziano, A.M. (1977). Parents as behavior therapists. In M. Hersen, R.M. Eisler, & P.M. Miller (Eds.), *Progress in behavior modification* (Vol. 4). New York: Academic.

Green, L.W. (1979). Educational strategies to improve compliance with therapeutic and preventive regimens: The recent evidence. In R.B. Haynes, D.W. Taylor, & D.L. Sackett (Eds.), *Compliance in health care* (pp. 157–173). Baltimore: Johns Hopkins University Press.

Greenberg, R.N. (1984). Overview of patient compliance with medication dosing: A literature review. *Clinical Therapeutics, 6*(5), 592–599.

Greene, B.F., Willis, B.S., Levy, R., & Bailey, J.S. (1978). Measuring client gains from staff-implemented programs. *Journal of Applied Behavior Analysis, 11,* 395–412.

Griffiths, R.D.P. (1974). Videotape feedback as a therapeutic technique: Retrospect and prospect. *Behavior Research and Therapy, 12,* 1–8.

Haefner, D.P., & Kirscht, J.P. (1970). Motivational and behavioral effects of modifying health beliefs. *Public Health Reports, 85,* 478–484.

Haynes, R.B. (1976). A critical review of the "determinants" of patient compliance with therapeutic regimens. In D.L. Sackett, & R.B. Haynes (Eds.), *Compliance with therapeutic regimens.* (pp. 26–39). Baltimore: Johns Hopkins University Press.

Haynes, R.B. (1979a). Determinants of compliance: The disease and the mechanics of treatment. In R.B. Haynes, D.W. Taylor, & D.L. Sackett (Eds.), *Compliance in health care* (pp. 49–62). Baltimore: Johns Hopkins University Press.

Haynes, R.B. (1979b). Strategies to improve compliance with referrals, appointments, and prescribed medical regimens. In R.B. Haynes, D.W. Taylor, & D.L. Sackett (Eds.), *Compliance in health care.* (pp. 121–143). Baltimore: Johns Hopkins University Press.

Haynes, R.B., Taylor, D.W., & Sackett, D.L. (1979). *Compliance in health care.* Baltimore: Johns Hopkins University Press.

Heifetz, L.J. (1977). Behavior training for parents of retarded children: Alternative formats based on instructional manuals. *American Journal of Mental Deficiency, 82,* 194–203.

Heinzelmann, F. (1962) Factors in prophylaxis behavior in treating rheumatic fever: An exploratory study. *Journal of Health and Human Behavior, 3,* 73–81.

Herbert, E.W., & Baer, D.M. (1972). Training parents as behavior modifiers: Self-recording of contingent attention. *Journal of Applied Behavior Analysis, 5,* 139–149.

Hoehn-Saric, R., Frank, J., Imber, S., Nash, E., Stone, A., & Battle, C. (1964). Systematic preparation of patients for psychotherapy: Effects on therapy behavior and outcome. *Journal of Psychiatric Research, 2,* 267–281.

Hoffman, P.B., & Rockhart, J.F. (1969). Implications of the no-show rate for scheduling OPD appointments. *Hospital Progress, 50,* 35–40.

Hulka, B.S., Kupper, L.L., Cassel, J.C., Efird, R.L., & Burdette, J. (1975). Medication use and misuse: Physician-patient discrepancies. *Journal of Chronic Diseases, 28,* 7–21.

Hulka, B., Cassel, J., Kupper, L., & Burdette, J. (1976). Communication, compliance, and concordance between physicians and patients with prescribed medications. *American Journal of Public Health, 66,* 847–853.

Hutchinson, J.M., Jarman, P.H., & Bailey, J.S. (1980). Public posting with a habilitation team: Effects on attendance and performance. *Behavior Modification, 4,* 57–70.

Iwata, B.A., Bailey, J.S., Brown, K.M., Foshee, T.J., & Alpern, M. (1976). A performance-based lottery to improve residential care and training by institutional staff. *Journal of Applied Behavior Analysis, 9,* 417–431.

Jay, M.S., Durant, R.H., Shoffitt, T., Linder, C.W. & Litt, I.F. (1984). Effect of peer counselors on adolescent compliance in use of oral contraceptives. *Pediatrics, 73*(2), 126–131.

Johnson, C.A., & Katz, R.C. (1973). Using parents as change agents for their children: A review. *Journal of Child Psychology & Psychiatry, 14,* 181–200.

Jones, F.H., Fremouw, W., & Carples, S. (1977). Pyramid training of elementary school teachers to use a classroom management "skill package." *Journal of Applied Behavior Analysis, 10,* 239–253.

Kazdin, A.E. (1977). Assessing the clinical importance of behavior change through social validation. *Behavior Modification, 1,* 427–452.

Kazdin, A.E. (1980). Acceptability of alternate treatments for deviant child behavior. *Journal of Applied Behavior Analysis, 13,* 259–273.

Kazdin, A.E. (1981). Acceptability of child treatment techniques: The influence of treatment efficacy and adverse side effects. *Behavior Therapy, 12*, 493–506.

Kelley, M.L., Embry, L.H., & Baer, D.M. (1979). Skills for child management and family support: Training parents for maintenance. *Behavior Modification, 3*, 373–396.

Kirscht, J.P., Haefner, D., Kegeles S., & Rosenstock, I. (1966). A national study of health beliefs. *Journal of Health and Human Behavior, 7*, 248–254.

Kluger, M.P., & Karras, A. (1983). Strategies for reducing missed initial appointments in a community mental health center. *Community Mental Health Journal, 19*(2), 137–143.

Koegel, R.L., Glahn, R.J., & Neiminen, G.S. (1978). Generalization of parent training results. *Journal of Applied Behavior Analysis, 11*, 95–109.

Koegel, R.L., Russo, D.C., & Rincover, A. (1977). Assessing and training teachers in the use of behavior modification with autistic children. *Journal of Applied Behavior Analysis, 10*, 197–205.

Komaki, J. (1977). Using behavioral self-control strategies in the training of beginning counseling skills. *Behavior therapy, 8*, 99–101.

Korsch, B.M., & Negrete, V.F. (1972). Doctor-patient communication. *Scientific American, 227*, 66–74.

Larsen, D.L., Nguyen, T.D., Green, R.S., & Attkisson, C.C. (1983). Enhancing the utilization of outpatient mental health services. *Community Mental Health Journal, 19*(4), 305–320.

Latiolais, C.J., & Berry, C.C. (1969). Misuse of prescription medications by outpatients. *Drug Intelligence & Clinical Pharmacy, 3*, 270–277.

Lebow, J. (1982). Consumer satisfaction with mental health treatment. *Psychological Bulletin, 91*, 244–259.

Leistyna, J.A., & Macaulay, J.C. (1966). Therapy of streptococcal infections. Do pediatric patients receive prescribed oral medication? *American Journal of Diseases of Children, 3*, 22–26.

Lima, J., Nazarian, L., Charney, E., & Lahti, C. (1976). Compliance with short-term antimicrobial therapy: Some techniques that help. *Pediatrics, 57*(3), 383–386.

Linkewich, J.A., Catalano, R.B., & Flack, H.L. (1974). The effect of packaging and instruction on outpatient compliance with medication regimens. *Drug Intelligence & Clinical Pharmacy, 8*, 10–15.

Litt, I.F., & Cuskey, W.R. (1980). Compliance with medical regimens during adolescence. *Pediatric Clinics of North America, 27*:2, 3–15.

Litt, I.F., & Cuskey, W.R. (1984). Satisfaction with health care: A predictor of adolescents' appointment keeping. *Journal of Adolescent Health Care, 5*(3), 196–200.

Loeber, R., & Weisman, R.G. (1975). Contingencies of therapist and trainer performance: A review. *Psychological Bulletin, 82*, 660–688.

Lowe, K., & Lutzker, J.R. (1979). Increasing compliance to a medical regimen with a juvenile diabetic. *Behavior Therapy, 10*, 57–64.

MacDonald, M.E., Hagberg, K.L., & Grossman, B.J. (1963). Social factors in relation to participation in follow-up care of rheumatic fever. *Journal of Pediatrics, 62*, 503–513.

Marston, M. (1970). Compliance with medical regimens: A review of the literature. *Nursing Research, 19*, 312–323.

Mathews, R.M., & Fawcett, S.B. (1979). Assessing dissemination capability: An evaluation of an exportable training package. *Behavior Modification, 3*, 49–62.

Mattar, M.E., Markello, J., & Yaffe, S.J. (1975). Pharmaceutic factors affecting pediatric compliance. *Pediatrics, 55* (1), 101–108.

McMahon, R.J., & Forehand, R.L. (1978). Nonprescription behavior therapy: Effectiveness of a brochure in teaching mothers to correct their children's inappropriate mealtime behaviors. *Behavior Therapy, 9*, 814–820.

McMahon, R.J., & Forehand, R.L., (1980). Self-help behavior therapies in parent training. In B.B. Lahey & A.E. Kazdin (Eds.). *Advances in clinical child psychology* (Vol. 3). New York: Plenum.

McMahon, R.J., & Forehand, R.L. (1983). Consumer satisfaction in behavioral treatment of children: Types, issues, and recommendations. *Behavior Therapy, 14,* 209–225.

McMahon, R.J., Forehand, R.L., & Griest, D.L. (1981). Effects of knowledge of social learning principles on enhancing treatment outcome and generalization in a parent training program. *Journal of Consulting and Clinical Psychology, 49,* 526–532.

McMahon, R.J., Forehand, R.L., & Griest, D.L. (1982). Parent behavioral training to modify child noncompliance: Factors in generalization and maintenance. In R.B. Stuart (Ed.), *Adherence, compliance, and generalization in behavioral medicine* (pp. 213–238). New York: Brunner/Mazel.

Meyers, A.W., Thackwray, D.E., Johnson, C.B., & Schleser, R. (1983). A comparison of prompting strategies for improving appointment compliance of hypertensive individuals. *Behavior Therapy, 14,* 267–274.

Mindlin, R.L., & Densen, P.M. (1971). Medical care of urban infants: Health supervision. *American Journal of Public Health, 61,* 687–697.

Mitchell, J.H. (1974). Compliance with medical regimens: An annotated bibliography. *Health Education Monographs, 2,* 75–87.

Montegar, C.A., Reid, D.H., Madsen, C.H., & Ewell, M.D. (1977). Increasing institutional staff-to-resident interactions through in-service training and supervisor approval. *Behavior Therapy, 8,* 533–540.

Moreland, J.R., Schwebel, A.I., Beck, S., & Wells, R. (1982). Parents as therapists: A review of the behavior therapy parent training literature—1975 to 1981. *Behavior Modification, 6,* 250–276.

Morse, D.L., Coulter, M.P. ,Nazarian, L.P., & Napadono, R.J. (1981). Waning effectiveness of mailed reminders on reducing broken appointments. *Pediatrics, 68,* 846–849.

Moser, M., Rafter, J., & Gajewski, J. (1984). Insurance premium reductions: A motivating factor in long-term hypertensive treatment. *Journal of the American Medical Association, 251*(6), 756–757.

Moulding, R., Onsted, G.D., & Sbarbaro, J.A. (1970). Supervision of outpatient drug therapy with the medication monitor. *Annals of Internal Medicine, 73,* 559–564.

Mushlin, A.I., & Appel, F.A. (1977). Diagnosing potential noncompliance: Physicians' ability in a behavioral dimension of medical care. *Archives of Internal Medicine, 137,* 318–321.

Nay, W.R. (1975). A systematic comparison of instructional techniques for parents. *Behavior Therapy, 6,* 14–21.

Nazarian, L.F., Mechaber, J., Charney, E., & Coulter, M.P. (1974). Effects of a mailed appointment reminder on appointment keeping. *Pediatrics, 53,* 349–352.

Nelson, R.O. (1977a). Assessment and therapeutic functions of self-monitoring. In M. Hersen, R.M. Eisler, & P.M. Miller (Eds.), *Progress in behavior modification* (Vol. 5). New York: Academic.

Nelson, R.O. (1977b). Methodological issues in assessment via self-monitoring. In J.D. Cone & R.P. Hawkins (Eds.), *Behavioral assessment: New directions in clinical psychology* (pp. 217–240). New York: Brunner/Mazel.

Norell, S.E. (1979). Improving medication compliance: A randomized clinical trial. *British Medical Journal, 2,* 1031–1033.

O'Dell, S. (1974). Training parents in behavior modification: A review. *Psychological Bulletin, 81,* 418–433.

O'Dell, S.,Flynn, J., & Benlolo, L. (1977). A comparison of parent training techniques in child behavior modification. *Journal of Behavior Therapy and Experimental Psychiatry, 8,* 261–268.

O'Dell, S.L., Mahoney, N.D., Horton, W.G., & Turner, P.E. (1979). Media-assisted parent training: Alternative models. *Behavior Therapy, 10,* 103–110.

Ossip-Klein, D.J., Vanlandingham, W., Prue, D.M., & Rychtarik, R.G. (1984). Increasing attendance at alcohol aftercare using calendar prompts and home based contracting. *Addictive Behaviors, 9*(1), 85–89.

Park, L.C., & Lipman, R.S. (1964). A comparison of patient dosage deviation reports with pill counts. *Psychopharmacologia, 6,* 299–302.

Parkin, D.M., Henney, C.R., Quirk, J., & Crooks, J. (1976). Deviation from prescribed drug treatment after discharge from hospital. *British Medical Journal, 2,* 686–688.

Parrish, J.M., Charlop, M.H., & Fenton, L.R. (in press). Use of a stated waiting list contingency and reward opportunity to increase appointment keeping in an outpatient pediatric psychology clinic. *Journal of Pediatric Psychology.*

Patterson, E.T., Griffin, J.C., & Panyan, M.C. (1976). Incentive maintenance program for nonprofessional personnel. *Journal of Behavior Therapy and Experimental Psychiatry, 7,* 249–253.

Peed, S., Roberts, M., & Forehand, R. (1977). Evaluation of the effectiveness of a standardized parent training program in altering the interaction of mothers and their noncompliant children. *Behavior Modification, 1,* 323–350.

Peterson, G.M., McLean, S., & Millingen, K.S. (1984). A randomized trial of strategies to improve patient compliance with anticonvulsant therapy. *Epilepsia, 25*(4), 412–417.

Podell, R.N. (1975). *Physician's guide to compliance in hypertension.* West Point, PA: Merck.

Porter, A.M. (1969). Drug defaulting in a general practice. *British Medical Journal, 1,* 218–222.

Rapoff, M.A., & Christophersen, E.R. (1982). Compliance of pediatric patients with medical regimens. In R.B. Stuart (Ed.), *Adherence, compliance, and generalization in behavioral medicine* (pp. 79–124). New York: Brunner/Mazel.

Rapoff, M.A., Lindsley, C.B., & Christophersen, E.R. (1984). Improving compliance with medical regimens: A case study with juvenile rheumatoid arthritis. *Archives of Physical Medicine and Rehabilitation, 65*(5), 267–269.

Reiss, M.L., & Bailey, J.S. (1982). Visiting the dentist: A behavioral community analysis of participation in a dental health screening and referral program. *Journal of Applied Behavior Analysis, 15,* 353–362.

Reiss, M.L., Piotrowski, W.D., & Bailey, J.S. (1976). Behavioral community psychology: Encouraging low income parents to seek dental care for their children. *Journal of Applied Behavior Analysis, 9,* 387–397.

Resnick, L.B., Wang, M.C., & Kaplan, J. (1973). Task analysis in curriculum design: A hierarchically sequenced introductory mathematics curriculum. *Journal of Applied Behavior Analysis, 6,* 679–710.

Rice, J.M., & Lutzker, J.R. (1984). Reducing noncompliance to follow-up appointment keeping at a family practice center. *Journal of Applied Behavior Analysis, 17,* 303–311.

Rockart, J.F., & Hofmann, P.B. (1969). Physician and patient behavior under different scheduling systems in a hospital outpatient department. *Medical Care, 7,* 463–470.

Rosenstock, I.M. (1974). Historical origins of the health belief model. *Health Education Monographs, 2,* 328–335.

Roth, H.P., & Caron, H.S. (1978). Accuracy of doctors' estimates and patients' statements on adherence to a drug regimen. *Clinical Pharmacology and Therapeutics, 23,* 361–370.

Roth, H.P., Caron, H.S., & Hsi, B.P. (1971). Measuring intake of a prescribed medication: A bottle count and a tracer technique compared. *Clinical Pharmacology Therapy, 2,* 228–237.

Sackett, D.L. (1976). The magnitude of compliance and noncompliance. In D.L. Sackett & R.B. Haynes (Eds.), *Compliance with therapeutic regimens* (pp. 9–25). Baltimore: Johns Hopkins University Press.

Sackett, D.L. (1979). A compliance practicum for the busy practitioner. In R.B. Haynes, D.W. Taylor, & D.L. Sackett (Eds.), *Compliance in health care* (pp. 286–294). Baltimore: Johns Hopkins University Press.

Sackett, D.L., & Haynes, R.B. (1976). *Compliance with therapeutic regimens.* Baltimore: Johns Hopkins University Press.

Sackett, D.L., & Snow, J.C. (1979). The magnitude of compliance and noncompliance. In R.B. Haynes, D.W. Taylor, & D.L. Sackett (Eds.), *Compliance in health care* (pp. 11–22). Baltimore: Johns Hopkins University Press.

Sanders, M.R., & Glynn, T. (1981). Training parents in behavioral self-management: An analysis of generalization and maintenance. *Journal of Applied Behavior Analysis, 14,* 223–237.

Sanson-Fisher, R.W., Seymour, F.W., & Baer, D.M. (1976). Training institutional staff to alter delinquents' conversation. *Journal of Behavior Therapy and Experimental Psychiatry, 7,* 243–247.

Schinke, S.P. (1979). Staff training in group homes: A family approach. In L.A. Hamerlynck (Ed.), *Behavioral systems for the developmentally disabled* (Vol. 2). New York: Brunner/Mazel.

Schroeder, S.A. (1973). Lowering broken appointment rates at a medical clinic. *Medical Care, 11,* 75–78.

Sepler, J.J., & Myers, S.L. (1978). The effectiveness of verbal instruction on teaching behavior modification skills to nonprofessionals. *Journal of Applied Behavior Analysis, 11,* 198.

Shepard, D.S., & Moseley, T.A. (1976). Mailed versus telephoned appointment reminders to reduce broken appointments in a hospital outpatient department. *Medical Care, 14,* 268–273.

Smiley, J., Byres, S., & Roberts, D.E. (1972). Maternal and infant health and their associated factors in an inner city population. *American Journal of Public Health, 62,* 476–482.

Smith, S.D., Rosen, D., Trueworthy, R.C., & Lowman, J.T. (1979). A reliable method for evaluating drug compliance in children with cancer. *Cancer, 43* (1), 169–173.

Smith, N.A., Seale, J.P., & Shaw, J. (1984). Medication compliance in children with asthma. *Australian Journal of Paediatrics, 20(1),* 47–51.

Stern, M.R., & Golden, F. (1977). A partial evaluation of an introductory training program in behavior modification for psychiatric nurses. *American Journal of Community Psychology, 5,* 23–32.

Stokes, T.F., & Baer, D.M. (1977). An implicit technology of generalization. *Journal of Applied Behavior Analysis, 10,* 349–367.

Stuart, R.B. (Ed.) (1982). *Adherence, compliance, and generalization in behavioral medicine.* New York: Brunner/Mazel.

Svarstad, B.L. (1974). Physician-patient communication and patient conformity with medical advice. In D. Mechanic, (Ed.), *The growth of bureaucratic medicine* (pp. 220–235). New York: Wiley.

Turner, A.J., & Vernon, J.C. (1976). Prompts to increase attendance in a community mental health center. *Journal of Applied Behavior Analysis, 9,* 141–145.

Twardosz, S., Cataldo, M.F., & Risley, T.R. (1974). An open environment design for infant and toddler day care. *Journal of Applied Behavior Analysis, 7,* 529–546.

Vessel, E.S. (1974). Factors causing interindividual variations of drug concentrations in blood. *Clinical Pharmacology and Therapy, 16,* 135–148.

Wahler, R.G. (1980). The insular mother: Her problems in parent-child treatment. *Journal of Applied Behavior Analysis, 13,* 207–219.

Wahler, R.G., & Graves, M.G. (1983). Setting events in social networks: Ally or enemy in child behavior therapy. *Behavior Therapy, 14,* 19–36.

Webb, K.L., Dobson, A.J., O'Connell, D.L., Tupling, H.E., Harris, G.W., Moxon, J.A., Sulway, M.J., & Leeder, S.R. (1984). Dietary compliance among insulin-dependent diabetics. *Journal of Chronic Diseases, 37(8)*, 633–643.

Webster-Stratton, C. (1981a). Videotape modeling: A method of parent education. *Journal of Clinical Child Psychology, 10,* 93–98.

Webster-Stratton, C. (1981b). Modification of mothers' behaviors and attitudes through a videotape modeling group discussion program. *Behavior Therapy, 12,* 634–642.

Webster-Stratton, C. (1982). The long-term effects of a videotape modeling parent-training program: Comparison of immediate and 1-year follow-up results. *Behavior Therapy, 13,* 702–714.

Weintraub, M., Au, W., & Lasagna, L. (1973). Compliance as a determinant of serum digoxin concentration. *Journal of the American Medical Association, 224,* 481–485.

Willner, A.G., Braukmann, C.J., Kirigin, D.A., Fixsen, D.L., Phillips, E.L., & Wolf, M.M. (1977). The training and validation of youth preferred social behaviors of child-care personnel. *Journal of Applied Behavior Analysis, 10,* 219–230.

Wolf, M.M. (1978). Social validity: The case for subjective measurement or how applied behavior analysis is finding its heart. *Journal of Applied Behavior Analysis, 11,* 203–214.

Wood, H.F., Feinstein, A.R., Taranta, A., Epstein, J.A., & Simpson, R. (1964). Rheumatic fever in children and adolescents: A long-term epidemiologic study of subsequent prophylaxis, streptococcal infections, and clinical sequelae. Part III. Comparative effectiveness of three prophylaxis regimens in preventing streptococcal infections and rheumatic recurrences. *Annals of Internal Medicine, 60(2),* 31–46, supp.

Yokley, J.M., & Glenwick, D.S. (1984). Increasing the immunization of preschool children: An evaluation of applied community interventions. *Journal of Applied Behavior Analysis, 17,* 313–325.

Zifferblatt, S.M. (1975). Increasing patient compliance through the applied analysis of behavior. *Preventive Medicine, 4,* 173–182.

21

Long-term Adherence to Health Care Regimens in Pediatric Chronic Disorders

JAMES W. VARNI AND LINA BABANI

Present trends in research and clinical practice suggest that the role of health-related behaviors in the prevention, development, maintenance, and/or exacerbation of disease is increasingly being recognized in pediatrics. With advances in biomedical science and technology, much of the threat of acute or infectious disease has been eliminated. As acute and infectious diseases have become more preventable and more easily treated, the focus of clinical research and practice has shifted toward the prevention and management of chronic disorders (Russo & Varni, 1982) and related behavioral and psychosocial factors (Nader, Ray, & Brink, 1981; Starfield, 1982; Sumpter, 1980). Consequently, pediatric practice is gradually moving from a focus on acute, infectious diseases, for which medical treatment is of singular importance, to chronic diseases, disorders, and problems, in which somatic factors represent only one component of comprehensive care (Varni, 1983).

502

With this shift towards disorders for which chronic symptomatic management, rather than cure, represents a primary focus of treatment, issues concerned with health care behaviors, coping, life quality, and optimal functional independence become key concerns. As a result of this emphasis on the interrelationship between health-related behaviors and chronic disease prevention and management, the child and his or her family become increasingly more instrumental in the health care system. Issues concerned with long-term adherence to therapeutic regimens, parent-child interactions, peers/siblings, and clinician-parent-child interactions become highly relevant, particularly in complex and long-term interventions. Simply prescribing a medical or exercise regimen is not a sufficient condition to assure the implementation of the regimen; behavioral and psychosocial factors may prevent or impede the therapy process. Attention to the biomedical, biobehavioral, and psychosocial dimensions inherent in chronic disease prevention and management requires integrated input from the various disciplines specializing in these areas, preferably within the interdisciplinary biobehavioral health team model (Varni, 1983).

The concept of the health team model of care has been proposed as the means by which prevention, diagnosis, treatment, habilitation, and rehabilitation might be provided in a coordinated, comprehensive manner by specialists representing several disciplines (Halstead, 1976). Comprehensive care of the patient within the health team model requires consideration of the biomedical, biobehavioral, and psychosocial factors which might influence the patient's health status. The ideal format for the health team model involves an interdisciplinary, integrated approach to patient care (Rothberg, 1981; Varni, 1983). Awareness of the difference between an interdisciplinary and a multidisciplinary approach is essential to optimal health care delivery (Melvin, 1980). The multidisciplinary approach entails the involvement of professionals from a number of disciplines and approaches the patient primarily in an uncoordinated, discipline-specific fashion. This approach requires that each professional only know the skills specific to their own discipline. In contrast, the interdisciplinary approach requires that physicians, nurses, physical therapists, psychologists, and other health care professionals have a working knowledge of the skills and specialties of the other team members. Thus the interdisciplinary approach is synergistic, integrating the knowledge and skills from the various disciplines into a coordinated plan for patient care. Particularly in pediatric chronic disorders for which the medical treatment is but one component of comprehensive care, the child's and parent's active involvement in the day-to-day management of the chronic condition is essential, and requires integrated interdisciplinary team planning.

Although the total prevalence of chronically ill and handicapped children has been estimated at more than 10 percent (Pless & Douglas, 1971), many pediatric chronic disorders have a low incidence. However, the impact of these disorders is not accurately reflected in their incidence, since their chronicity imposes a disproportionately greater strain on the patient and families, and on medical resources and society (Holroyd & Guthrie, 1979; Meenan, Yelin, Nevitt, & Epstein, 1981; Zwagg, Mason, Joyner, & Runyan, 1980). In 1976 alone, 31 million school days were lost secondary to a chronic disease or disability (Department of Health, Education and Welfare, 1979).

Although biologically very diverse, pediatric chronic disorders have in common the features of significant duration and potential long-term and significant impact on the daily lives of the children and their families (Gortmaker & Sapenfield, 1984; Pless, 1984; Stein & Jessop, 1982). The potential disruptions in school attendance, academic achievement, social relationships, lifestyle, and personal and financial costs necessitate ongoing coping/adaptation and long-term adjustment on the part of the child and his or her family (Drotar, 1981; Masters, Cerreto, & Mendlowitz, 1983; Varni & Jay, 1984). In pediatric chronic disorders, a family-oriented approach is now advocated (McAndrew, 1976; Murphy, 1982; Stein & Riessman, 1980). The literature suggests that the siblings of chronically ill and handicapped children may be at risk for psychosocial adjustment problems (Breslau, 1983; Breslau, Weitzman, & Messenger, 1981; Ferrari, 1984; Lavigne & Ryan, 1979). Maternal psychosocial distress (depression, anxiety) and marital discord have been suggested as additional variables in the psychosocial adjustment of children and their management (Breslau, Staruch, & Mortimer, 1982; Friedrich, 1979; Griest, Forehand, Wells, & McMahon, 1980; Porter & O'Leary, 1980; Sabbeth & Leventhal, 1984). In addition the successful mainstreaming of chronically ill and handicapped school-aged children may depend on their social competence skills and social acceptance (Gresham, 1982; O'Moore, 1980). Although most families with chronically ill and handicapped children receive traditional biomedical care, gaps in and barriers to psychosocial and behavioral management services continue to exist (Stein, Jessop, & Reissman, 1983), and may result in parent dissatisfaction and noncompliance with the medical regimen (Lau, Williams, Williams, Ware, & Brook, 1982).

Given that the difficulties of chronically ill and handicapped children and their families are similar regardless of the cause of the disability (Stein & Jessop, 1982), interdisciplinary biobehavioral strategies may be designed which can in many ways be generalized across different pediatric chronic disorders; for example, therapeutic adherence, behavioral parent training, child self-management training, and health care staff behavior training (Varni, 1983).

Pediatric chronic care requires multiple and comprehensive assessment and management over long periods of time, routine long-term follow-up, and ongoing family involvement. Adherence to therapeutic regimens in pediatric chronic disorders encompass a broad spectrum of health-related behaviors, including correct consumption of prescribed medications, clinic appointment attendance, appropriate eating, exercise, and diet patterns, correct performance of home-based therapeutic regimens (e.g., factor replacement therapy in hemophilia), and avoidance of health risk behaviors such as smoking, and drug and alcohol abuse. Improving adherence to therapeutic regimens may produce as great an impact upon disability and death as the development of new biomedical treatment techniques, and may result in greater cost effectiveness in the provision of health care services. Patient noncompliance with prescribed therapeutic regimens seriously undermines the effectiveness of therapy in preventive, curative, and management situations and results in unnecessary morbidity, mortality, and cost. For instance, the effectiveness of a treatment program may be misjudged, with undetected noncompliance leading to unnecessary diagnostic tests, alternative treatments, increased or additional medications, and eventually hospitalization.

The most important determinants of noncompliance have consistently been found to be the complexity and duration of the treatment regimens (Dunbar & Agras, 1980). Although age, gender, personality, health care professional/patient relationship, health beliefs, socioeconomic status, community support systems, clinic structure, and attitude have been investigated as determinants of noncompliance (Anderson & Kirk, 1982; Eraker, Kirscht, & Becker, 1984; Friedman & DiMatteo, 1982; Jones, 1983), this chapter will focus only on the following three modifiable dimensions: (1) the patient education instructional method, (2) the therapeutic regimen implementation, and (3) the functional analysis of the antecedents and consequences of adherence and noncompliance (Varni, 1983). Hemophilia, juvenile diabetes, and spina bifida have been selected as exemplary disorders to illustrate the application of these three dimensions.

HEMOPHILIA

A major breakthrough in the management of hemophilia occurred in the early 1960s with the discovery and separation of the essential clotting factors from the plasma of normal blood (Buchanan, 1980). Freeze-dried plasma concentrates of the clotting factor proteins obtained from a pooled source of multiple donors can easily be reconstituted with sterile water and injected intravenously. The intravenous infusion of the missing clotting factor temporarily corrects the clotting status and allows a functional blood clot to form (Dietrich, 1976).

The recognition of the advantages of prompt factor replacement therapy for each bleeding episode on functional independence has served as a stimulus for the creation of the hemophilia home care program (also called supervised self treatment) in an attempt to minimize or prevent the crippling effects of internal hemorrhaging, such as hemophilic arthropathy, chronic arthritic pain in the joints, and restriction of mobility (Dietrich, Luck, & Martinson, 1982; Guenthner, Hilgartner, Miller, & Vienne, 1980; Varni,

1981a,b; Varni & Gilbert, 1982; Varni, Gilbert, & Dietrich, 1981). The home care program, which has been adopted nationally through hemophilia comprehensive care centers, facilitates the prompt administration of factor concentrate at home when a bleeding episide begins, potentially resulting in earlier recovery of joint function, greater self-sufficiency for the patient and family, fewer absences from school or work, and a decrease in the cost of treatment (Kaufert, 1980; Lazerson, 1972; Levine & Britten, 1973; Sergis & Hilgartner, 1972; Smith, Keyes, & Forman, 1982). The home care program consists of teaching the hemophiliac, the parents, and other family members the techniques necessary for the administration of factor replacement products. Since the life expectancy of patients with severe hemophilia is now that of the general male population (Ikkala et al., 1982), the issue of long-term adherence to correct factor replacement therapy techniques has become increasingly important (Varni & Wallander, in press). If proper adherence to factor replacement procedures and sterile technique is not followed during the reconstitution, administration, and disposal process, then the following problems may result and adversely affect the patient and family: loss of potency of the factor concentrate, infection, damage to the veins selected for venipuncture, and spread of hepatitis to family members.

Sergis-Deavenport and Varni (1982, 1983) investigated the effectiveness of behavioral techniques and instructional strategies in increasing parental adherence to factor replacement therapy. The instructional strategies included providing the information in incremental quantities over time, organizing the information into specific categories, and combining verbal and written instructions. The behavioral techniques consisted of the modeling of correct factor replacement procedures by the pediatric nurse practitioner, with the parent of a hemophilic child observing these modeled behaviors (observational learning). The parent's behavioral rehearsal of the observed techniques were recorded on a reliable and valid behavior checklist of factor replacement procedures. This assessment instrument was designed to represent standard content for factor replacement therapy, and consisted of the behaviors considered essential for the safe administration of concentrate to maintain asceptic technique and minimize the spread of hepatitis and damage to the veins.

Three classifications of factor replacement were delineated: (1) reconstitution consisted of 20 behaviors; (2) syringe preparation consisted of 20 behaviors; and (3) infusion consisted of 36 behaviors. The parent's behavioral responses on each task performed were recorded on an occurrence/nonoccurrence basis on the behavior checklist, with proper sequencing required for the correct responding of certain behaviors. Specific criteria were required before learning each subsequent classification within a multiple-baseline across factor replacement behaviors design (Sergis-Deavenport & Varni, 1982). In addition to a treatment group of parents who received factor replacement training for the first time, a comparison group of parents who had been on the home care program for an average of 5 years was also tested on the behavior checklist (Sergis-Deavenport & Varni, 1983). The performance of the treatment group increased from 15 percent during baseline to 92 percent by the end of the treatment condition, maintained at 97 percent correct adherence over a long-term follow-up assessment. In contrast the comparison group showed only 65 percent correct adherence when tested. These initial findings demonstrate the necessity and the potential of these techniques in improving long-term adherence to a complex treatment regimen for this pediatric chronic disorder. Recently this methodology has been developed into a self-management training program for teaching and maintaining long-term adherence to proper factor replacement techniques by children with hemophilia (Gilbert & Varni, 1985).

For most hemophiliacs, repeated hemorrhages into the joint areas result in the development of a pathophysiological condition similar to osteoarthritis, marked by articular cartilage destruction, pathological bone formation, chronic arthritic pain, and impaired function (Arnold & Hilgartner, 1977; Pettersson, Ahlbert, & Nilsson, 1980; Varni, 1981a,b), with progressive hemophilic arthropathy evident even with appropriate factor replacement therapy (Guenthner et al., 1980; Helske, Ikkala, Myllyla, Nevanlinna, & Rasi, 1982; Soreff & Blomback, 1980). The knees, elbows, and ankles are the joint sites most commonly involved (Aronstam, Rainsford, & Painter, 1979; Helske et al., 1982).

Although intensive physical therapy has been suggested as an essential rehabilitation modality in hemophilia comprehensive care (Boone, 1975; Koch, Cohen, Luban, & Eng, 1982; Weisman, 1977), children with hemophilia have been found to demonstrate poor exercise performance when compared to normal standards, possibly as a result of lack of physical conditioning (Koch, Galioto, Kelleher, & Goldstein, 1984). The potential benefits of regular therapeutic exercise by children with hemophilia include enhanced psychological and functional status, and may even have a positive influence on coagulation parameters (Koch et al., 1984). However, even with these potential benefits, Greene and Strickler (1983) found that adherence to even a simple daily modified isokinetic exercise regimen was extremely low in a six-month study of thirty-two patients with homophilia (mean age = 20.8 years, range 7-51 years). During the six-month treatment period, 37.5 percent of the patients exercised for less than 60 days, 31.25 percent for 60 to 100 days, and 31.25 percent for longer than 100 days. Thus, only 31.25 percent of these patients adhered to the daily regimen for even 100 days out of the total six-month treatment period.

While adherence to therapeutic exercise as a component in treatment programs for cardiovascular risk modification, obesity, and diabetes in adults has received increasing attention (Dishman, 1982; Martin & Dubbert, 1982), adherence to therapeutic exercise in children has not been widely investigated, and has been typically studied as only one component of a pediatric weight control intervention (Epstein, Wing, Koeske, Ossip, & Beck, 1982; Killam, Apodaca, Manella, & Varni, 1983).

Greenan, Powell, and Varni (1985) studied the relationship between long-term adherence to therapeutic exercise by hemophilic children and their functional independence within both a preventive and rehabilitative approach to musculoskeletal disability in these children. Greenan et al. (1985) conducted a 12-session group behavioral physical therapy program for ten children with hemophilia (ages 8 to 15). The children were instructed in therapeutic exercises such as swimming and water polo, which provide optimal musculoskeletal conditioning without potentiating a joint or muscle bleed. They were also instructed in a strengthening regimen, which involved modified and individualized progressive weights. The musculoskeletal status of the knees, elbows, and ankles were obtained with an isokinetic instrument (Cybex II exerciser-dynamometer). This instrument measures strength in foot pound torque. Ambulation, school attendance, hospitalizations, pain, bleeding frequency, and factor replacement units prescribed were measured. A contingency contract was developed and signed by the children, their parents, and the physical therapists, and was periodically renegotiated. The contingency contract specified the behaviors required of each party, and the reciprocal consequences for each behavior. Thus the contingency contract provided a clear, written specification of the target health-related behaviors and the negotiated contingencies which would be available for their performance (Varni, 1983). Designated points were given for adherence and exchanged for reinforcers within a token exchange system. Adherence parameters included the percent of the correct performance of the prescribed therapeutic exercises, the percent of the self-monitoring forms completed by the children and returned, the percent of the parents' initialling of the children's self-monitoring data sheets, and the percent of the sessions attended. Working under the hypothesis that therapeutic exercise can become a habit response or life-style pattern over time, Greenan et al. (1985) initially programmed very powerful reinforcers for the children to earn during the early phases of the program, thus attempting to *prevent* noncompliance from becoming a significant problem. Thus the study was conducted under the model that noncompliance to complex and long-term regimens in pediatric chronic disorders may be expected to occur without systematic behavioral intervention, and the aim was to prevent, or at least greatly reduce, its occurrence. The initial six-month follow-up data demonstrated substantial adherence on all the parameters, with overall therpeutic adherence averaging 81 percent.

JUVENILE DIABETES

The successful management of insulin-dependent diabetes mellitus (IDDM) requires strict adherence by the pediatric patient and his or her parents to a long-term and complex regimen, consisting of insulin injections, collection of urine and/or serum specimens, specific diet behaviors, exercise, and hygiene behaviors. As reviewed by Simonds (1979), studies of children's and adolescents' adherence to the diabetes regimen indicate that noncompliance is a pervasive and serious problem. The complexity and the life-long duration of the regimen provide many occasions for noncompliance, such as giving insulin injections at wrong or irregular time intervals, skipping prescribed snack intervals, not regularly and systematically testing urine/serum specimens, not appropriately adjusting insulin dose and diet during changes in activity level, and not checking and cleaning feet on a regular basis (Varni, 1983).

In a review of the literature, Surwit, Scovern, and Feinglos (1982) confirm the high incidence of noncompliance with diabetic regimens. They suggest that a lack of clear intrinsic consequences in achieving adequate metabolic control plays an important role in the difficulty of maintaining compliance. While a state of hypoglycemia will almost immediately be noticed by the patient because of the aversive autonomic reaction it creates, symptoms of hyperglycemia are noticeable only when blood glucose levels reach extremely high levels. Thus the young diabetic patient may choose to err on the side of hyperglycemia, in an attempt to avoid the immediate aversive symptoms of hypoglycemia.

Lowe and Lutzker (1979) described a therapeutic adherence program incorporating parental home monitoring and contingency management procedures with a 9-year-old child with IDDM. Three behaviors were selected for intervention: adherence to foot care, diet, and urine testing. Adherence was calculated by dividing the number of times the child performed the required behaviors by the total number of prescribed behaviors required to be completed for the day. Within a multiple-baseline across behaviors design, the token exchange point system which was implemented for adherence was highly effective in enhancing therapeutic adherence by this child.

Accurate patient self-monitoring of urine glucose and/or blood glucose concentrations is an essential component of an overall diabetes self-management regimen (Tattersall & Gale, 1981). Several studies have investigated adherence to the self-monitoring of glucose levels by insulin-dependent diabetics. Epstein et al. (1981) designed a study to decrease the amount of urine glucose in insulin-dependent diabetic children by regulating eating and exercise behaviors and adjusting insulin dosage through a combination of self-management training for the children and behavioral parent training. Within a multiple-baseline across groups design, the intervention for 19 families included instructions in insulin adjustment, decrease in intake of simple sugars and saturated fats, an increase in exercise, self-monitoring of urine glucose, and a point system for the children's self-management behaviors. The results of the study indicated a significant increase in the percent of negative urine glucose tests. However, the findings on the parameters of metabolic control were equivocal. A study by Schafer, Glasgow, and McCaul (1982) with three diabetic adolescents utilized an approach similar to Epstein's et al. (1981), but demonstrated better metabolic control.

The equivocal metabolic control findings by Epstein et al. (1981) may be partially explained by the urine testing procedure. Urine testing has been found to have a relatively poor correlation with blood glucose levels and is a relatively poor prior warning system of potential hypoglycemia (Tattersall & Gale, 1981). More recent developments in biomedical science and technology have now made home self-monitoring of blood glucose levels possible, with patients obtaining their blood samples using a spring-loaded finger lancer and measuring their blood glucose concentrations either by reagent-impregnated strips of filter paper alone or in conjunction with a reflectance meter (Geffner, Kaplan, Lippe, & Scott, 1983; Miller, Stratton, & Tripp, 1983; Schiffrin, Desrosiers, & Belmont, 1983; Tamborlane & Sherwin, 1983). A more recent behavioral study on therapeutic adherence incorporated the self-monitoring of blood glucose levels in the diabetic regimen. Carney, Schechter, and Davis (1983) utilized a multiple-baseline across subjects design for three children with diabetes. The intervention consisted of contingent praise by the parents, and a point system in which points were awarded for the self-monitoring of blood glucose levels at designated times during each day. Self-monitoring of blood glucose levels increased for all three children, and was accompanied by improvements in metabolic control measures.

One of the most important components in the treatment of diabetes is the dietary regimen. The dietary regimen recommended by the American Diabetes Association (1979) is widely used and consists of five to six meals per day, a fixed schedule for meals, well balanced meals (in terms of carbohydrates, fat, and protein), and a fixed amount of daily caloric consumption. It is generally believed that long-term adherence to the dietary regimen will have a positive effect in achievement of metabolic control in children with IDDM (Arky, 1984). Nevertheless, there are no experimental studies conducted with children that can provide information as to the specific components in a dietary regimen that will enhance metabolic control. Thus there is much controversy in the literature in regards to the importance of recommending strict adherence to the dietary regimen (Nuttall, 1983; Wing, Epstein, Nowalk, & Hyg, 1984). In an assessment study of 97 insulin-dependent diabetics (age ranges 3 to 57, mean age 16.03), Christensen, Terry, Wyatt, Pichert, and Lorenz (1983) reported that only 10 percent of the sample was adherent to the complete dietary regimen. The dietary regimen was explained to the subject in terms of an exchange system, which facilitates quantitative assessment of dietary adherence. It was found that the subjects who were in good metabolic control were more compliant with regard to exchanges added or deleted and to total deviations of exchanges than were patients in poor metabolic control, and that adherence to the diet schedule and to the caloric intake recommended did not differ between patients in good and poor metabolic control.

Unquestionably, given the complexity of the knowledge needed for diabetes self-management (Johnson et al., 1982; Pennebaker et al., 1981), any study on therapeutic adherence must assess and implement a patient education phase to assure the patient's accurate understanding of the complex diabetic regimen. An education program with IDDM adults conducted by Webb et al. (1984) consisted of individual dietary recommendations, instruction in food composition and carbohydrate counting, problem-solving discussions, and suggestions in preparation of high-carbohydrate, low-fat meals. A six-month follow-up assessment revealed significant changes in compliance with dietary composition (from 13.9 percent to 38.9 percent), which was positively related to two measures of metabolic control (glycosylated hemoglobin and fasting blood glucose levels). These results are encouraging in that patient education can begin to improve adherence as well as metabolic control in diabetic adults; similar studies are needed with IDDM children in combination with specific child self-management training and behavioral parent training with the identification of the potential psychosocial and behavioral barriers to long-term therapeutic adherence (Schafer, Glasgow, McCaul, & Dreher, 1983).

SPINA BIFIDA

Spina bifida (myelomeningocele) is the most common congenital central nervous system defect in children. This chronic disorder is characterized by myelodysplasia and cystic distension of the meninges, with associated neurogenic deficits (for example, neurogenic incontinence) and lower extremity paralysis (Austin, Lindgren, & Dietrich, 1972; Shurtleff, 1980). The development of improved medical and surgical techniques has resulted in dramatically increased survival rates, with Dietrich (1979) reporting an 86 percent survival rate out of a total of 500 patients seen over a 16-year period. With such a high survival rate, opportunities now exist to focus on the habilitation and rehabilitation of associated chronic dysfunction in children with spina bifida (Akins, Davidson, & Hopkins, 1980; Morrissy, 1978; Varni & Wallander, in press).

As stated by Sumpter (1980), "Myelodysplasia is the prototype of the multiple-system disability, calling on the skills of a variety of medical professions, community agencies, and special educators. Unless there is a carefully planned convergence of these resources, care may be fragmented, and these various elements may at times find themselves working at cross-purposes." Such a multiple-system handicapped child population certainly requires a coordinated interdisciplinary health care team approach to comprehensive care (Varni, 1983).

In children and adolescents with spina bifida, marked developmental delays in self-help skills such as dressing, grooming, feeding, meal preparation and hygiene have been found, resulting in much longer periods of time to achieve functional independence (Sousa, Gordon, & Shurtleff, 1976). Recently behavioral parent training has been successfully utilized in teaching the parents of children with spina bifida the necessary behavioral techniques to increase the level of self-help skills in their children (Feldman, Manella, Apodaca, & Varni, 1982; Feldman, Manella, & Varni, 1983; Feldman & Varni, 1983). Behavioral programs have also been applied to promoting functional ambulation (Manella & Varni, 1981, 1984) and managing neurogenic incontinence (Jeffries, Killam, & Varni, 1982; Killam, Jeffries, & Varni, in press; Whitehead, Parker, Masek, Cataldo, & Freeman, 1981). Thus far, obesity and pressure sores have received specific empirical attention in terms of long-term therapeutic adherence.

Obesity has been well recognized as a chronic problem in myelomeningocele (Hayes-Allen, 1972; Hayes-Allen & Tring, 1973). Factors that may place these children at high risk for becoming overweight include a reduced energy expenditure secondary to relative inactivity. Even when the children begin walking with bracing and/or crutches, the combination of the greater expenditure of energy/effort and excessive weight often results in a gradual confinement to a wheelchair (Williams et al., 1983), which further increases the propensity toward obesity (Evans & Tew, 1983). An incidence study of obesity in children with myelomeningocele demonstrated that girls at each lesion level have a higher incidence of obesity than boys and that the more severely paralyzed boys and girls have a higher incidence of obesity than their less paralyzed peers (Shurtleff, Lamers, Goiney, & Gordon, 1982). Because of reduced energy expenditure and a lower body potassium content which affects the basal metabolic rate, these children may require a much lower caloric intake, perhaps even 50 percent less than that of children without myelomeningocele (Llenado & Grogan, 1978). In one clinic population, over 90 percent of the teenagers with myelomeningocele exceeded the 75th percentile (Rickard, Brady, & Gresham, 1977). In another clinic study, 60 percent of the children with myelomeningocele exceeded the 75th percentile, even though the caloric intake of 80 percent of the children was lower than the recommended levels for nonobese children of comparable chronological age (Farrel, Layton, Ford, & Tervo, 1981). For the child with myelomeningocele, obesity may cause additional problems; for example, ambulation becomes increasingly harder, orthopaedic surgeries are more difficult, scoliosis may be negatively affected, perineal hygiene and catheterization may be more difficult, and the potential for pressure sores is greater. The sum of these findings points to the importance of pediatric weight rehabilitation programs in myelomeningocele.

Killam et al. (1983) designed a weight control group program for children with myelomeningocele and their parents. At treatment initiation, the children averaged 52 percent overweight (range, 28 to 76 percent overweight). The children and their parents received specific instruction on selected aspects of eating, exercise and diet modification (see Varni, 1983, for a detailed description of the program). Nutritional instruction included discussions of the four basic food groups, servings required, nutrients available, and considerations of calorie value and cost. In order to further increase the children's awareness of the caloric densities of specific foods, foods were divided into red, yellow, and green groups, corresponding to high, medium, and low caloric density, respectively, and were explained in relationship to the colors of a traffic light. "Green" foods could be eaten freely, caution was required for "yellow" foods, and "red" foods signalled "stop!". Information regarding the effects of exercise and caloric expenditure upon weight management was presented, as well as individualized exercise techniques and group participation in adapted sports activities (for example, wheelchair track, tennis and racing, horseback riding).

The behavioral techniques emphasized included stimulus control, specific changes in eating behaviors, and reinforcement of the prescribed eating, exercise, and diet patterns. The stimulus control techniques focused on the management of the antecedents of eating behaviors. For example, the children were asked to separate eating from other activities (such as television viewing), and to eat only in one place at home and to schedule meals and snacks. Reinforcement of gradual changes in eating, exercise, and diet behaviors was emphasized rather than weight change per se.

To assess therapeutic adherence, data were compiled on the number of self-monitoring forms completed and returned in relation to the number assigned. In addition the number of treatment and follow-up sessions attended by each family was recorded. As a subjective measure of adherence, a questionnaire was administered during follow-up. This questionnaire described 21 eating, exercise, and diet behaviors related to weight control that had been introduced during the program (Varni, 1983). A final assessment tool used was a social validity questionnaire administered during follow-up. Two dimensions of social validity were addressed: social appropriateness (i.e., acceptability of the treatment procedures) and social importance (i.e., satisfaction with the results).

Although there was wide variability in the change in percent overweight, four of the five children evidenced a therapeutic effect, averaging a 13 percent overweight loss at the six-month follow-up. The measures of therapeutic adherence also showed wide differences among the children, with greatest adherence tending to be positively related to overweight loss. Finally, the measure of social validity was also positively related to overweight loss, with the larger social validity ratings associated with the larger percent overweight loss.

The impact of pressure sore lesions in terms of patient morbidity and habilitation/rehabilitation, and health care expenditures is considerable (Reuler & Cooney, 1981). Particularly in children and adolescents with spina bifida who are wheelchair bound, the potential for pressure-sore formation is an ongoing chronic problem, potentially resulting in long-term hospitalization and plastic surgery, further disruption of schooling, and poor psychosocial adaptation (e.g., peer relations).

Manella, Jeffries, and Varni (1985) designed an outpatient program to improve the health care behaviors of adolescents with spina bifida, targeting skin care, nutrition, general hygiene, and pressure relief through position change. The aim of the program was to teach health care behaviors which might prevent the occurrence or reoccurrence of pressure sores. The patients were instructed in the self-monitoring of wheelchair push-ups, and received points for wheelchair push-ups performed every 15 minutes. These points were then exchanged for reinforcers from an individually tailored reinforcement list. The adolescents also received points for other adherence behaviors, such as self-monitoring forms completed and returned, and session attendance.

Ten adolescents were initially identified for the treatment program. Of the ten patients, five went through the entire treatment program (adherent group) and five were noncompliant from the very beginning of the treatment program (noncompliant group). At the six-month follow-up, the adherent group continued to demonstrate adherence to the treatment regimen (wheelchair push-ups = 96 percent correct adherence; self-monitoring forms completed/returned = 83 percent; follow-up session attendance = 75 percent), and on skin check did not exhibit any pressure sore formation or hospitalizations for pressure sore lesions. In contrast, the noncompliant group demonstrated no adherence (0 percent) to the treatment regimen at the six-month follow-up, and three of the surviving four patients had been hospitalized for pressure sore rehabilitation. Hospitalization lasted from three weeks to several months, resulting in considerable personal and financial cost for the noncompliant group.

CONCLUSION

The studies reviewed in this chapter included one or more of the following components of the model proposed by Varni (1983) to enhance long-term therapeutic adherence: (1) child self-management training, (2) behavioral parent training, and (3) health care staff behavioral training. Future investigations across chronically ill and handicapped childhood populations will likely replicate and further develop this three component model, given the current family-oriented and interdisciplinary biobehavioral approach increasingly being recognized as required in the comprehensive care of chronically ill and handicapped children.

Finally, as emphasized by Varni and Wallander (1984), it is extremely important to differentiate between short-term therapeutic adherence in pediatric acute illnesses and *long-term* therapeutic adherence in pediatric chronic illnesses and handicapping conditions. Acute illnesses typically can be cured within a short (one or two week) time period, with relatively immediate improvement in the condition serving as a powerful intrinsic reinforcer in maintaining short-term adherence. However, the management of pediatric chronic disorders requires long-term adherence to health care regimens which may not have immediate beneficial results, such as an immediate reduction in physical symptoms, or may be required primarily to prevent further morbidity. Thus immediate intrinsic reinforcement may not exist for the child and family to engage in a routine long-term health care regimen. Consequently interventions which provide more immediate, powerful extrinsic reinforcers for the child within a point system may increase the child's motivation to perform the necessary health-related behaviors when administered within the behavioral parent training and health care staff training format. The successful comprehensive care of chronically ill and handicapped children requires life-long lifestyle modifications, and parents and health care professionals must provide the necessary socioenvironmental support structure so as to optimize the child's successful daily self-management life-style as a habit pattern, which if established early in life,may generalize to adulthood.

REFERENCES

Akins, C., Davidson, R., & Hopkins, T. (1980). The child with myelodysplasia. In A.P. Scheiner & I.F. Abroms (Eds.), *The practical management of the developmentally disabled child.* St. Louis: Mosby.

American Diabetes Association. (1979). Principles of nutrition and dietary recommendations for individuals with diabetes mellitus. *Diabetes, 28,* 1027–1029.

Anderson, R.J., & Kirk, L.M. (1982). Methods of improving patient compliance in chronic disease states. *Archives of Internal Medicine, 142,* 1673–1675.

Arnold, W.D., & Hilgartner, M.W. (1977). Hemophilic arthropathy: Current concepts of pathogenesis and management. *Journal of Bone and Joint Surgery, 59,* 287–305.

Arky, R.A. (1984). Nutrition therapy for the child and adolescent with type I diabetes mellitus. *Pediatric Clinics of North America, 31,* 711–719.

Aronstam, A., Rainsford, S.G., & Painter, M.J. (1972). Patterns of bleeding in adolescents with severe hemophilia A. *British Medical Journal, 1,* 469–470.

Austin, E.S., Lindgren, W.D., & Dietrich, S.L. (1972). Spina bifida and myelomeningocele. *American Family Physician, 6,* 105–111.

Boone, D.C. (1975). Physical therapy management. In K.M. Brinkous & H.C. Hemker (Eds.), *Handbook of hemophilia.* Amsterdam: Excerpta Medica.

Breslau, N. (1983). Siblings of disabled children: Birth order and age-spacing effects. *Journal of Abnormal Child Psychology, 10,* 85–96.

Breslau, N., Staruch, K.S., & Mortimer, E.A. (1982). Psychological distress in mothers of disabled children. *American Journal of Diseases of Children, 136,* 682–686.

Breslau, N., Weitzman, M., & Messenger, K. (1981). Psychological functioning of siblings of disabled children. *Pediatrics, 67,* 344–353.

Buchanan, G.R. (1980). Hemophilia. *Pediatric Clinics of North America, 27,* 309–326.

Carney, R.M., Schechter, K., & Davis, T. (1983). Improving adherence to blood glucose testing in insulin-dependent diabetic children. *Behavior Therapy, 14,* 247–254.

Christensen, N.K., Terry, R.D., Wyatt, S., Pichert, J.W., & Lorenz, R.A. (1983). Quantitative assessment of dietary adherence in patients with insulin-dependent diabetes mellitus. *Diabetes Care, 6*(3), 245–250.

Department of Health, Education, and Welfare, Public Health Service. (1979). *Public Policy and Chronic Disease* (NIH Publication No. 79-1896). Washington, DC: U.S. Government Printing Office.

Dietrich, S.L. (1976). Medical management of hemophilia. In D.C. Boone (Ed.), *Comprehensive management of hemophilia*. Philadelphia: F.A. Davis.

Dietrich, S.L. (1979). Death and survival of spina bifida patients. Orthopaedic Hospital, unpublished manuscript.

Dietrich, S.L., Luck, J.V., & Martinson, A.M. (1982). Musculoskeletal problems. In M.W. Hilgartner (Ed.), *Hemophilia in the child and adult*. New York: Masson Press.

DiMatteo, M.R., & DiNicola, D.D. (1982). *Achieving patient compliance: The psychology of the medical practitioner's role*. New York: Pergamon Press.

Dishman, R.K. (1982). Compliance/adherence in health-related exercise. *Health Psychology, 1*, 237–267.

Drotar, D. (1981). Psychological perspectives in chronic childhood illness. *Journal of Pediatric Psychology, 6*, 211–228.

Dunbar, J.M., & Agras, W.S. (1980). Compliance with medical instructions. In J.M. Ferguson & C.B. Taylor (Eds.), *Comprehensive handbook of behavioral medicine* (Vol. 3). New York: Spectrum.

Epstein, L.H., Beck, S., Figueroa, J., Farkas, G., Kazdin, A.E., Daneman, D., & Becker, D. (1981). The effects of targeting improvements in urine glucose on metabolic control in children with insulin dependent diabetes. *Journal of Applied Behavior Analysis, 14*, 365–375.

Epstein, L.H., Wing, R.R., Koeske, R., Ossip, D., & Beck, S. (1982). A comparison of lifestyle change and programmed aerobic exercise on weight and fitness changes in obese children. *Behavior Therapy, 13*, 651–665.

Eraker, S.A., Kirshct, J.P., & Becker, M.H. (1984). Understanding and improving patient compliance. *Annals of Internal Medicine, 100*, 258–268.

Evans, E.P., & Tew, B. (1983). Energy expenditure and movement among children with myelomeningocele. *Spina Bifida Therapy, 4*, 43–52.

Farrell, S.R., Layton, M.S., Ford, F., & Tervo, R.C. (1981). Obesity and diet in a spina bifida clinic: Associated factors and management. *Journal of the Canadian Dietetic Association, 42*, 160–166.

Feldman, W.S., Manella, K.J., Apodaca, L., & Varni, J.W. (1982). Behavioral group parent training in spina bifida. *Journal of Clinical Child Psychology, 11*, 144–150.

Feldman, W.S., Manella, K.J., & Varni, J.W. (1983). A behavioral parent training program for single mothers of physically handicapped children. *Child Care, Health, and Development, 9*, 157–168.

Feldman, W.S., & Varni, J.W. (1983). A parent training program for the child with spina bifida. *Spina Bifida Therapy, 4*, 77–89.

Ferrari, M. (1984). Chronic illness: Psychosocial effects on siblings—I. Chronically ill boys. *Journal of Child Psychology and Psychiatry, 25*, 459–476.

Friedman, H.S., & DiMatteo, M.R. (Eds.) (1982). *Interpersonal issues in health care*. New York: Academic.

Friedrich, W.N. (1979). Predictors of the coping behaviors of mothers of handicapped children. *Journal of Consulting and Clinical Psychology, 47*, 1140–1141.

Geffner, M.E., Kaplan, S.A., Lippe, B.M., & Scott, M.L. (1983). Self-monitoring of blood glucose levels and intensified insulin therapy: Acceptability and efficacy in childhood diabetes. *Journal of the American Medical Association, 249*, 2913–2916.

Gilbert, A., & Varni, J.W. (1985). Behavioral techniques in teaching factor replacement therapy to children with hemophilia. Manuscript submitted for publication.

Gortmaker, S.L., & Sappenfield, W. (1984). Chronic childhood disorders: Prevalence and impact. *Pediatric Clinics of North America, 31*, 3–18.

Greenan, E., Powell, C., & Varni, J.W. (1985). Adherence to therapeutic exercise by children with hemophilia. Manuscript in preparation.

Greene, W.B., & Strickler, E.M. (1983). A modified isokinetic strengthening program for patients with severe hemophilia. *Developmental Medicine and Child Neurology, 25*, 189–196.

Gresham, F.M. (1982). Misguided mainstreaming: The case for social skills training with handicapped children. *Exceptional Children, 48*, 422–433.

Griest, D.L., Forehand, R., Wells, K.C., & McMahon, R.J. (1980). An examination of differences between nonclinic and behavior-problem clinic-referred children and their mothers. *Journal of Abnormal Psychology, 89*, 474–500.

Guenthner, E.E., Hilgartner, M.W., Miller, C.H., & Vienne, G. (1980). Hemophilic arthropathy: Effects of home care on treatment patterns and joint disease. *Journal of Pediatrics, 97*, 378–382.

Halstead, L.S. (1976). Team care in chronic illness: A critical review of the literature of the past 25 years. *Archives of Physical Medicine and Rehabilitation, 57*, 507–511.

Hayes-Allen, M.C. (1972). Obesity and short stature in children with myelomeningocele. *Developmental Medicine and Child Neurology, 14*, 59–64.

Hayes-Allen, M.C., & Tring, F.C. (1973). Obesity: Another hazard for spina bifida children. *British Journal of Preventive and Social Medicine, 27*, 192–196.

Helske, T., Ikkala, E., Myllyla, G., Nevanlinna, H.R., & Rasi, V. (1982). Joint involvement in patients with severe haemophilia A in 1957-59 and 1978-79. *British Journal of Haematology, 51*, 643–647.

Holroyd, J., & Guthrie, D. (1979). Stress in families of children with neuromuscular disease. *Journal of Clinical Psychology, 35*, 734–739.

Ikkala, E., Helske, T., Myllyla, G., Nevanlinna, H.R., Pitkanen, P., & Rasi, V. (1982). Changes in the life expectancy of patients with severe hemophilia A in Finland in 1930-79. *British Journal of Haematology, 52*, 7–12.

Jeffries, J.S., Killam, P.E., & Varni, J.W. (1982). Behavioral management of fecal incontinence in a child with myelomeningocele. *Pediatric Nursing, 8*, 267–270.

Johnson, S.B., Pollak, R.T., Silverstein, J.H., Rosenbloom, A.L., Spillar, R., McCallum, M., & Harkavy, J. (1982). Cognitive and behavioral knowledge about insulin-dependent diabetes among children and parents. *Pediatrics, 69*, 708–713.

Jones, J.G. (1983). Compliance with pediatric therapy: A selective review and recommendations. *Clinical Pediatrics, 22*, 262–265.

Kaufert, J.M. (1980). Social and psychological responses to home treatment of hemophilia. *Journal of Epidemiology and Community Health, 34*, 194–200.

Killam, P.E., Apodaca, L., Manella, K.J., & Varni, J.W. (1983). Behavioral pediatric weight rehabilitation for children with myelomeningocele. *MCN: American Journal of Maternal Child Nursing, 8*, 280–296.

Killam, P.E., Jeffries, J.S., & Varni, J.W. (in press). Urodynamic biofeedback treatment of urinary incontinence in children with myelomeningocele *Biofeedback and Self-Regulation*.

Koch, B., Cohen, S., Luban, N.C., & Eng, G. (1982). Hemophiliac knee: Rehabilitation techniques. *Archives of Physical Medicine and Rehabilitation, 63*, 379–382.

Koch, B., Galioto, F.M., Kelleher, J., & Goldstein, D. (1984). Physical fitness in children with hemophilia. *Archives of Physical Medicine and Rehabilitation, 65*, 324–326.

Koch, B., Luban, N.L.C., Galioto, F.M., Rick, M.E., Goldstein, D., & Kelleher, J. (1984). Changes in coagulation parameters with exercise in patients with classic hemophilia. *American Journal of Hematology, 16*, 227–233.

Lau, R.R., Williams, H.S., Williams, L.C., Ware, J.E., & Brook, R.H. (1982). Psychosocial problems in chronically ill children: Physician concern, parent satisfaction, and the validity of medical records. *Journal of Community Health, 7,* 250–261.

Lavigne, J.V., & Ryan, M. (1979). Psychologic adjustment of siblings of children with chronic illness. *Pediatrics, 63,* 616–627.

Lazerson, J. (1972). Hemophilia home transfusion program: Effect on school attendance. *Journal of Pediatrics, 81,* 330–332.

Levine, P.H., & Britten, F.H. (1973). Supervised patient-management of hemophilia. A study of 45 patients with hemophilia A and B. *Annals of Internal Medicine, 78,* 195–201.

Llenado, M., & Grogan, D. (1978). Myelomeningocele. In S. Palmer & S. Ekvall (Eds.), *Pediatric nutrition in developmental disorders.* Springfield, IL: Charles C Thomas.

Lowe, K., & Lutzker, J.R. (1979). Increasing compliance to a medical regimen with a juvenile diabetic. *Behavior Therapy, 10,* 57–64.

Manella, K.J., Jeffries, J.S., & Varni, J.W. (1985). Adherence to health care behaviors in the prevention of pressure sores by adolescents with spina bifida. Manuscript in preparation.

Manella, K.J., & Varni, J.W. (1981). Behavior therapy in a gait-training program for a child with myelomeningocele. *Physical Therapy, 61,* 1284–1287.

Manella, K.J., & Varni, J.W. (1984). Behavioral treatment of ambulatory function in a child with myelomeningocele. *Physical Therapy, 64,* 1536–1539.

Martin, J.E., & Dubbert, P.M. (1982). Exercise applications and promotion in behavioral medicine: Current status and future directions. *Journal of Consulting and Clinical Psychology, 50,* 1004–1017.

Masters, J.C., Cerreto, M.C., & Mendlowitz, D.R. (1983). The role of the family in coping with childhood chronic illness. In T.G. Burish & L.A. Bradley (Eds.), *Coping with chronic disease: Research and applications.* New York: Academic.

Mazzuca, S.A. (1982). Does patient education in chronic illness have therapeutic value? *Journal of Chronic Diseases, 35,* 521–529.

McAndrew, I. (1976). Children with a handicap and their families. *Child Care, Health and Development, 2,* 213–237.

Meenan, R.F., Yelin, E.H., Nevitt, M., & Epstein, W.V. (1981). The impact of chronic disease: A sociomedical profile of rheumatoid arthritis. *Arthritis and Rheumatism, 24,* 544–549.

Melvin, J.L. (1980). Interdisciplinary and multidisciplinary activities and the ACRM. *Archives of Physical Medicine and Rehabilitation, 61,* 379–380.

Miller, P.F.W., Stratton, C., & Tripp, J.H. (1983). Blood testing compared with urine testing in the long-term control of diabetes. *Archives of Disease in Childhood, 58,* 294–297.

Morrissy, R.T. (1978). Spina bifida: A new rehabilitation problem. *Orthopaedic Clinics of North America, 9,* 379–389.

Murphy, M.A. (1982). The family with a handicapped child: A review of the literature. *Journal of Developmental and Behavioral Pediatrics, 3,* 73–82.

Nader, P.R., Ray, L., & Brink, S.G. (1981). The new morbidity. Use of school and community health care resources for behavioral, educational, and social-family problems. *Pediatrics, 67,* 53–60.

Nuttal, F.Q. (1983). Diet and the diabetic patient. *Diabetes Care, 6*(2), 197–207.

O'Moore, M. (1980). Social acceptance of the physically handicapped child in the ordinary school. *Child Care, Health and Development, 6,* 317–337.

Pennebaker, J.W., Cox, D.J., Gonder-Frederick, L., Wunsch, M.G., Evans, W.S., & Pohl, S. (1981). Physical symptoms related to blood glucose in insulin dependent diabetes. *Psychosomatic Medicine, 43,* 489–500.

Pettersson, H., Ahlbert, A., & Nilsson, I.M. (1980). A radiologic classification of hemophilic arthropathy. *Clinical Orthopedics and Related Research, 149,* 153–159.

Pless, I.B. (1984). Clinical assessment: Physical and psychological functioning. *Pediatric Clinics of North America, 31,* 33–45.

Pless, E.V., & Douglas, J.W.B. (1971). Chronic illness in childhood: Part 1. Epidemiological and clinical characteristics. *Pediatrics, 47,* 405–414.

Porter, B., & O'Leary, K.D. (1980). Marital discord and childhood behavior problems. *Journal of Abnormal Child Psychology, 8,* 287–295.

Reuler, J.B., & Cooney, T.G. (1981). The pressure sore: Pathophysiology and principles of management. *Annals of Internal Medicine, 94,* 661–666.

Rickard, K., Brady, M.S., & Gresham, E.L. (1977). Nutritional management of the chronically ill child: Congenital heart disease and myelomeningocele. *Pediatric Clinics of North America, 24,* 157–174.

Rothberg, J.S. (1981). The rehabilitation team: Future direction. *Archives of Physical Medicine and Rehabilitation, 62,* 407–410.

Russo, D.C., & Varni, J.W. (1982). Behavioral pediatrics. In D.C. Russo & J.W. Varni (Eds.), *Behavioral Pediatrics: Research and Practice.* New York: Plenum.

Sabbeth, B.F., & Leventhal, J.M. (1984). Marital adjustment to chronic childhood illness: A critique of the literature. *Pediatrics, 73,* 762–768.

Schafer, L.C., Glasgow, R.E., & McCaul, K.D. (1982). Increasing the adherence of diabetic adolescents. *Journal of Behavioral Medicine, 5,* 353–362.

Schafer, L.C., Glasgow, R.E., McCaul, K.D., & Dreher, M. (1983). Adherence to IDDM regimens: Relationship to psychosocial variables and metabolic control. *Diabetes Care, 6,* 493–498.

Schiffrin, A., Desrosiers, M., & Belmont, M. (1983). Evaluation of two methods of self blood glucose monitoring by trained insulin-dependent diabetic adolescents outside the hospital. *Diabetes Care, 6,* 166–169.

Sergis, E., & Hilgartner, M.W. (1972). Hemophilia. *American Journal of Nursing, 72,* 2011–2017.

Sergis-Deavenport, E., & Varni, J.W. (1982). Behavioral techniques in teaching hemophilia factor replacement procedures to families. *Pediatric Nursing, 8,* 416–419.

Sergis-Deavenport, E., & Varni, J.W. (1983). Behavioral assessment and management of adherence to factor replacement therapy in hemophilia. *Journal of Pediatric Psychology, 8,* 367–377.

Shurtleff, D.B. (1980). Myelodysplasia: Management and treatment. *Current Problems in Pediatrics, 10,* 7–41.

Shurtleff, D.B., Lamers, J., Goiney, T., & Gordon, L. (1982). Are myelodysplastic children fat? Anthropometric measures: A preliminary report. *Spina Bifida Therapy, 4,* 1–21.

Simonds, J.F. (1979). Emotions and compliance in diabetic children. *Psychosomatics, 20,* 544–551.

Smith, P.S., Keyes, N.C., & Forman, E.N. (1982). Socioeconomic evaluation of a state funded comprehensive hemophilia-care program. *New England Journal of Medicine, 306,* 575–579.

Soreff, J., & Blomback, M. (1980). Arthropathy in children with severe hemophilia A. *Acta Paediatrica Scandinavica, 69,* 667–673.

Sousa, J.C., Gordon, L.H., & Shurtleff, D.B. (1976). Assessing developmental daily living skills in patients with spina bifida. *Developmental Medicine and Child Neurology, 18,* 134–142.

Starfield, B. (1982). Behavioral pediatrics and primary health care. *Pediatric Clinics of North America, 29,* 377–390.

Stein, R.E.K., & Jessop, D.J. (1982). A noncategorical approach to chronic childhood illness. *Public Health Reports, 97,* 354–362.

Stein, R.E.K., Jessop, D.J., & Riessman, C.K. (1983). Health care services received by children with chronic illness. *American Journal of Diseases of Children, 137,* 225–230.

Stein, R.E.K., & Riessman, C.K. (1980). The development of an impact-on-family scale: Preliminary findings. *Medical Care, 18,* 465–472.

Sumpter, E.A. (1980). Behavioral aspects of pediatrics and chronic illness. In A.P. Scheiner & I.F. Abrons (Eds.), *The practical management of the developmentally disabled child.* St. Louis: Mosby.

Surwit, R.S., Scovern, A.W., & Feinglos, M.N. (1982). The role of behavior in diabetes care. *Diabetes Care, 5,* 337–342.

Tamborlane, W.V., & Sherwin, R.S. (1983). Diabetes control and complications: New strategies and insights. *Journal of Pediatrics, 102,* 805–813.

Tattersall, R., & Gale, E. (1981). Patient self-monitoring of blood glucose and refinements of conventional insulin treatment. *American Journal of Medicine, 70,* 177–182.

Varni, J.W. (1981a) Self-regulation techniques in the management of chronic arthritic pain in hemophilia. *Behavior Therapy, 12,* 184–194.

Varni, J.W. (1981b) Behavioral medicine in hemophilia arthritic pain management. *Archives of Physical Medicine and Rehabilitation, 62,* 183–187.

Varni, J.W. (1983). *Clinical behavioral pediatrics: An interdisciplinary biobehavioral approach.* New York: Pergamon Press.

Varni, J.W., & Gilbert, A. (1982). Self-regulation of chronic arthritic pain and long-term analgesic dependence in a hemophiliac. *Rheumatology and Rehabilitation, 21,* 171–174.

Varni, J.W., Gilbert, A., & Dietrich, S.L. (1981). Behavioral medicine in pain and analgesia management for the hemophilic child with factor VIII inhibitor. *Pain, 11,* 121–126.

Varni, J.W., & Jay, S.M. (1984). Biobehavioral factors in juvenile rheumatoid arthritis: Implications for research and practice. *Clinical Psychology Review, 4,* 543–560.

Varni, J.W., & Wallander, J.L. (1984). Adherence to health-related regimens in pediatric chronic disorders. *Clinical Psychology Review, 4,* 585–596.

Varni, J.W., & Wallander, J.L. (in press). Pediatric chronic orthopaedic disabilities: Hemophilia and spina bifida as exemplary disorders. In D.K. Routh (Ed.), *Handbook of pediatric psychology.* New York: Guilford.

Webb, K.L., Dobson, A.J., O'Connell, D.L., Tupling, H.E., Harris, G.W., Moxon, J.A., Sulway, M.J., & Leeder, S.R. (1984). Dietary compliance among insulin-dependent diabetics. *Journal of Chronic Diseases, 37,* 633–643.

Weissman, J. (1977). Rehabilitation medicine and the hemophilic patient. *Mount Sinai Journal of Medicine, 44,* 359–370.

Whitehead, W.E., Parker, L.H., Masek, B.J., Cataldo, M.F., & Freeman, J.M. (1981). Biofeedback treatment of fecal incontinence in patients with myelomeningocele. *Developmental Medicine and Child Neurology, 23,* 313–322.

Williams, L.O., Anderson, A.D., Campbell, J., Thomas, L., Feiwell, E., & Wiker, J.M. (1983). Energy cost of walking and of wheelchair propulsion by children with myelodysplasia: Comparison with normal children. *Developmental Medicine and Child Neurology, 25,* 617–624.

Wing, R.R., Epstein, L.H., Nowalk, M.P., & Hyg, M.S. (1984). Dietary adherence in patients with diabetes. *Behavioral Medicine Update, 6,* 17–21.

Zwaag, R.V., Mason, W.B., Joiner, M.B., & Runyan, J.W. (1980). Cost of chronic disease care. *Journal of Chronic Diseases, 33,* 713–720.

22

Chronicity and Normalcy as the Psychological Basis for Research and Treatment in Chronic Disease in Children

DENNIS C. RUSSO

Pediatrics has been, since the turn of the century, among the most successful branches of medicine. Advances in prenatal care, sanitation, nutrition, immunization, and disease management have resulted in great reductions in child morbidity and mortality. It is precisely this success which serves as the evaluative base for this paper. In science, success as well as failure must serve as the stimulus for reappraisal and modification of research and practice.

As we shall see the unequivocal success of pediatrics in managing acute disease has led to the need for the revision of modern pediatric practice. Recognition of resultant gaps has led medicine to collaborative endeavor with physics, electronics, and newer approaches to biochemistry which have generated new directions for the management of chronic disease. In areas where the infusion of new approaches has been successful, it has resulted in the inclusion of such methods in medical curriculum, and to the development of new professions as complements to medicine.

This atmosphere of collaboration has, in the past decade, facilitated, as well, a merger of medicine and psychology. The potency of psychological variables in the maintenance of health and the production and exacerbation of illness is increasingly recognized (Engel, 1977) as an important area for the training of physicians and a valid point of convergence for medical and psychological research (Schwartz, 1982; Schwartz & Weiss, 1978).

It is the purpose of this paper to provide an exposition of the trends which have supported the position that psychological variables have potent impact in disease production and maintenance and to suggest that collaborative relationships between medicine and psychology are necessary for improved understanding and management of chronic disease. To accomplish this goal, one must first review the context of current research and practice through its historic and demographic roots, as well as consider the current context of care. The success of pediatric medicine has created new morbidity (Haggerty, Roghman & Pless, 1975), an understanding of which may serve to guide joint medical/psychological research aimed at improved management of chronic disease in children.

Changes in the Demography of Disease

From Galen to Descartes and beyond, prominent thinkers have pondered the mysteries of the relationships between the body and the mind. The recognition that thoughts, feelings, and actions could influence susceptibility to disease as well as its course was evidenced in the folklore of both the East and West, prior to and coincident with improved scientific understanding of somatic function. Cartesian dualism, however, forced separation between aspects of mind and body and allowed for little progress in their joint study. The methods of science applied to the somatic aspects of disease, as evidenced in the work of Pasteur and others, created a vast increase in knowledge. Psychological aspects of disease, on the other hand received little attention.

Indeed at the start of the twentieth century mind and body were more concretely separated than ever before. A number of factors such as the development of psychoanalysis, the science revolution in medical training whereby physicians in training received initial instruction in the natural sciences, and the brief course of most diseases of the day, focused attention away from the systematic study of behavior/disease relationships. Despite this dualism, instances of such relationships continued to be recognized, with Freud, for example, commenting that depressed affects, as in the propensity of defeated armies to contact typhus and dysentary, could influence health and shorten life (1905).

Despite awareness of these psychological factors, the undivided effort of science began to elucidate the nature of disease at the outset of the twentieth century. In the ensuing 80 years this approach has brought forth a vast amount of knowledge about somatic aspects of disease and their treatment. Indeed, as Dubos (1965) and others have demonstrated, the epidemiology of disease has changed radically since the turn of the century, due primarily to advances in medicine, sanitation and immunization.

Today, increasing numbers of persons suffer from chronic, debilitating diseases which produce limitations in activity and mobility (Cataldo, Russo, Bird & Varni, 1980). Disease itself has changed as well. Acute germ-based illness such as cholera and typhoid have been all but eradicated as a result of scientific advances in disease etiology and treatment. Disease present in our society today is of a different nature: chronic and with, as yet, a poor understanding of etiology.

Changes in the Philosophy of Science

As Schwartz (1982) has suggested, previous advances in the knowledge base of medicine have occurred largely as a result of the adoption of particular epistemologies. These methods of inquiry may be, under the rubric of Pepper (1942), classified as being dominated by formistic or mechanistic thinking. These approaches are characterized by linear, "either-or" logic, in which single entities (e.g., germs) produce single outcomes (e.g., disease). Such a view of disease has been quite successful, as can be seen in the altered disease epidemiology of the twentieth century. The value of such a "model" in the history of medicine is clear. The primary point here is that given changes in our knowledge base and disease epidemiology, such a model may be too simplistic to deal with the current context of disease treatment.

Schwartz (1982) suggests that current models of care be based on more relational forms of thinking which incorporate multiple factors. Contextual or organismic methodologies, he proposes, which allow consideration of multiple causative factors as well as the inclusion of multiple setting and outcome variables, represent more adequate methodologies for the study of contemporary disease. Such approaches are characterized as biopsychosocial (Engel, 1977; Leigh & Reiser, 1980) and suggest that understanding of disease requires evaluation of the context or system as well as biological aspects of both the patient and the disease.

It is important to note that such a shift in focus is a result of the success of medicine. The value of the germ theory is undisputed, and resulted in many advances. These advances, however, suggest that the model must be revised. Such changes are common in science: consider the complement a relativistic approach provided the science of physics in moving beyond the universe of Newton. Einstein's notions had much in common with current medicine in that they required consideration of multiple "relativistic" and contextual factors. As we shall see, such a relational view of medicine is justified, given the current status of disease treatment, chronic care, and the patient in current practice.

The History of Pediatrics

The evolution of pediatrics has mirrored the course of medicine as a whole. More complex explanatory mechanisms may be required in pediatrics to provide adequate care of patients as well as to promote advances in the knowledge of disease.

Kenney and Clemmens (1975) suggest that an appreciation of this process can be obtained by evaluating the development of pediatrics since the turn of the century. At that time a new model of the teaching of medicine was being promulgated. While previous medical training had focused primarily on a mentor-apprentice model, medical students at the turn of the century were receiving initial training in the basic sciences as a precursor to clinical practice.

The development of a science-based curriculum in the teaching of medicine may be viewed as an important first step, allowing medicine to become proficient in the laboratory study of disease as well as in practical technique. This new curriculum led in the 1900s to a period of descriptive pediatrics, in which science developed an improved understanding of the etiology, course, and pathophysiology of disease. This resulted in the 1920s in what is referred to as curative pediatrics. Because of advances in basic understanding of disease, new treatments became possible to prevent or defeat many of the killers of children through the discovery of antibiotics, improvements of sanitation, and the synthesis of hormones. The resultant decrease in morbidity and mortality was furthered by the development of prophyllactic pediatrics in the early 1950s, which provided methods for preventing many diseases in children.

One can see, therefore, that during the 1960s pediatrics had indeed been successful: killing diseases of the century had been largely eradicated, providing for reduced death risk in children and a longer life span. Advances in surgical care as well allowed many children who previously would have died to continue to live without total cure of disease or defect.

Primary care of the well child (Starfield & Pless, 1980) has become a major task for modern pediatric practice. The pediatrician, as opposed to any other health provider, is most appropriate for this function. Through periodic patient visits over the course of childhood, the pediatrician is able to monitor development, facilitate the early identification of disease, and help to insure adequate care for the child. Interest in biological aspects of disease is now complemented by recognition of the importance of social, developmental, and behavioral factors in the growing child (Russo & Varni, 1982; Varni, 1983). The problems of living, learning, and growing have resulted in the expansion of medical curriculum and require conceptual approaches to integrate these psychosocial issues into modern practice.

Advances in neonatology, surgery, and management of the child with congenital anomalie or birth defect have likewise created a new area of speciality. With increasing numbers of children surviving despite serious initial defect or mental retardation, problems of management increasingly require attention to educational, social, and behavioral factors to assist the child in development (Cataldo & Russo, 1979). Management of spina bifida, cerebral palsy, and mental retardation, for example, suggest the need for continued joint psychological and medical management, despite medical stability of the primary disorder.

With respect to noncongenital disease of children, the literature suggests medicine's success in the cure of many diseases. As can be seen in Table 22.1, over the past 100 years, the disorders which afflict our children have changed drastically. This has been in large part due to improvements in medical care, sanitation, and the development of new medicines and medical technologies. Children today simply do not die in significant numbers of acute infectious disease. Rather, they suffer from long-term, chronic, overt and symptomatic diseases for which medicine provides no cure. Chronic disease treatment is now focused on the management of the disease process. Reduction of symptomatology, maintenance of internal homeostatis, and improved comfort for the patient represent major goals of such an approach. Pediatric medicine has been very successful in maintaining life in children with chronic diseases such as end-stage renal disease, that only a few years ago would have been quickly fatal (Russo, Bennett, Harmon & Brown, 1981).

TABLE 22.1.   MOST COMMON SOURCES OF ADMISSION: CHILDREN'S HOSPITAL MEDICAL CENTER, BOSTON, 1882 AND 1982

1882	1982
Rickets	Asthma
Cholera infantum	Seizure disorders
Diphtheria	Cancer/Abdominal tumors
Scarlet fever	Cystic fibrosis
Whooping cough	Ventricular septal defect
Bone infections	Otitis media
Tuberculosis	Scoliosis
Congenital syphilis	Gastroenteritis/Colitis
Measles	Fever
Scurvy	Failure to thrive

Source: *Children's World*, the Children's Hospital Medical Center, Spring 1982.

In each of these three areas—well-child care, congenital disorders, and chronic disease—a major area of concern is the child's growth, development, and behavior, and the relationship between behavior and the exacerbation or maintenance of disease. It has become increasingly the case that pediatric medicine, in its concern for the continued follow-up of the patient, is also involved with aspects of child management and parental concerns over behavior. The process of chronic disease itself entails a number of potential threats to the development and behavior of children (Russo & Varni, 1982). Physical side effects of treatment, altered social histories, the presence of continued symptomatology, and other factors, all contribute to the perception of the chronically ill child as different. We shall review these areas below as a basis for discussion of the psychological impact of chronic disease in children.

BEHAVIORAL PERCEPTIONS OF CHRONIC DISEASE IN CHILDREN

As a basis for evaluating behavioral perceptions of the treatment of pediatric chronic disease it is important to evaluate the current context of care of the chronically ill child. Behaviorally the context of care may provide us with a good deal of information about learning characteristics of the hospital environment, potential areas for maladaptive learning, and some potential alterations for improving the comprehensiveness of care for the child with chronic disease.

Currently, management of the child with chronic disease is perhaps best viewed from a biopsychosocial model (Engel, 1977) of pediatric care. Such a model assumes contributants ot the disease process arise in the social and psychological as well as biological spheres. For the first time, advances in the areas of biology, medicine, biochemistry, and psychology have come together to allow the simultaneous assessment of the impact of disease on children. A simple germ-based model is no longer sufficient to deal adequately with the overall requirement of care for the chronically ill child. Much of medical procedure in the past has been dedicated to the identification of etiologic variables which, when identified, have produced cure of a particular disease. Many of the diseases from which children suffer today, such as cancer, cystic fibrosis, renal disease, and diabetes, are not sufficiently understood to allow for etiologic management. Under such circumstances, the goal of medicine becomes management and symptom reduction as opposed to cure. As a result of medical success in symptom management, children are currently living for long periods with chronic medical diseases. These diseases place systematic stresses upon the lives of the children, potentially impair their learning ability, and may significantly alter social and environmental circumstances. Under these conditions, it is appropriate to revise traditional models of disease management.

A number of factors must be considered in the comprehensive formulation of treatment strategies for children with chronic disease. Indeed, such formulation requires the input of a number of trained individuals in addition to those in medicine. Table 22.2 provides an elucidation of some of these areas. As can be seen in Table 22.2, comprehensive treatment and management formulation requires attention to the disease itself, the environment of care, significant others in the environment, the patient's behavior, the patient's biochemistry, and beliefs of the patient. It is important to consider the relevant characteristics of each of these dimensions in the development of improved services.

With respect to diseases, it is appropriate to consider that most diseases from which children suffer today are chronic, overt, and symptomatic. Disorders such as cystic fibrosis and diabetes represent life long alterations in the physiology and capability of children. Treatment of these diseases requires ongoing regimens in which behavior plays a significant part. In many diseases, children and their families are required to adhere to long-term regimens, such as dietary and exercise modification and medication taking. Additionally, physical therapy, periodic painful treatments such as

TABLE 22.2. FACTORS IN THE MANAGEMENT OF CHRONIC ILLNESS IN CHILDREN

Factors	Characteristics
Disease	Overt
	Symptomatic
	Chronic
Environment	Hospital
	Home
	School
Others	Parents
	Hospital staff
	Teachers
Behavior	Lack of activity
	Dependency
	Social deficit
Biochemistry	Endorphins
	Immune function
	Hormones
Belief	Self-esteem
	Value?
	Depression

hemodialysis, or periodic surgeries may be required for management. Each of these factors, with respect both to the disease and the treatment, sets potent occasions for learning. Further, learning due to painful symptoms or treatment may be the occasion of development of maladaptive behaviors which, in the long run, may result in decreased success in management of the disorder.

With respect to the environment of care, chronically ill children are treated repeatedly in hospitals, clinics and doctors' offices. The unique characteristic about such environments is that they are largely standardized from hospital to hospital and clinic to clinic. The benefit of consistency in the medical environment is that it allows for the implementation of treatment and diagnostic procedures and, in its present design, assures for competent physical care procedures. Such environments do, however, pose a difficulty. That is, hospitals were originally designed to manage children with acute disease. In past years, the hospitalization of children with acute diseases were brief, often one-time affairs. Under such circumstances, consistency served to promote quality and care. Under conditions of chronicity, however, the medical environment sets a potent stage for the learning of behavior. Such factors as changing shifts, the provision of certain treatments in certain environments, and the attention paid to somatic distress all potentially provide the basis for maladaptive learning. It is important to note that hospitals, particularly pediatric hospitals, in recognition of these iatrogenic characteristics have attempted to change. It is now common for child activity programs or surgical preparation programs to exist in many hospitals to help ease the burden of hospitalization (Melamed, 1977).

A third area of consideration is the significant others in the child's environment. This includes not only parents, but also hospital staff and school teachers. These individuals interact with the child on a frequent and periodic basis throughout the course of his or her illness. The attention provided by these individuals to certain aspects of symptom presentation, positive behavior, or maladaptive responding may significantly shape the behavior of the child.

Fourthly, the behavior of the patient is also notable in its consistency. In many cases the behavior of the chronically ill child is denoted by passivity, dependence, and a low level of activity. In many cases the child perceives himself or herself to be different from peers, less capable than them, and potentially less able to affect his or her world. The effects of the illness may produce an individual who becomes increasingly passive and dependent or an individual who may develop significant coping skills. In such circumstances, the systematic behavior of the patient plays an important role, not only in the production of disease symptoms, but also in the reactions of others in the environment to the individual.

In recent years, two additional areas have become scientifically assessable. The first of these areas, physiology and biochemistry, is particularly important because of recent work demonstrating the ability of learning to produce significant alterations in body chemistry. Early studies (Ader, 1971; Anderson & Brady, 1979) demonstrated the ability to produce chronic physiological changes as a result of altered environmental circumstances in animals. These studies showed changes in immune system function, the production of hormones, and the alteration of homeostatic mechanisms as a result of exposure to certain structured learning tasks. Over the past ten years, research on brain peptides, such as beta endorphin, and research on conditioned alteration of immune function in humans have extended this argument to the point where it must be considered in the production, exacerbation, and maintenance of disease. That is, it is a reasonable possibility that the behavior of individuals in reaction to chronic disease may exacerbate or maintain physical aspects of that disease. Such is clearly the case in diabetes, where chronic stress may alter the body's need for insulin.

The second area, belief, is one in which medicine has traditionally had difficulty integrating into theory and practice. Relegating the mind to psychological provinces has been the characteristic position of dualistic thinking. In the present context, consideration of the belief and behavior of the patient forms a necessary additional component in the management of chronic disease. As is suggested above, and has been suggested in various studies (Levine, Gordon, & Fields, 1978), the beliefs and behavior of the patient may provide significant alteration in the physiological response of the individual. Over and above this is the simple fact that the belief of the patient may motivate much behavior. Particularly, since much of medical care involves behavior, issues such as medication compliance, dietary adherence, and the exchange of information between patient and doctor may be strongly altered under conditions of inappropriate perception of the patient.

What is clear from the data found in Table 22.2 is that the management of chronic disease, for which etiologic treatment is unavailable, is a complex affair. Over the course of the disease, a number of factors will appear which require consideration. Indeed, chronic disease strongly sets the stage for learning. For the patient with chronic disease, the consistency and predictability of care practices, treatment procedures, the learning effects of symptoms themselves, and the reactions of others in the environment, all combine to create a powerful and consistent learning environment. Typically, the beneficial or iatrogenic effects of this environment have not been extensively considered in treatment formulation. Rather, problems such as noncompliance have been identified post hoc. Given the consistent and logical environment of medical care, it would seem reasonable to consider learning aspects of chronicity as important variables. Quite simply put: chronicity teaches. What is clearly required in this area are studies which explicitly postulate this notion and assess the impact of chronic disease on children via learning characteristics of the environment. It may be quite possible to provide minor alterations (Cataldo, et al. 1980) of treatment environments which have a facilitative effect on the behavior of children. Likewise, the iatrogenic effects of current medical practices may be identified by simultaneously considering their medical and psychological impact. Psychological intervention in current medical care requires the understanding of this process of development and behavior as a result of chronic disease. The mission of chronic care teams in this area should be seen as the prevention of secondary psychopathology arising out of the chronic disease condition, its environment, and the reactions of individuals to the child with the disease. Given that the psychosocial aspects of disease may well dictate the adherent behavior of the child and, therefore, the effectiveness of medical management, consideration of these factors at an early stage appears warranted.

THE CHILD WITH CHRONIC DISEASE

Under such circumstances the behavior of patients may be viewed as a lawful process of learning and a normal outcome of the process of chronicity. The patient with chronic disease is exposed to a systematic learning environment which places continued attention on aspects of disease and illness. Indeed many of the children require special education programs because of limitations in mobility and activity, or because of the schedule required for chronic disease treatments (for example, dialysis patients). Many of them also have further limitations placed on physical activities. Likewise the effects of many diseases may be to alter growth patterns, so that the children feel physically different from their peers. Such are the *normal* characteristics of living with a chronic disease. Within this context, it is important to recognize that the way in which the children are approached psychologically may have profound impact on the outcome of therapy.

Historically the psychological evaluation of children and adults with chronic disease has been guided by contemporary theoretical formulations in psychology. For example, the theories of psychosomatic medicine were largely derived from traditional notions of psychodynamic theory (Alexander, 1950). These approaches to the patient were based on psychological assessment of deviancy of the individual, which deviancy was felt to be responsible for the maladaptive behavioral patterns identified.

Under such circumstances the child experiencing difficulty in reaction to chronic disease was seen as an individual with potentially significant psychopathology. Treatment was derived from this perception, typically involving remediation of the underlying psychopathological condition.

It is appropriate to consider another more parsimonious alternative: that the child who suffers from chronic disease should first be considered as a normal individual. Such an assumption suggests that a normal individual placed in a chronically altered learning environment in which aspects of illness and dependency are reinforced may develop behaviors consistent with that environment. Such a normalcy notion (Russo & Varni, 1982) is reflected in Stein and Jessop's (1982) elucidation of a noncategorical approach to chronic disease. Stein and Jessop proposed that individuals with chronic disease be looked at in terms of the burden that the chronic disease inflicts upon the child, as opposed to the disease itself. They suggest that such non-categorical formulation will allow assessment of psychological impact and potential remediation based upon the burden of the disease.

These notions are further supported when one reviews existing studies of the impact of chronic disease on the psychological adjustment of children. When reviewing studies in this area, it is important to consider not only the population under study, but also the theoretical view of those conducting the study, and in addition, the rigor of the assessment methodology provided. Varni (1983) suggests that when these studies are considered as a whole, those employing more subjective clinical impression and projective assessment have posited increased probability of psychological disturbance as a result of chronic disease. On the other hand, those studies which have been based on more objective measures of function have documented lesser instances of psychopathology. For example, Zeltzer, Kellerman, Ellenberg, Dash and Rigler (1980), in their study of adolescents with four different chronic diseases, suggest that the chronic disease population exhibits psychopathology at a rate consistent with the population as a whole.

Pelcovits (1983), in studying the psychological adaptation of adolescents with heart disease, likewise suggests that these children are similar to matched controls seen in an outpatient clinic for nonspecific problems. Her study is notable in that it included a large number of measures of social function and self-perception. Koocher (1983) underscores these notions by suggesting that the process of adaptation to chronic disease is likely to produce periodic conflict in the developing child. When viewed from this perspective, it is clear that while the conflicts exist and that certain diseases will produce problems to the developing child at different periods, the attempt at the solution of conflict is an appropriate focus for psychological study and intervention.

This does not mean that severe psychopathology does not exist in this population or that, for some children, the process of learning in chronic disease will not produce markedly aberrant behavior. It merely suggests that as a default mode, we should assume that children do not, a priori, have psychological problems. The process of the development of such problems may be tied to the process of treatment, coping, and chronicity itself.

What the above rationale suggests is that the child with chronic disease may best be viewed psychologically under two primary dimensions: chronicity and normalcy. Chronicity suggests that, in the evaluation of the burden of chronic disease on children, attention be focussed on the alterations in behavior produced by symptom expression, the behavior of others in the environment, and the alterations in social and environmental contingencies. It suggests, most importantly, that management be based on the normalization of those characteristics of behavior and by the imposition of appropriate contingencies. The concept of normalcy supports this idea. If the child with chronic disease is viewed as a basically normal learner, it follows that the individual may be taught altered patterns of behavior which should allow for increased adaptation, coping, and overall function.

Under this approach adaption and maladaption are looked at in the framework of current context of care and the disease process, as opposed to being indicative of some underlying pathology. This perception of patient and process is likely to have many advantages. First, it is likely to bring into sync treatments for medical and psychological manifestations of chronic disease. Under assumptions of chronicity and normalcy, disease management requires alteration of behavior and environment within the context of care, as opposed to the utilization of the extracontextual methods of traditional psychological treatment. Secondly, it suggests that the time-frame of change may well fit within current medical management efforts. Under these circumstances, the child who, for example, is noncompliant may be trained in adherence strategies within the context of his or her ongoing medical care. Additionally fears or anxiety arising from medical treatment may likewise be treated with those issues proposed to have caused them: namely, the medical procedures themselves. Most importantly, viewing the child as an active, developing, and capable learner provides benefit in psychological adaptation. Control of the process of the disease and the process of care may therefore be perceived by the child to be within his or her ability to manage significantly. Under this set of assumptions, the child with chronic disease can assume control over certain aspects of disease or care, thereby increasing his or her mastery of the environment and perception of control over at least some aspects of the disease process.

Such a changed view of the patient provides not only for improving congruency between psychological and medical care and in improving patient perception of control, but, additionally, suggests that ongoing psychological care should focus on the reduction of the iatrogenic effects of the disease and of medical treatment, as opposed to the remediation of underlying pathology. Such a base calls for collaborative endeavor between psychologically oriented practitioners and medicine, allowing for continued and ongoing management of both disease and chronicity.

FUTURE AREAS FOR PSYCHOLOGICAL ASSESSMENT OF THE EFFECTS OF CHRONICITY

With these factors in mind, the assessment of the impact of chronicity on children becomes a primary area of psychological intervention. As such it allows the phrasing of a number of questions for future inquiry. Foremost among these is the potential value of the noncategorical/normalcy based approach in management of the child with chronic disease. Such an approach has a number of advantages, since it allows specific research aimed at separating the generic effects of chronicity from those of specific diseases. As Russo and Varni (1982) and Stein and Jessop (1982) suggest, generic factors related to the burden of chronic disease may have profound impact over and above the specifics of individual disease. Clear understanding needs to be formulated of the impact of chronic disease upon development, learning, and behavior. At the present time, few studies exist in this area and it would appear logical that this would comprise an area of value in future research.

Bibace and his colleagues (Bibace & Walsh, 1980) conducted a series of studies regarding the perceptions of illness among normal children at varying developmental levels. They find, as with most other factors, that knowledge and explanation of disease tends to be consistent with the level of cognitive development of the individual. These studies, while informative, have traditionally been conducted with normal populations. Studies do exist evaluating the impact of chronic disease and development on the knowledge of children with chronic disease (Neuhauser, Amsterdam, Hines & Steward, 1978). These studies, however, have treated knowledge within the framework of a singular disease. We do not know, for example, whether a given child's knowledge of his or her own disease process influences the ability to cope with and adapt to that disease process. Sergis-Deavenport and Varni (1983) have demonstrated that in the case of adherence to self-infusion in children with hemophilia, knowledge is an essential first step to adequate self care. They further suggest that many children do not have sufficient knowledge to produce adequate compliance with regimen. By breaking the process of disease management into discrete components, such as knowledge, behavior, developmental impact, new research may be generated to facilitate both the understanding and the management of the child with chronic disease.

Adherence is largely a psychological phenomenon. That is, adherence is likely to be determined by the knowledge, belief set, motivation, and behavior of the individual, rather than by the disease process itself. Therefore, it is well within the purview of psychological study. Studies are required which assess the interrelationship among these dimensions in the production of patient difficulties. We at present know little as to whether the compliance is mediated by belief, by parent contingency management, by developmental level, by understanding of the disease process, or by simple operant processes such as reinforcement. Further research is clearly indicated to assess the parameters of compliance in children. Such research should involve not only the development of an understanding of the relationship between adherence and child development, but also the evaluation of methodologies by which improved adherence may be facilitated. In this regard, a primary strategy would be to evaluate the potential of a "train for compliance model," in which children, at the early stages of chronic disease, were taught via specific behavioral mechanisms to comply with adherence prescriptions in the area of medication, diet, and activity. Early training in adherence so that habitual patterns might be developed may well facilitate chronic disease management from a medical perspective. For example, the diabetic child trained at an early age to comply carefully might well experience significant reduction in symptom burden as a result of these behaviors.

A second area for the application of psychological assessment is terminal care. Traditional formulations of terminal care have typically involved the development of a relationship between the psychological care giver and the patient of a warm, trusting, and supportive nature (Kubler-Ross, 1975). These formulations ignore the essential behavioral realities that children must cope with increasing anxieties, frustrations, and significant alterations in family and peer relationships in the terminal phases of disease. Spirito, Russo and Masek (1984) have outlined a behavioral approach to terminal care in the cystic fibrosis patient. They argue that the terminal phase of illness represents a period in the child's life for which behavioral strategies may have a profound impact in assisting the child to cope with decreased function, increased symptomatology, and the extreme anxiety around symptom episodes. While terminal care represents a difficult and sensitive area for psychological work, it is likely that psychological intervention during this time may well reduce patient anxiety, may well reduce the appearance of stress-related symptomatology, and may improve patient/family interaction patterns (Koocher, 1983).

A third area of study dictated by the notions of chronicity and normalcy is the assessment of placebo effect in health care. For many years, the placebo effect was a little studied phenomenon in medicine (Kanigel, 1983). Studies of the placebo effect as a specific psychological phenomenon are required. Such studies may lead to the improved understanding of the role of belief and knowledge in symptom management and disease exacerbation. Under such circumstances psychological understanding of the placebo effect may allow manipulation of belief variables to reduce symptom burden and decrease patient anxiety.

The areas outlined previously—a noncategorical approach to childhood disease; improved studies of adherence; improved understanding of the relationship between child development, behavior, and illness; behavioral methods in terminal care; and studies of the placebo effect—all represent questions which may be directly phrased from the view of the chronically ill child as a normal individual under chronically altered learning environment. The purpose of this chapter has been to suggest that such a view should be paramount in the production of efficacious research. Russo and Newsom (1982) have suggested that traditional theory-based psychological approaches have provided little in the way of empirically verifiable successes in treatment of traditional psychological disorders. In light of Schwartz's (1982) call for the extension and improvement of research paradigms in health to consider contextual variables and multiple factors in disease development, exacerbation, and maintenance, this finding might profitably be extended to the child with chronic disease. Arguably, the development of treatments for the child with chronic disease should follow from an inductive/constructive approach in which an attempt is made to separate the psychological impact of chronic disease from its physical manifestations. Assessment of the learning characteristics, development, and finally the interaction of the child with his or her world and disease are required to accomplish such an undertaking.

REFERENCES

Ader, R. (1971). Experimentally induced gastric lesions. *Advances in Psychosomatic Medicine, 6,* 1–39.

Alexander, F.G. (1950). *Psychosomatic medicine: Its principles and application.* New York: Norton.

Anderson, D.E. & Brady, J.V. (1979). Experimental analysis of psychosomatic interactions: behavioral influences upon physiological regulations. In R.S. Davidson (Ed.), *Modification of pathological behavior* (pp. 198–231). New York: Gardner.

Bibace, R. & Walsh, M.E. (1980). Development of children's conceptions of illness. *Pediatrics, 66,* 912–917.

Cataldo, M.F., & Russo, D.C. (1979). Developmentally disabled in the community: behavioral/medical considerations. In L.A. Hamerlynck (Ed.), *Behavioral systems for the developmentally disabled: II institutional, clinic, and community environments* (pp. 105–143). New York: Brunner/Mazel.

Cataldo, M.F., Russo, D.C., Bird, B.L., & Varni, J.W. (1980). Assessment and management of chronic disorders. In J. Ferguson & C.B. Taylor (Eds.), *Comprehensive handbook of behavioral medicine: Extended applications and issues* (Vol. 3, pp. 76–95). New York: Spectrum.

Dubos, R. *Man adapting.* (1965). New Haven, CT: Yale University Press.

Engel, G.L. (1977). The need for a new medical model: A challenge for biomedicine. *Science, 196,* 129–136.

Freud, S. (1905). Psychological (mental) treatment. In *The complete psychological works of Sigmund Freud.* Vol. 7, 1953. London: Hogarth.

Haggerty, R.J., Roghman, K.J., & Pless, I.B. (1975). *Child health and community.* New York: Wiley.

Kanigel, R. (1983, August). Magic medicine: The placebo. *Johns Hopkins Magazine,* 12–16.

Kenney, T.J. & Clemmens, R.L. (1975). *Behavioral pediatrics and child development.* Baltimore: William & Wilkins.

Koocher, G.P. (1983). Promoting coping with illness in childhood. Paper presented at the Vermont Conference on the Primary Prevention of Psychopathology.

Kubler-Ross, E. (1975). *Death: The final stage of growth.* Englewood Cliffs, NJ: Prentice-Hall.

Leigh, H., & Reiser, M.F. (1980). *The patient biological, psychological and social dimensions of medical practice.* New York: Plenum.

Levine, J.D., Gordon, N.C., & Fields, H.L. (1978). The mechanisms of placebo analgesia. *Lancet, 8091(2),* 654–657.

Melamed, B.G. (1977). Psychological preparation for hospitalization. In S. Rachman (Ed.), *Contributions to medical psychology* (Vol. I). New York: Pergamon.

Neuhauser, C., Amsterdam, B., Hines, P., & Steward, M. (1978). Children's concepts of healing: cognitive development and locus of control factors. *American Journal of Orthopsychiatry, 48,* 334–341.

Pelcovits, M. (1983). Emotional and interpersonal adjustment in adolescents with congenital heart disease. Unpublished doctoral dissertation. State University of New York at Stony Brook.

Pepper, S.C. (1942). *World hypotheses.* Berkeley: University of California Press.

Russo, D.C., Bennett, A.K., Harmon, W.E., & Brown, D. (1981). Behavioral medicine issues in the management of children with end-stage renal disease. *Behavioral Medicine Update, 3,* 15–19.

Russo, D.C., & Newsom, C.D. (1982). Psychotic disorders of childhood. In J. Lachenmeyer & M. Gibbs (Eds.), *Psychopathology in childhood* (pp. 120–154). New York: Gardner.

Russo, D.C., & Varni, J.W. (1982). *Behavioral pediatrics: research and practice.* New York: Plenum.

Schwartz, G.E. (1982). Testing the biopsychosocial model: The ultimate challenge facing behavioral medicine? *Journal of Consulting and Clinical Psychology, 50,* 1040–1053.

Schwartz, G.E., & Weiss, S.M. (1978). Yale conference on behavioral medicine: A proposed definition and statement of goals. *Journal of Behavioral Medicine, 1,* 3–12.

Sergis-Deavenport, E. & Varni, J.W. (1983). Behavioral assessment and management of adherence to factor replacement therapy in hemophilia. *Journal of Pediatric Psychology, 8,* 367–377.

Spirito, A., Russo, D.C., & Masek, B.J. (1984). Behavioral interventions and stress management training for hospitalized adolescents and young adults with cystic fibrosis. *General Hospital Psychiatry, 6,* 211–218.

Starfield, B., & Pless, I.B. (1980). Physical health. In O.G. Brim, Jr, & J. Kagan (Eds.), *Constancy and change in human development* (pp. 272–324). Cambridge: Harvard University Press.

Stein, R.E.K., & Jessop, D.J. (1982). A noncategorical approach to chronic childhood illness. *Public Health Reports, 97,* 354–362.

Varni, J.W. (1983). *Clinical behavioral pediatrics: An interdisciplinary biobehavioral approach.* New York: Pergamon.

Zeltzer, L., Kellerman, J., Ellenberg, L., Dash, J., & Rigler, D. (1980). Psychological effects of illness in adolescence II. Impact of illness on adolescents' crucial issues and coping styles. *Journal of Pediatrics, 97,* 132–138.

23

Pediatric Gastrointestinal Disorders

WILLIAM E. WHITEHEAD

INTRODUCTION

Table 23.1 lists the most common pediatric gastrointestinal disorders and gives estimates of their prevalence. There are three striking aspects to this table: (1) Gastrointestinal disorders are very common; they affect 10 to 15 percent of children. (2) Psychological factors—learning, stress, psychopathology—are believed to play a role in the etiology or course of all these disorders. (3) With the exception of peptic ulcer disease, none of these disorders is very effectively managed with drugs or surgery.

These data indicate that there is a major need for behavioral treatments of pediatric gastrointestinal disorders. Unfortunately this need is not now being met. There is very little research on the behavioral treatment of these

Preparation of this manuscript was supported in part by Research Career Development Award MH00133 from the National Institute of Mental Health.

TABLE 23.1. PEDIATRIC GASTROINTESTINAL DISORDERS

Disorder	Prevalence	Reference
Rumination syndrome	6–10% retarded	Ball, Hendricksen & Clayton, 1974; Singh, 1981
Peptic ulcer disease	.04%	Sultz, Schlesinger, Feldman & Mosher, 1970
Recurrent abdominal pain	11–18%	Apley & Naish, 1958; Miller Court, Knox & Branden, 1974
Ulcerative colitis and Crohn's Disease	.01%	Mendeloff, 1975; Korelitz, 1982
Fecal incontinence Overflow/incontinence	1.5% at 7–8 yrs	Schaeffer, 1979
Incompetent sphincter	60% myelo-meningocele	Lorber, 1971
Imperforate anus	Unknown	

disorders, and neither psychologists nor pediatricians are normally trained to use the techniques which have been developed.

The purpose of this chapter is to summarize the psychophysiological mechanism for symptom development in these disorders and to describe the treatment outcome research which is available. Areas where additional research is most needed will also be identified.

RUMINATION SYNDROME

Rumination syndrome refers to the voluntary regurgitation of previously ingested food into the mouth where it may be rechewed and either reswallowed or spit out. It is a form of self-stimulation which is very common in retarded individuals (see Table 23.1), but it also occurs in children and adults of normal intelligence (Kanner, 1936).

Johnson (1980) investigated the mechanism of the regurgitation which precedes rumination in adults and found it to be a voluntary response sequence. In most cases the patient stimulates the palate with a finger or tongue to elicit a gag reflex, which opens the upper esophageal sphincter. In all instances there is a brisk contraction of the striated abdominus rectus muscles to force the stomach contents up the esophagus and into the mouth. Regurgitation occurs in a controlled fashion which ordinarily results in no loss of vomitus from the mouth.

Several observations suggest that rumination is a form of self-stimulation engaged in because it brings pleasure. The adult ruminators described by Kanner (1936) sometimes reported that rumination first occurred unintentionally (e.g., when bending over after a large meal) but that the action was pleasurable and came to be repeated with increasing skill and increasing frequency. In children (Richmond, Eddy, & Green, 1958), rumination often coexists with other self-stimulatory behaviors, such as head-banging and genital play. Sometimes the behavior can be interrupted by distracting the child.

Unlike most bad habits, however, rumination can be life-threatening. It can become so absorbing that the child seems oblivious to other stimuli, and rumination may preempt eating in some children (Lang & Melamed, 1969). From 15 percent (Kanner, 1972) to 20 percent (Einhorn, 1972) of ruminating children die as a result of malnutrition, dehydration, or aspiration of vomitus into their lungs.

There are two common hypotheses about the psychological mechanism for the etiology of rumination syndrome, and each is associated with an apparently successful behavioral treatment.

One hypothesis, termed the maternal deprivation hypothesis, is that rumination syndrome results from separations from the mother early in life or from inappropriate behaviors on the part of the mother. In support of this hypothesis, rumination syndrome is more common in institutionalized children and in children who have been hospitalized for the first few weeks of life because of medical complications at birth than it is for other children. Einhorn (1972) has described the mothers of ruminating infants as impoverished, often unmarried women who are emotionally immature and sometimes mentally ill. They are observed to hold their infants infrequently and to hold them at arms' length facing away from them (to avoid having their clothes soiled) when they do hold them. Thus, there is strong support for the maternal deprivation hypothesis.

The treatment following logically from the maternal deprivation hypothesis is increased mothering. This is usually operationalized as increased holding of the infant, especially at mealtimes, by a mother substitute. The holding is done regardless of whether the infant regurgitates. A total of 22 case studies (Whitehead & Schuster, 1985) have been published in which ruminating children were treated in this fashion. Fifteen of the patients (68 percent) ceased ruminating, and an additional four patients (18 percent) showed at least a 75 percent reduction in frequency. Nine of the eleven patients (82%) for whom follow-up of six months or longer was reported continued not to vomit. This simple approach appeared to be effective. It produced no adverse side-effects and was easy to teach to parents.

The alternative theory of the etiology of rumination syndrome is that this behavior is an operant response which is learned and maintained because it is reinforced with increased attention from adults (Cunningham & Linscheid, 1976; Sheinbein, 1975; Toister, Condron, Worley, & Arthur, 1975). This operant hypothesis is not necessarily incompatible with the maternal deprivation hypothesis, but it does suggest a different approach to treatment—namely, punishment. In 12 published case studies (Whitehead & Schuster, 1985) regurgitation was punished with electric shock to the leg or other parts of the body. This resulted in elimination of the regurgitation in seven cases (58 percent) and at least a 75 percent reduction in frequency in the remaining five. Results were well-maintained in four of six patients for whom follow-up of at least six months was reported. However, in one case the patient was noted to increase the frequency of other self-stimulatory behaviors.

In 11 cases, regurgitation was punished by injecting lemon juice or tabasco sauce into the child's mouth or by brushing the child's teeth with an astringent (Listerine). This approach seemed particularly promising because of animal research suggesting that gustatory stimuli are readily associated with gastrointestinal responses (Garcia, Hankins, & Rusiniak, 1974). However, only 3 of 11 patients (27 percent) ceased ruminating while an additional 7 showed a 75 percent reduction in frequency. Recurrences of vomiting were noted in two of the six children who had follow-up of at least six months, and two showed increases in other self-stimulatory behaviors as rumination decreased.

The most effective, and the least ethically objectionable, of the punishment procedures was time out from positive reinforcement. This consisted of placing the child in social isolation (that is, alone in a room or in a chair turned to the wall) for 3 to 10 minutes (depending on age) immediately after regurgitation occurred. Four of five children treated in this manner ceased ruminating, and the other child showed at least a 75 percent reduction in frequency. These results were well maintained in three of the four children for whom follow-up of at least six months was available. No adverse side-effects have been reported.

Reviews and evaluations of the published case studies (Davis & Cuvo, 1980; Whitehead & Schuster, 1985) strongly support the efficacy of two types of behavioral interventions for children with rumination syndrome: noncontingent holding at mealtimes and punishment of regurgitation. However, there are no controlled experiments demonstrating the efficacy of either technique, and case studies are known to overestimate the efficacy of therapies by selectively reporting successful cases. They may also underestimate the frequency of undesirable side effects, such as increases in other self-stimulatory behaviors. Controlled studies comparing holding and punishment with an untreated control group are urgently needed, as are studies which identify the characteristics of patients which predict to which treatment they are most likely to respond. However, the available data warrant the following tentative conclusions:

1. In infants and young children whose history suggests an interruption of the mother-infant relationship, holding should be the first treatment tried. It is effective in approximately 80 percent of cases; it

involves no risks, and it will begin to have an effect within about four days if it is going to work at all.

2. In children who seem to receive normal amounts of holding and in children who fail to respond to holding, punishment should be tried.

3. The most effective and least ethically objectionable punishment procedure is contingent time out from social interaction. However, time out may require a few weeks to be effective. If the child's medical status requires immediate control of rumination, electric shock may be the treatment of choice. Punishment with aversive tastes is not recommended.

PEPTIC ULCER DISEASE

Peptic ulcer disease, which was once thought to be rare in children, is now recognized to have a prevalence of approximately 3.6 per 100,000 in the United States (Sultz, Schlesinger, Feldman, & Mosher, 1970). Approximately two-thirds of these cases are primary ulcers, the rest being attributable to trauma or drug reactions (Deckelbaum, Roy, Lussier-Lazaroff, & Morin, 1974; Seagram, Stephens, & Cumming, 1973). As in adults, primary ulcers occur in the duodenum in three-fourths of instances, and ulcers are 2.5 to 4 times as common in males as in females.

The clinical presentation of peptic ulceration is different for children than for adults. The first symptoms noted in preadolescents are usually vomiting or bleeding from the gastrointestinal tract (Deckelbaum et al., 1974; Roy & Silverman, 1980). Abdominal pain is common but is not usually described in the manner typical of adults: Adults report epigastric or mid-abdominal pain which is related to meals and relieved by antacids or eating and which tends to awaken them at night. Infants and children up to age 3 years are unable to report pain, although they may display distress in the form of crying after meals. Preadolescents may give vague reports of abdominal pain.

Estimates of the age of onset of peptic ulcers in children suggest that the incidence of secondary (stress) ulcers is about equally distributed, across age groups but primary ulcers show increasing frequency with increasing age. There is also an age-related difference in the type of ulcers seen; in children younger than 7 years, primary ulcers are usually gastric, whereas duodenal ulcers predominate in the older age groups.

Children with primary duodenal ulcers (but not gastric ulcers) show a strong family history of ulcer disease, suggesting a genetic predisposition for the disorder. Deckelbaum et al. (1974) found a family history of peptic ulcer in 28 percent of children with duodenal ulcer, and Seagrams, Stephens, and Cumming (1973) found a family history of ulcers in 35 percent.

The pathophysiological mechanism for peptic ulcer development appears to be similar to that of adults. Christie and Ament (1976) reported that maximal gastric acid secretion and peak acid output were significantly greater in children with active duodenal ulcer disease than in children without duodenal ulcer, and Mohammed, Hearnes, and Crean (1982) found these rates to be comparable to those of adults with duodenal ulcer and greater than adults without ulcers.

There is, unfortunately, very little data on the psychological characteristics of children with peptic ulcer diseaes. Robb, Thomas, Orszulok, and Odling-Smee (1972) reported on the basis of uncontrolled interviews that 61 percent of male children and 50 percent of female children with duodenal ulcer "were living in a stress situation," but they did not characterize these children psychologically. Christodoulou, Gargoulas, Papaloukas, Marinopoulou, and Rabavilas (1979) reported a controlled study of psychoanalytic hypotheses about peptic ulcer disease in children. They blindly interviewed the families of 30 children with peptic ulcer and 30 matched controls, and they administered a projective test (Rorschach), an intelligence test (Wechsler Intelligence Scale for Children), and an objective personality test. They found the ulcer group to be more introverted, shy, and submissive although they were not significantly more anxious. Significantly more of the ulcer patients had parents who were judged to be anxious and overprotective. Psychologically traumatic separations from parents were said to precede the onset of peptic ulcer disease in 11 of 30 patients, and school adjustment was less satisfactory for the ulcer patients. Ulcer patients were significantly less intelligent than the controls.

There is no published data on the psychological treatment of peptic ulcer disease in children. This is a significant omission, since the data of Deckelbaum et al. (1974) and Puri, Boyd, Blake, and Guiney (1978) show that two-thirds of children with primary ulcers have recurring problems. Nonsurgical management of these children has usually been unsuccessful, and about half require surgery to cut the vagal innervation to the stomach (Seagram et al., 1976).

RECURRENT ABDOMINAL PAIN

Recurrent abdominal pain (RAP) is the most common pediatric gastrointestinal disorder. It is defined by the presence of at least three discrete episodes of periumbilical pain severe enough to result in a change in activities over a period of at least three months (Apley, 1975). Using this definition, Apley and Naish (1958) found a prevalence of 10.8 percent in a study of 1000 randomly selected children aged 4 to 18 years. Other investigators, using less strict criteria for the diagnosis, have arrived at prevalence figures ranging from 14 to 18 percent (Miller, Court, Knox, & Branden, 1974; Oster, 1972; Pringle, Butler, & Davie, 1966). The prevalence is slightly greater in females (12 percent versus 10 percent, Apley & Naish, 1958). The incidence varies with age, rising until about age 9 and declining thereafter (Oster, 1972). However, long-term follow-up studies show that approximately a third of the children with RAP will have similar symptoms as adults, which will in most cases be diagnosed as irritable bowel syndrome (Apley & Hale, 1973; Christensen & Mortensen, 1975). This frequency is significantly greater than would be expected by chance.

The diagnosis of RAP is made only after alternative diseases have been excluded. However, only 7 percent to 10 percent of children with the symptoms defined by Apley (1975) are found to have an organic basis for their symptoms. The most frequent alternative diseases are urogenital disease, lactase deficiency (intolerance to milk), peptic ulcer, ulcerative colitis, and Crohn's disease. Lactase deficiency deserves special mention because of the belief that intolerance to milk accounts for a large percentage of cases of RAP. Liebman (1979), for example, found evidence for lactase deficiency in 11 of 38 children with RAP he examined and noted that 10 of the 11 had pain relief with a lactose-free diet. Liebman interpreted his data as suggesting that lactase deficiency contributes to the etiology of RAP. However, other investigators who have used control groups have found that the incidence of lactase deficiency is not significantly greater in children with RAP than in the general population and that a lactose-free diet produces clinical improvement no more often in patients with RAP who are lactase deficient than it does in patients with RAP who are not lactase deficient (Lebenthal, Rossi, Nord, & Branski, 1981; Wald, Chandra, Fisher, Gartner, & Zitelli, 1982). The explanation for the high frequency of "cures" with the lactose-free diet used by Liebman (1979) is that children with RAP are prone to show a strong placebo response to treatment.

The physiologic mechanism for the symptoms of RAP is not definitely known, but the symptoms appear to be due, at least in part, to disturbances in the motility of the distal bowel. Several authors note an association of the symptoms with constipation or diarrhea (Dimson, 1971; Stone & Barbero, 1970). Dimson reported that constipation was present in 22 percent of 306 children with RAP, and he suggested on the basis of physical findings of a tender sigmoid colon that colonic spasm was responsible for attacks of pain in the remaining children. Dimson's data show delayed bowel transit time in 91 percent of those with constipation and in 44 percent of the remaining children with RAP. Kopel, Kim, and Barbero (1967) demonstrated that these children show significantly greater amounts of motility in the distal bowel in response to parasympathetic drug stimulation than do normal children or children with ulcerative colitis.

Early investigators postulated an abnormally low threshold for pain or low pain tolerance, but recent studies do not confirm this (Apley, Haslam, & Tulloch, 1971; Feuerstein, Barr, Francoeur, Houle, & Rafman, 1982). Similarly, early reports of disturbed autonomic recovery from a stressor (measured as the rate of habituation of the pupillary response to light following painful ice water stimulation) (Rubin, Barbero, & Sibinga, 1967) have not been supported by recent studies (Feuerstein et al., 1982). Thus motility disturbances of the gastrointestinal tract appear to be more clearly implicated in the pathophysiology of RAP than other physiological parameters investigated.

Psychological investigations of children with RAP suggest that at least two-thirds of them exhibit significant psychopathology (Apley & Naish, 1958; Astrada, Licamele, Walsh, & Kessler, 1981; McKeith & O'Neill, 1951; Stone & Barbero, 1970). They are described as anxious, shy, perfectionistic children who worry excessively, and who have a high frequency of nocturnal enuresis, sleep disorders, and appetite difficulties. The beginning of pain episodes can be related to psychological stressors in the family or at school in most of these children (Apley & Naish, 1958; Rubin et al., 1967; Stone & Barbero, 1970). Miller and Kratochwill (1979) describe a case in which pain complaints were maintained by social reinforcement from the mother.

A striking feature of RAP is the strong family history of chronic pain syndromes, especially gastrointestinal pain. Stone and Barbero (1970) found that 50 percent of mothers had gastrointestinal symptoms described by their physicians as functional and 46 percent of fathers had gastrointestinal disorders. Oster (1972) compared the families of 185 children with RAP or headache for three consecutive years to families of 166 children with no pain for five years. He found that parents of children with chronic pain were significantly more likely to report that they had had chronic pains during childhood or currently had them than parents of children without chronic pain (24 percent versus 14 percent). The association was stronger for current parental pains than for prior pains and was stronger for pains of mothers than for pains of fathers. These data are usually interpreted as reflecting the contribution of learning via modeling rather than the contribution of heredity to the etiology of RAP.

The usual recommendation to pediatricians for treating RAP is to provide reassurance that there is no serious or life-threatening disease present and to explain the effects of emotional arousal on the symptoms. The long-term effects of such supportive psychotherapy have been evaluated in three studies. Apley and Hale (1973) compared 30 children treated 8 to 20 years earlier with another 30 children who were medically evaluated but not treated 8 to 20 years earlier. Patients were 15 to 28 years old when the follow-up evaluation was done. The number in each group who still had abdominal pain was nearly identical (12 in the treated group and 11 in the untreated group), and equal numbers denied abdominal pains but complained of other chronic symptoms, such as headaches (9 versus 10 patients). Supportive psychotherapy thus seemed to have no long-term benefit, although Apley and Hale felt that it resulted in more rapid symptom improvement for those who did improve.

Christensen and Mortensen (1975) reported 30-year follow-up for 34 patients treated with supportive psychotherapy. Eighteen of the 34 had suffered from recurrent abdominal pain as adults, of whom 16 had symptoms consistent with a diagnosis of irritable bowel syndrome and 7 had symptoms compatible with peptic ulcer disease (5 patients had symptoms of both ulcer and irritable bowel syndrome). The frequency of gastrointestinal disorders was significantly greater than for a control group who had not experienced recurrent abdominal pain as children. These data are consistent with those of Apley and Hale (1973) and imply that supportive psychotherapy did not have a significant impact on the long-term course of the disorder. However, there may be short-term benefits to supportive psychotherapy. Berger, Honig, and Liebman (1977) reported that counseling of the whole family resulted in symptom remission in 17 of 19 patients by the end of treatment. Some of these short-term benefits are due to a placebo response.

More elaborate treatment recommendations derived from a behavioral conceptualization of RAP have been offered by Michener (1981). He recommends: (1) Reassurance to the family and child that no serious disease is present. (2) Explanation of the effects of emotional arousal on the gastrointestinal tract. (3) Specific treatment of school avoidance if the symptoms have become the basis for avoiding school. (4) Extinction of somatic complaints by encouraging the family not to discuss the abdominal pain with the child and not to make the abdominal pain the basis for avoiding chores. Although there are no data on the outcome of such a comprehensive treatment program, Miller and Kratochwill (1979) describe a case study in which they used contingent time-out to eliminate symptoms of RAP in a child whose pain complaints appeared to be maintained by attention from her mother.

RAP represents a seriously understudied disorder of childhood. It is the most common somatic complaint in children, and there is suggestive evidence that social learning plays a major role in its etiology. However, there remain many unanswered questions about the interaction between psychological and biological variables, and there is almost no treatment outcome data to guide clinical practice.

INFLAMMATORY BOWEL DISEASE

Inflammatory bowel disease includes ulcerative colitis and Crohn's disease, two apparently related disorders which involve inflammatory changes in the walls of the intestine (Kirsher & Shorter, 1975). Ulcerative colitis, the more prevalent of the two, is restricted to the colon and rectum, and it is characterized by superficial ulcerations or polyps on the walls of the bowel. This disease produces symptoms of pain, rectal bleeding, and diarrhea; and it frequently progresses into colon cancer. Crohn's disease, the less frequent of the two inflammatory bowel diseases, may occur in any part of the gastrointestinal tract. It is characterized by inflammation under the mucosal lining and penetrating ulcers, and may result in abcesses or fistulous tracks to the bladder, skin, or other parts of the bowel. Crohn's disease rarely results in cancer, but scar tissue from the lesions may obstruct the bowel. Both ulcerative colitis and Crohn's disease frequently require removal of the colon and parts of the small intestine, leaving the patient with a colostomy or ileostomy.

The onset of inflammatory bowel disease is before the age of 21 for more than half of the patients with ulcerative colitis and Crohn's disease. These diseases appear to be more virulent in children than in adults. There is a greater need for surgery and a higher mortality rate (Korelitz, 1982). Besides mutilating surgery, these diseases frequently cause growth retardation. Korelitz (1982) attributes the psychological changes frequently seen in patients with inflammatory bowel disease to the occurrence of these physical disfigurements during adolescence.

There are no studies available specifically on the psychological characteristics of children with inflammatory bowel disease, but studies of older patients characterize them as shy, socially conforming individuals who are dependent on others and who are especially distressed by real or imagined separations from those on whom they are dependent (Engel, 1973; Hislop, 1974). Studies using the MMPI find elevations on the scales for hypochondriasis, depression, and hysteria, with normal scores on other scales (Ford, Glober, & Castelnuovo-Tedesco, 1969; Fullerton, Kollar, & Caldwell, 1962; McMahon, Schmitt, Patterson, & Rothman, 1973; West, 1970). This profile is shared by many other patients with chronic diseases or psychosomatic disorders and may represent a reaction to the disease. When patients with inflammatory bowel disease are compared to patients with irritable bowel syndrome, a more benign disorder, they show less severe psychopathology than the patients with irritable bowel disorder (Esler & Goulston, 1973). Patients with inflamatory bowel disease do not report that more stressful events happen to them than to people in general (Fava & Pavan, 1976/77; Mendeloff, Monk, Siegel, & Lilienfeld, 1970).

The available studies on the psychological characteristics of adults with inflamatory bowel disease suggest that they exhibit relatively mild psychopathology which could reasonably be explained as a reaction to their chronic physical disease. However, the objective studies have been criticized on the grounds that shy, conformist patients are unlikely to reveal the extent of their psychological distress to relative strangers. The benefits which have been reported for these patients when supportive psychotherapy is offered suggest that there is some truth to the belief that psychological stressors can precipitate exacerbations of these diseases.

Grace, Pinsky, and Wolff (1954) reported a controlled study in which 34 patients treated with "superficial psychotherapy" were compared with 34 patients matched for age and severity of illness who were treated with medications, diet, and antibiotics. The psychotherapy encouraged a dependent relationship on the therapist and aimed to alleviate stress through advice to patients. At follow-up a minimum of two years later, a larger proportion of the psychotherapy group were symptomatically improved (65 percent versus 32 percent), fewer had been hospitalized (47 percent versus 71 percent), fewer had received ileostomies (3 versus 10), and fewer had died (3 versus 6). Similarly favorable results were reported in uncontrolled studies by Groen and Bastiaans (1951) and Karush, Daniels & Flood, and O'Connor (1977).

There have been no reports of behavioral treatments for inflammatory bowel disease other than a series of four case studies treated successfully with autogenic training (Degossely, Koninckx, & Lenfant, 1975). Given the favorable results achieved with supportive psychotherapy, one could speculate that stress management training might produce comparable benefits at less cost. Stress management training might be easier to provide to children than psychotherapy.

Fecal Incontinence

Continence depends on a learned response which is under stimulus control (Whitehead, Orr, Engel, & Schuster, 1981). As stool moves into the rectum, it stimulates stretch receptors which give rise to a sense of urgency. This urgency is the cue (discriminative stimulus) to do two things: to immediately contract the external anal sphincter in order to prevent a bowel movement, and to look for a toilet. The requirements for continence can be inferred to be as follows:

1. Ability to perceive rectal distension.
2. Rectal compliance—the ability to store enough stool in the rectum to permit the child to reach the toilet.
3. Ability to contract the external sphincter with enough force to postpone a bowel movement.
4. Motivation to remain continent.
5. History of relevant learning.

Fecal incontinence can result from a deficit in any of these areas. When evaluating a child with fecal soiling, it is useful to do a behavioral and physiological analysis which considers each component, and not to rely on the classification of the problem as either functional (encopresis) or organic. There are many children (e.g., those with spina bifida) who have deficits in several areas, and appropriate treatment recommendations can be made only after evaluating each area.

Overflow Incontinence

The most prevalent type of fecal incontinence in children is overflow incontinence (Table 23.1). This is the type which occurs when the rectum becomes impacted with hard stool, causing a reflex dilation of the anal canal that permits small amounts of stool and liquid to leak out (Lowery, Srour, Whitehead, & Schuster, 1985). Fecal impaction also contributes to incontinence by reducing the child's ability to perceive the movement of additional stool into the rectum.

The cause of the fecal impaction in overflow incontinence is disputed. Some authors have pointed out that overflow incontinence is associated with other behavioral problems (Bemporad, Kresch, Asnes, & Wilson, 1978; Levine & Bakow, 1976), and have argued that this is a psychogenic disorder. However, other investigators argue that a congenital tendency toward constipation is the cause and that any behavioral disturbances are the result of social consequences for previous incontinence. The evidence for this somatopsychic point of view is (1) approximately 95 percent of children with incontinence who are neurologically normal have a fecal impaction, (2) parents often report a history of constipation dating from birth and preceding the recognition of incontinence, (3) more than half of encopretic children have a family history of constipation, (4) overflow incontinence can be effectively treated by a bowel training regimen without attending to psychological causes, and (5) problem behaviors frequently disappear spontaneously when the incontinence has been treated successfully.

Similar habit training procedures for the treatment of encopresis appear to have been developed independently by several people (Christophersen & Rainey, 1976; Schuster, 1977; Wright, 1975; Young, 1973). These treatment programs are based on bowel training regimens used in spinal-cord injured patients (White et al., 1972). The essential elements of the programs are as follows:

1. Begin by disimpacting the child's bowel with an enema or suppository.
2. Have the child attempt a bowel movement at the same time each day, preferably after a meal. The intent is to take advantage of the tendency for the bowel to be more active after a meal and to condition colonic evacuation to the meal stimulus.
3. Use an enema or suppository to produce a bowel movement if none occurs naturally for two days. The purpose is to prevent fecal impaction.
4. Laxatives, mineral oil, or stool softeners may be given if needed to facilitate bowel movements in the early stages of treatment.
5. Rewards in the form of prizes or special privileges may be provided for bowel movements in the toilet and/or for days without soiling.

Young (1973) reported that such a habit-training program was successful (success criterion unspecified) for 22 of 24 children treated; and that at follow-up an average of 29 months later, there were recurrences in only four children. Lowery et al. (1985) reported that 83 percent of the children showed substantial clinical improvements, consisting of continence in 60 percent and staining only in 23 percent. At follow-up an average of three years later, 51 percent were continent and 10 percent had staining only. In the only other large series of patients, Levine and Bakow (1976) reported that a combination of family counselling and habit training resulted in continence for 51 percent and in marked improvement for another 27 percent.

Several case studies have appeared in which encopresis was treated by rewarding self-initiated bowel movements and/or punishing soiling (Doleys & Arnold, 1975; Edelman, 1971; Keehn, 1965; Neale, 1963). These reports suggest that contingency management requires longer to be effective and is less consistent in its outcome than habit training. Habit training is now regarded as the treatment of choice for encopresis.

Sensory-Motor Incontinence

In our bowel control program neurological injuries or birth defects are the most common causes in children of sensory-motor incontinence, that is, incontinence due to reduced ability to perceive rectal distension and/or reduced ability to contract the external anal sphincter. Myelomeningocele, the most severe form of spina bifida, is assocaited with weak sphincter muscles in all cases and with gross fecal incontinence in at least 30 percent. Trauma or anorectal surgery (for example, for imperforate anus) may also lead to impaired sphincter function.

Biofeedback procedures for the treatment of sensory-motor fecal incontinence were first reported for adults by Engel, Nikoomanesh, and Schuster (1974). These investigators inserted a tube into the rectum which contained a balloon for distending the rectum and separate balloons to record contraction and relaxation of the internal anal sphincters. Patients watched a polygraph recording of external sphincter contractions and were taught to squeeze the external sphincter in response to rectal distension. Between biweekly biofeedback training sessions, the patient was instructed to exercise the sphincter by squeezing it approximately 50 times per day.

The biofeedback procedure described by Engel et al. (1974) can be modified to emphasize teaching the patient to discriminate weak distensions of the rectum when incontinence is due primarily to sensory loss, or to emphasize teaching the patient to augment the strength of sphincter contractions when incontinence is due primarily to weak sphincter muscles (Whitehead, Parker, Masek, Cataldo, & Freeman, 1981).

Studies of biofeedback training in adults have consistently found that 70 to 80 percent of patients with sensory-motor incontinence can be made continent or substantially improved with three to four biofeedback training sessions (Cerulli, Nikoomanesh, & Schuster, 1979; Engel et al., 1974; Wald, 1981a). Similar results were reported for children, including those with imperforate anus (Olness, McParland, & Piper, 1980).

Children with fecal incontinence secondary to myelomeningocle have been a more difficult group to help. Wald (1981b) reported a study of 14 children with myelomeningocele of whom 6 were not treated because their rectal sensation was too poor. In the group of 8 who were given biofeedback training, 4 (50%) showed elimination of soiling or at least a 75 percent decrease in frequency. Whitehead, Parker et al. (1981) found normal rectal sensation in 7 of 8 children tested and provided biofeedback to all of them. Four of the 8 became continent, and another two showed more than a 50 percent reduction in frequency. In follow-up studies, Wald (1983) reported that 7 of 15 children with myelomeningocele showed substantial clinical improvements, and Whitehead, Parker, Bosmajian, Morrill-Corbin, Middaugh, Garwood, Cataldo, and Freeman (in press) reported that 65 percent of 23 patients were substantially improved, including 30 percent who were continent. Whitehead et al. (in press) noted that most children with spina bifida have a fecal impaction as well as weak sphincters and have never been taught to defecate in the toilet; they therefore recommend a two-stage training procedure, beginning with a habit-training regimen like that for overflow incontinence and ending with biofeedback training.

The biofeedback procedure described by Engel et al. (1974), which employs a set of three rectal balloons, has certain disadvantages when used with children; the equipment is expensive, and the feedback provided from looking at a polygraph tracings is so complex that young children do not attend well to the task. MacLeod (1979, 1983) has described an EMG biofeedback procedure which appears to overcome some of these difficulties. MacLeod inserts a small, plastic plug which contains metal rings into the anal canal. These rings pick up the EMG activity from the sphincter muscles, and this activity is amplified and displayed to the patient as a meter reading or variable pitched tone by an EMG biofeedback unit. MacLeod (1983) reported that 74 percent of adult patients treated in this fashion became continent or substantially improved, but no children were included. The relative value for EMG biofeedback versus balloon biofeedback and the different indications for the two have not been studied. However, biofeedback to retrain external sphincter contractions is the treatment of choice for sensory-motor fecal incontinence.

Incontinence Due to Poor Rectal Compliance

Children with ulcerative colitis or imperforate anus sometimes present with a type of incontinence which is due to reduced compliance of the rectum. This may be due to inflamation, tonic contraction, or the development of scar tissue around the rectum as a result of disease in the children with ulcerative colitis or as a result of surgery in the case of children with imperforate anus. Reduced compliance contributes to incontinence in two ways: It reduces the storage capacity of the bowel so that fecal material passes through rapidly leaving little time for the patient to reach the toilet. Reduced compliance may also make it painful for the child to tolerate any fecal material in the rectum, so that immediate defecation occurs as an escape from pain.

There is no behavioral technique for increasing rectal compliance. However, it is sometimes possible to improve bowel control by encouraging the child to use a stool softener so that stools are less painful.

SUMMARY AND CONCLUSIONS

1. From 10 to 20 percent of children aged 5 to 18 have gastrointestinal complaints caused or exacerbated by psychological stressors.

2. With the exceptions of rumination syndrome and fecal incontinence, little is known about the treatment of these prevalent childhood disorders. For example, there are only three treatment-outcome studies dealing with recurrent abdominal pain even though this disorder affects 11 to 18 percent of children.

3. Behavioral treatments are accepted as the treatment of choice for rumination syndrome, encopresis due to constipation, and fecal incontinence secondary to neurological injury with sensory-motor impairment.

4. Behavioral investigations of the physiological mechanisms for bowel continence reveal that behavioral concepts such as stimulus control, learning, and motivation are essential to an understanding of physiology as well as overt behavior. This has lead to new and successful treatment applications for bowel incontinence, and it promises to be a useful model for the investigation of other disorders.

5. Research needs in the area of pediatric gastrointestinal disorders include the need for programs to develop effective behavioral treatments for recurrent abdominal pain, ulcerative colitis, Crohn's disease, and, possibly, peptic ulcer disease. The search for effective treatment techniques is likely to require additional basic research on the psychophysiological mechanisms by which environmental events modify physiological behaviors.

REFERENCES

Apley, J. (1975). *The child with abdominal pain.* London: Blackwell Scientific.

Apley, J., & Hale, B. (1973). Children with recurrent abdominal pain: How do they grow up? *British Medical Journal, 3,* 7–9.

Apley, J., Haslam, D.R., & Tulloch, G. (1971). Pupillary reaction in children with recurrent pain. *Archives of Disease in Childhood, 46,* 337–340.

Apley, J., & Naish, N. (1958). Recurrent abdominal pain: A field survey of disease in childhood. *Archives of Disease in Childhood, 33*, 165–170.

Astrada, C.A., Licamele, W.L., Walsh, T.L., & Kessler, E.S. (1981). Recurrent abdominal pain in children and associated DSM-III diagnosis. *American Journal of Psychiatry, 138*, 687–688.

Ball, T.S., Hendricksen,H., & Clayton, J.A. (1974). A special feeding technique for chronic regurgitation. *American Journal of Mental Deficiency, 78*, 486–493.

Bemporad, J.R., Kresch, R.A., Asnes, R., & Wilson, A. (1978). Chronic neurotic encopresis as a paradigm of a multifactorial psychiatric disorder. *Journal of Nervous and Mental Disease, 166*, 472–479.

Berger, H.G., Honig, P.J., & Liebman, R. (1977). Recurrent abdominal pain. *American Journal of Diseases of Children, 131*, 1340–1356.

Cerulli, M.A., Nikoomanesh, P., & Schuster, M.M. (1979). Progress in biofeedback conditioning for fecal incontinence. *Gastroenterology, 76*, 742–746.

Christensen, M.F., & Mortensen, O. (1975). Long-term prognosis in children with recurrent abdominal pain. *Archives of Disease in Childhood, 50*, 110–114.

Christie, D.L., & Ament, M.E. (1976). Gastric acid hyperscretion in children with duodenal ulcer. *Gastroenterology, 71*, 242–244.

Christodoulou, G.N., Gargoulas, A., Papaloukas, A., Marinopoulou, A., & Rabavilas, A.D. (1979). Peptic ulcer in childhood: Psychological factors. *Psychotherapy and Psychosomatics, 32*, 297–301.

Christophersen, E.R., & Rainey, S.K. (1976). Management of encopresis through a pediatric outpatient clinic. *Journal of Pediatric Psychology, 4*, 38–41.

Cunningham, C.E., & Linscheid, T.R. (1976). Elimination of chronic ruminating by electric shock. *Behavior Therapy, 7*, 231–234.

Davis, P.K., & Cuvo, A.J. (1980). Chronic vomiting and rumination in intellectually normal and retarded individuals: Review and evaluation of behavioral research. *Behavior Research of Severe Developmental Disabilities, 1*, 31–59.

Deckelbaum, R.J., Roy, C.C., Lussier-Lazaroff, J., & Morin, C.L. (1974). Peptic ulcer disease: A clinical study in 73 children. *Canadian Medical Association Journal, 111*, 225–228.

Degossely, M., Koninckx, N., & Lenfant, H. (1975). La recto-colite hemorragique: Training autogene. A propos de quelques cas graves. *Acta Gastro-Enterologica Belgica, 38*, 454–462.

Dimson, S.B. (1971). Transit time related to clinical findings in children with recurrent abdominal pain. *Pediatrics, 47*, 666–674.

Doleys, D.M., & Arnold, S. (1975). Treatment of childhood encopresis: Full cleanliness training. *Mental Retardation, 13*, 14–16.

Edelman, R.I. (1971). Operant conditioning treatment of encopresis. *Journal of Behavior Therapy and Experimental Psychiatry, 2*, 71–73.

Einhorn, A.H. (1972). Rumination syndrome. In H.L. Barnett (Ed.), *Pediatrics*. New York: Appleton-Century-Crofts.

Engel, B.T., Nikoomanesh, P., & Schuster, M.M. (1974). Operant conditioning of rectosphincteric responses in the treatment of fecal incontinence. *New England Journal of Medicine, 290*, 646–649.

Engel, G.L. (1973). Ulcerative colitis. In A.E. Lindner (Ed.), *Emotional factors in gastrointestinal illness*. Amsterdam: Exerpta Medica.

Esler, M.D., & Goulston, K.J. (1973). Levels of anxiety in colonic disorders. *New England Journal of Medicine, 288*, 16–20.

Fava, G.A., & Pavan, L. (1976/77). Large bowel disorders. I. Illness configuration and life events. *Psychotherapy & Psychosomatics, 27*, 93–99.

Feuerstein, M., Barr, R.G., Francoeur, T.E., Houle, M., & Rafman, S. (1982). Potential biobehavioral mechanisms of recurrent abdominal pain in children. *Pain, 13*, 287–298.

Ford, C.V., Glober, G.A., & Castelnuovo-Tedesco, P. (1969). A psychiatric study of patients with regional enteritis. *Journal of the American Medical Association, 208,* 311–315.

Fullerton, D.T., Kollar, E.J., & Caldwell, A.B. (1962). A clinical study of ulcerative colitis. *Journal of the American Medical Association, 181,* 463–471.

Garcia, J., Hankins, W.G., & Rusiniak, K.W. (1974). Behavioral regulation of the milieu interne in man and rat. *Science, 185,* 824–831.

Grace, W.J., Pinsky, R.H., & Wolff, H.G. (1954). The treatment of ulcerative colitis. II. *Gastroenterology, 26,* 462–468.

Groen, J., & Bastiaans, J. (1951). Psychotherapy of ulcerative colitis. *Gastroenterology, 17,* 344–352.

Hislop, I.G. (1974). Onset setting in inflammatory bowel disease. *Medical Journal of Australia, 1,* 981–984.

Johnson, L.F. (1980). 24-hour pH monitoring in the study of gastroesophageal reflux. *Journal of Clinical Gastroenterology, 2,* 387–399.

Kanner, L. (1936). Historical notes on rumination in man. *Medical Life, 43,* 27–62.

Kanner, L. (1972). *Child psychiatry* (4th ed.). Springfield, IL: Charles C Thomas.

Karush, A., Daniels, G.E., Flood, C. & O'Connor, J.F. (1977). *Psychotherapy in chronic ulcerative colitis.* Philadelphia: Saunders.

Keehn, J.D. (1965). Brief case-report: Reinforcement therapy of incontinence. *Behaviour Research and Therapy, 2,* 239.

Kirsner, J.B., & Shorter, R.G. (Eds.). (1975). *Inflammatory bowel disease.* Philadelphia: Lea & Febiger.

Kopel, F.B., Kim, I.C., & Barbero, G.J. (1967). Comparison of rectosigmoid motility in normal children, children with recurrent abdominal pain, and children with ulcerative colitis. *Pediatrics, 39,* 539–545.

Korelitz, B.I. (1982). Epidemiological and psychosocial aspects of inflammatory bowel disease with observations on children, families, and pregnancy. *American Journal of Gastroenterology, 77,* 929–933.

Lang, P.J., & Melamed, B.G. (1969). Case report: Avoidance conditioning therapy of an infant with chronic ruminative vomiting. *Journal of Abnormal Psychology, 74,* 1–8.

Lebenthal, E., Rossi, T.M., Nord, K.S., & Branski, D. (1981). Recurrent abdominal pain and lactose absorption in children. *Pediatrics, 67,* 828–832.

Levine, M.D., & Bakow, H. (1976). Children with encopresis: A study of treatment outcome. *Pediatrics, 58,* 845–852.

Liebman, W.M. (1979). Recurrent abdominal pain in children: Lactose and sucrose intolerance, a prospective study. *Pediatrics, 64,* 43–45.

Lorber, J. (1971). Results of treatment of myelomeningocele: An analysis of 524 unselected cases, with special reference to possible selection for treatment. *Developmental Medicine and Child Neurology, 13,* 279–303.

Lowery, S.P., Srour, J.W., Whitehead, W.E., & Schuster, M.M. (1985). Habit training as treatment of encopresis secondary to chronic constipation. *Pediatric Gastroenterology and Nutrition, 4,* 397-401.

MacKeith, R., & O'Neill, D. (1951). Recurrent abdominal pain in children. *Lancet, 2,* 278–282.

MacLeod, J.H. (1979). Biofeedback in the management of partial anal incontinence: A preliminary report. *Diseases of the Colon and Rectum, 22,* 169–171.

MacLeod, J.H. (1983). Biofeedback in the management of partial anal incontinence. *Diseases of the Colon and Rectum, 26,* 244–246.

McMahon, A.W., Schmitt, P., Patterson, J.F., & Rothman, E. (1973). Personality differences between inflammatory bowel disease patients and their healthy siblings. *Psychosomatic Medicine, 35,* 91–103.

Mendeloff, A.I. (1975). The epidemiology of idiopathic inflammatory bowel disease. In J.B. Kirsner & R.G. Shorter (Eds.), *Inflammatory bowel disease*. Philadelphia: Lea & Febiger.

Mendeloff, A.I., Monk, M., Siegel, C.I., & Lilienfeld, A. (1970). Illness experience and life stresses in patients with irritable colon and with ulcerative colitis. An epidemiologic study of ulcerative colitis and regional enteritis in Baltimore, 1960–1964. *New England Journal of Medicine, 282,* 14–17.

Michener, W.M. (1981). An approach to recurrent abdominal pain in children. *Primary Care, 8,* 277–283.

Miller, A.J., & Kratochwill, T.R. (1979). Reduction of frequent stomachache complaints by time out. *Behavior Therapy, 10,* 211–218.

Miller, F.J.W., Court, S.D.M., Knox, E.G., & Branden, S. (1974). *The school years in Newcastle-upon-Tyne.* Oxford: Oxford University Press.

Mohammed, R., Hearns, J.B., & Crean, G.P. (1982). Gastric acid secretion in children with duodenal ulceration. *Scandinavian Journal of Gastroenterology, 17,* 289–292.

Neale, D.H. (1963). Behaviour therapy and encopresis in children. *Behavior Research and Therapy, 1,* 139–149.

Olnes, K., McParland, F.A., & Piper, J. (1980). Biofeedback: A new modality in the management of children with fecal soiling. *Pediatrics, 96,* 505–509.

Oster, J. (1972). Recurrent abdominal pain, headache and limb pains in children and adolescents. *Pediatrics, 50,* 429–435.

Pringle, M., Butler, N.R., & Davie, R. (1966). *11,000 seven year olds.* London. Longmans.

Puri, P., Boyd, E., Blake, N., & Guiney, E.J. (1978). Duodenal ulcer in childhood. A continuing disease in adult life. *Journal of Pediatric Surgery,13,* 525–526.

Richmond, J.B., Eddy, E., & Green, M. (1958). Rumination: A psychosomatic syndrome of infancy. *Pediatrics, 22,* 49–55.

Robb, J.D.A., Thomas, P.S., Orszulok, J., & Odling-Smee, G.W. (1972). Duodenal ulcer in children. *Archives of Disease in Childhood, 47,* 688–696.

Roy, C.C., & Silverman, A. (1980). Gastrointestinal tract. In C.H. Kempe, H.K. Silver, & D. O'Brien (Eds.), *Current pediatric diagnosis & treatment* (6th ed.). Los Altos, CA: Lange Medical Publications.

Rubin, L.S., Barbero, G.J., & Sabinga, M.A. (1967). Pupillary reactivity in children with recurrent abdominal pain. *Psychosomatic Medicine, 29,* 111–120.

Schaeffer, C.E. (1979). *Childhood encopresis: Its causes and therapy.* New York: Van Nostrand Reinhold.

Schuster, M.M. (1977). Constipation and anorectal disorders. *Clinics in Gastroenterology, 6,* 643–658.

Seagram, C.G.F., Stephens, C.A., & Cumming, W.A. (1973). Peptic ulceration at the Hospital for Sick Children, Toronto, during the 20-year period 1949–1969. *Journal of Pediatric Surgery, 8,* 407–413.

Sheinbein, M. (1975). Treatment for the hospitalized infantile ruminator: Programmed brief social behavior reinforcers. *Clinical Pediatrics, 14,* 719–724.

Singh, N.N. (1981). Rumination. In N.R. Ellis (Ed.), *International review of research in mental retardation* (Vol 10). New York: Academic Press.

Stone, R.T., & Barbero, G.J. (1970). Recurrent abdominal pain in childhood. *Pediatrics, 45,* 732–738.

Sultz, H.A., Schlesinger, E.R., Feldman, J.G., & Mosher, W.E. (1970). The epidemiology of peptic ulcer in childhood. *American Journal of Public Health, 60,* 492–498.

Toister, R.P., Condron, C.J., Worley, L., & Arthur, D. (1975). Faradic therapy of chronic vomiting in infancy: A case study. *Journal of Behavior Therapy and Experimental Psychiatry, 6,* 55–59.

Wald, A. (1981a). Biofeedback therapy for fecal incontinence. *Annals of Internal Medicine, 95,* 146–149.

Wald, A. (1981b). Use of biofeedback in treatment of fecal incontinence in patients with meningomyelocele. *Pediatrics, 68,* 45–49.

Wald, A. (1983). Biofeedback for neurogenic fecal incontinence: Rectal sensation is a determinant of outcome. *Journal of Pediatric Gastroenterology and Nutrition, 2,* 302–306.

Wald, A., Chandra, R., Fisher, S.E., Gartner, J.C., & Zitelli, B. (1982). Lactose malabsorption in recurrent abdominal pain of childhood. *Journal of Pediatrics, 100,* 65–68.

West, K.L. (1970). MMPI correlates of ulcerative colitis. *Journal of Clinical Psychology, 26,* 214–229.

White, J.J., Suzuki, H., El Shafie, M., Kumar, A.P.M., Haller, Jr., A.J., & Schnaufer, L. (1972). A physiologic rationale for the management of neurologic rectal incontinence in children. *Pediatrics, 49,* 888–893.

Whitehead, W.E., Orr, W.C., Engel, B.T., & Schuster, M.M. (1981). External anal sphincter response to rectal distention: Learned response or reflex. *Psychophysiology, 19,* 57–62.

Whitehead, W.E., Parker, L., Bosmajian, L., Morrill-Corbin, E.D., Middaugh, S., Garwood, M., Cataldo, M.F., & Freeman, J. (in press). Treatment of fecal incontinence in children with spina bifida: Comparison of biofeedback and behavior modification. *Archives of Physical Medicine and Rehabilitation.*

Whitehead, W.E., Parker, L.H., Masek, B.J., Cataldo, M.F., & Freeman, J.M. (1981). Biofeedback treatment of fecal incontinence in patients with myelomeningocele. *Developmental Medicine and Child Neurology, 23,* 313–322.

Whitehead, W.E., & Schuster, M.M. (1985). *Gastrointestinal disorders: Behavioral and physiological basis for treatment.* New York: Academic.

Wright, L. (1975). Outcome of a standardized program for treating psychogenic encopresis. *Professional Psychologist, 6,* 453–456.

Young, G.C. (1973). The treatment of childhood encopresis by conditioned gastro-ileal reflex training. *Behavior Research and Therapy, 11,* 499–503.

PART VI

FUTURE DIRECTIONS

24

Research Strategies and Future Directions in Behavioral Pediatrics

MICHAEL F. CATALDO

OVERVIEW AND HISTORICAL PERSPECTIVE

In the broadest sense, behavioral pediatrics is the application of knowledge about human behavior and child development to the concerns of pediatric medicine and child health. In research and practice, behavioral pediatrics seeks to integrate two scientific bases, behavioral science and biomedical science.

If such activity defines behavioral pediatrics, then the subject matter of this area may be either behavioral or biological, or both. In addition, activities in behavioral pediatrics have been both clinical and scientific. While the concerns of clinical and scientific activities are similar, they are structured differently.

In clinical activities, the clinician may be concerned about how a child behaves, how well the child is developing, how his behavior may affect his health, and so on. The clinician may also be interested in avoiding the use of medical procedures which adversely affect a child's adaptive behavior or development, unless such procedures are absolutely necessary to avoid or ameliorate serious medical consequences. In clinical activity, the problem presented usually dictates the immediate and subsequent activity.

In the use of scientific methods of inquiry to obtain knowledge about phenomena, activities of the scientist are deliberate and structured to best understand the phenomenon under study. The scientist seeks to manipulate one set of conditions or variables (independent variables) while observing in as precise a way as possible the effect on other variables (dependent variables). Biomedical science, and its application to pediatrics, has been concerned with the study of the effects of biological independent variables on other biological dependent variables. Behavior has only been a consideration insofar as it is a sign or symptom of a biological dependent variable of concern.

Three Considerations in the Development of Behavioral Pediatrics

Behavioral pediatrics suggests that three other considerations should be of import: (1) the effects of behavioral independent variables on behavioral dependent variables, (2) the effects of biological independent variables on behavior, and (3) the effects of behavioral independent variables on biology.

The first of these three considerations, how behavioral procedures can be used to affect behavior, has been the concern of behavioral science. Behavioral pediatrics has merely asked how the pediatric service systems (pediatricians, nurses, clinics, private practices) may use knowledge about behavioral assessment and treatment to best help children and families. While scientific investigation to answer this question may also produce important basic knowledge about relationships between clinician's and patient's behavior when they interact with each other, the primary concern has been one of immediate application of behavioral science knowledge to pediatric clinical settings.

The second consideration, how biological independent variables affect behavior, is more than a logical outgrowth of adding measures to the study of how biological dependent variables are affected during medical procedures, for two important reasons. First, this consideration places increased emphasis on the importance of behavior as a primary outcome of medical intervention. Changes in the biological status of a patient are of little clinical value if the ability to function is not improved, or impaired. Second, the processes involved in behavior change (as opposed to exclusively biological change) are now an explicit area of inquiry. These processes may be either those of biobehavioral interaction (e.g., how drugs affect behavior) or behavioral-behavioral interaction (e.g., how aversive medical procedures affect behavior).

The third consideration, how behavioral procedures can affect biological conditions, has been the least studied of the three. The modification of the environment may have little effect on biological conditions of significance, especially in comparison to direct biological manipulation. Or, possibly, environmental manipulation may have a small immediate effect on biological status, but the consistency of the manipulation and properties of the environment which allow it to generalize across settings may greatly enhance effects over time. However, should behavioral independent variables have significant (clinical as well as statistical) effects on health status and biological function, then the specification of such biobehavioral processes and their subsequent elaboration into clinical practice affords an opportunity akin to other great advances in medicine.

Because of scientific and clinical contributions of the application of learning principles (operant conditioning) to pediatric problems, this approach has enjoyed increased enthusiasm and emphasis in behavioral pediatrics. This chapter will overview the broader area of behavioral pediatrics, and will highlight in greater detail this learning-based approach.

Behavioral Pediatrics as an Area for the Advancement of Knowledge

As an integrative effort behavioral pediatrics offers considerable promise. Indeed, the most significant advances in science and technology result either from the scientific demonstration of hitherto undocumented phenomena ("new" phenomena), or the integration of two scientific areas of inquiry. For example, in the past decade scientific demonstrations of phenomena which offer considerable generality to advances in medicine and health include investigations which detail the existence of slow growing viral diseases (e.g., Kuru and Creutzefeld-Jakob) and the discovery of endogenous opiates, to name but two. Advances resulting from the integration of medical science with nuclear physics have led to basic knowledge about cellular responses to radiation and radioactive tracing, with applications for radiation therapy and the use of short-lived isotopes in diagnosis; while integration of medical and computer sciences has resulted in such diagnostic and physiological mapping tools as the CAT and PET scanners and magnetic resonance imaging.

With regard to child health and human development, at least two events in science offer considerable promise for future advances. First, recent investigations on genetic anomalies and resultant medical and developmental sequelae have taken a significant leap forward with the discovery of restrictive enzyme analysis. Secondly, scientific and technological areas of inquiry concerned with child health have increasingly over the past two decades integrated aspects of medical and behavioral science, primarily with regard to the field of psychology (the scientific study of behavior).

Historical Development of the Area

The development of behavioral pediatrics has been spawned by (1) the changing nature of pediatrics from acute care and treatment of infectious diseases to well-child care and treatment of chronic disorders, and (2) the dramatic increase in basic knowledge and practical clinical techniques which has resulted from behavioral research, particularly research on learning principles.

In a 1951 statement, the American Board of Pediatrics pointed out the importance of pediatricians relating basic knowledge about growth and development to clinical practice (American Board of Pediatrics, 1951). Subsequent elaboration of the Board's recommendations included the development of the area of behavioral pediatrics (Christophersen, 1982). While this activity has most commonly been termed behavioral pediatrics, the integration of medical and behavioral science applied to pediatric problems has also occurred under the rubric of psychosocial pediatrics, pediatric psychology, medical psychology, psychosomatic medicine, somatopsychology, health psychology, behavioral medicine, child psychiatry, and developmental pediatrics.

Historically, behavioral pediatrics has evolved from three lines. One is based on liaison psychiatry and adaptation of some aspects of child psychiatry; another line evolves from psychosomatic medicine for adults that then lowers the age focus to children; the third line is the attempt to apply findings from psychological research to pediatric problems.

Independent of this changing emphasis in pediatrics has been the concurrent increase in knowledge about behavior gleaned from operant research. Based on extensive investigations with animals, the parameters of operant learning were well defined and replicated within and across species during the 1950s and 1960s. This resulted in principles of behavior that had generality across behaviors and organisms. These principles are founded on the observation that learning occurs from experience; or, more precisely stated: behavior is a function of its consequences. Beginning in the 1960s, this knowledge began to be broadly applied to study human behavior of social significance. The defining characteristics both of research procedures and practical applications are that environmental events are manipulated, contingent upon behavior, so as to increase, suppress, maintain, elaborate, or otherwise alter behavior occurring in the future (Baer, Wolf, & Risley, 1968).

Areas of Inquiry for Behavioral Pediatrics Research

Research trends in behavioral science indicate that interdisciplinary collaboration in behavioral pediatrics is likely to expand greatly in three areas, two of which are not likely to be known to the general pediatric community (Cataldo, 1982). The first area, the best known, is the use of behavioral procedures for *remediation of routine behavioral and developmental problems* identified through pediatric clinic and office visits. The second area concerns the analysis of the medical setting and its effect on children. Quality medical care often includes procedures which can have profound behavioral, psychological, and, thus, biological effects on the pediatric patient. Behavioral research is beginning to report procedures for the *identification and reduction of the behavioral iatrogenic effects of medical care*. The third area deals with the direct *modification of biological conditions* by behavioral means. The extension of this line of study to situations of daily living and prevention has resulted in research on *child health behavior*.

Accordingly, behavioral pediatrics has increasingly come to be an effort to apply theories of human behavior and learning to health and illness behaviors of children, and in some cases to those significant adults in their environment. The implication and promise of these activities, if widely adopted, is that a host of health promoting and health damaging behaviors could legitimately be studied.

SIGNIFICANT FINDINGS

Remediation of Routine Behavior and Developmental Problems

The decline in infectious diseases from advances in public health and immunization has changed the role of the practicing pediatrician. Increasingly this role has expanded to address problems in development, child rearing, and school (Green, 1980; Richmond, 1975; Starfield & Borkowf, 1969). With parental access to professional assistance for these problems limited by matters of economy, a pediatric office or clinic can provide excellent resources. However, as in all areas of pediatrics, professional aid for even nonmedical problems of growth and development should be based, when possible, on scientifically validated procedures. For this reason, considerable research has been conducted to determine the adequacy and cost effectiveness of pediatric services providing a focus for identification of and early intervention in problems of behavior and development, in addition to the more traditional concern for the health of the child. For example, investigations have looked at the primary care setting as an opportunity to identify early behavior patterns as predictors for later developmental problems (Chamberlin, 1982). With the exception of early developmental screenings and the identification of more gross behavioral and developmental pathology, this particular approach has not proved to be especially fruitful.

On the other hand, considerable research validating the application of learning principles to child behavior problems has been conducted. The result is an extensive experimental literature on procedures for treating a wide variety of problems, including noncompliance (Forehand et al., 1979), tantrums (Hawkins et al., 1966; Russo & Cataldo, 1977), enuresis (Azrin,

Sneed, & Foxx, 1974; Foxx & Azrin, 1973), encopresis (Christophersen &
Rainey, 1976), habit disorders (Azrin & Nunn, 1973; Varni, Boyd, & Cataldo, 1978), hyperactivity (O'Leary, 1980; O'Leary et al., 1976), and any
problems of children with developmental disorders such as feeding (Riordan, et al., 1980), rumination (Linscheid & Cunningham, 1977), and self-
injury (Russo, Carr, & Lovaas, 1980). While this literature addresses problems presented to pediatricians, with rare exceptions these studies have
not been conducted in the context of the restrictions of a pediatric practice.
Only within the past five years have clinical applications of this data base
begun to be experimentally demonstrated in pediatric practice settings
(Rapoff, Christophersen, & Rapoff, 1982).

Perhaps the most important aspect of behavioral research with great
generality to pediatric practice concerns the problem of noncompliance
with medical advice. Compliance is the one area which is singularly the domain of behavioral science dealing with learning principles (i.e., compliance is a learned behavior). Biomedical and epidemiological research can
recommend specific procedures to be followed, but ensuring patient compliance is a behavioral consideration amenable to the same principles that
affect all behavior. Basic operant research with animals, adults, and, more
recently, with young children has identified the parameters of behavioral
and environmental interaction that affect and, therefore, can modify compliance. While considerable research has been conducted on the demographic characteristics of noncompliers, (socioeconomic status, educational
level, prior contact with medical professionals, etc.), these variables are not
readily amenable to therapeutic manipulation. Fortunately, operant approaches to this problem have demonstrated that compliance is affected by
environmental consequences, many of which can be manipulated by pediatric professionals (Finney, Friman, Rapoff, & Christophersen, 1985). Further, compliance can develop as a class of behavior, so that an increase
in compliance in one situation can generalize to other situations. In this
sense, compliance can be considered as a generalizable response class
(Cataldo, 1984).

The application of behavioral procedures to pediatric behavior and developmental problems identified in office and ambulatory clinics is the
most extensive application of behavioral science to pediatric medicine. Addressing behaviorally related problems in such pediatric medical settings
has set the occasion for also considering the problem of the unwanted behavioral effects of medical care.

Identification and Reduction of Behavioral Iatrogenic Effects of Medical Care

With the decline in infectious diseases and increases in medical technology and heroics, there has also come an increase in chronic disorders
among children. Children who would have died a number of years ago are

now kept alive through advances in biomedical science, but often with permanent handicapping sequelae and the need for long-term medical treatment. This has provided the opportunity and challenge to study (1) the effects of medical treatments on children, (2) the methods that can be used to successfully mitigate detrimental effects of quality medical care (especially when medical procedures are particularly aversive, such as debridement of burn victims), and (3) the behavioral and developmental effects of chronic medical problems, especially those requiring long term medical care. To date the approach in behavioral science has been toward adaptive modification of behavior and away from deviancy-based theorizing. Such a normalcy-based approach fits well with the conceptualization of the developing child with chronic disease (Russo and Varni, 1982), and provides for real-time alteration of behavior.

Measures that have been considered in this research include symptoms of pain, anxiety, nausea, vomiting, and neuropsychological data; disruptions and aberrant behavior in nonmedical settings, such as the home and school; and a variety of behaviors of children while in the medical setting. As biomedical science has created treatments for childhood diseases that are sometimes worse than the disease itself, research has shown a variety of interesting and clinically important relationships. For many children the behavioral iatrogenic effects of medical procedures can be mitigated by a variety of procedures which prepare the child for medical treatment, such as the use of films (Melamed & Siegel, 1975; Melamed, Weinstein, Hawes, & Katin-Borland, 1975; Melamed, Yurcheson, Fleece, Hutcherson, & Hawes, 1978), puppets (Cassel, 1965), and relaxation techniques, including hypnosis (Redd, Andresen, & Minagawe, 1982; Zeltzer & LeBaron, 1979).

In general, research on clinical procedures with regard to the aforementioned problems can be considered to be a desensitization approach. In contrast, other research has focused on interventions with children undergoing intensive and often unanticipated medical treatment for which psychological preparation cannot be planned (Cataldo, Bessman, Parker, Pearson, & Rogers, 1979; Pearson, Cataldo, Tureman, Bessman, & Rogers, 1980). The data from this research has shown that on the average, one-third of the children in an intensive care setting were awake and alert and, therefore, able to be affected by the sights and sounds of the environment. While these children were capable of making a variety of responses, their behavioral repertoires were found to be markedly suppressed. The addition to the hospital environment of a simple behavioral intervention for brief periods was sufficient to result in more normal child behavior, such as increased attention, engagement with the environment, positive affect, and decreased inappropriate behavior. The behavioral intervention used play activities to provide both a positive environment and a period of time during which children were "safe" from medical interventions. This approach is based on operant learning theory and thus enables similar approaches to be tied to an extensive body of basic animal and human research. Particularly relevant to this line of study is the basic research on the effects on behavior of unpredictable and unavoidable aversive stimulation. Investigations with animals and healthy adults have shown profound suppression of behavior and dramatic biological effects which, for a hospitalized patient, would generally be considered undesirable, if not dangerous (Cataldo & Maldonado, in press).

Regardless of the theoretical orientation from which such scientific activity results, behavioral research on hospitalized children undergoing medical treatment provides the opportunity to significantly intervene in the traditional milieu of medical routine without compromising medical therapeutics. It also affords an extraordinary opportunity to study the behavioral and biological effects of aversive events on children, which otherwise would not be permitted outside the conduct of necessary medical treatment.

Chronicity represents another major problem in behavioral pediatrics. With the increasing prevalence of chronic disease, involving periodic, often painful symptomatology and the need for repetitive treatment, conditions exist for learning maladaptive behavior. Viewed as a cross-disease issue, chronicity may seem as a problem in disorders with overt, painful, or arousal-related symptomatology; with symptom management as the focus of medical treatment as opposed to cure; with necessary repetitive medical treatments; and with disease- or cure-imposed alterations in daily behavior. Under such circumstances, reliable antecedents and consequences may be identified that place the child *at risk* for increased symptomatology and potentially decreased impact of treatment. Research on chronicity falls into several areas: identification of at risk populations; evaluation of psychologic, biologic, or developmental variables which increase risk; identification of treatments which reduce maladaptive learning; and studies of successful patients (those without serious learning-produced reactions).

Modification of Biological Conditions

Behavioral principles have also been applied to directly alter biological responses, including those diagnosed as medical problems. Behavioral research studies have demonstrated the modification of acute and chronic medically related problems of both normal and developmentally delayed pediatric populations (Cataldo & Russo, 1979; Cataldo, Russo, Bird, & Varni, 1980; Russo & Varni, 1982). Basic and clinical research strongly suggest that behavioral procedures can now be added to the traditional armamentarium of medical and surgical procedures used for direct treatment of medical disorders. Carefully controlled animal experiments have demonstrated the majority of and most convincing evidence for behavioral science principles being directly related to changes in biological activity. Laboratory studies have shown experimental manipulation of endocrine, cardiovascular, and gastrointestinal responses, both by the scheduling of specific environmental contingencies and by systematically providing environmental consequences for the targeted biological response (Brady, 1966, 1979). Similarly, animal research has demonstrated the relationship of behavioral contingencies on changes in immune responses to viral, bacterial, and parasitic challenges, neoplastic responses, and antigen experiments (Ader, 1981).

That behavioral principles should be equally applicable regardless of the "behavior" modified, whether it be compliance, tantrums, seizures (Cataldo, Russo, & Freeman, 1979), or muscle activity (Bird & Cataldo, 1978; Cataldo, Bird, & Cunningham, 1978) constitutes the foundation for this use of behavioral procedures. The type of response is no longer the limiting factor for response change. Rather, the ability to provide precise signals or antecedent conditions and the ability to provide effective consequences for the exact response now define the possibility of response change. If the proper antecedents and consequences could be determined, even discrete physiological and biochemical responses should be pliant to modification by behavioral science methods.

Special equipment representing biological activity is often implemented when effecting antecedents and consequences. The use of biofeedback for the treatment of a variety of medically related disorders has recently been met with considerable enthusiasm. In this procedure, information concerning biological responses is provided to a motivated patient and pathological conditions are found to improve. Unfortunately, the scientific principles underlying the use of biofeedback are unproven. One possibility is that biofeedback represents the successful use of sophisticated transducers of biological activity to establish cues (discriminative stimuli) for the change of biological responses (Sidman, 1980). One excellent example of such an extension of behavioral science principles to medical problems is that of treatment for incontinence.

This application of principles of behavioral science to the modification of biological (biochemical, neurophysiological) events offers the promise of providing an additional investigative method for advancing basic knowledge about biological function and the pathogenesis of medical disorders.

Child Health Behavior

Studying behavioral procedures related to medical problems can be extended to address the question of how environmental learning affects children's health. This country's economy has reached the point where not all desired and necessary medical procedures can be afforded. Therefore, the most efficient and cost effective solution is the prevention of the onset of illness; that is, the maintenance of health. With the decline in the incidence of infectious and many forms of acute diseases, the preponderance of health risks now relate either directly or indirectly to behavioral lifestyle. Accidents are the leading cause of morbidity and mortality in children, exceeding the six most prevalent diseases combined. In many cases, the two disease entities with the greatest adult prevalence, cardiovascular disease and cancer, have contributory factors that are the result of unhealthy lifestyle habits acquired early in life. Unhealthy habits develop early in life and are modeled by adults in society. It therefore follows that the establishment of healthy lifestyles earily in life should serve as an important public health goal. Principles resulting from basic research on learning have provided the foundation for understanding and being able to design practical programs for the maintenance of healthy lifestyles.

GAPS IN KNOWLEDGE

The Effects of Behavioral Procedures on Behavior

Use of Behavioral Procedures in Pediatric Settings.   Applied behavioral research has demonstrated unequivocally the successful use of learning principles to remediate a variety of socially significant childhood behavior problems. The major gap of knowledge in this area of behavioral pediatrics concerns the methods by which proven effective procedures for remediating behavior problems of children can be applied with the same degree of success to pediatric service settings, such as well-child visits. Data that will need to be obtained include anlaysis of current methods employed by professionals in pediatric settings to direct and influence the behavior of parents and children, as well as the variables and the practical techniques which can be applied to ensure proper technology transfer. This type of research should not be considered purely technological. While the goals would include immediate improvement in clinical procedures and resolution of numerous childhood behavior problems, such research would also identify variables involved in physician/patient interaction, and as such would constitute an important contribution to basic knowledge about therapeutics affecting child health and development.

Adolescent Medicine.   Adolescent health and development has been an understudied area. Increased efforts must be made to study the development of the children of adolescent mothers and adolescent parenting strategies. At present it is not known whether parenting strategies of adolescents differ from those of their older counterparts; nor is it clear that the offspring of adolescent mothers are at any greater developmental or behavioral risk from factors other than those directly related to the biological risks of adolescent pregnancy.

Community Support.   Research is needed on supportive versus nonsupportive communities in terms of assistance to families in childrearing and support of appropriate child health and development practices. Such research will bridge the gap between individual subject and epidemiological investigative strategies. Further, supportive communities can facilitate professional assistance to families by ensuring that behavioral and adherence programs are successfully generalized to daily living situations and are sufficiently maintained to affect long-term health.

The Effects of Medical Procedures on Behavior

Iatrogenic Effects. With regard to the concern in behavioral pediatrics for the behavioral iatrogenic effects of quality medical care, the primary methodological gap is one of measurement of both "stress" and "coping." Expressed more operationally, the questions are (1) How does one measure the immediate and long-term sequelae of children's exposure to dramatic, aversive medical procedures? and (2) How does one ascertain the various methods by which children and their parents successfully or unsuccessfully respond to such exposure? In a sense, much of the research on behavioral iatrogenic effects has occurred through consideration of likely solutions to a problem before studying the nature and parameter of the problem. This research should include the study of normal populations (that is, those not exposed to medical procedures) in terms of how they adjust to dramatic and aversive events. Subsequently, a number of important investigations could proceed, including how to assess symptoms and symptom change as an indication of "coping" and "distress"; the cataloging and demonstration of children's adaptation styles; how adaptation (or coping) styles develop; whether children's styles are similar to adults; how children of various ages respond to medical information; and, of course, the longitudinal study of the effectiveness of behavior procedures in mitigating the unintended results of quality medical procedures (to date, research has been primarily related to immediate effects of behavioral procedures). Related to this approach is the lack of information on whether some diseases can cause cognitive and/or affective changes because of biological or behavioral/environmental interaction. This type of research will need to be conducted so that biological versus environmental variables can be separated with regard to the above considerations.

Drug Effects. We also lack knowledge about drug action with children. For example, research and clinical practices with children employing drugs (including drugs with significant side effects) are proceeding in the absence of carefully developed and agreed upon measures concerning the basic parameters of behavioral competency. Much of the drug recommendations for children are based upon either animal or adult human drug action studies. It is not clear whether such drug action data can be extrapolated to children (uptake, half-life, etc.). While the laboratory techniques for determining blood levels of these drugs is known in many cases, research employing blood-level data has not been conducted in most cases, nor is it a common practice to obtain these levels during clinical intervention. Such research must be conducted, and should be carried out with combined biological and behavioral measures, especially if the drug is to be recommended to treat behavioral disorders.

An excellent model is provided by the area of behavioral pharmacology. Operant learning tasks have been employed to serve as baseline condition(s) for the evaluation of various pharmacological agents and drug levels, primarily because performance characteristics during these tasks have been so extensively studied and are so highly replicable. The development of an agreed upon methodology that provides data on basic parameters of behavior for each subject would enable not only the study of the effects of various biological conditions (across drug agents, drug studies, pathological entities or progression), but would also allow for investigation of whether such biobehavioral interaction data are different across developmental levels.

The Effects of Behavioral Procedures on Biological Conditions

Potentially, the most far-reaching area of research to date in behavioral pediatrics is that related to biobehavioral interaction; that is, how behavioral/environmental contingencies can affect children's biological status. Such information has profound implications for child health and for changing how medicine is taught and practiced. To date, the medical approach to illness and health has been at the biological mechanism level. Only recently have we begun to understand the significant and often dramatic way in which environmental learning can affect biological change. This research is proceeding in a haphazard fashion. The clear importance of this line of investigation demands that a more systematic approach be taken.

Effects of Chronicity.   Research needs to be undertaken to determine the effects of limitations imposed by disease, symptomatology, and disease treatment on the course of child development. With increases in medical technology, children suffering disorders such as end-stage renal diseaes, cystic-fibrosis, diabetes, and cancer will experience increasing life spans, with subsequent stress to their development. The impact of such chronic disease on development is not yet known, as many medical advances (e.g., dialysis and transplantation) are relatively recent. Of particular importance would be the study of chronic disease impact *across* diseases. Primary questions involve the potency of developmental or cognitive level as opposed to specific disease-related parameters such as treatments or symptoms.

Biological Measures.   Methods need to be improved for obtaining biological baselines so that the effects of behavioral/environmental independent variables may be studied. For example, there is no generally agreed upon set of measures for studying the biological effects of extreme aversive events on children. The development of such measures would permit research on techniques for mitigating these effects to be conducted at the biological as well as behavioral level. This gap severely limits research on the iatrogenic effects of quality medical care.

Accident Prevention.   Accidents constitute *the* child health behavior problem of practical and *immediate* need of a research-based solution. Data need to be obtained on the conditions and behaviors that lead to the occurrence of accidents. Considering the prevalence of childhood morbidity and mortality due to accidents, the available knowledge on accident prevention is trivial. Had "accidents," been classified as a "disease," it would clearly be considered at epidemic proportions and be the subject of our highest priorities. This gap may exist in part because the professional group most closely involved in the sequelae of accidents (i.e., medicine) employs investigative methodologies that are not especially relevant to a solution of the problem. On the other hand, behavioral science does employ methodologies amenable to the study of this problem, but until recently behavioral science has not been sensitized to this important problem. Another possibility for the existence of this gap is that the critical variables (the behaviors to be studied) occur in situations that are difficult, or at least expensive to observe—natural daily-living environments of adults and children. However, behavioral science has, in the past, been able to address a number of important and socially significant problems in this domain of the everyday "natural laboratory."

Child Health Behavior.   Lastly, research is just beginning on child health behavior. The most important data to be obtained now are on the variables that influence the development of health behaviors, or conversely, how illness behaviors develop. Such research has occurred at a clinical level in such areas as childhood and adolescent hypertension, weight control and obesity, and adherence. Basic research is especially needed to identify the general principles involved in development of health or illness behavior.

In summary, such a line of research as suggested here would provide important information about normative behavior and development in relation to a variety of environmental conditions and biological states. It is somewhat of an anomaly that the majority of research in child health and development considers either environmental variables or biological variables, as if these two important effects on children were independent of each other. Behavioral pediatrics as an integrative activity has begun to change this practice.

ACKNOWLEDGMENTS

Preparation of this paper was supported in part by Grant 917 from the Maternal and Child Health Division of Health and Human Services.

Gratefully acknowledged are the contributions and assistance of Edward Christophersen, Robert Haggerty, Philip Nader, Dennis Russo and James Varni, who served as members of a subcommittee to prepare a five-year funding plan for NICHD, which preparation served as the basis for this chapter. Appreciation is also extended to John Parrish for his comments and to Fred Leebron for his editorial assistance.

REFERENCES

Ader, R. (1981). Behavioral influences on immune responses. In S.M. Weiss, J.A. Herd, & B.H. Fox (Eds.), *Perspectives on behavioral medicine*. New York: Academic.

Anderson, D.E., & Tosheff, J. (1973). Cardiac output and total peripheral resistance changes during pre-avoidance periods in the dog. *Journal of Applied Psychology, 34,* 650–654.

American Board of Pediatrics. (1951). Statement on training requirements in growth and development. *Pediatrics, 7,* 430–432.

Azrin, N.J., & Nunn, R.G. (1973). Habit reversal: A method of eliminating nervous habits and tics. *Behaviour Research and Therapy, 11,* 619–628.

Azrin, N.H., Sneed, T.J., & Foxx, R.M. (1974). Dry-bed training: Rapid elimination of childhood enuresis. *Behaviour Research and Therapy, 12,* 147–156.

Baer, D.M., Wolf, M.M., & Risley, T.R. (1968). Some current dimensions of applied behavior anlaysis. *Journal of Applied Behavior Analysis, 1,* 91–97.

Bergman, G.E., & Hiner, L.B. (1984). Psychogenic intractable sneezing in children. *Journal of Pediatrics, 105,* 496–498.

Bird, B.L., & Cataldo, M.F. (1978). Experimental analysis of EMG feedback in treating dystonia. *Annals of Neurology, 3,* 310–315.

Bollard, J., & Nettlebeck, T. (1982). A component analysis of dry-bed training for treatment for bedwetting. *Behaviour Research and Therapy, 20,* 383–390.

Boyce, W.T., Sprunger, L.W., Sobolewski, S., & Schaefer, C. (1984). Epidemiology of injuries in a large, urban school district. *Pediatrics, 74,* 342–349.

Brady, J.V. (1966). Operant methodology and the production of altered physiological states. In W. Honig (Ed.), *Operant behavior: Areas of research and application*. New York: Appleton-Century-Crofts.

Brady, J.V. (1979). Learning and conditioning. In O.F. Pomerleau & J.P. Brady (Eds.), *Behavioral medicine: Theory and practice*. Baltimore: Williams & Wilkins.

Casey, P.H. (1983). Failure to thrive: A reconceptualization. *Journal of Developmental and Behavioral Pediatrics, 4,* 63–66.

Cassel, S.E. (1965). The effect of brief puppet therapy upon the emotional responses of children undergoing cardiac catheterization. *Journal of Consulting and Clinical Psychology, 29,* 1–8.

Cataldo, M.F. (1982). The scientific basis for a behavioral approach to pediatrics. *Pediatric Clinics of North America, 29,* 415–423.

Cataldo, M.F. (1984). Clinical considerations in training parents of children with special problems. In R.F. Dangel & R.A. Polster (Eds.), *Parent training: Foundations of research and practice*. New York: Guilford.

Cataldo, M.F., Bessman, C.A., Parker, L.H., Pearson, J.E.R., & Rogers, M.C. (1979). Behavioral assessment for pediatric intensive care units. *Journal of Applied Behavior Analysis, 12,* 83–97.

Cataldo, M.F., Bird, B.L., & Cunningham, C.E. (1978). Experimental analysis of EMG feedback in treating cerebral palsy. *Journal of Behavioral Medicine, 1,* 311–322.

Cataldo, M.F., Jacobs, H.E., & Rogers, M.C. (1982). Psychosocial factors in pediatric intensive care. In D.C. Russo & J.W. Varni (Eds.), *Behavioral pediatrics: Research and practice.* New York: Plenum.

Cataldo, M.F., & Maldonado, A.J. (in press). Psychological effects of pediatric intensive care on staff, patients, and family. In M.C. Rogers (Ed.), *Pediatric intensive care.* Baltimore: Williams & Wilkins.

Cataldo, M.F., & Russo, D.C. (1979). Developmentally disabled in the community: Behavioral/medical considerations. In L.A. Hamerlynck, P.O. Davidson, & F.W. Clark (Eds.), *History and future of behavior modification for the developmentally disabled: Programmatic and methodological issues.* New York: Brunner/Mazel.

Cataldo, M.F., Russo, D.C., Bird, B.L., & Varni, J.W. (1980). Assessment and management of chronic disorders. In J. Ferguson & C.B. Taylor (Eds.), *Advances in behavioral medicine* (pp. 67–95). Hollinswood, NY: Appleton-Century-Crofts.

Cataldo, M.F., Russo, D.C., & Freeman, J.M. (1979). Behavioral analysis and treatment approach to myoclonic seizure control. *Journal of Autism and Developmental Disorders, 9,* 413–427.

Chamberlin, R.W. (1982). Prevention of behavioral problems in young children. *Pediatric Clinics of North American, 29,* 239–247.

Christophersen, E.R. (1982). Incorporating behavioral pediatrics into primary care. *Pediatric Clinics of North America, 29,* 261–296.

Christophersen, E.R., & Rainey, S. (1976). Management of encopresis through a pediatric outpatient clinic. *Journal of Pediatric Psychology, 1,* 38–41.

Finney, J.W., Friman, P.C., Rapoff, M.A., & Christophersen, E.R. (1985). Improving compliance with antibiotic regimens for otitis media: Randomized clinical trial in a pediatric clinic. *American Journal of Diseases of Children, 139,* 89–95.

Forehand, R., Sturgis, E.T., McMahon, R.J. et al. (1979). Parental behavioral training to modify child noncompliance. *Behavioral Modification, 3,* 3–25.

Foxx, R.M., & Azrin, N.H. (1973). Dry pants. A rapid method of toilet training children. *Behaviour Research and Therapy, 11,* 435–442.

Green, M. (1980). The pediatric mode of care. *Behavior Therapy, 3,* 7–8.

Hawkins, R.P., Peterson, F. Jr., Schweid, E., et al. (1966). Behavior therapy in the home: Amelioration of problem parent-child relations with the parent in therapeutic role. *Journal of Experimental Child Psychology, 4,* 99–107.

Linscheid, T.R., & Cunningham, C.E. (1977). A controlled demonstration of the effectiveness of electric shock in the elimination of chronic infant rumination. *Journal of Applied Behavior Analysis, 10,* 500.

Mason, J.W., Brady, J.V., & Tolson, W.W. (1966) Behavioral adaptations and endocrine activity. *Proceedings of the Association for Research in Nervous and Mental Diseases,* Baltimore: Williams & Wilkins.

Melamed, B.G., & Siegel, L.J. (1975). Reduction of anxiety in children facing hospitalization and surgery by use of filmed modeling. *Journal of Consulting and Clinical Psychology, 43,* 511–521.

Melamed, B.G., Weinstein, D., Hawes, R., & Katin-Borland, M. (1975). Reduction of fear-related dental management problems using filmed modeling. *Journal of the American Dental Association, 90,* 822–826.

Melamed, B.G., Yurcheson, R., Fleece, E.L., Hutcherson, S., & Hawes, R. (1978). Effect of filmed modeling on the reduction of anxiety-related behavior in individuals varying in levels of previous experience in the stress situation. *Journal of Consulting and Clinical Psychology, 46,* 1357–1367.

O'Leary, K.D. (1980). Pills or skills for hyperactive children. *Journal of Applied Behavior Analysis, 13*, 191–204.

O'Leary, K.D., Pelham, W.E., Rosenbaum, A., et al. (1976). Behavioral treatment of hyperkinetic children: An experimental evaluation of its usefulness. *Clinical Pediatrics, 15*, 510–515.

Pearson, J.E.R., Cataldo, M.F., Tureman, A., Bessman, C., & Rogers, M.C. (1980). Pediatric intensive care unit patients: Effects of play intervention on behavior. *Critical Care Medicine, 8* (2), 64–67.

Rapoff, M.A., Christophersen, E.R., & Rapoff, K.E. (1982). The management of common childhood bedtime problems by pediatric nurse practitioners. *Journal of Pediatric Psychology, 7*, 179–196.

Redd, W.H., Andresen, G.U., & Minagawe, R.Y. (1982). Hypnotic control of anticipatory emesis in patients receiving cancer chemotherapy. *Journal of Consulting and Clinical Psychology, 50*, 14–19.

Richmond, J.B. (1975). An idea whose time has arrived. In S.B. Friedman (Ed.) *Pediatric Clinics of North America, 22*, 517–524.

Riordan, M.M., Iwata, B.A., Wohl, M.K., et al. (1980). Behavioral treatment of food refusal and selectivity in developmentally disabled children. *Applied Research in Mental Retardation, 1*, 95–112.

Russo, D.C., Carr, E.G., & Lovaas, O.I. (1980). Self-injury in pediatric populations. In J. Ferguson & C.B. Taylor (Eds.), *Comprehensive handbook of behavioral medicine* (pp. 23–41). Hollinswood, NY: Spectrum.

Russo, D.C., & Cataldo, M.F. (1977). Issues in community based treatment programs for the handicapped: Tantrum control. *Journal of Practical Approaches to Developmental Handicap, 1* (3), 13–18.

Russo, D.C., & Varni, J.W. (1982). *Behavioral pediatrics: Research and practice.* New York: Plenum.

Sidman, M. (1980). *Some thoughts about biofeedback.* Paper presented at conference on Behavioral Interventions in Neurology, Baltimore, Maryland.

Starfield, B., & Borkowf, S. (1969). Physicians recognition of complaints made by parents about their children's health. *Pediatrics, 43*, 168–172.

Varni, J.W., Boyd, E., & Cataldo, M.F. (1978). Self-monitoring, external reinforcement, and timeout procedures in the control of high-rate tic behaviors in a 7-year-old male child. *Behavior Therapy and Experimental Psychology, 9*, 353–358.

Whalen, C.K., Henker, B., Collins, B.E., Finck, D., & Dotemoto, S. (1979). A social ecology of hyperactive boys: Medication effects in structured classroom environments. *Journal of Applied Behavior Analysis, 12*, 65–81.

Zeltzer, L., & LeBaron, S. (1979). Hypnosis and non-hypnotic techniques for reduction of pain and anxiety during painful procedures in children and adolescents with cancer. *Behavioral Pediatrics, 101*, 1032–1035.

25

Concepts for Training in Behavioral Pediatrics

BARBARA J. HOWARD AND JEAN SMITH

Progressive health care for children requires incorporation of current knowledge about child development and behavior into both preventive and therapeutic services. Training health professionals toward this goal continues to present a challenge, not only to pediatrics but also to programs preparing psychologists and other professionals to care for children and their families. What makes training in this area so difficult? The nature of behavioral pediatrics, its historical place in health care, multiplicity of professionals involved, and etiological factors affecting behavior, all contribute to the complexity of training and have implications for its improvement (Table 25.1).

NATURE OF BEHAVIORAL PEDIATRICS

A major source of difficulty in designing training in "behavioral pediatrics" is providing a uniform definition. The 1978 Task Force on Pediatric

TABLE 25.1.   CAUSES OF DIFFICULTY FOR TRAINING IN BEHAVIORAL PEDIATRICS

Nature of behavioral pediatrics
  Definition
  Universality
  Lack of specialty advocate
  Multiple sources of services
History of attention to behavior in health care
  Lack of defined curriculum
  Subspecialty orientation
  Psychoanalytic approach preceded psychology
  Tertiary training sites
Diversity of disciplines involved
  Different knowledge bases
Multiple etiologic factors
  Broad definition of health
  Preventive role
  Lifestyle choices
Inherent complexity of subject
  Conflicting theories
  Lack of trainee motivation and background
  Intense family involvement
  Personal life issues touched
  Societal mores change
  Emotional demands
  Interpersonal skills central
  Difficulties in measuring outcome

education defined biosocial problems as "health problems which are socially induced or complicated by social and environmental factors." This expanded the area to include more than was previously considered under developmental disabilities, which focused on more severe, chronic handicaps. Friedman (1975) has defined behavioral pediatrics as "an area within pediatrics which focuses on the psychological, social and learning problems of children and adolescents." These definitions focus on identification of problems and early intervention, rather than on etiology and prevention. At the turn of the century, Abraham Jacobi (Senn, 1946) wrote that "Pediatrics deals with the entire organism." This concept ushered in the era of expanding research and knowledge in the areas of normal growth and development and preventive medicine for children.

Needless to say, such broad definitions pose problems in delineating services and specifying curricula to adequately prepare health care professionals. As Christophersen (1982) pointed out in referring to the *Standards of Child Health Care* provided by the American Academy of Pediatrics "most providers do not disagree with the majority of the Academy's recommendations, [however] putting these recommendations into practice is an entirely different story." Behavioral pediatrics came to include preventive care with attention to anticipatory guidance, accident prevention and issues of compliance; early detection of problems; supportive intervention; and referral for children with psychosocial as well as developmental difficulties that have an impact on their total functioning. In contrast to psychiatry, it includes referral rather than treatment of psychopathology and uses eclectic, generally short-term interventions (Richmond, 1975).

PROVIDING BEHAVIORAL PEDIATRICS CARE

In considering training professionals to deal with children on a behavioral level it is important to keep in mind the changing pattern of service delivery in this country. Although parents come to their primary care physicians first for professional help with behavioral concerns they have about their children (Hessel & Haggerty, 1968; Yancy, 1975), other disciplines are not only available but often more suitable sources of assistance. Psychologists, behavioral pediatricians, psychiatrists, psychiatric social workers, parent educators, school counsellors, nurses, nurse practitioners, mental health counsellors and religious professionals, all have skills to assist families (Confort & Kappy, 1974; Wishingrad, 1963). Many of them are better trained, have more appropriate time available, are more interested in these problems, and are less expensive than primary care physicians. As the health needs, health financing, and expectations of the public change, the patterns of use of these disciplines are also likely to change. Primary care physicians, however, are likely to remain the point of first contact for defining problems, the most likely to make referrals to others, and are in the best position to coordinate and follow-up such care. In many locales the primary care physician—pediatrician, general practitioner, or family practitioner—may be the only one available to help. For these reasons physician training must include behavioral pediatrics to make this part of practice effective. The principles to be discussed for improving training in the future apply to trainees of *all* disciplines, with differences in content specific to their backgrounds rather than differences in concept.

TEACHING BEHAVIORAL PEDIATRICS

Behavioral pediatrics cannot *not* be taught, just as communication cannot not occur. There are emotional responses to all illnesses, and behaviors that lead to, avoid, or ameliorate any injury, stress or significant life event. Professionals develop attitudes and ways of dealing with behavioral aspects of medicine whether or not they receive instruction. The sensitivity and effectiveness of their dealings can be fostered by careful education,

however. Medical students may actually lose sensitivity to patient concerns as they go through training without attention to behavioral aspects of
their education (Werner, Adler, Robinson, & Korsch, 1979). The fact that
behavioral pediatrics addresses phenomena integrally entwined throughout medicine, and, in fact, inherent in human existence, makes identifying teaching goals and sites more difficult. No one may take responsibility
for seeing that education about behavior occurs, each assuming that because of its pervasiveness and the professional's own humanness, the basic knowledge of behavior has been acquired. Ideally, all teachers of professionals should understand the behavioral components of their topics,
and maintain awareness of these components among their students at
every level of training. In fact, the advantage of the teacher being of the
same profession as the student makes this even more important for later
application of what is taught. In spite of the universality of behavioral aspects in medicine, having no clear definition or subspecialty advocate in
charge of behavioral pediatrics teaching often results in a lack of assigned
time in crowded professional curricula.

A striking aspect of professional education in general, not just in medicine, is its lack of clearly defined goals and objectives. Each institution includes different subjects among its required courses, often determined by
the funding, prestige and power of the department faculty rather than by
the needs of its students. The Task Force on Pediatric Education (1978) was
formed to address this lack of consistency and found psychosocial pediatric
education and behavioral areas of training to be particularly in need of
greater emphasis. Behavioral aspects of the care of children have been perhaps more systematically addressed in nursing and nurse practitioner
training programs. In nurse practitioner programs three half- or full-semes-
ter courses are required covering family theory and communication skills
(Fond, 1983). Education of psychologists varies so much from institution to
institution that each institution declares itself to be "experimental" or "analytically oriented." Faculty orientation as well as course content often focuses on one theory to the virtual exclusion of others.

Ideally the department chairman sets an example of awareness and carefully monitors how and what (not whether) learning about behavior occurs. With the specialty orientation of academic faculties, however, this
may not occur.

Why does something so integral to the care of children require a special
training effort? In the not so distant past most of what physicians had to
offer was counsel and support. Training occurred through apprenticeship
at the clinician's side. With the advent of enormous progress in effective
therapeutics and information about disease, learning by observing clinicians with their patients has become a minor, sometimes nonexistent, part
of the training process.

At about the same time as the explosion of scientific knowledge in medicine, Freud's psychodynamic view of human psychology and psychopa-

thology came into ascendance. The science of psychology, most clearly beginning with the laboratory work of Wundt in 1879, did not work its way into the clinical care of patients until the late 1950s (Lang, 1980). Information from psychology relevant to patient care is thus relatively new and qualitatively different from the more entrenched psychodynamic view. Both views need to be taught, but psychologists, on the other hand, have had difficulty being accepted in medical faculty roles. All this comes at a time when trainees are expected to absorb vastly increased amounts of data from all other disciplines as well. Faculty, too, have more specialized areas of expertise, particularly in the tertiary care centers in which most medical training occurs. They tend to place emphasis on areas of personal interest and are often unaware of new knowledge in the behavioral sciences. Carrying out training of pediatricians largely in tertiary medical centers has been problematic for training in general. Whereas most graduates enter primary care practice, their training time is dominated by tertiary-care-level problems. Besides undertraining about topics of most common concern later, especially normal growth and development and behavioral problems in children, this method may also contribute to physician disillusionment with the pace and focus of practice.

Training of nurses and nurse practitioners often shares this problem of being largely sited in tertiary care centers. Psychologists actually face an even greater gap between experiences during training and later roles. Their education usually is based in a general academic center rather than one designed for health services. Faculty, while expert in the basic science of behavior, have had variable experience with children presenting with health concerns. Internships occur mainly in adult mental health centers and veteran's hospitals, providing little or no exposure to medically ill or normal range children.

Thus, both pediatric clinicians and behavioral scientists who later work at a primary care level with patients often have been trained with a tertiary orientation. Graduates who pursue research in behavioral aspects of child health, on the other hand, may learn excellent research skills through tertiary level training but are led to focus on uncommon conditions or therapies which cannot be generalized to children in their home settings. Thus, historically, training site biases both faculty and experiences away from a balanced view of children's health.

ETIOLOGICAL FACTORS THAT COMPLICATE TRAINING

While medical knowledge is becoming more detailed, the definition and scope of the health field is expanding. The World Health Organization defines health as "a state of complete physical, mental and social well-being and not merely the absence of disease or infirmity" (McKeown, 1976). With improvement in nutritional status and immunity and control of many infectious diseases in developed countries, more attention can be given to subtler manifestations of suffering, including emotional distress, and etiological factors, including social and environmental. While medicine will always have primary responsibility for biological aspects of health, families increasingly seek and expect assistance with psychological and social adjustment concerns. Duff, Rowe, and Anderson (1972) determined that only 12 percent of patients presenting to a pediatric clinic were there for purely physical concerns whereas 36 percent came for purely psychological ones and the majority with both. Furthermore, between 10 and 15 percent of children have significant emotional difficulties and require detection and referral. The traditional view that health is the absence of organic pathology may not prepare clinicians to manage such a preponderance of psychological concerns or inculcate the attitude that it is appropriate for them to do so. Their ambivalence about taking on this broader role and teaching it is intensified by the already enormous demands made on them by technical advances in medicine and the fact that skills for care of behavioral problems are difficult to acquire.

INTRAPERSONAL FACTORS THAT COMPLICATE TRAINING

Even when programs accept the importance of training for behavioral pediatrics, there are problems in doing this successfully. There is no standard approach, defined basic core content, or single theoretical basis that can be taught that adequately prepares a trainee. In fact several theories, often apparently conflicting, must be studied. Trainees, especially in medicine, may have no background in the social sciences and no interest in acquiring knowledge in this area. Only 6.9 percent of medical students major in social sciences in college and only 20 percent of medical schools require (with only 15 percent strongly recommending) behavioral science courses for admission (Stokes & Martin, 1983). Since a child's behavior is inherently part of an interaction with others, the professional must deal with family members, and often with emotionally charged issues that also touch his or her personal life. As the professional develops as an adult, personal issues change and new coping skills must be learned. Simultaneously, society's notions of appropriate parent-child roles are also in flux. One's own interpersonal skills and sensitivity are basic to discovering, interpreting and assisting parents in solving behavioral problems. Although success depends on the cooperation of parent, child and professional, failure may be experienced as personal, even though actual implementation of the plan is out of the professional's control. Just as this is difficult to come to terms with in practice, so is it difficult to learn and therefore frustrating to teach. Teaching may concentrate on the traditional didactic pathology-oriented model simply because it comes more easily. Even satisfactory indices of efficacy of behavioral teaching are rare because of the multiplicity of factors affecting change. The complexity of teaching in this area can deter even the most determined faculty and trainees.

PREVENTION AS PART OF HEALTH CARE

Beyond overt requests for assistance with psychosocial and emotional problems, pediatric practitioners have the opportunity and responsibility to help prevent such problems. Because of their role as monitors of health status and as first contact of patients, pediatric clinicians need to know how to *promote* health as well as how to identify, assess and manage health problems. McKeown (1976) points out that "it is nearer the truth to say that we are well and are made ill" than to focus on illness as the primary problem. A dramatic example of this concept is the fact that improvement in the life expectancy of mature males from 1938–54 to 1970 has been estimated to have been reduced by at least half by smoking alone—a voluntary behavior. All of the gains of modern medicine can be largely lost by failure to deal with health related behaviors. McKeown's conclusion was that, in considering health as a whole, "in technologically advanced countries behavioral influences are now more important than all others." Understanding and influencing lifestyle behavior has thus become a prime consideration for the health profession.

Preparing parents for the changing developmental needs of their children is appropriately called anticipatory guidance. Specific ideas for avoiding common problems, such as sleep disorders in the 8 to 10 month old infant, are possible in the context of routine health maintenence visits (Telzrow, 1978). Accidents currently are the leading cause of death for children from 1 to 14 years old in the U.S. (Dershewitz & Christophersen, 1984). Parent education in controlling child injuries as well as enhancing compliance with all health measures should be part of every pediatrician's practice. Professionals working in the behavior area should acquire the expertise to educate pediatricians in transmitting this guidance effectively. Behavioral pediatrics is thus enlarging its scope to include all behavioral factors affecting health.

CONTENT OF TRAINING

Certainly the range of information relating to children's behavior makes defining the content of training for work in behavioral pediatrics very difficult. In addition, professionals from different disciplines have very different bases of knowledge and therefore different needs. Preparation for clinical patient care versus patient care and teaching versus behavioral research have different requirements. Fortunately for the task of designing training programs, there are only a few basic levels that need to be ad-

TABLE 25.2.   FACTORS AFFECTING BEHAVIOR AND RELATED
TRAINING AREAS

Etiology	Related Discipline
Developmental	Normal and abnormal development, embryology, neuropathology, neurology, speech and language pathology, physical and occupational therapy, audiology, etc.
Biochemical	Psychoneuroendocrinology, nutrition, psychopharmacology
Environmental	Environmental studies, toxicology
Learned	Psychology, education and learning theory, psycholinguistics, psychiatry
Genetic	Genetics and metabolic disease
Social	Sociology, anthropology, epidemiology, social psychology, systems theory, hygiene and public health

dressed for training students of all disciplines. All trainees must acquire basic information, develop skills for using it, have experiences to refine and consolidate what they are learning, and evolve an orientation towards their patients and themselves that furthers the work.

What knowledge is basic to behavioral pediatrics? Certainly a broad perspective on human social as well as biological functioning is helpful. Expertise about the diverse factors affecting behavior comes from many fields not traditionally recognized as part of medicine, for example, psychology, sociology, anthropology and epidemiology. No one professional can have in-depth knowledge in all of these areas, but an awareness of the availability and organization of information in these related areas can provide useful perspective. In order to obtain this perspective faculty members must abstract core information and present it in a manner appropriate to the background, level, and needs of the trainee. Table 25.2 presents a nonexhaustive listing of disciplines related to behavioral pediatrics based on the diverse etiologies of health-related behavior. To fully deal with a child's development, each area of functioning must be understood and related to its *normal* evolution and pathology (Table 25.3). For example, appreciation of motor development and its deviations requires knowledge of normal and abnormal developmental neurology, embryology and neuropathology, including genetic and metabolic factors, and knowledge of physical and occupational therapies.

The study of language development involves neurology, audiology,

TABLE 25.3. AREAS OF CHILD FUNCTION AND RELATED AREAS OF STUDY

Motor development
  Developmental neurology—normal and abnormal
  Embryology
  Neuropathology
    Genetic and metabolic factors
  Physical and occupational therapies
Language development
  Neurology
  Audiology
  Speech and language pathology
  Psycholinguistics
  Social environment
Cognitive development
  Cognitive psychology—normal and abnormal
  Learning and education theories
  Piagetian psychology
  Psychoanalytic theory
    Psychiatric classification systems
    Psychological and educational testing methods
    Neurosensory and perceptual testing
    Group and family dynamics
    Theories of emotional development
    Theories of personality development
    Psychopathology with genetic and metabolic influences
    Therapeutic modalities
      Psychotherapy
      Psychoanalysis
      Family and group therapy
      Behavior modification
      Hypnotherapy
      Imaging
      Relaxation therapy
      Pharmacotherapy
      Biofeedback
Social and emotional development
  Anthropology
  Sociology
  Social psychology
  Epidemiology
  Systems theory
  Education
  Environmental studies
    Human ecology
    Toxicology
    Nutrition
    Hygiene
    Public Health
    Knowledge of community resources (schools, day care, religious institutions, political bodies, health agencies, recreational facilities)

speech and language pathology, psycholinguistics, and understanding of the role of social environment.

The complexity of cognitive function is reflected in the variety of approaches used to describe it. Trainees need to appreciate the different ways of explaining cognition in order to be flexible in their clinical approach to the patient. Thus the approaches offered by psychology and psychiatry, including cognitive psychology (normal and abnormal), learning and education theories, Piagetian psychology and analytic views, should be presented. Concerning these approaches, trainees should be aware of the psychiatric classification system, psychological and educational testing methods, neurosensory and perceptual testing, psychopharmacology, group and family dynamics, theories of emotional development and personality, and psychopathology, including genetic and metabolic influences. Trainees, regardless of their future clinical or research plans, should at least be aware of the variety of therapeutic modalities, including psychotherapy, psychoanalysis, group and family therapy, behavior modification, biofeedback, hypnotherapy, imaging, relaxation therapy and pharmacotherapy, even if they cannot be skilled in using them all.

The socioemotional development of children perhaps touches on the greatest variety of other fields. Here knowledge of the contribution of anthropology, sociology, social psychology, epidemiology, systems theory, education, and environmental studies, including human ecology, toxicology, nutrition, hygiene and public health is desirable. A knowledge of community resources, including schools, religious institutions, political bodies, health agencies, and recreational facilities is important for clinical care as well as for understanding influences on the child.

Appreciating the significance of the aforementioned areas for child behavior depends on the trainee's basic understanding of the interrelationships between biological and behavioral processes. Professionals who have not undergone training as physicians or nurses (including the courses required for admission to those professional schools) need additional background in the biological aspects of behavior (Table 25.4). This should include the central concepts of developmental neurology, psychoneuroendocrinology, psychopharmacology, genetics, nutrition, environmental influences, speech and language development, and pathology, audiology and psychiatry. The traditional focus in these areas is on the abnormal. Adequate focus on the range of normal is very important to realistic clinical work. Much of this kind of training is presently optional, even in training of clinical psychologists.

One of the key factors contributing to successful management of behavioral dysfunction in childhood is the ability to understand the perspective of other professionals. Medically trained professionals organize their approach to the patient based on formation of a differential diagnosis. This is a different way of thinking than that used by other disciplines. It orients

TABLE 25.4. TRAINING NEEDS OF HEALTH PROFESSIONALS ("NON-MEDICAL" BACKGROUND)

Developmental neurology—normal and abnormal
Psychoneuroendocrinology
Psychopharmacology
Genetics
Nutrition
Environmental influences
Speech and language development and pathology
Audiology
Psychiatry
Differential diagnosis

the physician to categories of dysfunction, probabilities of different etiologies, the order in which evaluation is most efficiently carried out, and anticipation of complications and outcome, rather than to making a diagnosis. It leads from diagnosis to therapy in a pragmatic fashion, which goes beyond the paucity of knowledge in the field in order to provide therapeutic intervention. Thus nonmedical professionals need to be aware that medical professionals, although they may speak in terms of a single diagnostic dysfunction, have not necessarily neglected to consider other etiologies. The psychologist may find it very helpful to ask what other diagnoses were considered, in order to maintain flexibility toward revising the working diagnosis during therapy. Additionally, the medically oriented professional more readily understands the recommendations generated by a consultation with the nonmedically oriented professional if the format of a differential diagnosis is used. That is, the nonmedically oriented consultant should generate diagnoses but suggest the most likely category of dysfunction and the best therapeutic regimen for that specific diagnosis to direct further evaluation.

Trainees who plan primarily to carry out investigative work in behavioral pediatrics must certainly have extensive knowledge of statistics and research design. Adequate knowledge in those areas, in order to read the literature and to communicate with research collaborators, is important also to trainees who plan primarily clinical or teaching roles. This is particularly true for behavioral pediatrics because of the inherent complexity of factors influencing research design. Of course nonmedical researchers must be completely familiar with detailed biological knowledge about their specific problem area. Similarly medical professionals doing research must be expert in behavioral techniques relevant to their topic. A practical appreciation of what constitutes a significant research question (and result) is perhaps the hardest but the most important thing to teach and to learn.

SKILL AREAS OF TRAINING

Not all of this vast smorgasbord of fields of study can be explored in detail by each trainee in a reasonable period of time. Each professional comes with his or her own background of strengths and weaknesses in content areas. What is most important is a core of topics presented with an interdisciplinary orientation that provides perspective on the variety of approaches possible. There should be a balance of micro, macro, and ecological level analyses. The micro level should include exposure to biochemical/neurophysiological processes; the macro a view of physical and emotional development of the individual; and the ecological an exposure to the transactional model of social systems. As the professional trainee personally investigates a few topics at all these levels, the value of the different approaches will become evident. Most important, perhaps, is that normal development be included along with the abnormal so that a model of individual variation in strengths and weaknesses will come to moderate the trainee's natural inclination towards labeling.

All of this basic knowledge about behavior must be translated into clinical skills if it is to be useful to children (Table 25.5). Trainees who will become clinicians need specific skills including: establishing relationships; examining the patient; testing abilities; observing interactions; interviewing for information about events, feelings, and expectations associated with problems; developing patient confidence and motivation; giving the patient information and direction for self-help; clarifying and restructuring family interactions; maintaining contact over time to allow for compliance, reinforcement, course correction and the evolution of insight and learning; and terminating relationships in a positive way.

Additionally, when behavioral pediatrics is practiced in the broader sense that includes attention to environmental influences on health, professionals need parallel interactional skills for dealing with institutions that affect children (Richmond, 1975; Dworkin & Dworkin, 1975). Providing consultation to schools, day-care centers, athletic teams, religious centers, housing and health authorities, courts and legislative committees, hospital boards (in determining visitation rights, confidentiality, and terminal-care policies, for example), and to organizations providing financing or political leverage can often make a great contribution to children's well being—sometimes more than individual therapies. Both institutional and patient-care skills need to be adaptable to direct person-to-person encounters and to situations of less direct contact, such as telephone calls and advising other professionals and paraprofessionals in their management of problems (Caplan, 1983). These skills too should be taught, along with practical experience.

The importance of learning how to collaborate with other professionals on behalf of a child cannot be overemphasized. The myriad of fields rele-

TABLE 25.5. SPECIFIC SKILLS FOR CLINICIANS

Establishing therapeutic relationship with child and family
Examining the child
Testing child's abilities
Ascertaining child's and family's feelings and expectations
  associated with the problem
Providing feedback and direction to help foster the family's
  self-help skills, motivation and self-confidence
Interviewing patient and observing interactions
Clarification of interactions
Restructuring of interactions
Maintaining continuity over time to allow:
  Compliance
  Revision of original therapeutic plan
  Evolution of insight and ability to generalize learning
Terminating the relationship in a positive fashion
Communicating with institutions
Use of telephone
Supervision of paraprofessionals
Consultation
Recording skills
Collaboration
Teamwork with parents
Statistics and research design familiarity
Teaching
Continuing self education—use of journals and library,
  obtaining consultation, peer teaching and support

vant to behavioral pediatrics makes it impossible for one person to master it all. Furthermore, people can communicate more freely and more effectively with one person than with another, whether that person is the most knowledgeable about their problem or not. Excellent care can result if the professional enlists advice from others as needed. In some programs for multiply handicapped children, for example, the "team leader" can be of any discipline and is backed up by colleagues who may even give the leader responsibility for teaching parents certain therapeutic methods from their area (Shonkoff, 1983).

Certainly skills for recording information that include careful wording for legal purposes, avoiding unnecessary labeling, attention to confidentiality and retrievability for research purposes are important (Weed, 1970). Such skills can make the professional's job more secure, protect the patient's interests, provide a model for patient respect, and facilitate continuing care and further knowledge.

Clinicians who will have a role in teaching other professionals can benefit from learning the basic principles of how to teach (Greenberg & Jewett, 1984). For example, one simple teaching principle is to organize information so that it is introduced, taught, practiced with feedback provided, summarized, and then learning evaluated. Illustrating concepts with concrete examples and aiming for only two or three points in one session are frequently ignored basics. These principles apply also to patient education and are therefore relevant to all clinicians. Clinicians especially need to learn how to work with parents on a problem, encouraging parent initiative and decision-making. Research workers in behavioral pediatrics need skill in research criticism, computer literacy, and grant writing, as well as teaching skills (Table 25.6). For them, attending to the clinical relevance of their research ideas is a particularly important skill.

Of course, modern education techniques should be used in teaching trainees. Providing feedback to the trainee about his or her progress should be an obvious component of training. Immediate feedback, with an equal focus on strengths and weaknesses, and concrete discussion of strategies for improvement are helpful to anyone. Patient simulators have been successfully used to give personal instruction (DaRosa, Majur & Markus, 1982). Videotapes have made individual faculty supervision more feasible by allowing better scheduling of discussions. Role playing allows for practice of verbal exchanges that are then more easily used in the real clinical situation, and evaluation is thereby incorporated into the teaching. Evaluation of interpersonal skills should be a requirement for advancement and continuing certification; interpersonal skills are central to pediatric care.

Professionals of all disciplines at all levels of academic involvement are sooner or later called upon for administrative duties. Not surprisingly the skills needed for accomplishing tasks with other adults in the work place, called administrative or personnel management skills, are similar to those needed for a family to function together. Much could be learned from this field that would be applicable and helpful to professionals in behavioral pediatrics (Procaccini & Kiefaber, 1983).

Since behavioral pediatrics is such a rapidly growing field, skills for continuing self-education of professionals are essential to professional integrity and quality patient care over time. Formal instruction and practice in the use of journals and the library, and in obtaining information from consultations are usually neglected in training. Awareness that faculty depend upon individual meetings and discussion groups for supervision and peer support can transmit to trainees a positive attitude toward continuing professional development.

ATTITUDINAL ASPECTS OF TRAINING

Assuring that professionals integrate knowledge and skills in behavioral pediatrics into their care of patients has been perhaps the most difficult

**TABLE 25.6.   ADDITIONAL SKILLS FOR
CLINICIAN-TEACHER AND RESEARCHER**

Advanced statistics
Research design
Research experience
Research criticism
Expertise in all aspects of problem area
Computer literacy
Teaching
Administration
Grant writing
Continuing self education—use of journals and library,
    obtaining consultation, peer teaching and support

training goal to attain. The many barriers to training in this area have already been discussed, including the difficulties presented by the heavy reliance on effective patient-clinician interaction. Acquisition of information about and aptitude for dealing with behavioral aspects of health require a high level of interest and a sense of the subject's importance. Helping children and families with this skill and knowledge, however, simply cannot be done optimally without a particular orientation toward the work. Clearly the professional must feel that it is part of his or her clinical responsibility to address the problems of patient and family. Furthermore, he or she must realize that the problem is important to the child and the family. Amelioration will require effort and desire to change on their part, both to carry out therapeutic plans effectively and to learn how to recognize and approach similar situations in the future. Since behavioral patterns have a history and serve a perhaps unconscious role in a person's life, the effort required to change them is often hampered by factors not readily apparent to the family. The clinician must be patient, tolerant of sometimes wavering application to the task at hand but specific and firm in correcting, generous with praise for small results, and appreciative of successes. In other words, the clinician's guidance should be a model for the kind of support the family members need to give the child and each other. Adaptation must be envisioned as possible, even if it is not perfect.

How can we give trainees such an orientation? (See Table 25.7.) The best way is through experience. Because of the universality of behavioral issues, particularly in dynamic situations such as a learning process, relevant experiences for trainees are readily available. Training is itself a developmental process (Brent, 1981). Trainees enter with vast differences in background. Such individual differences can be a source of competitiveness and anxiety or of stimulation and mutual support. The faculty themselves

TABLE 25.7.   ORIENTATION TO THE WORK

Accommodate individual differences in trainees
   Learn from them
   Encourage peer learning
   Accept faculty limitations
   Work at trainee's developmental level
      Gradually increase responsibility
      Vary supervision to needs
      Provide feedback
Consider progression-regression
   Faculty advisors
Provide experience with normal children with trainee in
   nontraditional role Day care, school, home visits
Assure experience with civic role and role models
   Schools, day care, health agencies, court, legislature,
   parent groups, funding sources
Provide a variety of faculty role models
Demonstrate faculty continuing education
   Peer teaching, support groups
   Nominal participation
Assure panel of well and problem patients
Involve in a variety of care settings
   Ward, clinic, NICU, PICU, committees

can foster the latter attitude by openly learning from the trainees and encouraging trainees to consult each other, showing awareness and acceptance of the faculty members' own limitations, and dealing with each trainee at his or her own developmental level. These are just the attitudes we hope parents will have toward their children. For example, initially trainees may be wise to watch a difficult patient being interviewed, even if they already have had experience with similar patients. They then should gradually be given increased responsibility for parts of the interview or management, with feedback on their effort provided frequently, for example, by videotaping, scoring, and group or individual discussion or supervision. Later they will work autonomously, but with the option of having the faculty member take over if necessary. Finally, the trainee will manage problems alone, with consultation available at their discretion. Even at this level, emotional support (often commiseration) can strengthen their ability to use their skills optimally. Putting trainees into difficult situations without this kind of support may actually make them more likely to *avoid* involvement in the future.

   Trainees will undergo regression as well as progressions in their professional development. Alert advisors can readily detect these down cycles and point out to the trainee that they can be expected to be transient. Fluctuations in the trainee's ability to cope can be a useful way of teaching about variability in children's growth. Supervised experience with normal children for all trainees, such as serving as teacher's aides in a day care center, is an excellent way for trainees to recognize individual strengths of children, become aware of the amazing impact they have on us as adults, gain respect for the complexity of the normal, and observe normal regressions and progressions (Fox, 1975). This role frequently helps highlight the trainee's own development as a professional, which can open useful discussions. Trainees planning research careers particularly need this kind of experience in order to plan appropriate studies for children of a given age and to deal with difficulties concomitant with normal behaviors.

EXPERIENCE ASPECTS OF TRAINING

Behavioral pediatrics often requires professionals to go beyond their traditional roles to best care for children. After many years of seeing themselves in a certain role, they may find this quite difficult. Experiences out of the medical setting force trainees to reevaluate their role and to test their skills of observation and interaction in situations where they lack power and responsibility and sometimes even competence. Such experiences can help trainees get a child's eye view of the environment and gain respect for the work of other professionals, such as teachers.

Similar lessons can be learned by visiting families in their homes, and by visiting their churches and their children's schools. Suddenly, learning is made concrete for the trainee. The reality of barriers to carrying out treatment plans—shared bathrooms, lack of privacy, poverty and so on—becomes clear. On the other hand, valuable suggestions may come from contact with family members, or from other professionals working with the child, which may not only help to solve problems but may well be used with other patients (Sharp, 1984).

Taking on civic advocacy roles may be particularly threatening to professionals who are unfamiliar with this mode of activism. Modeling, experience, time-allotment and support are needed to help trainees become involved in advising schools, evaluating day care centers, consulting for agencies, testifying in court, lobbying with legislators, organizing parent groups, or soliciting funds from granting foundations. Acquaintance with activist professionals from their own discipline with whom the trainee can identify can provide role models for community involvement.

Needless to say, faculty training in behavioral pediatrics should be an ongoing effort. To this end, peer teaching and support groups have been used successfully (Charney, 1983). In Scandanavia, videotape techniques have helped involve physicians in the learning and teaching process of behavioral pediatrics (Fenderson, 1983).

It is important that trainees be given the opportunity to manage a variety of behavioral problems and to promote health behavior in a number of normal children. Physicians need continuity of experience with patients (who can thus come to identify them as "their" doctor) to develop strategies for setting priorities for care. In such a setting they can learn to provide anticipatory guidance during well-child visits and to try out screening and testing tools to assess behavior, interaction and developmental abilities. Best of all, they can actually see the results of their efforts to solve patient and family problems. Through experience with a variety of normal as well as dysfunctional children, trainees can learn the important lesson that all children have strengths and that a problem, no matter how severe, does not necessarily imply a pathological family or child. Experiences with families with a chronically ill child are especially valuable. By keeping a log book of their patients, the trainee can develop a sense of the prevalence of various types of dysfunction, and an appreciation of the many skills involved in behavioral pediatrics. Faculty preceptors should monitor the mix of patients with which the trainee is involved to ensure that it is as widely representative as possible. A representative mix can be facilitated by use of the computerized systems which are now widely used for billing and appointments (Straus, 1985).

SPECIAL NEEDS OF NONMEDICAL PROFESSIONALS

Nonmedical professionals should also have a continuity of experience, even though they do not provide medical care. They can, for example, have ongoing involvement with parenting groups in the well-child setting as well as ongoing involvement with their own patients with behavioral problems.

Participation in ward rounds, intensive care unit support groups, parenting groups, specialty clinic teams, and acting as consultants to medical curriculum committees, help nonmedical trainees understand the medical approach to problems. It can also help them gauge the predisposition of various physicians to incorporating behavioral knowledge into practice, which can be particularly important in that nonphysicians are likely to be called upon to select physician-collaborators in their future work as clinicians or researchers. Appreciating the range of skills and interest in behavioral techniques among physicians will help trainees choose wisely.

With much research continuing to be needed in behavioral pediatrics, especially on the clinical level, trainees are very likely to be involved in research projects during their careers, including research involving patient participation. Participation in research is itself a modifying influence on attitudes and behavior (Stern, 1983). It can be a worrying, intrusive, meaningless experience or it can be therapeutic, enhancing self-esteem and understanding. Having trainees participate as subjects in research projects (or sham projects) can be a graphic way of illustrating the potential effects of involvement in research. Arrangements should be made for trainees to serve on human subjects committees or ethics committees, along with parents to help trainees understand what being involved in research means to parents and children. Of course, ethical issues are universal in clinical practice and are taught mostly by faculty example.

The child-care team often mirrors the dynamics of family interrelationships. This phenomenon can be utilized to the advantage of trainee education as a model for intervention techniques as well as for learning. Faculty are looked to for direction, often with unrealistic expectations of omnipotence (as are parents). Transference actually occurs. Trainees often vie with each other for praise and recognition from the faculty, sometimes to a point of competitiveness that interferes with care (as do siblings). Sexual issues come up in the guise of faculty favoritism and trainee interactions. Faculty often experience countertransference in their relationships with trainees. Stereotyped expectations may determine interactions among professionals and paraprofessionals. Religious biases may also come into play, especially in scheduling for holiday work. All of these "family" dynamics present opportunities for individual and group discussion. "Family conferences" can be held on the ward to clarify perceptions and mediate disputes (Allmond, Buckman & Gofman, 1979). Plans for behavior change can be formulated and the complexity of carrying them out experienced first hand. Experiencing the impact of behavior change techniques on their own problems can help trainees gauge their usefulness as tools to be used in clinical practice. Discussion of these experiences can take place in ward rounds, clinic team conferences, or even at retreats designated for this purpose. (Bergman, Rothenberg & Telzrow, 1979).

STRESS IN TRAINING

Training is a stressful experience, especially training that depends heavily on interactional skills. Not only are physician trainees worked to exhaustion but they are deprived of sleep, adequate income, healthful food, opportunities to be with their families, and opportunities to fully meet their religious obligations. They often find themselves in an unfamiliar location, distant from their supportive friends. They are sometimes put into positions of responsibility for problems beyond their level of expertise, then criticized for lack of success rather than praised for approximations to success. All of this takes place in the context of a voluntary decision to undertake a major role change. One might say that this is an optimal situation for brainwashing (Charney, 1983). Brainwashing, in fact, occurs whether it is intended or not. Siegel and Donnelly (1983) note that internship is critical in part "for the implicit expectation that this is the way medicine works and that this is how the life of a physician must be." Professionals may then carry over these demands on themselves into their posttraining years, perpetuating a highly stressful milieu in which, among other things, interpersonal sensitivity is diminished. For example, Knights and Folstein (1977) found that 30 percent of patient emotional and cognitive disorders were not detected by primary care physicians.

Certainly the concept of arranging a child's environment to reduce stress is better served when the professional's own well-being is attended to during training. The structure of the training program could itself be a model that respects individual differences, supports family life, and recognizes adult developmental needs. The program should individualize experiences for trainees of different backgrounds as much as possible. Arrangements should be made for professionals who are also parents to attend to family duties and to be present at important family events. Religious observances should be fostered by flexible scheduling. Exchange of duties among trainees to allow for special needs to be met should be encouraged. Of course, these modifications of training cost money, but ignoring them conveys an attitude antithetical to that being taught. The way in which professionals are treated during training may well be reflected in the way they eventually treat their patients.

Instruction in stress management and availability of mental health counseling should be part of professional training for the sake of the trainee, and indirectly, for his or her patients. Although most medical schools are providing counselling services for physicians in training, 35 percent of medical school deans recently surveyed and 45 percent of student representatives felt that the services were inadequate (Seigle, Schuckit & Plumb, 1983). Psychological support services, kept confidential by separation from school administration and including services for spouses, were recommended. One stress-control program involves parents of medical students, instructing them about the training process so that they can provide more appropriate support (DeVaul & Murphy, 1982). Given the estimated 30-percent prevalence of clinical depression in first year residents (Valko and Clayton, 1975), psychological services are not peripheral to training. Aside from their therapeutic value, such services can provide important lessons for trainees, who, having gone through the process of seeking and receiving help, are now more aware of the complexities involved in patient referral.

FACULTY CONSIDERATIONS

The need to develop training programs in behavioral pediatrics has become more apparent as changes in the field of pediatrics have evolved. Rothenburg (1949) notes that "By the second half of this century, 'curative' pediatrics comprised only one part of the speciality's growing commitment to total child care, while issues such as the emotional and intellectual development of both the sick and well child were receiving more and more attention." Researchers Hessel, Haggerty, and Richmond were among the first to note that pediatricians were being turned to by their patients' families for problems which included psychosocial dynamics, personality development, and community programs (Hessel & Haggerty, 1968; Richmond, 1959). The need to incorporate behavioral pediatrics teaching in child-health professional programs is now so widely recognized that the debate in the last decade has been over not whether teaching behavior is or is not important but, rather, in what manner it should be taught and who will do the teaching. (Anders, 1977; Felice & Friedman, 1982).

The child psychiatry-pediatric liason programs were among the first efforts to incorporate teaching of behavior into pediatric residency training. Although this would seem to be a natural marriage, the outcome of such programs has been less productive than expected. Numerous problem areas have been identified. Housestaff tend to be preoccupied with organic diseases rather than behavioral issues. Housestaff come to identify with a child psychiatrist rather than a practicing pediatrician. Department chairmen lack commitment to behavioral teaching. There is a lack of qualified teaching faculty in these areas. There has been resistance both by pediatricians and child psychiatrists to such a model (Felice & Friedman, 1982). There has been a focus on consultation/service rather than on a collaboration/teaching model. And yet, despite these obstacles, the advantages of sharing knowledge and skills between these two disciplines is so attractive that new programs are continually being developed in an effort to minimize the conflicts and maximize the training both for the child psychiatrist and the pediatrician.

Psychology has also been called upon as a source of teaching for pediatric housestaff. Haggerty (1982) points out that, in fact, there may be less resistance by the pediatricians to such a model than to the child psychiatrist model because of the pediatrician's perceived sense of control over a "nonmedical" professional. On the other hand, many psychologists still do not feel comfortable with this model. And once again we are faced with the problems of lack of role models and a focus on consultation services rather than collaborative teaching. Areas such as child development, research, behavioral modification, psychological testing and other specific treatment modalities within the expertise of psychologists are so important, however, that ways of utilizing this expertise continues to be sought.

The biosocial or behavioral pediatric fellowship models have also met with difficulties in the task of teaching pediatric trainees. Two major factors have led to complications. One is that many times these fellowships have been sought out by pediatricians who wish to fill a gap in their residency training by acquiring skills in dealing with issues of behavioral pediatrics in their clinical practice. Secondly, these fellowship programs vary greatly in the content emphasized, ranging from areas of developmental disabilities to programs concentrating on a more psychiatric approach (Sarles & Friedman, 1979). Both factors promote the "identity crises" noted in behavioral fellowship trainees. Additionally, the emergence of a subspecialty of "behavioral pediatrics" complicates attainment of the overall goal of teaching behavioral techniques to all clinicians.

For the trainee within each discipline there should be a "core" faculty with skills and knowledge in diagnosis and management of behavioral problems, normal growth and development, and psychological development of children. The faculty must be easily identified as role models in that they come from the same discipline as the trainee. Additionally, they need special skills in consultation in order to collaborate effectively with the other disciplines. The faculty can thus serve as a role model in how to work with professionals of other disciplines. When this type of training is provided at the residency training or internship level, we should see specialized training being sought mainly by individuals who wish to continue in academic teaching and research in the behavioral areas. At the teaching and research levels we would expect that the trainee will more readily seek out and use information provided by professionals from other disciplines.

We should not presume, however, that expertise is limited to any one particular discipline. Because of the importance of behavioral pediatrics to the care of children, its teaching must be coordinated and directed by individuals from many disciplines who are committed to assuring that each trainee has the best opportunity to learn the skills necessary to practice behavioral pediatrics.

What is needed is a core faculty with an interdisciplinary orientation and a resolve to bring in specialists from whatever discipline to teach on relevant topics. This requires a knowledge of local resources. It also requires briefing the specialist on how to address students who are possibly unfamiliar with the intricacies of the specialist's discipline so that the trainee can understand its relevance to the care of children. Having trainees visit sites of research or service of other disciplines is another approach that can broaden their perspective, especially if the objective for the visits are carefully laid out in advance. This has been found to be a particularly effective way of demonstrating opportunities for community involvement as well as for making the expertise of others relevant (Sharp, 1984). Teaching of this kind is usually volunteered by members of other disciplines free of charge in exchange for the opportunity to educate future referral sources, or as a contribution to education in general. When medical schools are affiliated with the behavioral pediatrics training program, the faculty will usually be willing to present overviews of various topics if adequately oriented to the course objectives. Schools of public health, for example, have sociologists and epidemiologists on their faculty who can be tapped for such overviews. State agencies, such as health departments, have officials whose jobs are by nature transdisciplinary who can be called upon.

Part-time practice of evaluation and counselling in behavioral and developmental problems as well as part-time practice in primary care can contribute significantly to faculty salaries. Paid consultation to schools, day care centers, and other community organizations can also add to faculty salaries. With grant funding in progressively shorter supply, these approaches are necessary. They are also desirable for testing the feasibility of the model they represent. Exchange of in-kind teaching services with other professionals may also be beneficial to all.

In summary, training professionals to provide comprehensive preventive and therapeutic health care for children requires incorporation of information about child development and behavior. In this chapter, we have discussed what is needed to train behavioral professionals at any level to provide this kind of care and to perform research furthering the field.

REFERENCES

Allmond, B.W., Buckman, W. & Gofman, H.F. (1979). *The family is the patient.* St. Louis: Mosby.

Anders T.F. (1977). Child psychiatry and pediatrics: The state of the relationship. *Pediatrics, 60*, 616–20.

Bergman A.F., Rothenberg, M.B. & Telzrow, R.W. (1979). A "retreat" for pediatric interns. *Pediatrics, 64*(4), 528.

Brent, D.A. (1981). The residency as a developmental process. *Journal of Medical Education, 56*, 417.

Caplan, S. (1983). The telephone in pediatric practice. In A.J. Moss (Ed.), *Pediatrics update* (p. 27). New York: Elsevier.

Charney, E. (1983). Child health care communications: Preparing physicians in training. In M.S. Thornton & W.K. Frankenburg (Eds.), *Child health care communications.* Skillman, N.J.: Johnson and Johnson.

Christopherson, E.R. (1982). Incorporating behavioral pediatrics into primary care. *Pediatric Clinics of North America, 29*(2), 261–296.

Confort, R.L., & Kappy, M.S. (1974). Pediatrician and socialworker as counseling team. *Social Work, 19*, 486.

DaRosa, D.A., Mazur, J., & Markus, J. (1982). Assessing patient evaluation skills: A structured versus traditional approach. *Journal of Medical Education, 57*, 472.

Dershewitz, R.A., & Christophersen, E.R. (1984). Childhood household safety. *American Journal of Diseases of Children, 138*, 85.

DeVaul, R.A. & Murphy, B. (1982). Parents of medical students: An underutilized support resource. *Journal of Medical Education, 57*, 563.

Duff, R.S., Rowe, D.S., & Anderson, F.P. (1972). Patient care and student learning in a pediatric clinic. *Pediatrics, 50*, 839.

Dworkin, A.L. & Dworkin, E.P. (1975). A conceptual overview of selected consultation models. *American Journal of Community Psychiatry, 3*, 151.

Felice, M.E., & Friedman, S.B. (1982). Teaching behavioral pediatrics to pediatric residents: The state of the art and description of a program. *Developmental and Behavioral Pediatrics, 3*(4), 225–231.

Fenderson, D. (1983). Paper presented at the National Behavioral Pediatrics Conference, St. Paul, Minnesota, June 23.

Fond, K. (1983). Practicing nurse practitioners. In M.S. Thornton & W.K. Frankenburg (Eds.), *Child health care communications*. Skillman, NJ: Johnson and Johnson.

Fox, E.M. (1975). Training pediatricians in mental health aspects of early child care. Paper presented at National Assoc. for the Education of Young Children Convention, 1975, Dallas, Texas.

Friedman, S.B. (1975). Symposium on behavioral pediatrics. *Pediatric Clinics of North America, 11*, 515.

Greenberg, L., & Jewett, L. (1984). Encouraging residents to be better teachers. Presented at Ambulatory Pediatrics Association, Region IV Meeting, Winston-Salem, North Carolina.

Haggerty, R.J. (1982). Behavioral pediatrics: Can it be taught? Can it be practiced? *Pediatric Clinics of North America, 29*(2), 391–398.

Hessel, S.J., & Haggerty, R.J. (1968). General pediatrics: A study of practice in the mid-1960's. *Journal of Pediatrics, 73*, 271.

Knights, E.B., & Folstein, M.F. (1977). Unsuspected emotional and cognitive disturbances in medical patients. *Annals of Internal Medicine, 87*, 723.

Lang, P. (1980). Foreward. In B.G. Melamed, & L.J. Siegel, *Behavioral medicine, practical applications in health care*. New York: Springer.

McKeown, T. (1976). *The role of medicine. Dream, mirage or nemesis*. London: Nuffield Provincial Hospitals.

Procaccini, J., & Kiefaber, M.W. (1983). *Parent burnout*. New York: Signet.

Richmond, J.B. (1959). Some observations on the sociology of pediatric education and practice. *Pediatrics, 23*,1175.

Richmond, J.B. (1975). An idea whose time has arrived. *Pediatric Clinics of North America, 22*,517.

Rothenberg, M.B. (1979). Child psychiatry-pediatrics consultation-liaison services in the hospital setting. *General Hospital Psychiatry, 1*(4), 281–6.

Sarles, R.M., & Friedman, S.B. (1979). Pediatric behavioral services. *Psychiatric Clinics of North America, 2*(2), 265–276.

Seigle, R.D., Schuckit, M.A., & Plumb, D. (1983). Availability of personal counselling in medical schools. *Journal of Medical Education, 58*, 542.

Senn, M.J.E. (1946). Relationship of pediatrics and psychiatry. *American Journal of Diseases of Children, 71*, 537.

Sharp, M. (1984). Development of community outreach training experiences for residents. Presented at Ambulatory Pediatrics Association Region IV meeting, Winston Salem, North Carolina.

Shonkoff, J. (1983). Personal communication.

Siegel, B., & Donnelly, J.C. (1978). Enriching personal and professional development: The experience of a support group for interns. *Journal of Medical Education, 53*, 908.

Stern, D. (1983) The place of affect in psychoanalysis and child development research: The need for convergence. Paper presented at Society for Research in Child Development, Biennial meeting, Detroit, Michigan.

Stokes, J. & Martin, M. (1983). Changes in medical school and admission requirements. *Journal of Medical Education, 58*(1), 58–9.

Straus, J. (1985). Personal communication.

Task Force on Pediatric Education, 1978, *The future of pediatric education*. Evanston, Ill.: American Academy of Pediatrics.

Telzrow, R. (1978). Anticipatory guidance in pediatric practice. *Journal of Continuing Education,* July, 14.

Valko, R.J., & Clayton, P.J. (1975). Depression in the internship. *Journal of Disorders of the Nervous System, 36,* 26.

Weed, L.J. (1970). Medical records. In *Medical education and patient care.* Chicago: Year Book Medical Publications.

Werner, E.R., Adler, R., Robinson, R., & Korsch, B.M. (1979). Attitudes and interpersonal skills during pediatric internship. *Pediatrics, 63,* 491.

Wishingrad, L. (1963). Role of a social worker in a private practice of pediatrics. *Pediatrics, 32,* 1125.

Yancy, S.W. (1975). Behavioral pediatrics and the practicing pediatrician. *Pediatric Clinics of North America, 22* (3), 685.

26

Future Directions and Behavioral Training Issues

MICHAEL F. CATALDO AND NORMAN A. KRASNEGOR

This book has presented the ideas and research efforts of pediatricians and behavioral scientists that address issues significant for the health of our nation's children. The preceding chapters have dealt with problems of health and development of children, how health and development relate to each other, different approaches to solutions, the implications of the problems and solutions for pediatrics, and other ways of addressing the problems—ways outside the pediatric profession but in collaboration with pediatrics.

Chapters by Morris Green and Robert Haggerty describe the current status of pediatrics and the child health challenges of the future. They point out that child health concerns have shifted from acute infectious, generally

Preparation of this chapter was supported in part by grants 917 and MCJ-243270-02-0 from Maternal and Child Health. We wish to thank Ruth Cargo and Fred G. Leebron for their editorial assistance.

short-term disorders, to chronic problems related to and with considerable impact on lifestyle. The list of challenges they identify is formidable: teenage pregnancy, infants born at risk, childhood injuries, compliance with medical regimens, immunological disorders, chronic illness, feeding disorders, depression, and suicide.

Because of the chronic nature of these child health problems, approaches to solutions and to assessing their impact must incorporate what is known about child development (see, for example, Chapter 9 by Horowitz and O'Brien). The knowledge base on child development is extensive and encompasses decades of descriptive and experimental research; major international journals and societies have been founded to advance the child development field; and an institute of the National Institute of Health—the National Institute of Child Health and Human Development, (NICHD)—has been devoted to this content area. Despite this progress, far too little integration has occurred between those concerned with child development and those concerned with child health, especially in terms of the interaction between health and development.

Similarly the nature of the "new morbidity" in pediatrics, with its emphasis on behavior, indicates that we must also look to the science of human behavior for a knowledge base and methodology. Potential solutions to problems such as proper nutrition during pregnancy, compliance with medical regimens, and injury control rest not only on identifying what people should do but also on how to get them to do it. Behavioral considerations are also a concern in pediatrics as behavior problems of children become a greater and greater portion of clinical practice. A relevant knowledge base appropriate to this new morbidity has been accumulating from the experimental analysis of behavior (see, for example, Chapters 13 to 24). Yet, as is the case with child development, these contributions of behavioral science have not easily nor readily been integrated into the problem-solving approaches to child health.

CHILD HEALTH AND BEHAVIORAL PEDIATRICS

The recognition of the complex nature of today's child-health problems that necessitate an integration of biological, developmental, and behavioral perspectives is currently articulated in the area of behavioral pediatrics. Numerous other disciplines that have been addressed in other volumes—disciplines such as child psychiatry, sociology, and other areas of psychology—are relevant to behavioral pediatrics and will certainly continue to be important to child health issues. And, to provide a comprehensive definition of the field is perhaps premature, as its nature, subject matter, and boundaries are still evolving; nevertheless, to proffer an operational perspective is appropriate. Our working definition is as follows: Behavioral pediatrics is a field of research that integrates the behavioral and biomedical sciences to study children's health. The discipline may be regarded as a branch of behavioral medicine, and its major distinguishing features include (1) an emphasis on observable behavior and measurable biological processes as both independent and dependent variables, (2) emphasis on the development period from conception to adulthood, and (3) extensive interdisciplinary collaboration among clinicians and behavioral and biomedical scientists. A hallmark of this field is the clinical application of principles of human learning and behavior to the behavior of children, their caregivers, and health care providers to promote health and ameliorate chronic illness.

Behavioral pediatrics is a rapidly evolving field of research and clinical practice, with a more comprehensive biobehavioral approach than any of its predecessors. Using a collaborative health team model, it attempts to integrate the medical, behavioral, psychosocial, and environmental dimensions of the child, the family, and the community for the primary purpose of health promotion. Within this context, multiple roles of behavior are recognized as both a determinant and a result of medical conditions and treatments. Behavior is viewed as a complex function of biological, developmental, and environmental variables. Behavioral pediatrics must, therefore, include the multiple foci of etiology, treatment, management,and prevention of disease.

CURRENT CONCERNS

Endeavoring to resolve contemporary child health problems identified by pediatrics can best be characterized as commerce across an interdisciplinary bridge. What weight must this bridge bear? It must be able to handle collaborative and cooperative efforts between clinicians and scientists, behavioral scientists and biological scientists, psychologists and pediatricians.

Like concrete and steel bridges, the interdisciplinary bridge should solve problems that exist because of the distance and lack of contact between two areas. But a few of the current concerns that could be addressed by a sufficiently broad interdisciplinary bridge are:

1. *What do we mean by behavioral pediatrics?* Despite the necessity of defining an area of endeavor at its inception, an area is ultimately defined by the activity of its participants. Bringing together the disciplines necessary to solve contemporary child health problems will lead to behavioral pediatrics being defined differently. The definition will come to encompass a broader range of activities that are increasingly proven to be functional in solving child health problems.

2. *How best can we address research, clinical, and guild issues to facilitate solutions to child health problems?* Research deals with the cumulative and gen-

erative advancement of knowledge. Clinical activities encompass the application of such knowledge for treating illness and promoting health. The "guild" issue pertains to which professionals should have the right to provide which services. Sorting out the roles of various professionals is an important issue. The degree to which we are able to use the methods and talents afforded by the research community in developing clinical solutions and then employing the sanctions of professional groups to ensure effective, ethical treatment implementation will be directly related to the success of our efforts to foster interdisciplinary collaboration.

3. *How can we develop solutions to the most pressing problems of children's health?* To the public, and certainly for the health of the nation, this issue is of prime importance. Additional questions that must be addressed include: To what extent can these problems be solved through the traditional medical system? How can we anticipate changes in the health care delivery system and use that knowledge to address problems of child health over the next two decades? These are difficult questions that can best be answered by interdisciplinary collaboration.

4. *How can we resolve the issue of multiple-factor versus single-factor solutions?* These two points of view—which in a sense reflect the perceived differences between the clinical approach and the scientific approach—are not necessarily incompatible. They represent different contingencies in dealing with health-related phenomena and both are essential. The clinician is faced with the need to help the patient and will therefore consider as many causes and corresponding treatments as might be relevant to the presenting problem. The result is a view of health problems as complex interrelationships among many factors and of solutions as correspondingly multifaceted. The scientist's charge is to understand phenomena, which is generally accomplished by identifying, describing, and quantifying as many factors as may be related to a phenomenon and then systematically determining, through further observation and experiment, their respective roles and limitations with respect to the occurrence of the phenomenon. The scientist's contributions to clinical solutions are at least twofold: (1) providing objective data on factors related to health problems and (2) identifying (occasionally) a factor so predominant and vital to the existence of a health concern that when properly controlled by the clinician, it will render the need for controlling other factors unnecessary and can greatly reduce health care costs. Interestingly the same health problems can serve to illustrate activities of both the clinician and the scientist. For example, tuberculosis in man is a disease resulting from multiple factors associated with the production and transmission of mycrobacterium—factors such as nutrition, population density, general health status, and, of course, presence of the bacteria. Before the research findings of Koch, clinical approaches included hygiene, diet, rest, and a host of other prescriptions. However, based on basic research, vaccine and antibiotics can now be used to control

the tubercle bacilli, making it unnecessary, in this instance, to control other factors.

5. *How should the government set research priorities?* As decision-makers who sponsor research, government officials play a significant role in shaping the direction of child health research and practice in this nation. There are two issues here: (1) How can the government, in this context the National Institute of Health, decide priorities for research that best advances formative knowledge about child health? and (2) How can this knowledge best be translated into practice to improve health and development?

6. *What should be the role of operant and other approaches in solving child health problems?* Operant research has demonstrated procedures for remediating a substantial portion of childhood problems currently addressed by clinical pediatrics, including childhood behavior problems (for example, tantrums, noncompliance) as well as medical problems (for example, migraine headaches, neuromuscular dysfunction). Despite this knowledge base and the existing service delivery system, operant behavioral approaches to pediatric problems, like many other approaches, have not been widely adopted in clinical pediatric practice. As with any characterization of a group's activities, the validity and utility of current approaches to child health problems, including operant psychology and a host of others, will be determined over time as a function of the practice of clinicians and the objective study of treatment outcomes. Incorporating the knowledge base of a number of disciplines within the objective rigor of scientific method will provide the foundation for future clinical approaches to child health.

OPERANT APPROACHES IN PERSPECTIVE

Two conclusions about behavioral pediatrics are evident from the preceding chapters: (1) that behavioral pediatrics is an area of clinical activity that encompasses (and therefore requires) a broad range of perspectives; and (2) that one especially emphasized perspective, operant psychology, may have significant applications to behavioral pediatrics and may be underrecognized and underutilized in behavioral pediatrics.

However, operant approaches need to be put into perspective. Elsewhere in this book, we have discussed when operant approaches should be considered, and the types of problems they can address. The basic rationales for operant approaches are (1) they are objective and replicable; (2) they are relevant to behavior, and behavior is central to the health of children; (3) they are based on nearly four decades of basic research; and (4) they are experimentally determined, rather than theory driven. The application of operant approaches to child health, development, and behavior has resulted in many solutions that have been applied by psychologists, parents, and teachers. The preceding chapters raise interesting clinical questions about the extent to which operant techniques can be effectively and economically employed in pediatrics and the extent to which operant methodologies can serve as one scientific approach employed by behavioral pediatrics.

Although operant approaches offer much promise, much of the promise has not yet been realized. We are just in the beginning stages of investigating the possibilities and acting on some of them, so near the beginning that we are still developing the advantages and have not taken the next, healthy step of listing limitations. The limitations of operant approaches include:

Operant approaches are based on the observation of behavior. Thus, if the behavior is difficult to observe—for example, studying or firesetting—then an operant approach is difficult to apply.

When a behavior is a low-frequency behavior (an extreme example is suicide), there are few occasions to modify the problem behavior and teach a different behavior, rendering an operant approach impractical unless it is directed at precursors that lead up to the problem behavior.

Operant approaches work on the basis of consequences. There are behaviors that pose great difficulty for health care professionals in determining effective consequences or in manipulating the consequences (for example, a parent who refuses to follow a program to comply with a child's medication regimen).

Thus there are circumstances that render operant principles difficult to apply—not theoretically unfeasible, but practically difficult. Therefore, in many instances we are several steps from working together on comparing and contrasting operant approaches with other approaches or in being able to specify for the pediatrician, who is charged with orchestrating continuity of care, a basis for choosing one approach as opposed to another.

CLINICAL TRAINING

Acknowledging both the yet-unfulfilled promises of operant approaches and the potential limitations, what opportunities are there for training? And, how should training differ for different members of the child health team?

Physicians

Pediatrics and family practice are the two specialty areas that relate most directly to child health and for whom operant approaches would be most helpful. The pediatrician or the family practitioner is often the first professional parents consult about children's problems. Thus pediatricians and family practitioners are in a position to (1) identify behavior-related problems; (2) provide appropriate interventions or refer parents to other professionals who are especially trained and have the necessary time to provide intervention program(s) to the parents and whose services are maximally cost effective; and (3) provide anticipatory guidance to parents to avoid or greatly reduce the severity of future problems.

Early in their training, pediatricians should be provided with information about basic operant principles and technical terms. Later, during their clinical rotations, appropriate and necessary training in operant approaches by skilled behavioral clinicians should focus on practical techniques and how to apply them. Training should also emphasize methods of assessing behavior problems, because the diagnostic approach of considering a problem from an operant point of view is substantially different from the traditional medical approach. In addition, information about identifying competent behavioral colleagues and successful methods for recruiting behaviorally trained professionals to staff positions should be conveyed.

Other Health Care Professionals

Other health care professionals—such as nurses, physician's assistants, and social workers—should also be trained to use operant approaches.

Nurses.   Nurses, in particular, are in an ideal position to assist parents and identify behavior-related disorders, especially given the many settings in which nurses work today. Through routine health-checks and history-taking, they can prompt parents to consider matters of behavior and development, can identify inappropriate behaviors and developmental delay, and can provide advice and brief office-based interventions. However, although many solutions to behavioral problems can be explained to parents and monitored in only a small amount of professional time, others require a greater commitment of time than is allotted for routine ambulatory care; thus, nurse practitioners with special training in operant behavioral approaches can provide effective behavioral services to parents at less cost than if the same effort had been provided by a physician or psychologist. In addition, the best place to observe a behavior and the conditions responsible for its existence is in the setting in which it occurs—the child's home, school, or other daily locales; thus, the visiting nurse program offers an exquisitely appropriate and potentially powerful mechanism for identifying, assessing, and intervening in child behavior problems.

Social Workers.   Social workers are another group of health professionals in a position to provide behavioral pediatric services. Most often, problem behaviors are supported by a variety of persons, all of whom need to work in concert if a behavior change program is to be employed with consistency. Further, behavior problems are sometimes established and maintained because of difficulties between significant adults in the child's life. The traditional role of the social worker in assessing interpersonal and family dynamics, providing support, and working with a wide variety of adults to ensure success are exactly the preconditions most important to a successful intervention program for a child behavior problem. Thus the social worker trained in operant behavioral approaches could combine the effective components provided by traditional social work training with the powerful behavior change techniques of operant psychology.

Psychologists. Psychologists are much less available and less sought out by parents—especially if parents have had no previous successful assistance from someone in the profession of psychology. Contact with psychologists almost always occurs through referrals. Yet the behavioral psychologist is the most extensively trained and should therefore be the most skilled at behavioral approaches to children's problems. The behavioral psychologist is also the most limited in formal training and skill in identifying and addressing nonbehavior-related health problems. Thus the current practice of parents finding their way to the psychologist through referral by another health care professional is appropriate, and entails the least degree of risk in that it ensures that sufficient and knowledgeable consideration has been given to the other possible causes of and solutions to a particular presenting problem. However, the vast majority of training programs in psychology do not prepare their graduates either to deal with the array of problems that might be referred by physicians and nurses or to sufficiently appreciate the circumstances, demands, and constraints faced by these other health care professionals. Therefore, behavioral psychologists should receive additional training in the application of their expertise to pediatric concerns. Specifically, psychologists must understand how physicians approach problems; how primary care is orchestrated as an interdisciplinary exercise (that is, it is not a singular approach to a problem); and, most important, how the medical system in general and the pediatric professional in particular operate as clinical and professional enterprises. Introductory courses in biochemistry and general mammalian physiology would be of considerable benefit, as would a basic understanding of childhood medical disorders and traditional medical approaches to their treatment.

RESEARCH TRAINING

In addition to training for clinical skills, operant research competencies could also be provided as part of a training program. Two distinct advantages offered by operant research approaches are (1) the means of identifying powerful environmental variables that modify and maintain behavior and (2) a set of experimental, data-based activities that are immediately applicable to accountable clinical services.

For the physician, measurement constitutes a critical area for focus in operant research training. The most important contribution to research methodology that the study of operant processes has produced is the reliable quantification of behavior by direct observation. This contribution both contrasts with and complements more traditional approaches that rely on reports about behavior and on the thoughts and feelings of the patient and the parent. For other health care professionals, this distinction should also be supplemented by specific training in the use of available observation and data-taking techniques as well as in the design of such systems. And, for all groups of health care professionals, operant science methodologies offer considerable economy for clinical research studies. In particular, single-subject and time-series designs provide for the identification of powerful variables and are particularly well suited to clinical practice approaches that are based on one-to-one contact between clinician and patient (in clinical, as opposed to public health models, the individual patient, rather than a societal population, is the primary focus of attention). Similarly, behavioral psychologists interested in child health research should receive additional training in measurement basic to biomedical research. Familiarity with considerations such as drug blood levels would be important to an investigator's ability to design biobehavioral research studies.

LOOKING TO THE FUTURE

During the past 100 years, the practice of medicine has increasingly been based on knowledge obtained from basic biological sciences about the mechanisms of normal and disease processes. The cumulative, objective, and replicable activities characteristic of scientific endeavor have allowed us to verify experimentally our empirical observations about the relationships of practices and treatment outcomes. The result has been unprecedented reductions in acute and infectious disease and an equally dramatic increase in the general health and longevity of the American people. Today, as the predominant activity in pediatric medicine shifts from diagnosis and treatment of acute and infectious diseases to problems such as developmental concerns, child rearing, school performance, adolescence, and injury control, we must begin to look to other scientific methodologies relevant to these problems in the same manner in which we looked to disciplines such as chemistry, microbiology, and nuclear physics in the past.

Our belief is that this book represents a beginning that has been long in the making. The rapprochement between behavioral scientists/clinicians and pediatricians is a natural one, which, if sensitively and properly fostered, can markedly enhance the likelihood that the child health issues articulated by our colleagues can be successfully addressed. We earnestly hope and urge that the dialogue and collaboration continue. The benefits from this alliance will speed advances in the field and, most importantly, will better the health of our nation's youth.

Author Index

Subject Index